PHARMACEUTICAL BIOTECHNOLOGY

S. CHAND & COMPANY PVT. LTD.

(An ISO 9001 : 2008 Company)

Head Office: 7361, RAM NAGAR, NEW DELHI - 110 055

Phone: 23672080-81-82, 9899107446, 9911310888 Fax: 91-11-23677446

Shop at: **schandgroup.com**; e-mail: **info@schandgroup.com**

Branches :

AHMEDABAD : 1st Floor, Heritage, Near Gujarat Vidhyapeeth, Ashram Road, **Ahmedabad** - 380 014, Ph: 27541965, 27542369, ahmedabad@schandgroup.com

BENGALURU : No. 6, Ahuja Chambers, 1st Cross, Kumara Krupa Road, **Bengaluru** - 560 001, Ph: 22268048, 22354008, bangalore@schandgroup.com

BHOPAL : Bajaj Tower, Plot No. 2&3, Lala Lajpat Rai Colony, Raisen Road, **Bhopal** - 462 011, Ph: 4274723, 4209587. bhopal@schandgroup.com

CHANDIGARH : S.C.O. 2419-20, First Floor, Sector - 22-C (Near Aroma Hotel), **Chandigarh** -160 022, Ph: 2725443, 2725446, chandigarh@schandgroup.com

CHENNAI : No.1, Whites Road, Opposite Express Avenue, Royapettah, **Chennai** - 600014 Ph. 28410027, 28410058, chennai@schandgroup.com

COIMBATORE : 1790, Trichy Road, LGB Colony, Ramanathapuram, **Coimbatore** -6410045, Ph: 2323620, 4217136 coimbatore@schandgroup.com **(Marketing Office)**

CUTTACK : 1st Floor, Bhartia Tower, Badambadi, **Cuttack** - 753 009, Ph: 2332580; 2332581, cuttack@schandgroup.com

DEHRADUN : 1st Floor, 20, New Road, Near Dwarka Store, **Dehradun** - 248 001, Ph: 2711101, 2710861, dehradun@schandgroup.com

GUWAHATI : Dilip Commercial (Ist floor), M.N. Road, Pan Bazar, **Guwahati** - 781 001, Ph: 2738811, 2735640 guwahati@schandgroup.com

HYDERABAD : Padma Plaza, H.No. 3-4-630, Opp. Ratna College, Narayanaguda, **Hyderabad** - 500 029, Ph: 27550194, 27550195, hyderabad@schandgroup.com

JAIPUR : 1st Floor, Nand Plaza, Hawa Sadak, Ajmer Road, **Jaipur** - 302 006, Ph: 2219175, 2219176, jaipur@schandgroup.com

JALANDHAR : Mai Hiran Gate, **Jalandhar** - 144 008, Ph: 2401630, 5000630, jalandhar@schandgroup.com

KOCHI : Kachapilly Square, Mullassery Canal Road, Ernakulam, **Kochi** - 682 011, Ph: 2378740, 2378207-08, cochin@schandgroup.com

KOLKATA : 285/J, Bipin Bihari Ganguli Street, **Kolkata** - 700 012, Ph: 22367459, 22373914, kolkata@schandgroup.com

LUCKNOW : Mahabeer Market, 25 Gwynne Road, Aminabad, **Lucknow** - 226 018, Ph: 4076971, 4026791, 4065646, 4027188, lucknow@schandgroup.com

MUMBAI : Blackie House, IInd Floor, 103/5, Walchand Hirachand Marg, Opp. G.P.O., **Mumbai** - 400 001, Ph: 22690881, 22610885, mumbai@schandgroup.com

NAGPUR : Karnal Bagh, Near Model Mill Chowk, **Nagpur** - 440 032, Ph: 2720523, 2777666 nagpur@schandgroup.com

PATNA : 104, Citicentre Ashok, Mahima Palace , Govind Mitra Road, **Patna** - 800 004, Ph: 2300489, 2302100, patna@schandgroup.com

PUNE : Sadguru Enclave, Ground floor, Survey No. 114/3, Plot no. 8 Alandi Road , Vishrantwadi **Pune** – 411015 Ph: 64017298 pune@schandgroup.com

RAIPUR : Kailash Residency, Plot No. 4B, Bottle House Road, Shankar Nagar, **Raipur** - 492 007, Ph: 2443142,Mb. : 09981200834, raipur@schandgroup.com **(Marketing Office)**

RANCHI : Flat No. 104, Sri Draupadi Smriti Apartments, (Near of Jaipal Singh Stadium) Neel Ratan Street, Upper Bazar, **Ranchi** - 834 001, Ph: 2208761, ranchi@schandgroup.com **(Marketing Office)**

SILIGURI : 122, Raja Ram Mohan Roy Road, East Vivekanandapally, P.O., Siliguri, **Siliguri**-734001, Dist., Jalpaiguri, (W.B.) Ph. 0353-2520750 **(Marketing Office)** siliguri@schandgroup.com

VISAKHAPATNAM : No. 49-54-15/53/8, Plot No. 7, 1st Floor, Opp. Radhakrishna Towers, Seethammadhara North Extn., **Visakhapatnam** - 530 013, Ph-2782609 (M) 09440100555, visakhapatnam@schandgroup.com **(Marketing Office)**

First Edition 2014

ISBN : 81-219-4247-0 Code : 22 040

PRINTED IN INDIA

By Rajendra Ravindra Printers Pvt. Ltd., 7361, Ram Nagar, New Delhi -110 055 and published by S. Chand & Company Pvt. Ltd., 7361, Ram Nagar, New Delhi -110 055.

PHARMACEUTICAL BIOTECHNOLOGY

Dr. V. Sreenivasulu
M.Pharm., Ph.D., FICCP, FICPHS
Professor and Principal
Lakshmi Venketeswara Institute of Pharmaceutical Sciences, Proddatur
Andhra Pradesh

Dr. K.N. Jayaveera
M.Sc., Ph.D., FIC, FICCP
Professor
Jawaharlal Nehru Technological University, Anantapur
Andhra Pradesh

Dr. K. Adinarayana
M.Sc., Ph.D., FICCP
Associate Professor
Annamacharya Collage of Pharmacy, Rajampet
Andhra Pradesh

S. CHAND & COMPANY PVT. LT

(AN ISO 9001:2008 COMPANY)

RAM NAGAR, NEW DELHI - 110055

PREFACE

Biotechnology as a fast developing technology as well as a science has already shown its impact on different aspects of day-to-day human life such as public health, pharmaceuticals, food and agriculture, industry, bioenergetics and information technology. Now it is very clear that biotechnology will be a key technology for the 21st century and the science of the future.

Biotechnology essentially and predominantly deals with the meticulous applications of living organisms or their corresponding products in a variety of large-scale industrial processes. It has its foundations and domain prominently spread in a wide spectrum of fields, such as pharmaceutical sciences, microbiology, biology, biochemistry, molecular biology, genetics, genomics, genetic engineering, chemistry, chemical and process engineering.

This book **Pharmaceutical Biotechnology** is based entirely on modern biotechnological techniques as to date and encompasses a wider range of altogether newer medical compounds, e.g. antibiotics, vaccines and monoclonal antibodies that may now be produced commercially using well-defined, optimized, and improved fermentative methodologies. In fact, genetic engineering has brought in a sea change by virtue of the directed construction of microorganisms resulting in a plethora of newer life-saving drugs.

In 1917, Karl Ereky, a Hungarian engineer, first coined the term 'biotechnology' when he wanted to describe the production of pigs that were fed with sugarbeets. It is indeed an altogether newer frontier charged with innovative ideas and approaches in modern-drug-discovery scenario to modify and improve upon the quality of life of human beings on this planet. Through the techniques of genetic engineering and molecular biology, microbes are being "tailor-made" to produce

There are several universities now offering graduate, postgraduate, doctoral and postdoctoral courses in biotechnology. Job prospects in different avenues are also expanding at a rapid pace with the entry of several pharmaceutical companies in India.

It is earnestly believed that students learning Pharmaceutical Biotechnology will certainly find this text not only useful but also a good companion for further pursuit of higher knowledge. Besides, research scientists, teachers, food technologists, industrial technical personnels, postgraduate students involved in industrial microbiology shall definitely be benefited from this practical approach to the broader horizons of biotechnology.

This book covers all the fundamental aspects of pharmaceutical biotechnology. It has been written in a very simple manner and explains the fundamental concepts and techniques in detail so that they are very easily understood, even by those without even a basic understanding of biology. Reading this textbook will give readers an idea of the relationship between biotechnology and health, nutrition, agriculture, environment, industry, etc. and will explain different pharmaceutical applications in biotechnology in everyday life.

First chapter covers the basic fermentation technology and fermentation products, means different types of bioreactors, methodologies and products like production of antibiotics and vitamins, etc. Second chapter also covers the production of organic acids, SCP. This chapter exclusively covers the microbial transformation, means biotransformation process and its improvements with special reference to steroids. Third chapter covers genetic recombination which includes transformation, transduction, conjugation and gene cloning. This chapter covers the development of hybridoma technology and drugs produced by biotechnology also. Fourth chapter covers the immunology and immunotechniques. It discusses the basic concepts of immunology and especially deals with the pharmaceutical immunology, which includes productions of monoclonal antibodies and different types of vaccines, etc. Fifth chapter on enzyme immobilization discusses the include basic concepts of enzymes, enzyme kinetics, production of some important of enzymes and immobilization of bacteria and plant cells. Sixth chapter on discusses the advent of biotechnology discusses the applications of biotechnology in different fields like food, environment, chemical and pharmaceutical industries. Seventh chapter on biosensor technology discusses the types of biosensors and biochips. Eighth chapter discusses the regulatory issues in biotechnology which includes biosafety, IPR, etc. Ninth chapter covers the safety in biotechnology, i.e. precautions while handling the chemicals, pathogenic microorganisms and fungi. Tenth chapter, on bioinformatics and data mining discusses the applications of computers in biotechnology. Now a days this topic is very hot science in the world.

This book is a must for every pharmacy student because it covers the basic biotechnology and applications of biotechnology in pharmaceutical industry. The book is exclusive for the pharmacy students. It covers the major fundamentals of biotechnology and importance of biotechnology in pharmaceutical research and industry.

This book covers the syllabi of all Indian Universities as well as of competitive examinations. Competitive exam purpose means GATE and GPAT also. It is meant for B.Pharm., M.Pharm., B.Tech., M.Tech., M.Sc. (Biotechnology, Microbiology, Biochemistry, Food Technology, Chemical Technology, and other Life Sciences) and B.Sc. Life Sciences degrees of India and abroad.

Dr. V. Sreenivasulu
Dr. K.N. Jayaveera
Dr. K. Adinarayana

CONTENTS

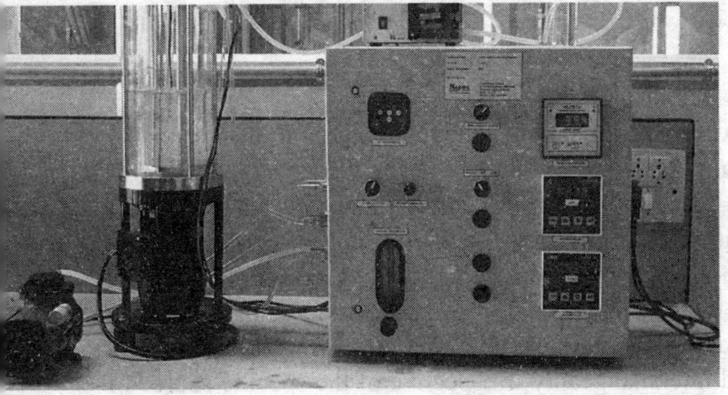

CHAPTER

1

Fermentation Technology and Fermentation Products

1.1 Historical Development of Antibiotics

Paul Vuilemin (1889) was the first and foremost scientist who vehemently promulgated the very concept of **'antibiotic'** activity to introduce the terminology *'influences antibiotiques' (or antibiotic influences)* in order to describe the prevailing negative interactions amongst the animals and plants.* Later on, Walksman (1940s) eventually coined the term **'antibiotic'** and also introduced a plausible definition as — *'a chemical substance derived from microorganisms which has the capacity of inhibiting growth, and even destroying, other microorganisms in dilute solutions'*.**

Another school of thought advocates that the **natural product antibiotics** essentially comprise of a specific category of chemical entities invariably termed as the **secondary metabolites.** Besides, on a rather broader perspective such substances may be characterized for possessing chemical structures which are found to be quite unusual when compared with those of the **intermediary metabolites.** Nevertheless, *such natural product antibiotics,* are being generated at an extremely low ebb specific growth rates, and also supported by the fact that these are not absolutely essential the growth of the **'producing organisms'** in a *pure culture medium.* In fact, the **'antibiotics'** are observed to be of highly critical nature with respect to the **producing organisms** in their usual natural environment because their presence is an absolute must not only for the *survival* but also for the *competitive advantage.*

However, the most widely accepted definition of an **'antibiotic'** promulgated by the scientific jargons is — *'a chemical substance produced by a microorganism that has the capacity, in low concentration, to inhibit or kill, selectively, other microorganisms'*.

Importantly, the aforesaid definition lays particular emphasis on the terminologies like **'selectively'** or **'selective toxicity'** that explicitly suggests that the *substance* either checks the growth of pathogens or exerts a bactericidal action on the microbes without displaying a similar action on the host organisms *i.e.,* the humans.

Interestingly, one may evidently observe from the above cited definition(s) that critically excludes the plethora of never medicinal compounds essentially having the pure synthetic genesis (origin). In reality and actual practice, these *'synthetic substances'* are virtually treated at par with the host of *natural compounds* together with their respective derivatives under the terminology **'antimicrobials'** that could be further sub-divided predominantly into *two* categories namely: **antifungal** and **antibacterial** depending on the specific type(s) of **microbe** undergoing *inhibition.* Therefore, in order to circumvent the practical aspects, both the terminologies, *viz.,* **'antibiotic'** and **'antimicrobial'** may be used effectively and interchangeably irrespective of the specific source of the *chemical entity.*

In general, the **'antibiotics'** are produced on a large scale by *three* well-known and defined methodologies, such as: (*a*) **fermentation process;** (*b*) semi-synthetic process; and (*c*) synthetic process. A tremendous quantum leap and qualified successful diversification in the specific field of **'biotechnology'** has helped the first two processes (*i.e.*, '*a*' and 'b') in accomplishing an enormous enhancement in the rate of production as well as improved upon their yield and purity.

Antibiotic Development: The latest progressive trend in the logistic aspects of **antibiotic development** may be observed vividly by the under mentioned sequence of goals and objectives, such as:

- To screen and evaluate different types of sources of microorganisms for the **detection of purposeful antagonism.**
- To identify and select modified versions of microbial mutants, establish optimal environmental and nutritional conditions, and to *develop suitable technique*(*s*) for the **recovery of antibiotics from cultures,**
- To induce the *production* of particular desired *metabolites,*
- To improve upon and modify the fermentative metabolites either by the aid of *biological* and *chemical* manipulations to accomplish **more useful antibiotic substances,**
- To develop an elaborated methods for the **'total synthesis'** of antibiotics from *ab initio* for a feasible economic advantage, and
- To make use of an '*adjunct agent*' to distinctly **enhance the impact or availability of an antibiotic.**

1.2 Antimicrobial Spectrum and Methods used for their Standardization

Microbiology, in particular *clinical medical microbiology*, is a scientific discipline chiefly concerned with the **isolation** and subsequent **identification** of causative disease-producing microorganisms (or **pathogens**): **bacteria, fungi** (including **yeast**), **viruses**, **rickettsia**, and **parasites.**

In general, there are well-defined specific as well as non-specific techniques available with regard to the *isolation* and *identification* of the **'suspect organisms'** as stated under:

- Propagation on an appropriate primary culture media,
- Selective isolation on special (specific) culture media,
- Application of appropriate living host material *e.g.*, mouse, *embryonated egg, tissue culture* and the like,
- Determination of morphological features of the organism,
- Determination of staining characteristics of the organism,
- Confirmation by biochemical analysis, and
- Confirmation by immunochemical analysis.

In actual practice, however, appropriate *'animal inoculation'*, wherever applicable, may be used to establish **pathogenicity**. It is pertinent to mention here that for accomplishing the **final differentiation** and **confirmation process** one has to take into consideration the *prime variables* directly associated, namely: *site, timing, technique* (*aseptic*), *instrumentation*, and *transportation of clinical specimens.*

Specific Tests*: There are *three* specific test that may be used to identify the pathogens, namely:

a. Enzymatic and Immunological Tests: The introduction of rapid manual enzymatic and immunological test kits have enormously enabled to identify the presence of **'pathogens'** in the **cerebrospinal fluid (CSF) analysis.**

b. Coagglutination Tests: In this specific tests, the particular antibody is bound to protein A on the surface of a *staphylococcal cell,* and the very presence of antigen causes agglutination, and

c. Latex-Agglutination Tests: In this particular tests a specific antibody gets coated onto the latex particles and when an antigen is present, the latex particles are visible distinctly. The various pathogenic organism(s), its type, occurrence and the identification tests have been duly summarized in Table 1 given below:

Antimicrobial Susceptibility Tests: It may be defined as — *'a determination of the least amount of an antimicrobial chemotherapeutic agent that will inhibit the growth of a microorganism in vitro, using a tube-dilution method, agar-cup method, or disk-diffusion method'.*

However, the **antimicrobial susceptibility test** may serve as a vital and critical help essentially needed by the physician in the judicious and precise selection of a chemotherapeutic agent. It is also pertinent to state here that the exact concentration of the **antimicrobial agent** in the **body fluids*** may be estimated by *'biological assay'* with the aid of an *'organism'* having a known susceptibility (predetermined) for the specific agent in question.

Table 1.1 *Identification Test of Various Pathogenic Organisms*

S. No	Organism	Type of Organisms	Occurrence	Identification Test
1.	***Staphylococcus aureus (Micrococcus pyrogens var aurens)***	Gram + ve	Normal human skin, mucous membranes frequently associated with abscesses septicemia, endo carditis, and osteomyelitis.	It is based on colonial (*pigmentation*) and microscopic morphology (*grape- like clusters*), positive catalase production, positive coagulase production (*staphylocoagulase plasma clotting factor*), and positive mannitol fermentation.
2.	***Streptococcus pyrogenes***	Gram + ve	Associated with tonsillitis or pharyn-gitis, erysipelas, pyoderma, and endocarditis.	Streptococcal groups are identified by **precipitin tests** with *group specific antisera for A, B, C, D, F* and *G*
3.	***Neisseria gonorrhoeae***	Grame – ve	Vinereal disease gonorrhoeae	It is based on the primary isolation of the gonococcus from urethral exudates on chocolate agar or Thayer-Martin medium. The microscopic examination of Gram – ve intracellular diplococci resembling the gonococcus supports a positive diagnosis of gonorrhea. The presence of oxidase enzyme activity of the gonococci is usually carried out by a reaction with ***p-dimethyl aminoaniline,*** that specifically changes oxidase – positive colonies balck.

4.	***Enteric bacilli*** (*Enterobacteriaceae*), such as: *Shigella* spp: dysentery: *Salmonella typhi*: typhoid fever; *Escherichia coli, Proteus* spp., And *Pseudomonas* spp: *urinary* tract and tissue infections; *Klebsiella* spp: pulmonary infections;	Grame – ve	Stated underorganism'	**Enteric bacilli** may be primarily isolated or *selective and differential infusion agar e.g.*, MacConkey and eosin-methylene blue (EMB); Besides, *enrichment media e.g.*, **tetrathionate and salenite broth.** **Leifson's deoxycholate citrate** agar (LCD) OR *Salmonella Shigella agar* (SS) **Brilliant green agar BG** And **Bismuth sulphite agar** (BS) Identification/confirmation of **enteric bacilli** may be carried out by a host of **serological tests** and **biochemical reactions** *e.g.*, *i.* H_2S — production (triple – sugar iron agar); *ii.* Acetylmethyl carbinol production; *iii.* Indole production; *iv.* Citrate utilization; *v.* Activity of various enzymes *e.g.*, urease, lysinase, and arginine decarboxylase; and phenylalanine deaminase.

Laboratory Diagnosis of Viral Infections: In actual practice, the laboratory diagnosis of several **viral infections** is exclusively based upon the following *five* cardinal factors, namely:

1. Examination of the infected tissues for actual **pathognomonic changes** or for the presence of **viral material.**
2. Isolation and identification of the viral agent.
3. Demonstration of an appreciable enhancement in the **'antibody titer value'** to a given virus in the span of the illness.
4. Detection of **viral antigens** present in lesions by employing **fluorescein-labeled antibodies.**
5. **Electron microscopic examination** of either the *tissue extracts* or the *vesicular fluids.*

Serological Tests: It is a common practice to use '*blood*' for carrying out the *serological tests*, but quite rarely for *virus isolation*. However, it is absolutely important and vital that both **acute** and **convalescent-phase blood specimens** should be examined thoroughly in parallel to estimate precisely whether **'antibodies'** have appeared, lowered or enhanced in the **'titer value'** in the span of the disease.

Examples: A few typical examples of **'human viral infections'** are as enumerated under:

- Respiratory infections (*e.g.*, **Adenovirus group)**
- Diseases of the nervous system (*e.g.*, **Polio** and **Coxsackie viruses of the picornavirus group)**
- Small pox (**Poxvirus group)**
- Measles (**Paramyxovirus group)**
- Chicken pox (**Herpesvirus group)**
- Influenza (**Myxovirus group)**

Clinical Parasitology: It is indeed a well-defined science that is exclusively concerned with the **parasitic protozoa** (*amoeba*), the **helminths** (*cestodes, tapeworms; trematodes, flukes; nematodes, roundwarms*), and the **arthopods.**

Identification of Protozoan Ova: It is based upon the **detailed microscopic morphological studies** (including *nuclei*) by making use of **wet mounts** (*e.g., saline* or *iodine*) or **strained preparations** (*e.g., iron, hematoxylin*) obtained from *fecal specimens* (fresh or preserved with polyvinyl alcohol) that have been *adequately concentrated* by **sedimentation, centrifugation,** or **floatation techniques.**

Example: Amebic Dysentry: Specifically, in the fecal specimens the presence of **trophozoite*** and/or **cystic stages** could be detected along with intestinal protozoa, as in the case of amebic dysentery usually caused by *Entamoeba histolytica.*

Serodiagnosis of Parasitic Diaseases: Serodiagnosis essentially concerns with the diagnosis by observing the reactions of blood serum. Importantly, the serodiagnosis of parasitic diseases includes the following critical 'tests', namely:

Immunodiagnositic Tests: *Complement-fixation* (trichinosis); *precipitin test* (schistosomiasis); *bentonite flocculation* (ascariasis); *hemagglutination* (echinococcosis); *latex agglutination* (trichinosis); *cholesterol flocculation* (schistosomiasis); *fluorescent antibody* (malaria); and *methylene-blue dye test* (toxoplasmosis).

Methods Used for Standardization of Antibiotics

Official compendia invariably make use of the terminology **'antibiotic'** that essentially designates a '*medicinal preparation*', containing an appreciable quantum of a *chemical entity* which is caused to produce naturally by a microorganism or by a semi-synthetic route artificially, and that possesses the inherent ability to either *destroy* (bactericidal effect) or *inhibit* (bacteriostatic effect) microorganisms in **relatively dilute solution.**

Following are some of the **standardization certification** of various '*antibiotics*' in a chronological order:

Year	Event
1938:	Federal Food, Drug and Cosmetic Act — Introduction in stages of the '*batch certification of antibiotics*' meant for human or veterinary applications.
1945:	Penicillin
1948:	Streptomycin
1949:	Aureomycin, Bacitracin and Chloramphenicol.
1962:	Kefauver-Harris Amendments — as part of these amendments it was mandatory for the **'batch certification'** of all **antibiotics** intended for human use.
1982:	Federal Drug Authority (FDA)-USA issued regulations which totally exempted the **'antibiotics'** from the *batch certification requirements* so long as the articles complied with standards; however, section 507 (*i.e.,* **related to certification of Antibiotics**) remains intact and hence applicable.

Federal Register (USA): It essentially incorporates the **'Standards of Potency and Purity for Antibiotics'** as established and determined by the FDA in the form of regulations published from time to time. It is, however, pertinent to mention here that as all **recognized antibiotics** are automatically subject to the provisions of the regulations; these eventually determine the **official standards.**

The following *three* cardinal points may be taken into consideration with regard to the '*assay*' *i.e., standardization of Antibiotics,* such as:

1. FDA-regulations governing all aspects of antibiotics testing are extremely detailed and are subject to periodic amendment,
2. FDA-regulations need to be referred to with regard to the **'prescribed methods'** for the *assay of individual antibiotics and their preparations,* and
3. While evaluating the potency of **'antibiotics substances',** the actual and apparent measured effect is the '*degree of inhibition*' of the growth of a suitable strain of microorganisms *i.e.,* the ultimate prevention of the multiplication of the **'test organisms'.**

The procedures usually employed in the **'microbial assay of antibiotics'** may be categorized under *two* heads, namely: (*a*) Cylinder-Plate Method; and (*b*) Turbidimetric Method, which shall now be treated briefly as under:

1.2.1 Cylinder-Plate Method

The **cylinder-plate method of assay** of *antibiotics potency* is solely based upon the measurement of the specific diameter of **'zones of microbial growth inhibition'** immediately surrounding cylinders containing various dilutions of the **'test compound'** *i.e.*, the substance under investigation, that are carefully placed on the surface of a solid nutrient agar medium previously inoculated with the **'culture'** of an *appropriate organism.* In actual practice the zone of inhibition caused by the **test compound** is meticulously compared with that produced by a known concentration of a pure **'Reference Compound'.**

1.2.2 Turbidimetric Method

The **turbidimetric method of assay** of *antibiotics potency* is exclusively based upon the inhibition of microbial growth as indicated by the corresponding measurement of the **turbidity** (*i.e.*, **transmittance**) of suspensions of an *appropriate organism* in a fluid medium into which the graded amounts of the **'test compound'** have been added duly. Consequently, the changes in the transmittance caused by the **'test compound'** are duly compared with those resulted by known concentrations of the **Reference Standard.**

Note:

1. Comprehensive account of appropriate microbial assays for specific antibiotic(s) (*viz.,* cylinder-plate or turbidimetric method) has been duly included in the 4th through 6th and 8th supplements of USP 23-NF 18.
2. The *'test organisms'* recommended for each antibiotic have been duly incorporated in these aforesaid supplements.

1.3 Screening or Soil for Organisms Producing Antiobiotics

'Soil' — is nothing but the upper layer of the earth. Ample studies and researches have substantially revealed and established the dictum that — **soil is the best available source** from which one may obtain ultimately a broad *spectrum of viable 'microorganisms'.*

Therefore, to ascertain the **'screening approach'** in an effective and justifiable manner, one may have to rigorously explore **'soil'** as a natural microbial source which essentially comprises of various kinds of microorganisms. It is absolutely immaterial whether a relatively large section of these organisms may or may not be recognized to exhibit the biosynthetic abilities of genuine interest. It is, however, pertinent to state here that there exists another unexplored possible source which could prove to be *'Meckenzie's Gold' i.e.,* an unbound source of microorganisms, such as: **ocean water** and **marine mud.** Interestingly, there are several other viable and enormous plausible sources of useful microorganisms, namely: compost, domestic sewage undergoing treatment, manure, rumen contents, and decomposed feed stuffs or foodstuffs.

At this juncture, one may raise a crucial and an extremely pivotal question that — *'why is soil invariably regarded to be the ideal source from which to obtain diverse types of microorganisms'* The various **logical explanations** to the above issue may be summarized as given below:

1. A sizable quantum, of the **'debris of the world'** finds its normal passage either *onto or into* the soil; and ultimately gets adequately decomposed by one microorganism or the other.
2. **'Soil'** may be thought of as being of a specified kind of **'huge natural fermentation vat'** wherein a plethora of organisms are actively engaged not only in the actual *decomposition* and *resynthesis* of simple to complex **organic materials,** but also in carrying out effectively the process of oxidation, reduction and other chemical changes pertaining to **inorganic materials.**
3. It has been duly demonstrated and established that more than one type, and often many types, of soil microorganisms are invariably capable of performing each of these individual **chemical or biochemical transformation.**

4. Though a large volume of different types of microorganisms do occur in the soil; however, it is not yet so clear and evident that actually upto what extent of these organisms, as on date, been pinned down and isolated in the form of **purest laboratory culture.**

Explanations: In fact, a host of researchers have more or less determined and established that both **plate counting** and **isolation procedures** as applicable to total numbers and types of the soil microorganisms, even though employing the best recognized media and incubation parmeters, perhaps would allow less than 1% of the **soil microorganisms** to be grown in the laboratory logistically. Obviously, these '*microorganisms*' urgently need the **'magic touch'** for someone to evolve a *suitable medium* and *cultural parameters* will permit their adequate growth in the laboratory environment ultimately. Evidently, it is of an immense interest and great value to one who wishes to isolate organisms having *predominant newer biosynthetic capabilities,* as it vividly indicates that, at least with **soil,** there exist a plethora of microorganisms not reported or described previously that are just waiting to be isolated and evaluated in the near future.

5. Importantly, **soil** also admits a certain extent of manipulation in the relative degrees of the various components of its microbial population just prior to the articulated procedures adopted for **screening** and **isolation.**
6. **Nutrients:** The availability of nutrients in **soil** is invariably found to be relatively at low ebb; and, therefore, the prevailing **microbial competition** for these nutrients is quite prevalent. In case, a highly desired and specific *nutrient* is timely incorporated to the **'moistened soil',** and the treated **soil** is duly incubated then a relatively much appreciable **larger growth response** takes place amongst the ensuing soil microorganisms that are capable of attacking this **specific nutrient** thereby rendering the isolation of these particular organisms much simpler and convenient. In other words, one may accomplish judiciously the **'enrichment in soil'** for specific microorganisms of our interest.
7. In the same vein, the resulting **soil** may be adequately incubated in a **particular liquid laboratory culture media** so as to cause enrichment for *specific organisms* before isolation is commenced. However, a natural phenomenon of enrichment invariably takes place in the **soil** located in the vicinity of plate roots; and, therefore, the prevailing microorganisms in the specified area may be found out to be quite different from those existing in the **'adjacent soil'** not duly penetrated by roots. In actual practice, this **'rhizosphere effect'** is afforded by root secretions and dead or sloughed debris of root would serve as microbial nutrients.

1.3.1 Screening

Screening may be defined as — *'the application of highly selective, specific and sophisticated sequential procedures to make the detection and isolation of only such microorganisms that are of genuine interest out of a large microbial population'.*

Concept of Screening: The various underlying concepts of screening essentially include:

1. *Segregation of Viable Microorganism:* It should be highly effective in the sense that either *a few steps* of *a single step* would be able to discard a major portion of the relatively not-so useful microorganisms; whereas, simultaneously allowing the rapid and fast detection of the small percentage of viable and useful microorganisms which are usually present in the population.
   Example: In industrial research programmes an attempt is made from a natural microbial source *e.g.,* **soil** is diluted to obtain a *'cell concentration'* in such a fashion that when aliquots spread, sprayed, or applied onto the surfaces of sterilized agar plates, in an asceptic condition, shall give rise to countable. Colonies not essentially touching the neighboring colonies.
2. *Detection of Microorganisms by Colour Change:* The various types of microorganisms yielding *organic acids* (attributing acidic characteristics) or *amines* (attributing basic features) generated from various carbon substrates quite often may be detected conveniently by the incorporation of a **pH indicating dye,** for instance: **bromothymol blue** or **neutral red,** into

a *slightly buffered agar nutrient medium.* In actual practice, the production of these aforesaid *'chemical entities'* is invariably indicative by exhibiting a definite change in colour of the previously incorporated indicating dye in the periphery of the ensuing colony to a **'colour'** showing either an alkaline or an acidic reaction. However, the usefulness of this *'specific methodology'* may be augmented appreciably if a media having much higher buffer capacity are utilized so that only such microorganisms which are responsible solely for producing significant quantum of either the **'amine'** or the **'acid'** can effectively induce characteristic changes in the colour of the dye.

Drawbacks: The various drawbacks of this technique are as enumerated under:

a. It fails to give a definite indication about which amine or organic acid has been produced actually. Hence, it should be immediately followed by further testing with the help of certain well-known analytical procedures *e.g.,* **paper chromatography, electrophoresis** so as to determine and establish whether the acidic or basic product really is one of interest.

b. Importantly, in such an event where colonies of microorganisms by virtue of this initial screening procedure, seem to possess **'appreciable fermentative potential'** must immediately be subjected to *purification;* and, therefore, sub cultured subsequently onto slants of an appropriate agar medium to be maintained adequately as *'stock cultures'* during further testing devices.

c. Sometimes, it is indeed quite discouraging to discover a specific organism exhibiting *'excellent fermentative potential'* only to observe that, *via* erroneous technique, either contamination or for other reasons, the culture in question has been lost ultimately.

3. **Microorganisms for Producing Antibiotics:** In the recent past, the **'screening approach'** has been exploited both extensively and intensively in the meticulous search for **viable and specific microorganisms** that are exclusively capable of producing **antibiotics** of interest to combat drea human diseases.

Crowded-plate Technique: It is one of the **simplest screening techniques** invariably employed by the *'antibiotic producers'.* In fact, this technique has an added advantage for exclusively looking for microorganisms which produce on **'antibiotic'** without any specific consideration whatsoever about the types of microorganisms that may be sensitive to the *antibiotic.*

Methodology: The various steps involved are as follows:

1. First of all, the **'soil'** or any other source of microorganisms is adequately diluted only to a cell concentration in such a manner that the agar plates normally prepared from these dilutions shall be crowded with individual colonies on the surface of the agar *i.e.,* approximately 300–400 or even more colonies per plate.
2. The **colonies** that are solely responsible for producing antibiotic activity are indicated by an area of agar around the colony which is usually free of growth of other colonies. It is a common practice to subculture such a colony further in an identical medium, and purified subsequently be streaking, just prior to making **'stock cultures'**. The *'purified culture'* thus obtained is now almost ready for testing to establish precisely the types of microorganisms that are sensitive to the **antibiotic** under investigation, by, means of the **'minimum inhibition concentration (MIC)'** or the **'microbial inhibition spectrum (MIS)'.**

Limitations of Crowded-plate Technique

There are several limitations that are noticeable in the crowded-plate technique, such as:

1. The crowded-plate technique does not necessarily aid in the precise selection of an antibiotic producing microorganisms by virtue of the fact that the inhibition area (or zone) immediately surrounding the colony may be attributed to other **vital reasons** quite frequently, such as:
   - Marked and pronounced alteration in the pH value of the medium caused due to the metabolism of the colony,
   - Rapid utilization of essential nutrients in the immediate vicinity of the colony.*

2. It essential has only limited application, because normally one is more inclined in finding a **microorganisms producing antibiotic activity** *Vs* **Specific microorganisms,** and certainly not against the **unknown microorganisms** which were present just as a stroke of luck on the agar plate in the vicinity of an *antibiotic-producing microorganisms.*
3. The **'antibiotic screening profile'** may, however, be improved by the strategic introduction into the laid-out procedure of a **'test organism'.**

The various **'screening'** aspects discussed under section 3.1 are usually referred to as the **'primary screening'** or the **'preliminary screening'.**

1.3.2 Secondary Screening

Primary screening (or **preliminary screening**) solely enables not only the *'detection',* but also the *'isolation'* of such viable microorganisms that essentially possess potentially interesting and commercially feasible applications. Nevertheless, this screening is invariably followed by a **secondary screening** so as to ascertain more useful information about these organisms, besides their actual inherent capabilities.

It is, however, pertinent to state here that the *primary screening* establishes exclusively the capability of microorganisms that are responsible for producing a compound without giving enough idea either with respect to the yield or production potential for the organisms. On the contrary, the **secondary screening** categorically enables the further **'sorting out'** of those specific microorganisms that essentially possess the *'real inherent value'* for feasible and gainful industrial processes; and distinctly eliminating those devoid of such a potential.

1.3.2.1 Methodology

The various steps involved are as follows:

1. **Secondary screening** is usually carried out on *agar plates* aseptically.
2. It may also be conducted in flasks or small fermentors containing liquid media, or as a combination of such available procedures.
3. However, one may use **'liquid culture'** as an alternative to **'agar plate'** in the *'secondary screening'* method. Following are some of the important *merits* and *demerits* of these two techniques stated briefly:

S.No	Agar Plate Method	Liquid Culture Method
1.	It is not so sensitive	It is very sensitive.
2.	More information is obtained.	Relatively provides less information.
3.	Usually occupies much lesser space in an incubator; besides, does not require enough degree of handling and work up effort.	Occupies relatively larger space in an incubator, and also requires sufficient procedural details.
4.	It essentially provides only a restricted knowledge with respect to the *actual product yield potentials* amongst the various isolates obtained.	It distinctly provides a much vivid idea with regard to the physical, nutritional and production responses of an organism in comparison to the actual fermentation production parameters.

1.3.2.2 Salient Features of Secondary Screening

The various vital and important **salient features of secondary screening** are enumerated below:

1. It may be either *qualitative* or *quantitative* in its approach.

a. Qualitative Approach: Provides valuable information(s) with regard to the *wide spectrum* or *ranges of microorganisms* that is significantly sensitive to an altogether newly discovered antibiotic.

b. Quantitative Approach: Gives authentic information(s) with regard to the specific yields of **'antibiotic substance'** that may be expected when the microorganisms is allowed to grow in various media having varying composition.

Special Notes

i. *There exists no clear cut and necessarily a distinct difference between the qualitative and the quantitative* ***secondary screening.***

ii. *In reality, a* ***qualitative screening*** *for the ensuing 'microbial inhibition spectrm' of an antibiotic essentially gives an ample idea with respect to the* ***'test organisms'*** *that are found to be sensitive to the antibiotic, whereas it may provide information pertaining to the comparative prevailing sensitivities of these organisms to the* ***respective antibiotic.***

2. It invariably promulgates a wide spectrum of highly valuable and authentic information(s) that are very much needed in order to evaluate the *precise* and *actual* (true) potential of particular microorganisms for industrial application.

Example: It must determine as well as establish the types of microorganisms that are involved, in addition to the fact whether these may be classified at least to various *genera* or *families*.

Note: The aforesaid information is of immense value, because it broadly makes possible a befitting comparison between the newly isolated organisms with those already reported either in the scientific journals or in the patent* literatures showing a adequate logical evidence to produce fermentation products of commercial value and interest.

3. ***Classification of Organisms:*** Interestingly, classification of the organisms due to secondary screening certainly makes a room for the much needed prediction of whether they **(organisms)** do own any genuine pathogenicity for *humans, animals* or *plants* that would necessarily warrant special precautions in the handling of such organsisms. Besides, it gives a probable prediction of the *growth characteristic features* in the intensive studies of these microorganisms.

4. ***Establishing a More Economically Variable Process:*** The secondary screening must provide adequate information(s) with respect to the fact whether the microorganisms (isolated and identified) are virtually giving rise to **'newer chemical entities'** not reported earlier or, alternatively, for such **fermentation procedures** which are already reported.

Highlights: A few highlights are as given below:

i. In case, the resulting product happens to be an altogether newly discovered compound then an attempt must be made to establish its real genuine usage.

ii. In actual practice, the **patents** are usually granted for exclusively *new as well as useful products**.

5. ***Real Differences in Product Yield Potentials:*** The secondary screening must be able to detect the real differences in product yield potentials amongst the various isolates irrespective of the fact whether the outcome of the **'ultimate fermentation product'** is or is not a *new chemical entity* (*i.e.,* compound). Therefore, in order to save on valuable resources, such as: manpower, time, energy and money, it is almost mandatory to allow the organisms to grow upon different media in liquid-culture for various length of time so as to accomplish quantitative assays effectively. Nevertheless, the aforesaid studies may be carried out only after the complete rejection (or elimination) or *useless cultures* previously ascertained by agar-plate procedures.

6. ***Critical Requirements for Specific Microorganisms:*** The secondary screening should articulately reveal whether the *two* cardinal phenomena, namely: (*a*) *growth of the organism;* and (*b*) *formation of chemical products,* are dependent on pH, aeration or other critical requirements associated with specific microorganisms. Importantly, it must also detect **'gross genetic instability'** present in various *microbial cultures.*

Therefore, **secondary screening** essentially expatiates the following relevant facts:

- a microorganisms is of practically little importance if it takes care of to either **mutate** or **change** in some manner thereby drastically losing its inheret ability to accumulate high yields of product.

- It must reveal evidently whether some **'medium constituents'** are either missing or perhaps prove to be too toxic to the growth of the organism or to its in-built capacity to accumulate fermentation products.
- it should exhibit the **chemical stability profile** of the product; and consequently, the **product's solubility profile** in different organic solvents.
- it must adequately establish whether the resulting product bears a **simple, complex** or rather a **macro-molecular structure.**
- it should demonstrate explicitely whether the **'ultimate isolated product'** possesses either *typical physical characteristic properties,* for instance: UV-absorption, fluorescence; or *typical chemical characteristic properties* which may be judiciously exploited to detect the **compound** *via* various sophisticated analytical techniques or by the aid of elaborated paper chromatographic studies, and which ultimately be of immense value is predicting and assigning the most probable chemical structure of the **'compound'.**
- adequate determinations must be made so as to ascertain whether *gross human, animal or plant toxicity* can be attributed to the *fermentation product(s)* obtained specifically during the **secondary screening,** in case it is be utilized (*e.g.,* **antibiotics**) exclusively in the treatment of human ailments. Therefore, the compound must be in its **purest form** so as to obtain both valid and reliable information's. Importantly, for studying the detailed toxicity tests of an **impure compound,** one should resort to a qualified and educated **'guess'** with respect to the various types of contaminating substances which may be intimately associated with the compound, and ultimately provide appropriate *experimental parameters* for such **identified contaminants** in the ensuing **toxicity testing.**
- it must reveal clearly whether the **'final product'** obtained from a microbial fermentation occurs in the culture broth in a **racemic form** *i.e.,* as a mixture of *optically active d-* and *l*forms of which one may turn out to be a biologically active material. Besides, there may also exist two or even more compounds of variant nature that could be obtained from a **'single fermentation'.** Hence, in the *ultimate fermentation broth* one may come across frequently one to several **intermediate chemical entities** in the prevailing *'metabolic pathways'* leading to product formation; besides absolutely **unrelated chemical entities.** Importantly, the presences of additional minor as well as major products are of **distinct interest,** because their subsequent recovery and commercial value as viable by-products may substantially improve upon the economic status of the **'prime fermentaion'.**
- it should adequately ascertain the fact whether the ensuing microorganisms are capable of undergoing changes under the influences of chemical compounds or even cause destruction of their self-generated fermentation products. Thus the microorganisms may, by virtue of the relatively high-level accumulation of product present in the culture broth, generate enough **adaptive enzymes** that would grossly destroy the potential value and usefulness of the product.

Examples

a. A microorganisms may be able to produce a **'racemes enzyme'** which in turn shall alter the *L*-configuration of an amino acid product to an equimolar mixture of the corresponding *D*- and *L*-isomers, with the *D*-isomers exhibiting almost little biological value.

b. A microorganism may strategically respond to the accumulation of an amino acid by adaptively influencing the production of a **'decarboxylase enzyme'** which would specifically remove CO_2 from the resulting molecule, thereby rendering an **organic amine** at the end.

- **Secondary screening** thus may give rise to a broad-spectrum of valuable information, such as:

(*i*) it helps in deciding precisely which of the various **microbial isolates** possess probable useful potentialities as a **viable industrial organism.**

(*ii*) it immensely helps most articulately in predicting the approaches to be utilized justifiably in persuing further productive, aggressive and meaningful research on the selected microorganism and its corresponding fermentation process.

1.4 Fermentors [or Bioreactors]

The most articulate, manipulative and progressive industrial (commercial) usag of microorganisms invariably needs that they be allowed to grow in large vessels essentially loaded with considerable quantum of highly nutritive cultur media. These specially designed vessels are universally and commonly termed as **fermentors** or **bioreactors.** In reality, these bioreactors (fermentors) could be quite complicated in design by virtue of the fact that most abundantly they should cater for the precise control and meticulous observation of the innumerable facets of microbial growth and the biosynthesis.

Another school of thought has rightly baptized the above mentioned phenomenon as the **bioprocess** or **fermentation technology.** In a rather broader perspective the *fermentation technology* or, as it is now widely recognised, *bioprocess technology* were conspicuously were derived in part from the use of microorganisms for the generous production of various important and vital products, for instance: *pharmaceutical drugs* [*e.g.,* **antibiotics,** diagnostic agents (enzymes, monoclonal antibodies MABs), enzyme inhibitors, steroids, vaccines]; *food products* [*e.g.,* cheeses, yoghurts, sauerkraut (chopped pickled cabbage), fermented pickles and sausages, soy sauce, tempeh, miso, mushroom products, starch products, vitamins and amino acids, glucose and high fructose syrups, functional modifications of proteins and pectins]; *beverages* [*e.g.,* beers, wines, derived spirits]; *organic chemicals* [*e.g.,* ethanol, acetone, acetic acid, citric acid, itaconic acid, *n*-butanol, perfumeries, enzymes, polymers (mainly polysaccharides)]; *inorganic chemicals* [*e.g.,* metal beneficiation, bioaccumulation and leaching (Cu, U)]; *energy* [*e.g.,* ethanol (gasohol), methane (biogas), biomass]; *agriculture products* [*e.g.,* animal feed stuffs (SCP)*, veterinary vaccines, ensilage and composing processes, microbial pesticides, *Rhizobium* and other N-fixing bacterial inoculants, *Mycorrhizal* inoculants, plant-cell and tissue culture (vegetative propagation), embryo production, genetic improvement].**

The aforesaid divergent and highly specific forms of **bioprocessing technology** were overwhelmingly long regarded as spectacular piece of *'arts'* or splendid *'crafts'*, but most interestingly these are now attracting wide recognition world wide besides increasingly being subjected to the full array of **modern science** and **magic touch of technological advancements.** Besides, the aforesaid innumerable highly beneficial product formations was the legitimate cognizance of the critical and specific roles of the **'microorganisms'** essentially utilized in the removal of extremely obnoxious and unhealthy waste products, that has resulted in the world-wide service industries intimately associated with water purification, effluent treatment, and above all the solid waste management efficaciously.

Biofermentors (bioprocessing technology) in its several recognized variants essentially embrances a relatively large multitude of *complex enzyme-catalyzed biochemical reactions* within the **specific microorganisms.** Nevertheless, these reactions are exclusively and critically dependent upon the broad spectrum of physical and chemical parameters which predominantly exist in their immediate vicinity. Importantly, the categorical success of the bioprocessing phenomenon will take place only when all the vital experimental conditions are duly brought together.

Bioprocessing technology, in the recent time, has spread its tentacles in several *major commercial byproducts* solely *derived from microbial fermentations,* such as:

(a) Primary Metabolites: *i.e.,* to overproduce certain essential primary metabolites, for instance: citric acid, lactic acid, acetic acid, glycerine, *n*-butanol, amino acids, vitamins, polysaccharides, perfumeries etc.

*(b) **Secondary Metabolities:*** *i.e.,* to produce most important and life-saving **'antibiotics'** (*pharmaceutical drugs*) *via* well defined *fermentative procedures,* for instance: Giberellins, Pencillins, Cephalosporins, Streptomycin etc.

*(c) **Enzymes***: *i.e.,* to produce a large variants of industrially viable and useful enzymes *e.g.,*
(a) intracellular enzymes: invertase, asparaginase, restriction endonucleases etc.;
(b) exocellular enzymes: amylases, pectinases and proteases.

1.4.1 Salient Features of Bioreactors

The various salient features of **'bioreactors'** or **'biotechnological processes'** are as enumerated under:

1. In the recent past, biotechnological processes (bioprocess technology) is found to use both *aggressively* and *progressively* **specific cells** derived exclusively from higher plants and animals to give rise to several useful and vital products.

Examples:

a. **Plant Cell Culture:** It is largely aimed at the adequate formation of **secondary products solely,** for instance: **drugs** (antibiotics), **flavours,** and **perfumes.**

b. **Animal Cell Culture (Mammalian Cell Culture):** It is mainly concerned with the production of extremely potent and life-saving products, such as:

(*i*) **Vaccines;** (*ii*) **antibody formation;** and (*iii*) protein molecules *e.g., interferon, interleukins* etc.

2. It has been amply demonstrated, proved and established beyond any reasonable doubt that the aforesaid **'bioproducts'** cannot be produced economically *via* other *chemical processes.*

Besides, with the advent of latest developments in the specific fields of *genetic engineering* (or **'organisms'**) and *technological advances* (in **processing modes**) one may accomplish wonderful viable economies in the production of **'bioproducts'.**

Examples:

(*a*) Huge quantum of cells are magnificently grown under *well-defined stringent controlled conditions,* whereby the *'organisms'* may be adequately *cultivated* and *motivated* to produce the desired products by the help of a **precise physical/technical containment system (*i.e.,* bioreactor)** in addition to the *appropriate medium composition* and the *specific environment growth regulating parameters,* for instance: **aeration** and **temperature.**

(*b*) Articulated optimization of various streams of the **'bioprocess'** spans not only the prevailing *biosystems* but also the ensuing *technical systems.* In actual practice, the careful and proper exploitation of an **organism's potential** to produce apparently *distinct divergent products* having *well-defined characteristic features, quality parameters* and in *huge quantum* will necessarily require the **in-depth knowledge of the biochemical mechanisms of product generation** duly.

3. Importantly, the same apparatus, of course with certain modifications, may be used to bring into being several vital products *e.g.,* **antibiotic, enzyme, amino acid** or **single-cell protein.** One may look at the *bioprocess phenomenon* as comprising of several sequential modes of operation, such as: mixing microorganisms with a nutrient broth, allowing the components of react (*e.g.,* yeast cells with a nutrient broth) to give rise to the formation of **ethanol.**
4. Most *biotechnological procedures* are meticulously carried out very much within *bioreactors* or *containment systems'* whereby large excess of cells that are actually involved in these processes and the **bioreactor** essentially secures their intimate involvement with the suitable correct dium as well as experimental parameters for the *actual growth* and *product formation.*
5. One of the most desired and major functional criterion of a **'bioreactor'** is to reduce drastically the cost involved in *producing a product* or *providing a service.* A few typical examples having the diverse product categories being produced on a commercial scale in **bioreactors** are summarized as under:

Category	Examples
Cell mass	Baker's yeast, single-cell protein
Cell components	Intracellular proteins
Biosynthetic products	Antibiotics, vitamins, amino and organic acids
Catabolic products	Ethanol, lactic acid, methane
Bioconversion	High fructose corn syrup, 6-amino pencillanic acid
Waste treatment	Activated sludge, anaerobic digestion.

1.4.2 Classifications

Evidences from the literature survey amply justifies that **'bioreactors'** are invariably classified in *two* broad categories, namely:

a. Based on the **'agent used'**, and *b.* Based on the **'process requirements'**

Bioreactors that are exclusively based on the **'agent used'** may be further sub-divided into *two* groups, such as:

i. Those based on *living cells,* and *ii.* Those *employing enzymes.*

On the contrary, **'bioreactors'** that are solely based upon the **'process requirements'** may be further classified into *four* prominent groups, for instance:

i. Solid-state fermentation,
ii. Anaerobic fermentation,
iii. Aerobic fermentation, and
iv. Immobilized cell bioreactors.

The aforesaid *four* groups of **'bioreactors'** based on the *'process requirements'* shall now be treated individually in the sections that follow:

1.4.2.1 Solid State Fermentation

In true sense, such fermentation procedures are usually governed by both *microbial growth* and *product formation* predominantly taking place at the surface of the solid substrates, such as: *mold ripened cheeses; starter cultures; mushroom cultivations* etc.

Importantly, in the recent past, the solid state fermentation approach has been judiciously and skilfully extended for the production of certain high-value products of interest, namely: *extracellular enzymes, valuable chemical entities, fungal toxins,* and *fungal spores* (exclusively employed for **biotransformation processes**).

However, the usual *traditional substrates* essentially comprise of a plethora of **'agricultural products'** like rice, maize, wheat, soybean etc. It has been observed duly that the prevailing substrate predominantly caters for a *rich* and *complex* source of nutrients that either may or may not require to be supplemented. Interestingly, *'substrates'* belonging to this specific class selectively support the **mycelial organisms** that are capable of growing even at an elevated nutrient concentrations, and ultimately give rise to variety of **extra cellular enzymes,** such as:

(*a*) A huge number of **filamentous fungi;** and

(*b*) A relatively small number of bateria (*e.g.,* **actinomycetes** and one strain of *Bacillus*).

It is, however, pertinent to mention at this point in time that according to the physical characteristic state, the *solid state fermentations* are invariably categorized into *two* major heads, namely:

(*i*) **Low moisture solids** fermented either without or with occassional/continuous agitation, and

(*ii*) **Suspended solids** fermented in packed columns through which liquid is circulated.

In actual practice, the fungi which are exclusively employed for carrying out the **solid state fermentations** are normally that **obligate aerobes.** The following table summarizes a few typical examples of the solid state fermentations which are used extensively in Japan for large-scal products of **food, enzyme** and **organic acid(s).**

S.No	Product	Substrate	Primary Genus	Product Used As	Comments
1.	Amylase	Rice *A.*	*Oryzae*	Enzyme	–
2.	Cellulose	Wheat Bran	*Trichoderma reesei* [Synonym:Viride]	Enzyme	–
3.	Citric acid	Cooked vegetable residues	*Aspergillus niger*	Organic acid	Occasionally in Japan
4.	Hamanatto	Soybean; Wheat	*Aspergillus sp.*	Food	Processed Further
5.	Miso	Rice/Barey; Soybean	A. *Oryzae*	Food	do
6.	Soy Sauce (Shoyu)	Soybean, Wheat	*Aspergillus Soyae* or *Oryzae*	Food	do
7.	Sufu	Tofu	*Actinomucor* sp.,	Food	do
8.	Tempeh	Soybean	*Rhizopus* spp., [*R.Oligosporus*]	Food	Further processing not required

Special Remarks: Following are some of the special remarks with respect of the solid state fermentation procedures, namely:

1. They make use of either stationary or rotary trays,
2. Invariably both *temperature* and *humidity* controlled air is being circulated through the entire stacked solids,
3. *rotary-drum type fermentors* are used rather less frequently,
4. They usually offer certain **unique advantages** besides some vital disadvantages also, and
5. Major commercial application of this phenomenon for the biochemical production is solely confined to Japan.

1.4.2.2 Anaerobic Fermentation

It is quite evident that in anaerobic fermentation a provision for 'aeration' is absolutely not required as shown in Fig. 1.1.

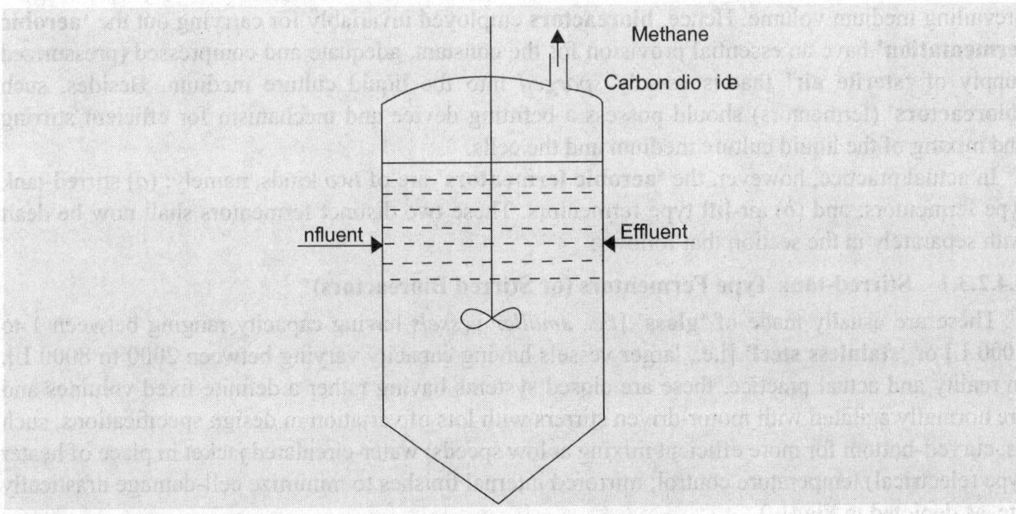

Fig. 1.1 *Anaerobic Digester or Bioreactor.*

Salient Features: The salient features of *'anaerobic fermentation'* are as follows:

1. Certain specific instances do require aeration at initial stages only to build-up inoculums.

2. Large number of cases do not essentially need a *'mixing device'*, whereas a few of them the initial mixing of the inoculums is an absolute necessity.
3. Once the fermentation commences the CO_2 generated in the reaction vessel generates sufficient mixing (*i.e.,* causes agitation).
4. **Air** present in the headspace of the fermentor must be adequately replaced by CO_2, N_2, H_2 or an appropriate mixture of these; and this specific operation is absolutely vital and important for critical **obligate anaerobes** *e.g., Clostridium.*
5. Process of **'fermentation'** invariably gives rise to CO_2 and H_2, that are carefully collected in pressurized cylinders and used accordingly in various commercial and production utilities, namely:
   i. CO_2 - for making dry ice and methanol,
   ii. CO_2 - for making carbonated beverages *e.g.,* beers, soft-drinks, shandies, club-sodas, etc., and
   iii. CO_2 - for slowly bubbling into freshly inoculated fermenters.

Note

1. Acetogens plus other gas-utilizing organisms it is necessary to bubble through the medium either oxygen free sterile CO_2 or other mixture of gases.
2. Acetogens may be cultured successfully in 400 L fermentors by carefully bubbling sterile CO_2; and thus 3 *kg cells* could be harvested in every individual operation.
3. Recovery of *'desired final products'* from the anaerobic fermentors does not essentially need anaerobic environments anymore. However, several **'enzymes'** belonging to such organisms are **high oxygen-sensitive.** Hence, the sole objective for the recovery of such enzymes may be accomplished by harvesting the *'cells'* strictly under **anaerobic conditions.**

1.4.2.3 Aerobic Fermentation

The apparent cardinal and most distinct features of the **'aerobic fermentation'** is the essential and critical provision of constant adequate *aeration.** It has been observed that in certain specific instances the *actual quantum of air required per hour is almost 60 folds* in comparison to the prevailing medium volume. Hence, **bioreactors** employed invariably for carrying out the **'aerobic fermentation'** have an essential provision for the constant, adequate and compressed (pressurized supply of **'sterile air'** that is usually *sparged* into the liquid culture medium. Besides, such **'bioreactors'** (fermentors) should possess a befitting device and mechanism for efficient stirring and mixing of the liquid culture medium and the cells.

In actual practice, however, the **'aerobic fermentors'** are of *two* kinds, namely: (*a*) stirred-tank type fermentors; and (*b*) air-lift type fermentors. These two distinct fermentors shall now be dealt with separately in the section that follows:

1.4.2.3.1 Stirred-tank Type Fermentors (or Stirred Bioreactors)

These are usually made of **'glass'** [*i.e., smaller vessels* having capacity ranging between 1 to 1000 L] or **'stainless steel'** [i.e., larger vessels having capacity varying between 2000 to 8000 L]. In reality and actual practice, these are closed systems having rather a definite fixed volumes and are normally agitated with motor-driven stirrers with lots of variation in design specifications, such as: curved-bottom for more efficient mixing at low speeds; water-circulated jacket in place of heater type (electrical) temperature control; mirrored internal finishes to minimize cell-damage drastically etc. as depicted in Fig. 1.2.

Advantages: The various vital advantages of stirred-tank type fermentors are as stated below:

1. Several **heteroploid cell-lines** may be grown successfully in such vessels.
2. Small scale reactors (cap. 2–50 L) fulfil the need for research *biochemicals* from cells.

3. Large scale reactors (cap. 100–5000 L) are largely employed for growing hybridoma cells for the production of *monoclonal antibodies* (MABs); whereas, their yields from the *'cultured cells'* ranges meagerly between 1–2% of those obtained by passing the cells *via* peritoneal cavity of mice.

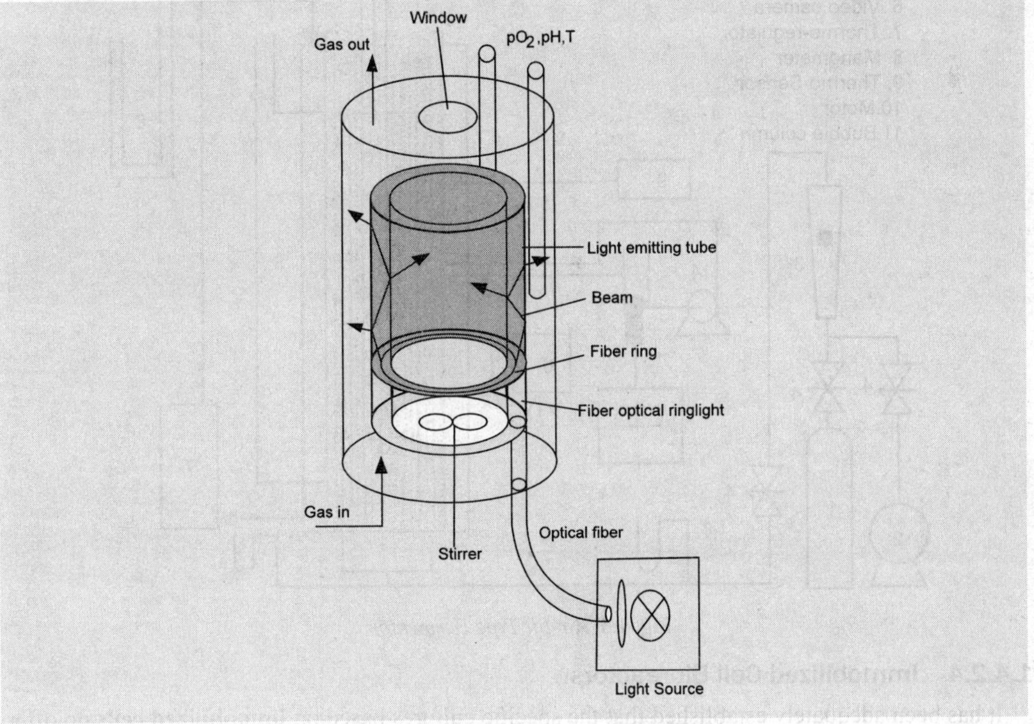

Fig. 1.2 *Stirred-Tank Type Fermentor.*

Note: Namalva cells grown for 'interferon'; but in actual practice the maximum size of the 'stirred bioreactor' is 20L only because larger vessels are rather not-so-convenient and difficult to handle, to autoclave, and also to agitate the culture medium effectively.

1.4.2.3.2 Air-lift Type Fermentors

The cultures in an **air-lift type fermentor** are not only subjected to *'aeration'* but also *'agitation'* by passing sterilized compressed air bubbles introduced strategically at the bottom of vessel as shown in Fig. 1.3.

Salient Features of Air-lift Type Fermentors: The various vital salient features of an air-lift type fermentor are as follows:

1. The fermentor has an inner draft tube *via* which the *air bubbles* as well as the *aerated medium* rise, because this effectively gives rise to through mixing of the culture and aeration simultaneously.
2. The air bubbles being lighter lift to the top of the medium and the air subsequently gets released through on outlet.
3. In this process, importantly the cells and the medium which eventually lift out of the draft tube usually move downwards outside the tube and are recirculated duly.
4. Air-lift type fermentors with a capacity of 2–90L are invariably available for large-scale production. However, 2000L fermentors are being employed specifically for the production of monoclonal antibodies (MABs).

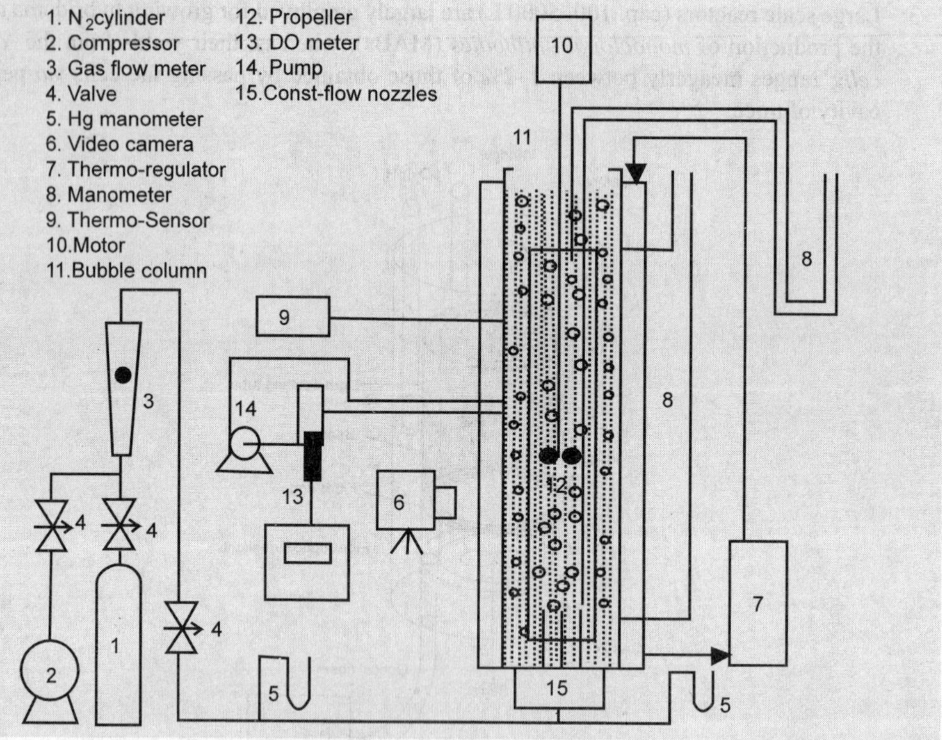

Fig. 1.3 *Air-lift Type Fermentor*

1.4.2.4 Immobilized Cell Bioreactors

It has been adequately established that the specific cultures based on **immobilized cells** do offer several important and vital advantages, namely:

1. Possess relatively *higher cell densities* to the tune of 50 – 200 × 10^{-6} cells. m L^{-1},
2. Retain evidently greater *stability* and *longevity* of cultures,
3. Possess *wider applicability* to both suspension and monolayer cultures,
4. Afford a plethora of systems that essentially *protect the cells from shear forces* by virtue of the medium flow, and
5. Provide comparatively *less dependence of cells at higher densitites* on the external supply of growth factors that eventually saves culture cost significantly.

In actual practice, there exist *two* basic approaches to cell immobilization, such as: (*a*) immurement; and (*b*) entrapment. These two different aspects shall now be treated individually in the section that follows:

1.4.2.4.1 Immurement Cultures

Obviously, in such type of cultures, cells are invariably confined within a medium permeable barrier. In actual practice, one may make use of the clustre of **'hollow fibers'** usually packed in an appropriate cartridge offer one such system. In this particular instance, the medium gets circulated through the fiber whereas the cells in suspension are normally present in the cartridge outside the fiber.

Advantages: The various cardinal advantages of this technique are as follows:

1. an extremely effective technology for scales upto 1 L, and affords cell densities upto 1 – 2 × 10^8 cells . mL^{-1},
2. Sophisticated units may yield even upto 40g MABs per month,

3. Interestingly, *membranes permitting medium* and *gas diffusion medium* are also employed to develop **bioreactors** of this particular type, and
4. Commercial availability of both small and large scale versions of **membrane bioreactors.**

1.4.2.4.2 Entrapment Cultures

In this particular instance, the cells are very much retained within an **'open matrix'** *via* which the medium flows freely.

Examples:

1. **Opticell** is the most befitting example wherein the cells are extrapped well within the porous ceramic walls of the unit. In actual practice, opticell units of upto 210 m^2 surface are generally available that may give rise upto 50g MABs per day.

The opticell units can also be enmeshed in **cellulose fibres,** such as: DEAE, TLC, QAE, TEAE. All these fibres are adequately autoclaved (sterilized), and washed subsequently as prescribed. Ultimately these are carefully incorporated into a **stirred/spinner bioreactor** at a concentration of $3g.L^{-1}$.

2. **Porous Microcarriers:** These are rather small beads (having diameter ranging between 170 to 600 μm) made up of gelatin, collagen, glass or cellulose that predominantly possess a network of interconnecting pores. In fact, these pores afford remarkable advantages, namely:
   i. Provide a tremendous enhancement in surface area *Vs* volume ratio,
   ii. Allow adequate and efficient diffusion of medium and product that are absolutely suitable for scaling up, and
   iii. Found to be equally beneficial for both *monolayer* and *suspension* cultures. Interestingly, these plus points may be amalgamated and arranged in **different variants of bioreactors** *e.g., fixed-bed reactors, fluidized-bed reactors,* and *stirred reactors.*

Future Scopes: It is, however, earnestly believed that future developments in this direction would probably render the **immobilized cell systems the most prevalent and dominant production systems of the twenty-first century.**

1.4.3 Design and Bioreactors (Fermentor Variants)

It is, however, pertinent to state here that the various design and types of **bioreactors (fermentors)** invariably employed either in *small-scale* or in *large-scale* (commercial) utilities and production are essentially of *twelve* types, namely:

(*a*) Fermacell (laboratory) fermentor, (*b*) Bubble-cap fermentor,
(*c*) Loop (recycle) bioreactor, (*d*) Tower bioreactor,
(*e*) Activated sludge bioreactor, (*f*) Continuous flow stirred-tank bioreactor
(*g*) Packed bed bioreactor, (*h*) Trickling film bioreactor,
(*i*) Mist Bioreactor, (*j*) Rotating drum bioreactor
(*k*) Bubble column bioreactor, and (*l*) Commercial fermentation plant.

The aforesaid twelve types of **bioreactors** (fermentors) shall now be described in the section that follows individually:

1.4.3.1 Fermacell (Laboratory) Fermentor

The **fermacell** or **laboratory fermentor** essentially makes use of the phenomena based on **'continuous fermentations'.** In actual practice, these specific fermentations are practically operated on a continuous mode without emptying the **'fermentor'** at each and every harvest of microbial cells or biosynthetic products. To accomplish this *'objective'* the fresh medium is either added *intermittently* or *continuously* to the **fermentor (bioreactor)** so as to replace spent nutrients, and a portion of the fluid, that invariably comprises of either cells or biosynthetic products, from the **'bioreactor'** is intermittently or continuously withdrawn for recovery of the product.

Nevertheless, **'continuous fermentation'** (or **continuous cultivation**) predominantly gives rise to near-balanced growth, with almost negligible fluctuation of nutrients, metabolites, and cell numbers or biomass. Thus, the ensuing practice solely depends upon the fresh medium gaining entrance into a batch system at the particular exponential phase of growth, as shown in Fig. 1.4, having a corresponding withdrawal of medium *plus* cells.

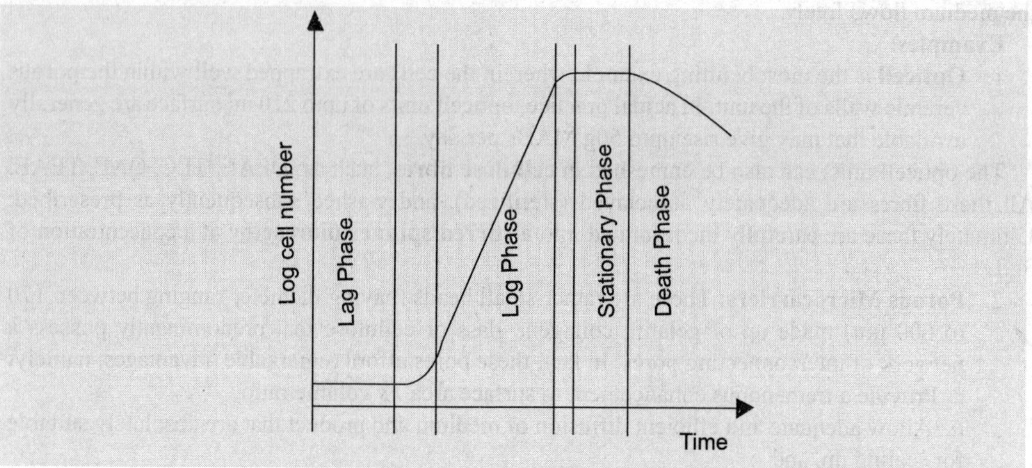

Fig. 1.4 *Growth Factor in a Batch Culture of a Microorganism*

The above graphic representation illustrates the *six* different phases that are encountered in the span of **'growth factor'** in a batch culture of a microorganism, such as:

1. [Lag Phase]: The initial **lag phase** designates a time of no apparent growth, but actual *biochemical analyses* reveal metabolic turnover thereby indicative of the fact that the cells are in the process of adaptation to the prevailing environmental conditions, and also suggest that new growth will commence eventually.

2. [Transient Acceleration Phase]: In this subsequent **transient acceleration phase**, in fact, the inoculum's beings to grow.

3. [Exponential Phase]: In the **exponential phase** the microbial growth specifically proceeds at the maximum possible attainable rate for that organism by virtue of *three* vital reasons *e.g.*, (*a*) absence of growth inhibitors; (*b*) excess of nutrients; and (*c*) ideal experimental conditions. Nevertheless, particularly in the batch cultivations the exponential growth phase is of very limited duration.

4. [Deceleration Phase]: It has been duly observed that when the nutrient parameters start depleting, growth rate decreases first gradually and then drastically thereby gaining entry into the **deceleration phase.**

5. [Stationary Phase]: The prolongation of the deceleration phase ultimately leads to the **stationary phase** whereby the growth rate virtually comes to a stand still.

6. [Death Phase]: The final phase of the growth cycle is termed as the **death phase** when eventually the growth rate has ceased completely.

Caution: A plethora of important biotechnological batch processes are arrested completely before reaching the 'death phase' on account of two vital reasons, namely:

a. Cell lysis and *b.* Decreased metabolism.

Figure 1.5 represents the flow-diagram of a not-so-complicated **'continuous laboratory fermentor'** or **'farmacell fermentor'**. **Methodology:** In an absolutely **mixed continuous culture system** the sterile medium is made to pass directly into the previously sterilized **'bioreactor'** at a steady flow rate, and the culture broth (containing medium, waste products and organisms) usually gets released from it at the same rate thereby maintaining the total volume of the culture in the **'bioreactor'** almost constant.

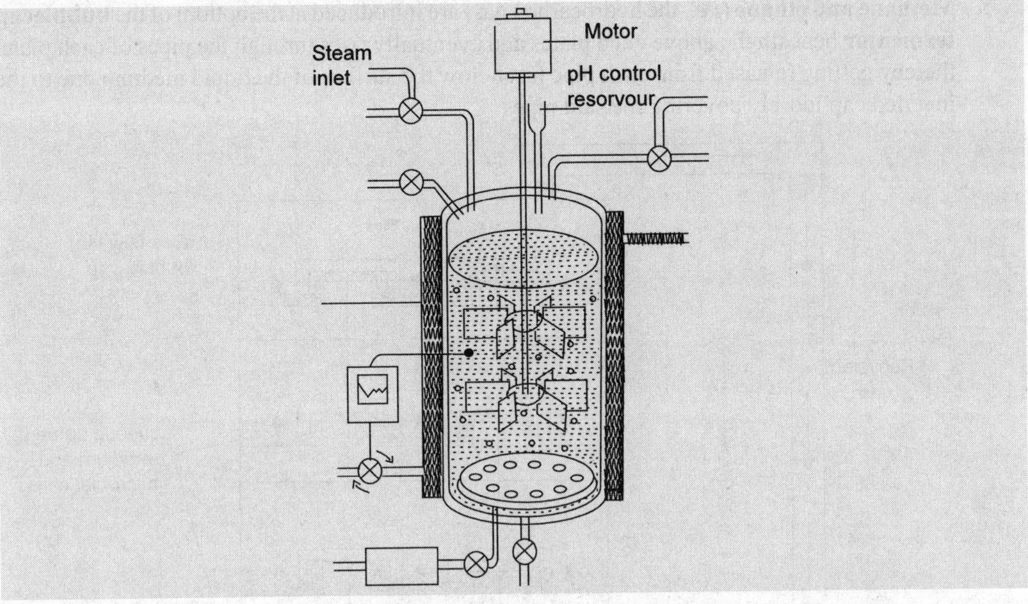

Fig. 1.5 *Diagramatic Representation of a Continuous Laboratory Fermentor*

Advantage: The most prominent advantage of it is that various factors, such as: (*a*) pH of the medium; and (*b*) concentrations of the nutrients as well as the metabolic products, which invariably undergo undue alternations in the course of batch cultivation may be held almost near constant in a continuous cultivation process.

Limitations: In industrial practice, however, the ensuing continuously operated systems are of almost limited application; and essentially include exclusively such operations as: (*a*) single-cell protein and ethanol productions; and (*b*) certain aspects of waste-water treatment phenomena.

1.4.3.2 Bubble-Cap Fermentor

In actual practice, the critical and specific **'gaseous-carbon nutrients'** serving as components of the fermentation media invariably pose *special articulated problems* with respect to the **'design'** of fermentation equipment.

Examples: Methane and **ethane** (gaseous-carbon nutrients) usually represent as two typical and befitting examples, and to circumvent these types of gaseous-carbon nutrients the **'Bubble-Cap Fermentor'** has been designed meticulously to allow the proper utilization of such substrates.

Salient Features: The various salient features of a **'bubble-cap fermentor'** are as follows:

1. It essentially comprises of a tank provided with a series of horizontal plates, as illustrated in Fig. 1.6.
2. Each plate supports nutrient medium devoid of a *carbon* source, and subsequently the medium are duly inoculated with the **'required microorganism'.**
3. Furthermore, each plate is provided with *several short vertical pipes* that are strategically connected to its upper surface, and duly projecting just above the surface of the liquid culture medium.
4. Each short vertical pipe has *two* important provisions, namely: (*a*) a **hole** in the bottom of this pipe allows legitimate contact with the atmosphere above the medium in the next immediate

lower plate; and (*b*) the **top** of the lower rim of the inverted cap extends beneath the surface of the nutrient medium.

5. **Methane and ethane** (*i.e.,* the hydrocarbon gas) are introduced at the bottom of the **bubblecap fermentor** beneath the above cited plates and eventually rises through the pipes of each plate, thereby getting released from each pipe just below the surface of the liquid medium due to the inverted cap loosely covering the said pipes.

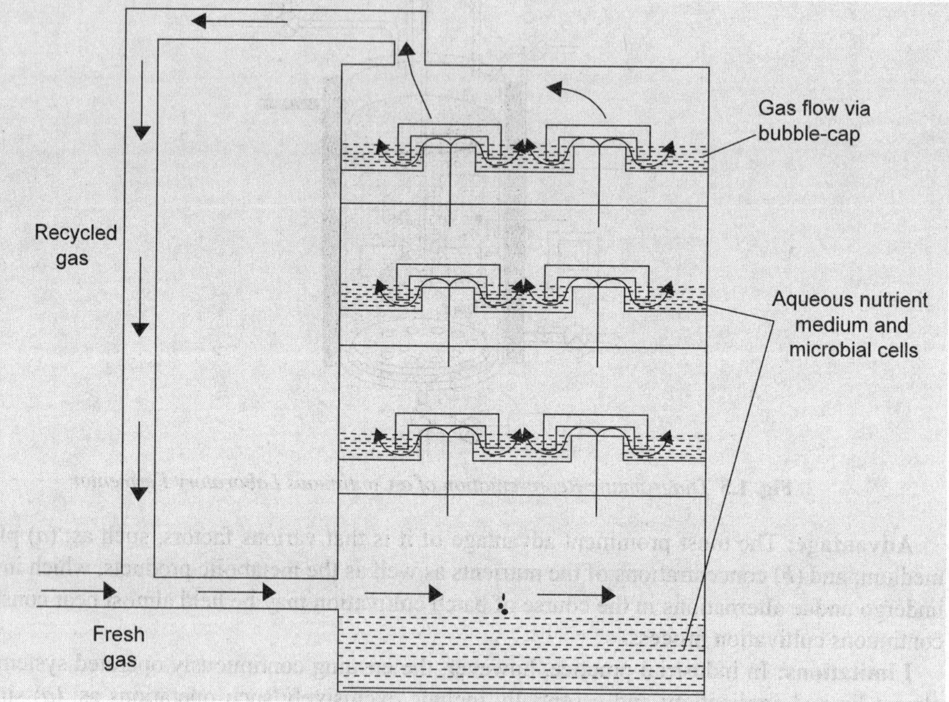

Fig. 1.6 *Bubble-Cap Fermentor Illustrating Microbial Attack on Gaseous Substrates e.g., Gaseous Hydrocarbons*

6. In this manner, the *'quantum of gas'* which fails to get oxidised at a particular plate level in the fermentor usually rises to the next plate to get exposed once again to the prevailing microbial oxidation. However, the **'gas'** rising completely through the *fermentor* may be recycled conveniently to the bottom of the *fermentor* for another passage, and hence usage consequently.
7. Evidently, an **'alternate procedure'** for carrying out the fermentation of **'gaseous substrates'** is to introduce them along with **'air'** *via* the **sparger** into a **submerged aerated fermentation device.**

Caution. It is absolutely necessary to adhere for special stringent precautionary measures, otherwise a good proportion of the *'gaseous substrate'* (*i.e.,* methane and ethane) shall go as a waste along with the air exhausted from the fermentor simultaneously.

Fermentations with Liquid Carbon Substrates: In actual manufacturing operational procedures it has been observed that the fermentations employing solely liquid carbon substrates together with water *e.g.,* liquid hydrocarbons which usually float on the surface of the aqueous medium, may be handled conveniently and effectively in one of the following *three methods,* namely:

(a) Vigorous Impeller Agitation: In reality, the SS or MS tanks for submerged aerated fermentations are employed quite frequently, accompanied by **vigorous impellar agitation** thereby helping to disperse the *'liquid hydrocarbons'* in the form of small oil droplets throughout the aqueous medium. It is, however, pertinent to state here that an *'emulsifying agent'* may also be incorporated so as augment the phenomenon of **dispersion** adequately.

(b) Lift (Cyclic) Fermentor: In this particular process, the required *'liquid hydrocarbon'* substrate is permitted to float upon the surface of the aqueous medium. The latter comprising of requisite/desired microorganisms is now withdrawn continuously from the bottom of the fermentor upto a small-bore lift pipe strategically located at the side of the fermentor. At this juncture, the column of the liquid medium in this very pipe is raised adequately to *two* different modes: (*i*) by introducing sterile air under pressure (*i.e.,* compressed sterile air); and (*ii*) by employing mechanical pumps, — right upto the top of the fermentor where it is duly sprayed over the entire surface of the *'liquid hydrocarbon'*. In fact, the spraying as well as the introduction of the **sterile-air** either into the *life-pipe* or the *head-space* of the fermentor accomplishes the following important aspects, namely: (*i*) maintains the liquid medium well aerated; (*ii*) passage of the condensed aqueous spray down the floating liquid hydrocarbon layer renders the prevailing microorganisms present in the spray into continuous contact with the liquid hydrocarbons; and (*iii*) a forceful spray may tend to break up the **layering effect** of the liquid hydrocarbons upon the **'liquid surface'** predominantly. (*c*) **Baffle Arrangement:** In this **'fermentor design',** the immiscible liquid substrates is duly pumped right into a mixture of *aqueous culture medium* and an *immiscible substrate* from the main reservoir of the fermentor, which is subsequently forced *via* a nozzle against a **baffle rearrangement.** Thus, the resulting thoroughly mixed and aerated splash falls back into the culture reservoir located right below.

1.4.3.3 Loop (Recycle) Bioreactor

Another vital and major approach to **aerobic bioreactor design** essentially makes use of air distribution (having reasonably much lower power consumption) to create both forced and controlled liquid flow in a **loop (recycle) bioreactor.** In this manner, the actual contents of the fermentor are adequately subjected to a **controlled recycle flow,** either involving the *external recycle loop* or very much *within the bioreactor.* Importantly, the process of stirring has been judiciously replaced by a pumping device that could be either *pneumatic* or *mechanical*, as may be observed in the instance of **airlift bioreactor.** Fig. 1.7 depicts a *loop bioreactor.*

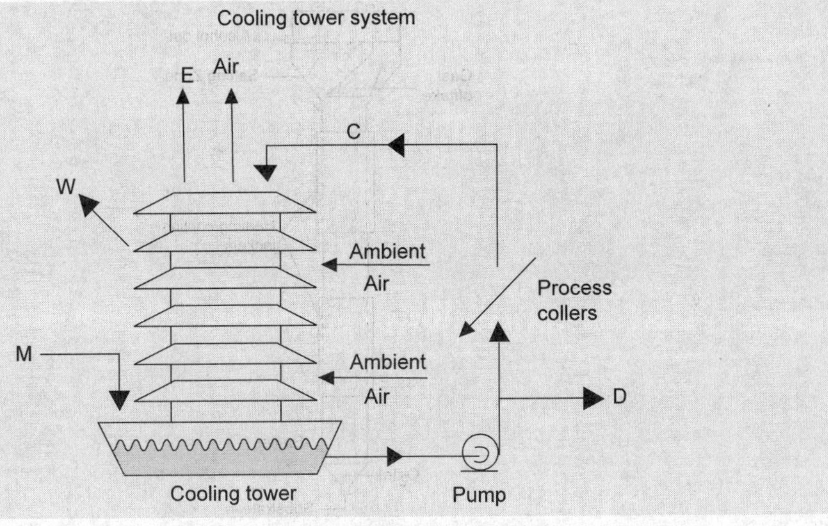

Fig. 1.7 *Loop (Recycle) Bioreactor*

1.4.3.4 Tower Bioreactor

The industrial fermentor *e.g.,* **tower bioreactor** is meticulously designed to provide the best feasible as well as possible growth and biosynthesis conditions meant for industrially vital microbial cultures; besides, to allow ease of manipulation virtually for almost all operations that are associated with the use of the fermentors. Thus, a tower bioreactor should be strong enough to withstand not only the pressures of large volumes of aqueous medium, but also the material of construction of the fermentor *i.e.,* it should not be either *corroded by the fermentation product* or even *contribute severe toxic ions* to the prevailing **growth medium**. Therefore, in an event when the growth of the fermentation microorganism is to take place aerobically, then a subsequent provision should be rendered for rapid introduction of sterile-air into the medium in such a fashion that the **oxygen (O2)** of this air is suitably dissolved in the medium. In short, the oxygen is readily and adequately available to the microorganism, and that the resulting CO_2 obtained from the **'microbial metabolism'** is mostly flushed out from the medium accordingly through a vent provided at the top-end of the **tower bioreactor** as illustrated in Fig. 1.8. The sample is introduced into the **tower bioreactor** from the bottom, and the finished fermented product is removed from the top-end outlet as and when required.

1.4.3.5 Activated Sludge Bioreactor

In actual practice, a huge quantum of **organic waste waters** obtained from either *industrial* or domestic sources, across the globe, are routinely subjected to aerobic and anaerobic systems. In this very context, the **activated sludge bioreactors** are being employed extensively for the specific oxidative treatment of sewage and other liquid wastes. To accomplish such objectives and processes one may utilize effectively either the *batch* or *continuous* **agitated bioreactor systems** to enhance categorically the **'adequate entrainment of air'** to optimize the oxidative breakdown of the organic material. However, these **activated sludge bioreactors** are relatively large in dimensions, and, therefore, to facilitate optimum functioning may have a battery of **'agitator units'** so as to accomplish thorough mixing as well as oxygen uptake. They are mostly and abundantly used in **municipal sewage treatment plants**. Fig. 1.9 depicts the diagram of a typical **activated sludge bioreactor.**

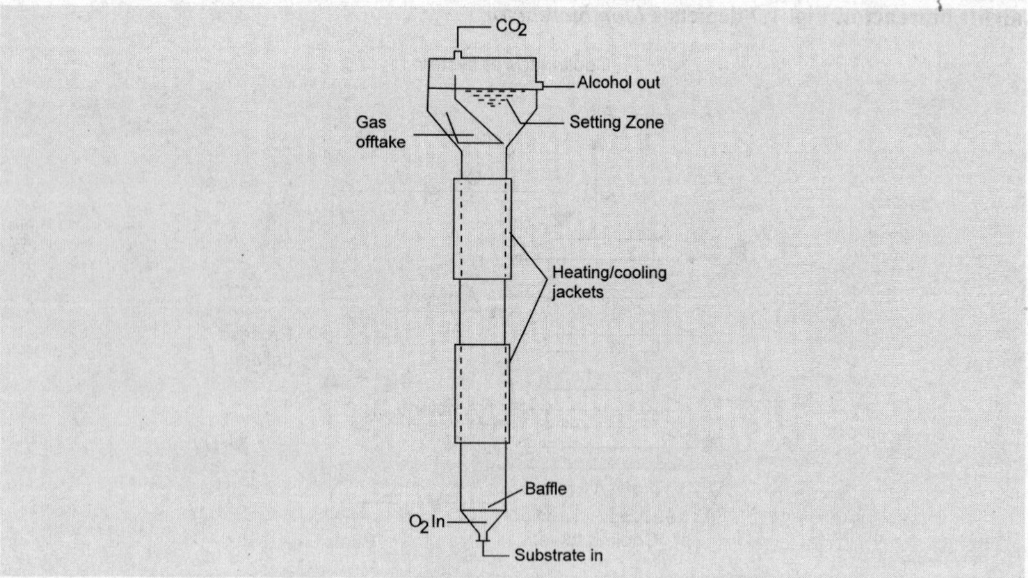

Fig. 1.8 *Tower Bioreactor*

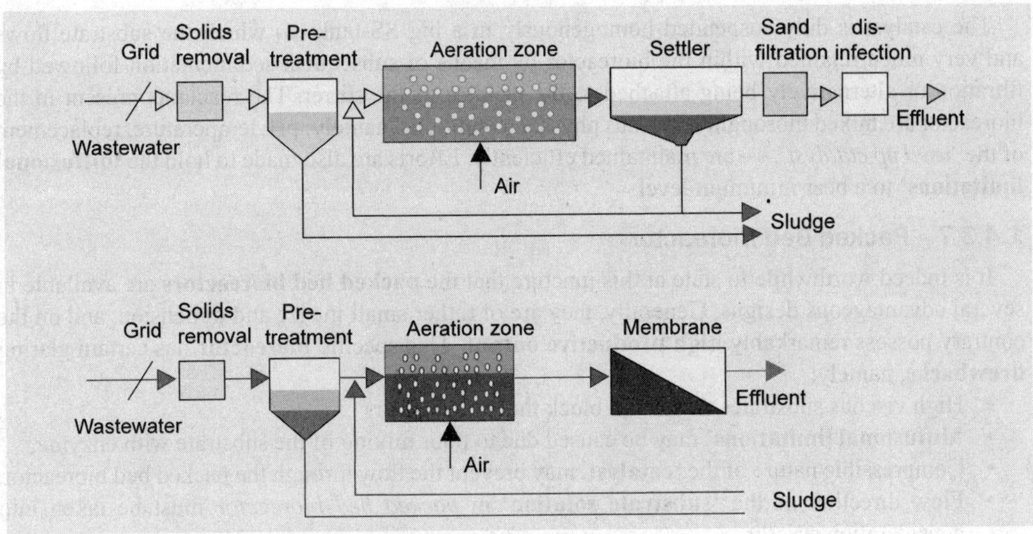

Fig. 1.9 *Activated Sludge Bioreactor.*

1.4.3.6 Continuous Flow Stirred Tank Bioreactor

In general, the **continuous flow stirred tank bioreactors** are of huge dimensions; and, therefore, these are obviously *less productive* and the overall percent conversion of substrate stands at a low level, however, the concentration of the end-product is relatively high. Consequently, the high concentration of the product reasonably inhibits the prevailing activity of the *'catalyst' that* may drastically reduce productively. Perhaps this very fact amply explains the ensuing low rate of conversion of the substrate. In actual practice, however, it is absolutely uneconomical for having a conversion factor of more than 90%. Importantly, the *continuous flow bioreactors* are basically of *two* different types, namely:

(*a*) **Continuous flow stirred tank bioreactor** having adequate provision of thorough mixing; and (*b*) **Plug flow bioreactor** having no mixing arrangement. Nevertheless, the various experimental parameters very much within a **continuous flow stirred tank bioreactor** predominantly remain identical to those prevailing at its outlet.

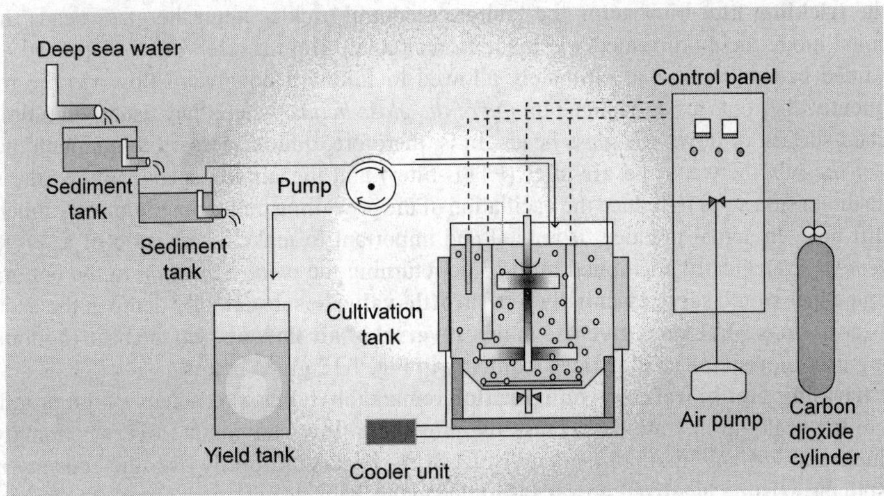

Fig. 1.10 *Continuous Flow Stirred Tank (CFST) Bioreactor*

The catalyst is duly suspended homogenously in a big SS-tank *via* which the substrate flows and very much retained within the bioreactor by means of subsequent sedimentation followed by filtration or alternatively being attached to the paddles of the stirrer. The reactants present in the bioreactor are mixed thoroughly. Various physical conditions, namely: pH, temperature, replacement of the *'used up catalyst'*, — are maintained efficiently. Efforts are also made to hold the **'diffusional limitations'** to a bear minimum level.

1.4.3.7 Packed Bed Bioreactor

It is indeed worthwhile to state at this juncture that the **packed bed bioreactors** are available in several advantageous designs. Generally, they are of rather small in size and dimension, and on the contrary possess remarkably **high productive output**. This specific **bioreactor** has certain glaring **drawbacks**, namely:

- High viscous substrates do tend to block these bioreactors
- **'diffusional limitations'** may be caused due to poor mixing of the substrate with enzyme.
- Compressible nature of the **'catalyst'** may prevent the flow through the packed bed bioreactor.
- Flow direction of the **'substrate solution'** in *packed bed bioreactor* must be taken into consideration strictly.

Fig.1.11. depicts the simple **packed bed bioreactor** wherein the flow of the **'substrate solution'** is indicated upwards. Evidently, the downward flow of the ensuing *'substrate solution'* invariably gives rise to the compression of the bed of enzyme columns. Hence, it is absolutely important and necessary that the said flow of *'substrate solution'* is preferably maintained in the upward direction particularly when *'gas'* is generated during the enzyme reaction. The **enzymes** may be advantageously incorporated into the **PBbioreactor** in *two* different forms, for instance: (*a*) **immobilized enzyme fibre skins**; and (*b*) **spirally rolled-up sheets of immobilized enzymes.**

Advantages of these enzymes are as stated below:

– Ease of handling procedures,

– Possess 'automatic control' and operational modes',

– Extremely cost-effective, and

– Quality control of end-products very easy and convenient.

Fig. 1.11 *Packed Bed Bioreactor*

1.4.3.8 Trickling Film Bioreactor

In the **trickling film bioreactor** the 'culture medium' trickles upon the glass beads. In actual operational mode the culture media is made to recirculate from a reservoir and sprayed carefully on the fixed bed of roots; and ultimately allowed to follow a downward flow *via* the root bed. Subsequently, the roots are inoculated on *top of the glass beads,* where they usually multiply either on the bed-surface or down the glass beads. In is, therefore, quite necessary to maintain the *actual length of the pipe* between the **air-inlet** (PTFE-filter) and the **air-lift** specifically to the shortest possible dimension so as to reduce the oscillation of the prevailing culture medium very much within the airlift tube. In actual practice, it is vital and important to make a provision of a *screw-clamp arrangement* strategically positioned in the pipe returning the *culture medium* to the bottom of the *air-lift* pipe that would serve essentially as a **throttle-valve** to substantially dampen the oscillations that otherwise may sometimes give rise to the **'reversal of air flow up'** *via* the base (bottom) of the **trickling film bioreactor** as illustrated explicitly in Fig. 1.12 given below.

The **trickling film bioreactor configuration** remarkably holds a reasonably high promise with regard to the scale-up operations because the prevailing flow patterns are overwhelmingly under the influence of *'gravity'* that predominantly acts more or less uniformly over the bed very much in contrast to the existing **localized power input** due to mechanized agitation. However, the harvesting of the ensuing roots is relatively difficult on account of their intimate adherence to the glass beads.

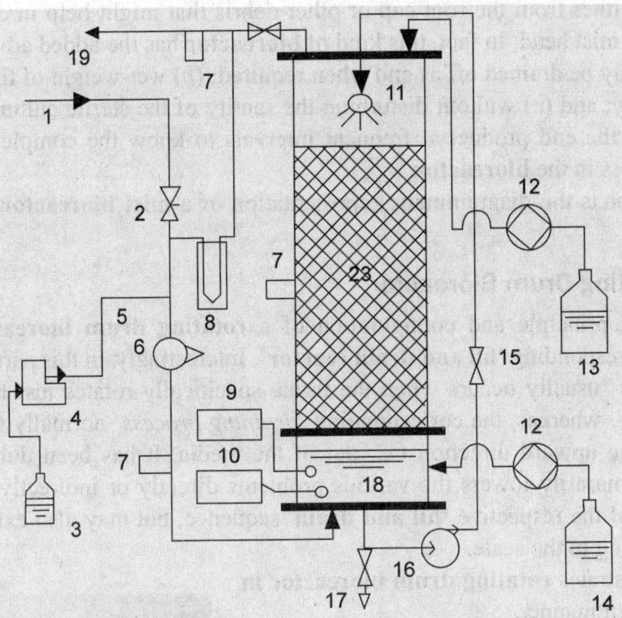

Schematic diagram of the trickle-bed filter: 1. air inlet, 2. needle valve, 3. pure styren solution, 4. syringe pump, 5. capillary, 6. rotameter, 7. sampling ports, 8. liquid manometer, 9. thermometer, 10. pH-meter, 11. spray nozzle, 12. peristaltic pump, 13. nutrient solution tank, 14. sodium hydroxide solution tank, 15. choke valve, 16. medium circulating pump, 17. drain valve, 18. drain vessel, 19. outlet gas

Fig. 1.12 *Trickling Film Bioreactor*

1.4.3.9 Mist Bioreactor

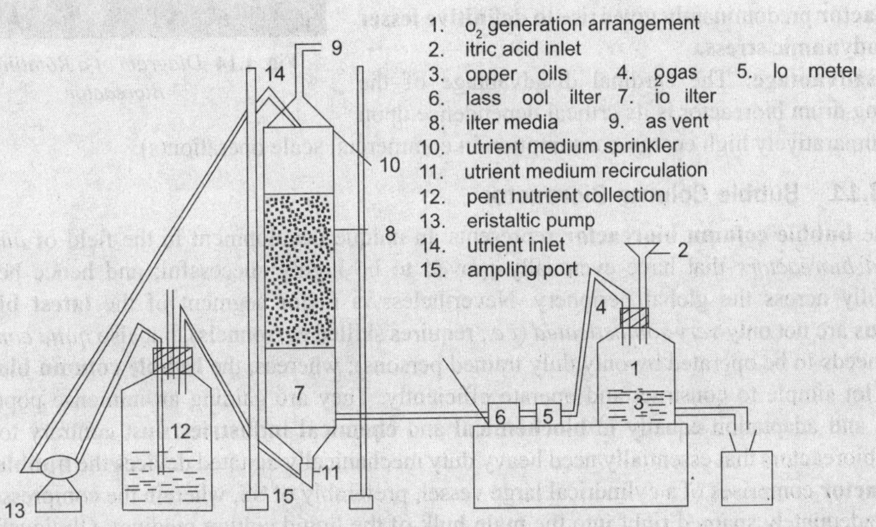

Fig. 1.13 *Diagram of Mist Bioreactor*

In the **mist bioreactor** the culture medium is strategically pumped *via* the provided **'mist head'** by adequately making use of a *peristaltic pump* fitted at the bottom of the reactor along with a *pump limer.* The base of the bioreactor is inserted with a **glass-wool fibre** to enable the filtration of cells shed out either from the root cap or other debris that might help in clogging the pin-hole (jet) located in the mist head. In fact, this kind of **bioreactor** has the added advantages, such as: (*a*) culture medium may be drained off as and when required; (*b*) wet-weight of the **'antibiotic'can** be determined directly; and (*c*) without disturbing the santity of the sterile cultures one may estimate the wet-weight of the end product at frequent intervals to know the completion of the on-going fermentative process in the **bioreactor.**

Figure 1.13 depicts the diagrammatic representation of a **mist bioreactor** showing its various essential parts.

1.4.3.10 Rotating Drum Bioreactor

The underlying principle and configuration of a **rotating drum bioreactor** are very much identical to the corresponding **'fill and drain reactor'**. Interestingly, in this particular configuration, the *'filling process'* usually occurs when the tissue specifically rotates just below the surface of the *'culture media'*; whereas, the corresponding *'draining process'* normally takes place when the tissue rotates in the upward direction *i.e.,* out of the media. It has been duly observed that this configuration summararily lowers the various problems directly or indirectly associated with the scheduled timing of the respective **'fill and drain'** sequence, but may also exhibit certain obvious limitations pertaining to the scale.

Figure 1.14 illustrates **rotating drum bioreactor** in a simple and explicit manner.

It essentially comprises of a horizontal rotating drum strategically filted on rollers. It is, however, pertinent to state here that the rotating motion of the drum markedly facilitates the proper as well as intimate mixing of gas and liquid phases in the bioreactors, whereby accelerating the promotion of efficient oxygen transfer to the respective cells specifically at high values of densities. Importantly, the **rotating drum bioreactor** predominantly gives rise to **definitive lesser hydrodynamic stress.**

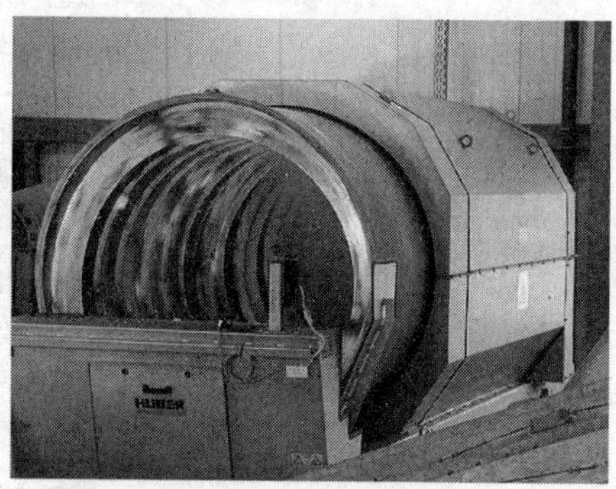

Fig. 1.14 *Diagram of a Rotating Drum Bioreactor*

Disadvantage: The cardinal disadvantage of the rotating drum bioreactor is its critical dependence upon its comparatively high energy consumption in commercial scale operation(s).

1.4.3.11 Bubble Column Bioreactor

The **bubble column bioreactor** represents an unique development in the field of *air-sparged stirred bioreactors* that have eventually proved to be highly successful; and hence being used gainfully across the global periphery. Nevertheless, a major segment of the **latest bioreactor designs** are not only *very sophisticated* (*i.e.,* requires skilled personnels), but also *quite complicated* (*i.e.,* needs to be operated by only duly trained persons); whereas, the **bubble column bioreactors** are a lot simple to construct and operate efficiently. They are gaining an immense popularity in usage and adaptation equally in **biochemical** and **chemical industries.** Just contrary to most of other bioreactors that essentially need heavy duty mechanically agitated devices the **bubble column bioreactor** comprises of a cylindrical large vessel, preferably of SS, wherein the compressed sterile air is adequately sparged right into the main bulk of the liquid culture medium. Obviously, it does not possess any moving parts because a relatively high and efficient degree of mixing could be accomplished with the duly sparged gas (air). Besides, these **bioreactors** the requisite quantum of energy needed for thorough agitation, and also the much required O_2 supplementation exclusively for the *'culture medium'* is duly provided by the sparged air itself.

Advantages: A number of cardinal and noteworthy advantages of a **bubble column bioreactor** are as stated below:

1. It is basically a highly simple arrangement for producing biochemical products *e.g.,* **antibiotics.**
2. It does not require energy for driving any mechanically operative devices whatsoever.
3. Complete elimination of sealing arrangement of the usual stirrer-shaft assembly (in other **'bioreactors'**) is achieved.
4. Absence of any shaft in the head-space of the fermentation vessel invariably provides enough room for various entry ports essentially required in such **bioreactors** that are mostly having rather small sizes and dimensions.
5. Complete freedom from any sort of *'mechanical arrangements'* does help tremendously to maintain the high degree of sterility over extended periods (5–6 days).
6. Absence of shafts also eliminates risk-prone, expensive, highly vulnerable and process unreliability factors to a great extent.

Limitations: The various limitations of the **bubble column bioreactor** are enumerated as under: It is less suited specifically for such processes that essentially make use of highly viscous liquids. It has been observed that the analogous environment in a bubble column bioreactor results in more aggressive homogenous mixing whereby the *'bubbles'* emerging at the sparger-head invariably coalesced instantly to give rise to relatively large bubbles usually termed as **'slugs'**. These *slugs* eventually rose quickly all along the **'axis of the column'** thereby setting the whole body of the liquid into circulation with distinct movement in the **upward direction** in the vicinity of the axis of the cylindrical vessel, and movement in the **downward direction** near the walls of the same vessel.

Sparger Specifications: The **'sparger'** actually determines the initial bubble *size, shape* and *dimension* in a given liquid. Interestingly, a sparger having small-sized diameter holes *e.g.,* sintered glass plate, perforated plate, produces appreciably **'much smaller bubbles'** in comparison to a **'singleorifice sparger'**; and, therefore, provide a distinct, advantageous, and stratgegic **higher interfacial gas-liquid contact surface area** in the close approximity of the *'sparger'*.

Choice of Cultures: Importantly, a host of large-scale fermentative bioprocesses make utilization of **shear-sensitive cultures.** Besides, the **hairy-root cultures,** which are also shear-sensitive, have been grown quite successfully and gainfully in the **bubble column bioreactors.** Ample evidences based on several experimental procedures duly revealed that the usual growth of **plant-cell cultures** in various **bioreactors,** namely: **bubble column bioreactors, stirred-tank bioreactors,** and **shake flasks** was almost identical. Finally, the **bubble column bioreactor** depending on its various excellent characteristic features, such as: **O_2-transfer at low shear, low hydrodynamic stress,** and **low operative cost** render it an exceptional attractive choice for a plethora of articulated scale-up investigative studies in **biotechnology.**

1.4.3.12 Commercial Fermentation Plant

Commercial fermentation plants (or industrial fermentors) are usually designed in such a manner so as to provide the following *three* cardinal objectives, namely:

a. Best possible growth,
b. Biosynthesis parameters for industrially important microbial cultures, and
c. Permit ease of manipulation associated with various operations of the fermentors.

In reality, these **'fermentation vessels'** (*i.e.,* **bioreactors**) should be strong enough to withstand the ensuing pressures of huge volumes of aqueous medium. As most industrial fermentations invariably make use of relatively **'pure cultures'**, the bioreactors should provide adequate provision and means for the control of or prevention of the growth of *possible contaminating microorganisms.* It is quite obvious at this juncture to take cognizance of the fact in the instance whereby growth of the microorganism responsible for fermentation is to take place in an *'aerobic environment'*, it is absolutely necessary to provide adequate and rapid introduction of enough **sterile-compressed air** right into the culture medium so that the oxygen present in this air gets dissolved appropriately in the medium and, hence, simultaneously available to the microorganism. Besides, the CO_2 released from the ensuing microbial metabolism is mostly flushed out from the prevailing medium constantly.

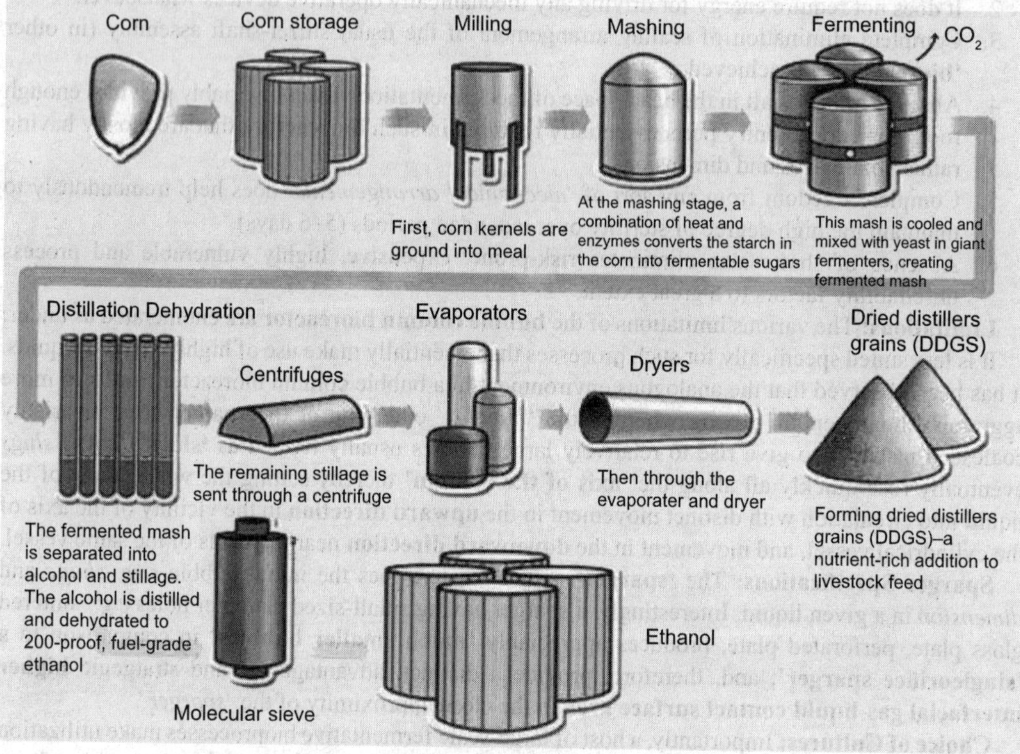

Fig. 1.15 *Flow Sheet Depicting Layout of a Commercial Fermentation Plant*

Highlights of Commercial Fermentation Plant: These are as follows:

1. Must have an adequate provision for the intermittent introduction of *'antifoaming agents**, as and when required by the actual foaming status of the medium.
2. Maintenance of a constant predetermined temperature in the fermentor for optimum growth of the microorganisms.
3. Adequate provision and means for the necessary withdrawal of culture samples in the course of fermentation process; besides, the introduction of inoculums at the initiation of the fermentation process.
4. A suitable aseptic-device for withdrawing sample(s) from the on-going fermentation process in the fermentor to ascertain pH values of the prevailing culture medium; and also for appropriate adjustment of these values by the addition of a calculated amount of alkali/acid to the fermentation medium.
5. Provision of seed tanks or additional innoculum wherein innoculum is produced and introduced directly to the fermentor without making use of extensive pipe-lines, that may usually not only magnify but also give rise to **serious contamination problems.**

1.5 Mutants

Mutants may be defined as — **'variations of genetic structures that eventually breed true'.** Nevertheless, the actual usage of metabolically blocked mutants of certain microorganisms is relatively quite recent, but do possess an immense importance and recognition. In reality, the extensive and intensive study of the **'genetic blocks'** has vividly unravelled largely and specifically the present-day- knowledge of *microbial genetics.* Besides, it has more or less paved the ways and means for directing microorganisms to accumulate comparatively *huge quantum of metabolic intermediates* which usually by virtue of their *'transient existence'* in the metabolic pathways, otherwise fail to get accumulated to any extent in cultures precisely. Interestingly, the actual mechanisms that are intimately associated with a few specific metabolic blocks are being decephered aggressively and progressively nowadays across the globe.

It has been adequately observed that the ensuing *mutation* of the fermentation organism poses a serious problem in a situation when the resulting **mutants** exert a *selective growth advantage* in the course of a prolonged incubation; and simultaneously give rise to an appreciably lesser amount of the desired fermentation product. Therefore, in order to circumvent the phenomenon of *'mutation'* it is always preferred to make use of **multistage-continuous fermentation procedures**, whereby the first fermentor (bioreactor) in the prevailing sequence being reinoculated periodically. In short, the real overall solution to curtail *mutation* is to minimise their incidences of occurrence whereby the offending cells may be flushed from the bioreactors before they get an opportunity to multiply once again.

1.5.1 Isolation of Mutants

In true sense, one may have to look into the means and ways whereby **'mutants'** are actually formed *i.e.,* the phenomenon of **mutagenesis**. In its simplest way one may explain mutagenesis as an essential process in the course of *genetic engineering experiments* that specifically lead to regulate a region of the gene of interest in order to be able to manipulate it in a highly desired manner. Therefore, to accomplish such manipulation(s), it is absolutely vital as well as necessary that the **'desired gene'** must be fully isolated and subsequently characterized meticulously. One must also have a clear picture with regard to its various important information's, such as: *restriction map; sequence of the entire gene;* and *sequence of the 'target region'.*

1.5.1.1 Method of Causing a Mutation

Evidently, the most common methodology usually adopted for effectively causing a mutation is to adequately expose the *'culture of the organism'* to a particular **mutagen.** For this, nitrous acid (HNO_2), is considered to be one of the most widely employed mutagens (chemicals). The culture of the bacteria on being exposed profusely to the respective mutagen, the former may be allowed to grow and multiply under several experimental parameters; and, thus the resulting mutants having **desired phenotypic* characteristic features** are isolated. Consequently, the genotype of these organisms is subjected to an elaborate characterization so that the *'specific gene'* actually responsible for the altered characteristic features in mutants may be scored without any ambiguity. Nevertheless, such mutations are found to be quite random and the resulting **mutants** are invariably recognized by the phenotypic changes in desired characteristic features.

1.5.1.2 Somaclonal Variation

It may be defined as — *'the genetic variability present amongst the cultured cells, plants derived from such cells, and progeny of such plants'.*

In general, the terminology is broadly employed for describing genetic variability invariably present among all types of cells/plants derived from cells that are cultured *in vitro.* It has been duly observed that the plants generated from either *tissue* or *cell* cultures exhibit predominant heritable variants associated with both *qualitative* as well as *quantitative* characteristic features.

Examples: A few typical examples wherein somaclonal variation has been described duly are: potato, tomato, sugarcane etc. There are, in fact, *two* types of variants, namely:

(a) R0 Generation: *i.e.,* those which are obtained in specific homozygous** condition in the plants usually *regenerated from cells cultured in vitro,* and

(b) R1 Generation: *i.e.,* those that are recovered in the *selfed progeny of tissue-culture-regenerated* plants.

1.5.1.2.1 Isolation of Somaclonal Variants

It has been well established that **mutants** for several characteristic features may be far more conveniently and easily isolated from respective cell cultures rather than from whole plant populations. Perhaps the above mentioned analogy holds good because a plethora of cells, approximately say 106–109, may be screened for **'mutant traits'** both effectively and conveniently.

However, in actual practice screening of as many plants would prove to be real herculian task, and may turn out to be virtually impossible. Importantly, **mutants** could be selected effectively to serve a host of definitive aims and objectives, namely: improvement in nutritional quality and aspects; disease resistance; adaptation of specific plants to several well-defined stress parameters *e.g.,* low temperature, soil conditions (salinity), toxic metals (*e.g.,* Al); resistance to various herbicides (chemicals); and to enhance particularly the biosynthesis of plant products usually employed for *industrial* or *medicinal* purposes.

In short, the major acceptable approaches put forward towards the isolation of **somaclonal variants** may be broadly categorized into *two* heads, namely: (*i*) screening; and (*ii*) cell selection, which shall now be dealt with individually in the sections that follows:

1.5.1.2.1.1 Screening

It is solely based upon the observation of a substantial quantum of cells or regenerated plants for the ultimate detection of variant individuals. Perhaps this particular approach is considered to be the only plausible and feasible technique employed for the isolation of **mutants** not only confined to yield exclusively but also the corresponding ensuing yield traits. Generally, as a common practice the *specific* R1 *progeny* (*i.e.,* the progeny of regenerated R0 plants) are invariably scored for the identification of variant- plants, and their *corresponding R2 progeny lines* are mostly evaluated for confirmation.

Advantages: Screening has been exploited both profitably and extensively for the categorical isolation of **'cell clones'** which evidently give rise to certain higher amounts of some biochemical's; besides, computer-aided automated cell sorting devices (CAACSDs) have also been introduced overwhelmingly to aid the screening of upto **1000–2000 cells per second** from the assorted cell-pool the desirable variant cells were segregated *via* automatic means.

1.5.1.2.1.2 Cell Selection

The wonderful **cell selection** *modus operandi* essentially makes use of an appropriate applied **'selection pressure'** that allows the preferential survival or growth of the ensuing variant cells solely.

Examples: A few typical examples of the **cell-selection** are, namely: high-salt concentration, presence of herbicides (chemicals), adequate selection of cells resistant to different toxins, and the like. However, **cell-selection** may be of *two* types, such as:

a) Positive Selection. In this particular instance the selection pressure largely permits only the *mutant cells* to either **survive** or **divide,** and

b) Negative Selection. In this specific case the wild-type of cells usually undergo division; and, therefore, get killed by a **counter selection agent,** such as: arsenate or 5-BUdR*. Obviously, the *mutant cells* fail to undergo division and consequently they escape the possibility of any interaction with the **counter selection agent.** Naturally, the prevailing cells may be rescued by timely removal of the **counter selection agent.** However, in actual practice the **negative-selection** *modus operandi* is employed exclusively for the **isolation** of **autotrophic** mutants.** Nevertheless, the **positive selection** methodology may be further categorized into *four* groups, namely:

(*i*) Direct selection; (*iii*) Stepwise selection; and
(*ii*) Rescue method; (*iv*) Double selection.

The four groups of positive selection shall now be discussed individually in the section that follows:

(a) Direct Selection: In this case, the cells that are resistant to the prevailing selection pressure survive and divide to form **colonies;** while the wild type of cells are eventually killed by the selection agent. It is, however, pertinent to state here that it is one of the most abundant common selection methods; and, therefore, is being employed for the **isolation** of cells that are specifically resistant to herbicides (chemicals), toxins (caused by **pathogens***), increased salt concentrations, amino acid analogues, antibiotics, and the like.

(b) Rescue Method: In this particular instance, the *wild type cells* are virtually **killed** by the corresponding selection agent; whereas, the *variant cells* do remain very much **alive,** but fail to undergo division by virtue of the ensuing unfavorable environment. Subsequently, attempt is made to remove the *selection agent* specifically so as to recover the prevailing **variant** cells. The rescue method has been employed frequently to recover the **low-temperature** as well as **aluminum resistant variant cells.**

(c) Stepwise Selection: In this specific instance, the ensuing **selection pressure** *viz.,* salt concentration, may be enhanced slowly from a relatively *low level* to the *Cytotoxic level;* and, thus, the *resistant clones* **isolated** at each and every progressive state are appropriately subjected to the higher selection pressure. In actual practice, **stepwise selection** approach may invariably **favor gene amplification** (an *unstable phenomenon*) or subsequent **mutations** in the *organelle DNA.*

(d) Double Selection: In **double selection** approach, it may be absolutely feasible to select cells for usual survival and/or growth on one hand, and affording resistance to the selection pressure on the other.

Example: Sterptomycin (an antibiotic): It illustrates *double selection* explicitly *i.e.,* the selection was based on **cell survival** as well as **colony formation** (*first aspect*); and specific **development of green colouration** in the aforesaid colonies (*second aspect*) — only green colonies were selected. Interestingly, the double selection approach has been judiciously applied for the selection of cells that are found to be resistant to such substances as: amitrole *a* herbicide; tobacco mosaic virus (TMV); and aluminium (Al).

1.5.1.2.1.3 Variant Traits

It has been observed that the soma clonal variants isolated *via* cell selection approach are invariably **unstable;** whereas, the percieved frequency of **stable** variants may vary between 8–62%, most probably depending on the species and the selection agent. Besides, there are several **selected clones** that do not exhibit their due resistance in the course of further selection or screening. Evidently, these emerged clones are fairly susceptible, and were wrongly classified as resistant; and, therefore, rightly termed as **escapes.** Nevertheless, there exists a plethora of *clones* which eventually lose their resistance to the prevailing selection agent after a certain span of growth in the absence of the ensuing selection pressure. Thus, the clones obtained in this manner are commonly known as **unstable variants.** However, the *unstable variants'* may be duly accomplished from valid and legitimate alterations achieved from **gene expression*** and from **gene amplification.**

1.5.1.2.1.4 Molecular Foundation of Somaclonal Variation

The **somaclonal variation** may come into being by virtue of any of the following events that occur at **molecular level exclusively,** such as: gene mutation; plasmagene mutation; gene amplification; changes in gene expression; mitotic crossing over; alterations in chromsome number and/or structure; rearrangements in cytoplasmic genes; and transposable element activation.

It has been observed that a majority of mutants isolated from cell cultures may essentially engage **single-gene mutations,** whereas the *mutant allele* could be either recessive or in dominant form.

Salient Features: A few salient features with respect to the molecular foundation of somaclonal variation are as follows:

(1) Gene amplication has been duly observed in certain variants which are normally recovered *via* stepwise selection of plant cell *in vitro*.

(2) Deamplication may often take place in somaclonal variants, *e.g.,* for rRNA genes.

(3) Transposable elements may be activated during *in vitro* culture.

(4) Cleavage and fusion of chromosomes that take place during culture may aid in augmenting the Ac activity and/or other controlling factors.

1.5.1.2.1.5 Somaclonal Variations and Induced Mutations

In certain specific instances, *mutagenesis* was observed to be absolutely vital and necessary for the adequate recovery of the specific variant that is being **isolated.** Nevertheless, the phenomenon of *mutagenesis* must be kept at an arm's length in view of the undesirable features intimately associated with such treatments.

It is pertinent to state here that the somaclonal variations are most preferable for the induction of mutations based on a plethora of widely acceptable valid reasons as enumerated below:

1. **Chimaerism** is a predominant and serious problem in the *induced mutations,* but not so in *somaclonal variations.*
2. **Induced mutations** are frequently linked with undesirable characteristic features *e.g.,* sterility.
3. Both *'newer breed of mutations'* and *'newer alleles'* have been legitimately **isolated** *via* somaclonal mutations.
4. Degree of **frequency-useful mutations** is found to be at a reasonably high level in somaclonal variations.
5. Applicability of **highly specific and effective selection** may be accomplished *in vitro* for a large number of economically viable and important characteristic features which is virtually impossible in the particular instance of **mutation breeding.**
6. Astronomically huge number of individuals may be screened quite effectively *in vitro.*

Special note: Precisely the *somaclonal variation* is exclusively applicable to those species whereby the whole plants may be reproduced from the cultured cells; whereas, *mutation breeding* may be applicable to all species in general. Furthermore, the somaclonal variation is solely dependent upon highly modernized and sophisticated facilities for the *tissue culture* as well as the *greenhouse.*

1.5.2 Factor Influencing Rate of Mutation

After having grasped sufficient understanding of the various aspects of **mutation** it is quite necessary and important to know the various factors that exert their specific influence upon the different types of mutation. A few such aspects are as stated under, namely:

i. Conditional mutation,
ii. Radiation induced mutation,
iii. Effect of UV radiation,
iv. Chemically induced mutation, and
v. Beneficial mutation.

These aforesaid aspects shall now be treated individually in the section that follows:

1.5.2.1 Conditional Mutation

It has been observed that sometimes the **mutation** is strategically taking place in such a *'genetic locus'* that under one particular experimental parameters the organism tends to grow normally, whereas under an altogether different experimental parameters, either the expected growth is far from being normal or the organism fails to grow at all. Thus, such not-so-steady mutations are usually termed as the conditional mutations. In actual practice, however, the prevailing conditions that invariably permits the *'normal growth'* are called the **'permissive conditions'**; and the other conditions are collectively referred to as either the **'non-permissive conditions'** or the **'restrictive conditions'**.

Now, if under the influence of **restrictive conditions** the organism is totally unable to grow, the **mutation** is known as a **conditional lethal mutation. Auxotrophic Mutation:** In this case, the *growth media* and the *metabolic conditions* are entirely responsible for the ensuing **expression of mutation.**

Examples: A few specific mutants have the capability to grow very conveniently in the presence of **'glucose'** but a possible replacement of glucose with any other sugar entity would virtually cause the growth to a complete stand-still (*i.e.,* stop).

Mutants may be either *temperature sensitive* (hot or cold) or supressor sensitive. In the latter instance the organism is found to be viable in the presence of a suppressor, whereas the mutation becomes lethal in the absence of a suppressor.

1.5.2.2 Radiation Induced Mutations

A plethora of **'electromagnetic radiations'**, particularly the electromagnetic waves having 100 nm or even smaller wave lengths may give rise to the phenomenon of **'ionization'**.

Examples: The various typical examples are: X-rays, γ-rays, and cosmic rays.

Muller (1927) observed the ultimate effect of these rays and concluded that an excessive exposure to X-rays enhanced the incidence of sex-linked **recessive-lethal mutation** in Drosophila particularly. It was further doctrined that there exists a direct relationship between the **'radiation dose level'** and the **'incidence of mutation'** articulately.

Examples: The following are some concrete evidences:

Exposure (r)	Occurrence of Mutation (%)
500	15
1000	3

Besides, there are some other vital factors that invariably govern the **incidence of mutation,** for instance:

1.5.2.2.1 Duration of Exposure to Radiation

It has been duly observed that certain mutations may even occur at very low exposure dose but for a relatively longer duration or at high exposure dose but for much shorter span. Therefore, one may infer that there is 'no **safe-level of radiation'**, and even a very small dose could be unsafe practically for causing **mutation.** It has been found that the probability of mutation in experimental rats is comparatively much less if a **'chronic radiation'** with a low dose is administered than if the **'same dose of radiation'** is given in one-go.

1.5.2.2.2 Environmental Conditions

In reality, the affect of **environmental conditions** exert a positive effect on **ionization.**

Example: Lower the presence of O_2-tension gives rise to lower incidence of mutation. Likewise, the presence of **higher O2-tension** at the time of irradiation affords **higher incidence of mutation,** even if the animal is subjected to lower O_2-tension at a later stage. All kinds of mutations are adequately accommodated by ionic radiation. Incidences of chromosome *aberration* of all kinds are duly observed *via* ionic radiation, such as: *duplication, deletion, inversion,* and *transversion.*

1.5.2.2.3 State of Cellular Metabolism

Both the *state of cellular metabolism* and the *phase of cell-cycle* do play a cognizable major role on the remarkable effect of **ionizing radiations.**

Example: In response to the given irradiation to the plant *Trillium,* the observed mutations were **60 times** more prevalent specifically at the **metaphase** in comparison to the **interphase** of the cell cycle.

1.5.2.3 Effect of UV Radiation

It has been well established that UV-radiation serves as a **'weak mutagen'.** Besides, the usual normal strengths of UV-radiation in the sun light are not strong enough to initiate and produce mutation.

Interestingly, any extent of damage caused to DNA is repaired instantly by the cell. Nevertheless, the exposed UV radiation gets adequately absorbed by both the **purine** and the **pyrimidine bases** respectively; and, thus, are converted into their corresponding **excitable state** that eventually render them **more reactive** ultimately.

Importantly, the UV range of either 254 nm or even lower is found to be highly damaging for **mutation.** In general, the prevailing relationship between the **degree of UV radiation** and the **rate of mutation** is predominantly variable in nature.

Mechanism of Action: Though the **'mutagenic'** effect of UV radiation has been known for quite sometime, but its exact mechanism whereby it causes **mutations** has been understood only recently. In fact, the irradiation of DNA with UV rays usually gives rise to the actual formation of covalent bonds between **thymine molecules** on the same strand of DNA yielding thereby the **thymine-thymine** dimmers as shown in Fig. 1.16.

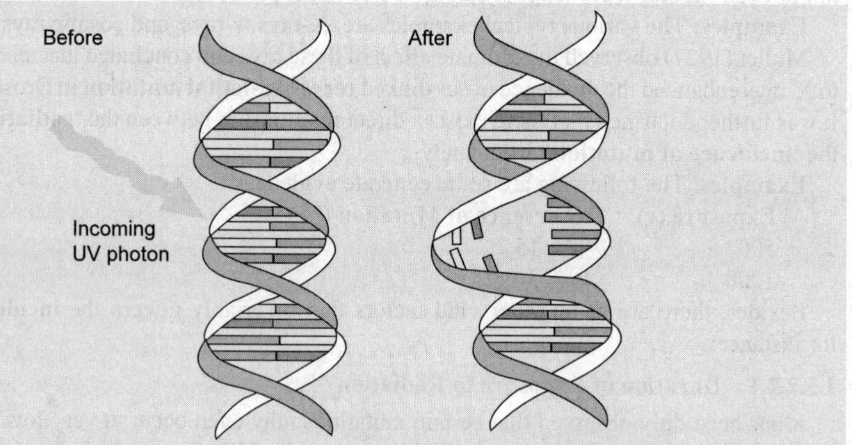

Fig. 1.16 *Formation of Thymine-Thymine Dimer by UV Radiation*

It has been observed that several microorganisms have enzymes which can affect this damage in the *dark* (*i.e.*, **dark repair**). In certain instances the **'repair-phenomenon'** is not *done correctly,* and this gives rise to **mutation(s).** Interestingly, as opposed to **dark repair,** the covalent bonds joining the **thymine dimers** may also be eliminated by the help of light of longer wavelength, which process is usually termed as **photo-reactivation.** In nut shell, most UV **mutations** are more or less *nonsense type of mutations;* and, therefore, are the ultimate result of a change in one or few bases in the structure of DNA.

Besides, X-rays and γ-rays are nothing but **'ionizing radiations'** and may cause damage to the prevailing DNA, but no dimer formation takes place at all. The overall net damage frequently caused by these radiations and improper follow up repairs may categorically lead to either *addition* or *deletion of* bases present in the DNA. This finally gives rise to a change in the *reading frame* (*i.e.*, **frame-shift mutations**).

1.5.2.4 Chemically Induced Mutations

There are a host of pure **'chemical substances'** that are *mutagenic* in nature. A few such chemicals are used frequently by humans while the others are not so common at all. On a broader perspective the **'chemical substances'** may be classified into *two* categories depending upon their inherent mode of action, such as:

(*a*) **Chemicals affording mutation to replicating and non-replicating DNA:** A few typical examples of this class are: nitrous acid (HNO_2) and alkylating/hydroxylating agents which would be discussed briefly depending upon their precise *'mechanism of action'* as stated under:

(1) Nitrous Acid (HNO2): It essentially exerts its mode of action *via* the oxidative deamination of bases in DNA. Consequently, 'A' gets converted to the corresponding hypoxanthine that may base pair with 'C' during the process of *'replication'* and, hence, finally converts on **'A-T pair'** into a **'G-C pair'.** Likewise, 'C' is converted to 'U' that may subsequently base pair with 'A', thereby converting a **'C-G pair'** to an **'A-T pair'.** Thus, 'G', on the other hand gets converted to **Xanthine** finally, that may also base pair with 'C'. Therefore, this very change fails to cause a **'mutation'.** In short, because the net effect of HNO_2 is to afford a plausible conversion of an **'A-T pair'** to a **'G-C pair'**; and eventually a **'G-C pair'** to an **'A-T pair'**, it may be gainfully employed to revert a **mutant** back to the corresponding *wild-type.*

(2) Alkylating/Hydroxylating Agents: It has been observed that both the alkylating and the hydroxylating agents help in the transference of a methyl ($-CH_3$) or ethyl ($-C_2H_5$) functional moiety to the corresponding bases.

Examples: Mustard gas (I) and ethyl methane sulphonate (II) usually affect the *'ethylation'* at the N-7 and C-6 positions respectively.

Consequently, these **'modified bases'** usually form a base pair with a wrong base:

Examples:

(*i*) **N-Methyl-N′-nitro, N-nitroso guanidine (NTG)** — is a highly potent alkylating agent and affords a good number of multiple as well as related mutations in DNA.

(*ii*) **Ethylene Sulphonate (EES)** — is another alkylating agent. These two *'chemicals'* help in 7 ethyl 'G' base pair with 'T', thereby converting a **'G-C pair'** to an **'A-T pair'.**

(*iii*) **Hydroxylamine (NH_2OH)** — is a hydroxylating agent that specifically converts a **'GC base pair'** to an **'A-T pair'.**

In general, these chemicals, besides effectively a base change may also bring about the following modifications in **mutants:**

- Cross-linking in mutants
- Occasional chromosomal breakage and aberrations
- Activate the repairing mechanism of the cell.

(b) Chemicals affording mutagenic activity to replicating DNA: A few befitting examples of this category are acridine dyes and base analogs that would be briefly described along with their respective mechanism of actions as given under:

(1) Acridines: It has been observed that the acridine dyes invariably give rise to the **'frameshift mutations'.** In other words, these dyes *e.g.,* acridine orange, proflavin, ICR 170 and 190 usually interchelate particularly between the stacked base pairs in the DNA and eventually are strategically sandwiched between two predominant bases. Consequently, *DNA possesses an enhanced rigidity* and its confirmation gets altered. In fact, the ensuing conformational change gives rise to the ultimate *deletion* and *addition* of one or more bases in the course of replication; and finally emerges with the **'frameshift mutation'.**

(2) Base Analogs: Extensive and intensive research has made it virtually possible to incorporate several **'modified bases'** in place of a **'normal base'** in the course of *DNA replication* by virtue of the fact that the prevailing **DNA polymerase** fails to afford critical differentiation between the normal base and its corresponding structural analog. Nevertheless, quite frequently the analog is capable of forming a *'base pair'* with an *'alternate base'* and thereby gives rise to a replacement change during the next cycle of replication.

Examples:

(*i*) 5-Bromo-deoxyuridine (BRDU) represents a thymidine analog; and, hence, may convert a **'G-C pair'** to an **'A-T pair'** only when it is present in an *enol*-form and thereby converts an **'A-T pair'** to a corresponding **'G-C pair'** in its *keto*-form as depicted in Fig. 1.17. Interestingly, identical mutation may be brought about by **2-amino purine.** These chemical entities may be strategically and gainfully employed for reverting a possible mutation.

(*ii*) Another set of examples for the **'base analogs'** are: **N4-hydroxy CTP** which is invariably replicated either as a 'G' or an 'A' and results into the replacement of 'G' to 'A' or 'C' to 'T' in 30% of the available molecules.

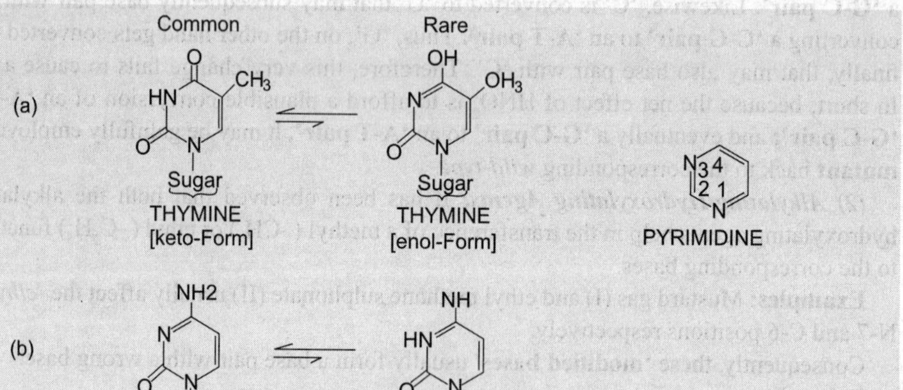

Fig. 1.17 *Representation of Tautomeric Isomeric Forms of four common bases in DNA e.g., Thymine; Cytosine; Adenine; and Guanine.*

It is, however, pertinent to state here that the base-pairing potentials of the above bases, namely: **pyrimidines;** and **purines,** which cause the effective change ultimately.

1.5.2.5 Beneficial Mutation

It has been well established that a major proportion of the **'spontaneous mutations'** are harmful to the organism because they invariably render an organism relatively lesser efficient with respect to its activity profile. In fact, the overall phenomenon of evolution could be made feasible exclusively by virtue of the ensuing rather slow **mutations.** It has been amply demonstrated that a plethora of **mutations** normally permit an organism to be more appropriate for effective survival in an altogether *unfriendly environment.* Therefore, these *newer developed mutations* critically allow the development of certain *newer characteristic features* that ultimately give rise to greater and befitting degree of adoptability to their immediate surrounding environment.

The actual applicability of such **'beneficial mutations'** have been duly extended and exploited in the domain of *plant sciences:*

Examples:

1. Induction of useful characteristic features in an organism *e.g.,* high-yielding seeds, stress resistance plants, and pest resistance species.
2. Development of specific variety of **Penicillium** that would yield definitely higher yields of **penicillin** (an antibiotic), obviously a highly viable and commercially feasible propositions.

1.6 Design of Fermentation Processes

The very **'design'** of fermentation processes essentially require the most predominant component of the *media i.e.,* **water,** wherein the microorganisms tend to grow. The aforesaid phenomenon holds good in several well-defined **'biotechnological processes'** leading to the commercial production of antibiotics, industrial alcohols, acetic acid, beer, wines and the like. It is, however, pertinent to state here that once the *liquid fermentation processes* have accomplished optimum production, it is absolutely necessary to remove **water** as far as possible because it evidently attributes to a major factor in the *'cost'* of **bioproduct recovery** and **downstream processing.**

In reality, there are several vital and critical factors that invariably govern as well as play an important role in the media design of various fermentation processes, such as:

i. Quality of water,
ii. Quality control of raw materials,
iii. Nutritional requirements,
iv. Sterilization practices, and
v. Media preparation.

The above mentioned factors shall now be treated individually in the section that follows:

1.6.1 Quality of Water

The prevalent quality of water is obviously of the greatest importance by virtue of the fact that it not only affects predominantly the ensuing **microbial growth,** but also the essential production of **specific bioproducts.**

In the past, it was actually a practice to erect and establish the so called **'traditional brewing centers'** particularly in such locations that more or less provided natural springs (*i.e., natural sources*) so as to obtain very high quality of soft, sweet and potable water without the cumbersome need to resort to *extensive* and *expensive* **'pretreatment'.**

However, the present day practice essentially needs the utilization of commercial-scale demineralized water plants (*i.e.,* DM-Plants), reverse-osmosis plants (*i.e.,* RD-Plants) etc., to obtain pure water required for the fermentation processes.

1.6.2 Quality Control of Raw Materials

Besides, water the other chemical constituents *e.g.,* pasteurized wort (malt extract solution), salts, acids etc., must be of relatively better grade and quality so as to obtain flawless optimized fermentation yielding specific bioproducts.

1.6.3 Nutritional Requirements

It has been duly observed that the required fundamental essential nutritional requirements of the microorganisms are, namely: an *energy* or *carbon* source, an available nitrogen source, inorganic elements, and for certain particular cell-types specific growth factors. Interestingly, most *biotechnological* processes invariably derive both carbon and nitrogen sources from rather complex admixtures of cheap natural by-products or products, for instance: glucose, lactose, starch and sucrose (as sources of carbohydrates providing carbon); and barley, beet molasses, corn-steep liquor, groundnut meal, oat flour pharmamedia, rye flour, soyabean meal, and whey powder (as sources of nitrogen), which have been duly summarized in the following table:

S. No	Source of Carbohydrate	S. No	Sources of Nitrogen [% Nitrogen by Weights]
1.	Glucose: Pure glucose monohydrate; hydrolyzed starch;	1.	Barley: [1.5 to 2.0]
2.	Lactose: Pure lactose; whey powder;	2.	Beet Molasses: [1.5 to 2.0]
3.	Starch: Barley; oat flour; rye flour; groundnut meal; Soya bean meal;	3.	Corn Steep Liquor [4.5]
4.	Sucrose: Sugarcane molasses; beet molasses; crude brown sugar; pure white sugar;	4.	Groundnut Meal: [8.0]
		5.	Oat Flour: [1.5 to 2.0]
		6.	Pharmamedia: [8.0]
		7.	Rye Flour: [1.5 to 2.0]
		8.	Soya bean Meal: [8.0]
		9.	Whey Powder: [4.5]

1.6.4 Sterilization Practices

The various conventional, time-tested and widely adopted sterilization practices solely meant for the **'biotechnological media'** should accomplished maximum kill of contaminating microorganisms, thereby maintaining almost bare minimum damage caused to the medium components. Of the two **sterilization practices** frequently employed the **'batchwise sterilization'** in the bioreactor is still regarded to be the most widely used method, whereas the various prevalent **'continuous sterilization'** methods are virtually gaining not only enhanced *acceptability* but also *adaptability.*

1.6.5 Media Preparation

The **media preparation** is precisely the backbone of the entire *'bioprocess operation'*; and, therefore, must be carried out with utmost care and precaution. Importantly, the improper and inadequate media design may ultimately give rise to both impaired efficiency of growth as well as concomitant significantly poor product formation.

Based on the enormous evidences available in the literatures the **design of fermentation processes** may be categorized into the following *five* techniques, namely:

a. Solid substrate fermentation,
b. Submerged fermentation,
c. Downstream processing,
d. Technology of mammalian and plant-cell culture, and
e. Cell-recycle technique.

The above stated techniques shall now be treated individually as under:

1.6.5.1 Solid Substrate Fermentation

There are a plethora of **'biotechnological processes'** which predominantly make use of the appreciable growth of desired microorganisms on particular *solid substrates* either in the **absence** or **near absence** of free availability of water. The **solid substrate fermentation** techniques are exploited abundantly for the specific production of fungal enzymes that essentially includes growth of filamentous fungus on a water-sprayed wheat or rice bran loaded with requisite nutrients to serve as **'substrates'** to yield *allulases, amylases, proteases* and *penctinases.* However, in the course of the fermentative phenomenon the effective management and control of **pH, temperature** and **humidity** is a little difficult task, but nevertheless should be maintained as prescribed as far as possible. The following Table records certain typical examples of solid substrate fermentations:

S.No	Example	Solid Substrate	Microorganisms (S) Utilized
1.	Mushroom production (Western and Eastern)	Straw; Organic manure;	*Araricus bisporus; Lentinula edodes; Volvariella volvalaceae;*
2.	Sauerkraut	Cabbage;	Lactic acid bacteria;
3.	Soy sauce	Soyabeans; Wheat;	*Aspergillus oryzae;*
4.	Tempeh	Soyabeans;	*Rhizopus oligosporus;*
5.	Ontjom	Peanut press cake;	*Neosporin sitophila;*
6.	Cheese(s)	Milk curd;	*Penicillium roquefortii;*
7.	Organic acid(s)	Cane sugar; Molasses;	*Aspergillus niger;*
8.	Enzymes	Wheat bran; Maize bran;	*Aspergillus niger;*
9.	Composting	Mixed organic substances;	Fungi, Bacteria; Actinomycetes;
10.	Sewage treatment	Components of sewage;	Fungi; Bacteria; Protozoa;

It has been observed that the most regularly and frequently employed solid substrates are, namely; legume seeds, cereal grains, wheat bran, lignocellulose substances *e.g.,* sawdust, straws, or wood shavings; besides, a broad spectrum of animal and plant materials. A good number of such typical chemical entities are mostly **'polymeric molecules'** that are essentially either insoluble or sparingly water soluble; but are, however, invariably inexpensive, easily obtainable, and do represent largely a concentrated source of nutrients strategically required for the microbial growth.

The **Western world** makes use of the solid substrate fermentation processes rather confined to the production of cheese and sauerkraut, silage and mushroom cultivation; besides, the composting of both animal and plant wastes. In contrast, the **Eastern world** the fermentation processes have virtually centered upon the very production of a wide array of food fermentations, such as: soy sauce, tempeh; besides, several huge industrial enzyme processes both profitably and effectively.

1.6.5.2 Submerged Fermentation

The **submerged fermentation** process essentially makes use of **bioreactors** which are very much identical both in *design* and *function* to those employed in the antibiotic production. It is mostly made of stainless steel having a capacity ranging between 10 to 15 m^3 and adequately provided with such devices as: *mechanical internal agitator* — for mixing the contents of the bioreactor; *external pumps* — for circulation, loading and evacuation; *bubble columns* — for aeration of the medium; and the *air-lift* loop. Cultivation progessively involves the suspension growth of microorganisms in the liquid environment. Nevertheless, the **sterilization** as well as the **process control** in the **submerged fermentation** is relatively easy and convenient to accomplish.

In general, the pH of the prepared culture medium is first optimized and then pumped right into the previously steam-sterilized bioreactor via HTST* sterilization devices. The thermobavile additives are carefully introduced individually into the sterile medium at an ambient temperature. Adequately *propogated inoculum* must be transferred into the production-stage vessels through sterilized SS pipes/ pumps with utmost care and precaution. At this particular stage *sterile-compressed air* is introduced into the *fermentation broth via* a strategically positioned sparger at the bottom of the

bioreactor. In commercial bioreactors the agitation is done by the aid of **multiple flat-bladed disc turbines** located onto a vertical shaft. Besides, other suitable devices, such as: *counter-current stirrers,* and *axial-flow* propellars, may also be employed as per the necessary requirements. It is, however, absolutely necessary to maintain the contents of the **bioreactors** (or **fermentors**) to an *ambient temperature* by two commonly used devices, namely: (*a*) *external* heat-exchangers; and (*b*) *internal* cooling-coils.

Note: The evolution of CO_2, as a byproduct, in fermentative procedures essentially generates adequate heat energy, which if not taken care of properly would cause serious unwanted microbial processes to triger off thereby lowering the yield of desired products.

Modern **bioreactors** are frequently provided with *in situ sophisticated probes* and *sensitive instrumental gadgets* to monitor as well as stringently control various physical parameters during development of the inoculums in the course of various production stages. It is, however, pertinent to mention here that the different physical parameters like: dissolved O_2, evolved CO_2, redox potential, and pH value must be monitored and simultaneously controlled adequately.

Factors Governing Submerged Culture: In fact, there are *three* major factors that essentially govern the submerged culture, namely: (*i*) temperature; (*ii*) pH; and (*iii*) dissolved oxygen tension (DOT). These factors would be treated individually in the section that follows:

(a) Temperature: Each fermentative process leading to a particular **bioproduct** essentially requires optimum temperature for the specific production of an *enzyme,* and hence the subsequent growth of the microorganism, which varies accordingly with the progressive stages of the entire process. Interestingly, the activity of an enzyme for an already utilized substrate gets remarkably influenced by temperature. It is, therefore, almost mandatory to closely monitor the range of temperature during fermentation in such a manner which would encourage cell growth appropriately.

(b) pH: The stability of an **'enzyme'** is exclusively guided by the pH optima. Therefore, it is quite evident to sustain and maintain pH optima so as to accomplish the maximum growth rate of the specific organism in question. In other words, it is absolutely vital and necessary that not only the *'pH profile in the course of fermentation alone'*, but also the *'enzyme production phase'* must be imposed as well as monitored in such a manner so as to achieve the **maximum growth** and **enzyme production** simultaneously.

(c) Dissolved Oxygen Tension (DOT): In actual practice, the **dissolved oxygen tension (DOT)** may be maintained stringently by controlling *three* most important physical conditions, such as: *adequate rate of aeration; agitation ratio;* and *gas-phase pressure.* It has been amply demonstrated that the *'level of O_2'* just lower than its **critical concentration** does affect the growth of microorganisms adversely. Therefore, it is very essential to maintain *'appropriate aerobic condition'* in the growth culture medium. Interestingly, the desired **'level of O_2'** predominantly in the **submerged microbial cultures** may be obtained by adopting either of the *two* following methods, namely:

(*i*) Enhancing the mass of O_2 being provided to the **bioreactor** per unit time by increasing the overpressure in the head-space of the **bioreactor,** and

(*ii*) Increasing the ensuing rate of air supply to the **bioreactor.**

Caution: Oxygen-enriched air could attribute to higher oxygen transfer rates.

1.6.5.3 Downstream Processing

The **downstream processing** is solely related to the extraction and purification of the desired end-product from the bioprocess based on the skills of bioscientists, chemists, chemical engineers, and process engineers.

The very design and absolute efficient operation of **downstream processing** methodologies essentially include *two* important aspects, namely:

(*a*) Vital elements in getting the required products into viable commercial usage, and

(*b*) Reflect the need to lose more of the desired product than is absolutely necessary.

Example: *Humulin(R) [Eli Lilly, USA]; Insulin:* More than 90% of the 200 staff members are actively engaged in the various recovery processes. Obviously, **downstream processing** of biotechnological processes truly represents a major portion of the overall costs directly involved in most processes, but at the same time is also the least glamorous aspect of biotechnology. Summararily, any improvements rightly afforded in the **downstream processing** would certainly benefit the overall efficiency and exhorbitant costs of processes.

The various stages of *'downstream processing operations'* are as stated below:

Stage 1: Separation — Filtration — centrifugation — flotation — disruption;

Stage 2: Concentration — Solubilization — extraction — thermal processing — membrane filtration — precipitation;

Stage 3: Purification — Crystallization — chromatographic methods;

Stage 4: Modification — Structural analogs;

Stage 5: Drying — Under vacuum — spray drying — freeze drying — fluidised — bed drying;

Salient Features: The salient feature variants of the **downstream processing** are as enumerated under:

1. Initial separation of the **bioreactor** broth into a *liquid phase* and a *solid phase,* and subsequent concentration and purification of the product.
2. Processing comprises of at least five stages as described above.
3. Methods either proposed or in use usually range from two extremes *i.e.,* conventional to almost mysterious that may predominantly comprise of such well-known techniques as: distillation, centrifugation, filtration, ultra filtration, solvent extraction, adsorption, reverse osmosis, molecular sieves, selective membrane technology, electrophoresis, and affinity chromatography.

Special Note: In fact, it is in this particular domain wherein a plethora of reasonably potential industrial applications of latest developments in biotechnology have virtually come to grief or rendered problematic by virtue of the following *two* important drawbacks, namely:

a. Extraction failed to achieve the ingenuity of the designers, and

b. Extraction procedure has virtually consumed so much excessive energy-input as to render it almost uneconomical.

It has been a practice to ascertain the final product of the ensuing downstream purification stages to possess some degree of **stability** for the ultimate commercial distribution. However, **stability** may be best accomplished for a wide range of products by affording some form of *drying,* for instance: **freeze-drying, spray-drying, fluidised-bed drying.** The method of choice is solely dependent on product quality and cost-effective measures.

Dry-form products: include — antibiotics, amino acids, organic acids, polysaccharides, single cell proteins, enzymes etc.

Liquid-form products: include — products which cannot be dispensed conveniently in a dried form.

Proteinacious products: to avoid possible changes of **'denaturation'.**

In general, special precautionary measures need to be taken 80 as to avoid any scope of either deterioration or microbial contamination.

Highlights of Downstream Processing: Operations indulging in downstream processing do possess quite a few outstanding features, namely:

1. It gives rise to several challenging and demanding aspects of a *wide spectrum of biotechnological processes.*
2. Hallmarks of *most high value biotechnological products* are solely based upon their **purity** and **stability.**
3. Ultimate success of a wide range of biotechnological processes shall entirely depend upon the correct well-defined area of choice and *modus operandi* of such established systems.

4. The commercial-scale operative measures will solely depend upon the economic viability/ feasibility without the least compromise on the final end-product; and for this the utmost understanding and cooperation should always prevail between the **'bioscientist'** and the **'process engineer'**.

1.6.5.4 Technology of Mammalian and Plant-cell Culture

Recent literatures have adequately substantiated the glaring fact that the mass cultivation of organisms for a host of biotechnological processes got evolved and subsequently developed invariably not only around the *bacteria, yeasts* and *filamentous fungi;* but also around the plant and animal cell cultures.

Plant-cell Culture: *Plant-cell Culture* may be defined as — **'a specific technique encompassing the *in vitro* culture of plant cells, tissues, organs, and even whole plantlets'.**

In actual practice, the application of plant-cell culture techniques have been abundantly extended and exploited for the micropropogation of certain plants. In such instances, plant-cell cultures would meticulously progress *via* several cardinal stages, namely: *organogenesis, plantlet amplification,* and eventual *establishment in soil.*

However, commercial-scale production of requisite suspension-cell cultures of several species has now been accomplished gainfully; and the ultimate yields of desired products very much akin and typical of the whole plant have been largely impressive and successful, such as: **alkaloids, ginseng,** and **nicotine.** Furthermore, the extension of the said technique to large-scale fermentation programmes may give rise to the legitimate production of commercially acceptable levels of some **high-value plant products,** for instance: **codeine, digitalis, jasmine, spearmint etc.**

Importantly, the plant-cell culture technique is relatively much slower in comparison to the microorganisms, through a large extent of the other characteristic features of fermentation are very much identical. Moreover, the operational volume of an average cultured plant cell could be upto 200,000 folds that of a bacterial cell. Although certain plant products are now being marketed; however, it is not expected to be commercially viable for several years from now.

Note: Animal or human cell cultures could give rise to a host of potentially vital and important organic compounds. Such break throughs have been mostly stalled or hampered due to several encountered problems together with exhorbitant scale-up operations.

Mammalian-Cell Culture: In reality, the culture of both mammalian cells and tissues representsa largely exploited and widely employed technique in the ever expanding domain of **modern cell biology** and **biotechnology.** In the recent past, the broad range of cells types now grown invariably in culture is both very extensive and progressively increasing; and essentially includes cells that are strategically derived from bone, liver, cartilage, lung, breast, skin, bladder, kidney, neurones, pituitary cells, and several types of cancers. In actual practice, there has been an enormous growth in the utilization of **animal-cell culture** cultivation for the commercial-scale production of a good number of **high-value products,** namely: life-saving **vaccines** (*e.g.,* polio, mumps, measles, rabies, chickenpox, cholera etc.,), **insulin, hormones, interferons, plasminogen,** and various **antibodies.**

Major Problems Encountered: The major problems that are mostly encountered in the mass cultivation of mammalians cells essentially include:

- Extreme sensitivity of cells to impurities in water.
- Cost effective measure.
- Stringent quality control of media.
- Need to discard contamination by more rapidly growing microorganisms completely.

Primary Cultures: Primary cultures may be defined as — **'freshly isolated cultures obtained from the mammalian systems'.**

The **primary cultures** are normally heterogeneous in nature but still closely designate and represent the parent cell types. They also exhibit and involve in the expression of tissue-specific characteristic features. It has been observed that after having passed through several sub-cultures upon fresh culture media, the ultimate **cell line** would either prove to be fatal (*i.e.,* die out) or get transformed into **continuous cell line.** It is, however, pertinent to mention at this juncture that the *continuous cell lines* exhibit a wide variation from the corresponding *primary cultures,* namely:

- Alternations in cytomorphology,
- Enhanced rate of growth,
- Increase in chromosome variation, and
- Increase in tumorigenicity.

Nevertheless, the *in vitro* transformation explicitly designates primarily the valid acquisition of an infinite extent of life span.

Cultivation of Anchorage-Dependent Cell Types: It has been amply demonstrated that specifically the animal cells may be grown either in an **unattached suspension culture** or **attached to a solid surface.**

Examples:

i. **Lymphoblastoid Cells** — usually grow in an unattached suspension culture,
ii. **Primary or Normal Diploid Cells** — normally grow only when they are attached duly to a solid surface, and
iii. **Hela Type Cells** — invariably can grow in either of the two states stated earlier.

It is duly apprehended that most of the future commercial development(s) with **animal cells** shall be predominantly guided by the prevailing cultivation of anchorage-dependent cell types.

Monolayer Cultivation of Animal Cells: Precisely the monolayer cultivation of animal cells is exclusively governed by the ensuing **'surface-area'** available for attachment. Importantly, the particular design considerations have been solely directed to methods of **increasing surface area.** The most recent sophisticated system has been developed that essentially supports the actual growth of cells strategically in coils of **gas-permeable TEFLON-tubing** (*i.e.,* each tubing with a surface area of 10,000 cm^2, and upto 20 such coils may be incorporated into an incubator chamber). A wide spectrum of cells has been cultured under these experimental parameters successfully.

In short, the **'suspension cultures'** have been developed so meticulously and successfully to substantially large **bioreactor** volumes thereby permitting the utilization of all the ensuing engineering advantages of the **stirred-tank bioreactor** that have eventually accrued from an elaborated microbial studies being presently employed to an added advantage. Such studies have been carried out only on batch culture basis.

Recent Innovative Breakthrough: The wonderful recent innovative breakthrough in biotechnological process has been duly accomplished *via* an unique combination of **attachment culture** and **suspension culture** by the application of *microcarrier beads.* The underlying principle essentially involves the strategic attachment of the *anchorage-dependent cells* to specially designed **DEAESephadex beads** (with a surface area of 7 $cm^2.mg^{-1}$) which are capable of floating in suspension. Thus, in this manner the engineering advantages of the designed stirred **bioreactor** may be employed with anchored cells overwhelmingly.

Examples: Many cell types have been meticulously grown in this way, namely: (*a*) *human interferon;* and (*b*) *viruses.*

Further developments entirely rest upon the **new bioreactor designs** based on the *microcarrierbead concept* that would certainly afford a much wider lage-scale development of both human and animal cell types.

1.6.5.5 Cell Recycle Technique

Ethanol has been exploited and used extensively not only as a **fuel supplement** but also as a **chemical feed stock** in the past 2 to 3 decades, thereby enhancing the overall global interest in seriously augmenting production in an extremely cost-effective manner and feasible way. Therefore, there are ample evidences in the literature that obviously show a broad spectrum of improvements affected in the *'traditional batch fermentation'*. Hence, one such methodologies researched in the recent past which has attracted tremendous attention is the **cell recycles technique**. In fact, it does not necessarily involve any appreciable additional expenditure.

The underlying principle of this newly evolved technique is that it essentially involves the *reuse of cell mass* which is critically produced in the *course of fermentation process*. Thus, it has been established that the aforesaid **cell recycle technique** gives rise to *three* prominent advantages, namely:

i. Net saving of nearly 5 to 10% of the entire substrate that would have been otherwise utilized for the ensuing cell growth,

ii. Significant saving in the cost of inoculums and time, and

iii. **Cell recycle technology** has virtually reduced the total fermentation time drastically upto 80% *viz.,* from 24–36 hours in a *batch fermentation* reduced to mere 5–6 hours.

1.7 Production of Antibiotics (Isolation of Fermentation Products)

Industrial fermentation industry, across the globe, commendably received its ever outstanding impetus for the most coveted strategic expansion as well as profits with the wonderful advent and exploitation of **antibiotics*** as potential well known **'chemotherapeutic agents'**.** During the World War II the actual demand for *penicillin* almost reached its peak to save the lines of millions of wounded soldiers; and later on followed by *streptomycin* and a host of other **antibiotics** in the domain of global scenario of pharmaceutical industry. These developments instantly triggered off extensive and intensive research programmes most articulately designed to look for useful microorganisms that are capable of producing highly effective, viable, and good antibiotics; and oriented a tremendous push towards the adequate research and development for producing antibiotic substances on a commercial scale. Thus, several altogether newer cultural procedures were devised, developed, and the state-of-the-art technique of submerged-agitated-aerated fermentation using deep-tank fermentors came into being with obvious high rate of success.

Primarily the antibiotics are produced by **bacteria** and **fungi;** besides, several other classes of microorganisms do possess at least limited liabilities in this aspect.

Examples: (*a*) *Bacteria; Streptomyces* species; *Bacillus* species;

(*b*) *Fungi (Mold)*: *Aspergillus* species; *Penicillium* species;

In genetal, a good many of the known *bacterial antibiotics* are *polypeptides that* have proved to be rather unstable, toxic, and difficult to purify. Likewise, the *fungal antibiotics,* with a few notable exceptions, generally have been observed to be too toxic for usage in medical practice. However, the **penicillins** (*i.e.,* the pencillin group of antibiotics) produced by various molds stand out to be an obvious exception. The earlier belief and conception that an **'antibiotic'** possesses toxicity, that invariably negates its **'internal administration'** both to the animal and human body, does not obviously restrict its medical usage, because in certain cases the antibiotic may even be judiciously recommended for use in **topical applications,** namely: dermatological preparations, treatment of burns, open cuts and injuries.

The following Table includes the names of certain known antibiotics, the related microorganisms, and therapeutic usages:

Antibiotic-Microorganisms-Therapeutic Usage

S. No	Antibiotics	Microorganisms	Therapeutic Usages (TN)
1.	Amphotericin B	*Streptomyces nodosus*	Deep-seated mycotic infections [Fungizone(R)]

2.	Bacitracin	*Bacillus subtilis*	Applied topically in ointment form.
3.	Chloramphenicol	*Streptomyces ven. Zuelae*	Broad spectrum agent useful in typhoid fever [Chloromycetin(R)]
4.	Erythromycin	*Streptomyces erythreus*	Many Gram +ve and some Gram –ve organisms [Illotycin(R)].
5.	Griseofulvin	*Penicillium griseofulvum P.nigricans; P.urticae;*	Oral antifungal antibiotic effective against ringworm.
6.	Kanamycin	*Streptomyces kanamyceticus*	Restricted to Gram –ve organisms; *viz., Klebsiella, Proteus, Serratia*, and *Enterobacter* spp.
7.	Neomycin	*Streptomyces fradiae*	Local infections *viz.*, burns, ulcers, wounds, impetigo, infected dermatoses, furunculosis, and conjunctivitis. [Fradiomycin(R)].
8.	Oxytetracycline	*Streptomyces rimosus*	Broad spectrum antibiotic for dysentery, gum infection etc. [Terramycin(R)].
9.	Penicillin	*Penicillium notatum, Penicillium chrysogenum*	Bactercidal, for most Gram +ve and certain Gram –ve organisms. [Crystaken(R)].
10.	Streptomycin	*Streptomyces griseus*	Treatment of tuberculosis in conjunction with drugs like: isoniazid and rifampicin [Streptomycin Sulphate(R)].

Based on the above statement of facts the isolation of fermentation products of the following substances shall be described individually in the section that follows:

a. Penicillins
b. Streptomycins
c. Tetracyclines
d. Vitamin B12.

1.7.1 The Penicillins

Penicillins, the β-lactam antibiotics, have indeed enjoyed the legendary of a long history of application as chemotherapeutic agents since 1929 by the epoch making discovery of Alexander Fleming; and, even today, they legitimately command the reputation for being prescribed more than 50% of all the known antibiotics across the globe. The most genuine and remarkable combination of unique *very effective bactericidal property* and *desirable levels of extremely low toxicity* are solely attributed by the ensuing **bacterial cell wall biosynthesis.** In reality, the relatively low cost of these therapeutic agents is exclusively based upon the tremendous acclaimed enhancement in fermentation yields which have been gainfully accomplished through years of dedicated researches as: strain improvement, fermentation optimization procedures, and above all meticulous refinement of downstream processing. It would be worth while to lay proper emphasis upon the current status of knowledge with regard to the genetics and molecular biology of penicillin biosynthesis.

1.7.1.1 Genes in Penicillin Biosynthesis

It has been observed that the biosynthesis of the penicillin group of antibiotics essentially involves a common pathway, having some *core activities* duly protected among all producer microorganisms which have been screened till date both intensively and extensively. Interestingly, most of these producer species embrace a plethora of *filamentous fungi,* such as: members of the genera *Penicillium, Cephalosporium, Aspergillus,* a number of **Actinomycetes** including *Streptomyces,* and *Nocardia* spp., and a few **bacterial species** *e.g., Flavobacterium* and *Lysobacter* spp. It is, however, pertinent to mention here that in every instance, the pathway essentially commences with the condensation of three prominent amino acids, namely: L-α-aminoadipic acid, L-Cysteine, and L-Valine to give rise to a corresponding tripeptide intermediate, δ-L-(α-aminoadipyl)-L-cysteinyl-D-valine (ACV). Now, ACV gets converted to **isopenicilln N** in the presence of the enzyme isopenicillin N synthase (pcbC), which in turn is duly modified to yield a variety of end product(s), for instance: **hydrophobic penicillins,** as depicted in Fig. 1.18.

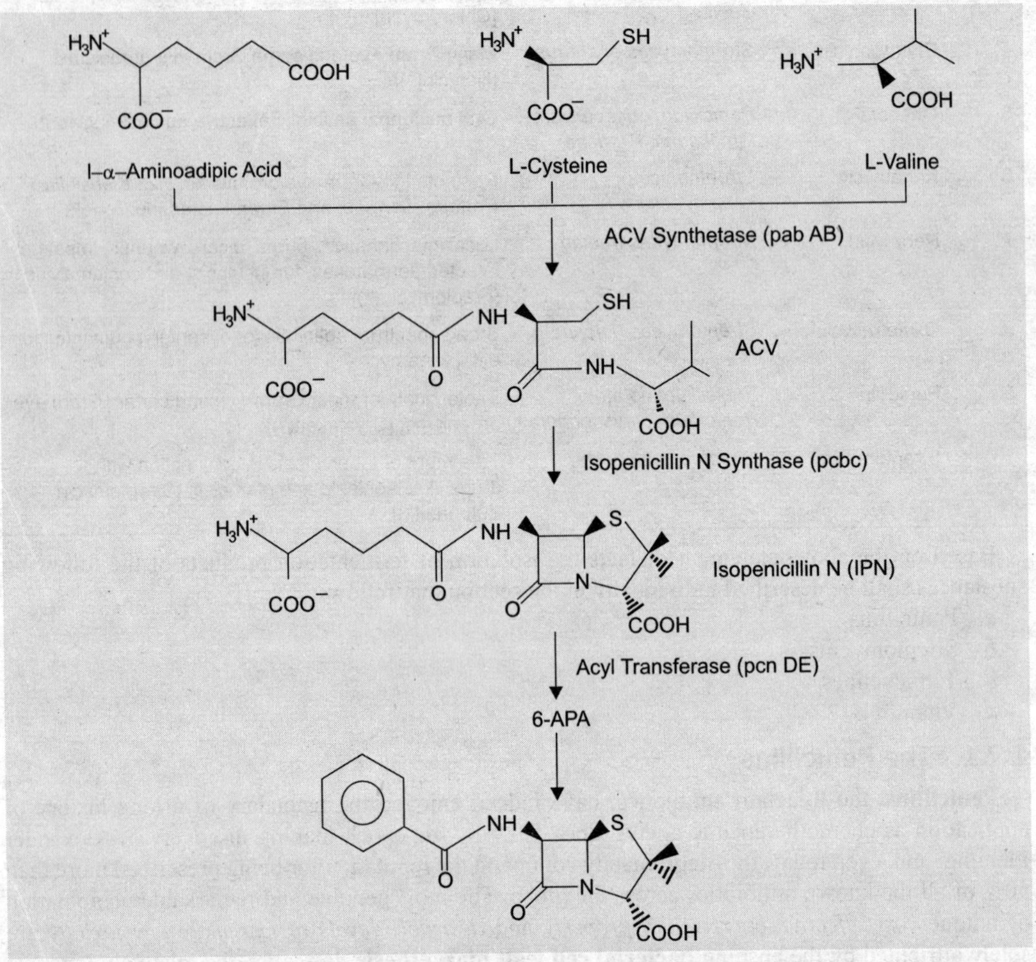

Fig. 1.18 *Pathway for Biosynthesis of Penicillin's*

A. L-α-Aminoadipic Acid: A common Precursor, but Different Biosynthetic Origins

Nevertheless, a predominant point of difference does exist between the *bacterial β-lactam* and *fungal* producer species with respect to the formation of L-α-aminoadipic acid, which is one of the three precursor amino acids of the **penicillins.** However, this difference actually comes into being *via* the two separate and distinct pathways specifically for the **lysine metabolism** as could be observed in *prokaryotes* and *eukaryotes.*

The two aforesaid routes of biosyntheses shall now be treated briefly:

In Prokaryotes: In this instance, lysine gets biosynthesized *via* a pathway without the utilization of L-α-aminoadipic acid; and, therefore, the **prokaryotic β-lactam producing species** have worked out an altogether different strategy to yield L-α-aminoadipic acid. It has been duly observed that in the two different species, namely: *Streptomyces* spp., and *Nocardia lactamdurans,* the production of L-α-aminoadipic acid by the **catabolism of lysine** occurs in a two-step phenomenon.

First, *lysine* gets converted to 1-piperidine-6-carboxylic acid, duly catalyzed by the enzyme *lysine-ε-amino transferase (LAT).* As LAT is exclusively present in **penicillin-producing actinomycetes,** and is apparently absent in *corresponding nonproducers,* and because the **'gene'** responsible for encoding this particular enzume (LAT) is eventually associated with other penicillin biosynthetic genes in *Streptomyces clevuligerus and Nocardia lactamdurans.* In reality, LAT is regarded to be an integral part of the ensuing penicillin biosynthetic pathway as illustrated in Fig. 1.19.

Secondly, 1-piperidine-6-carboxylic acid gets converted to α-amino-adipic acid by the prevailing reputed enzyme *piperidine-6-carboxylate dehydrogenase.*

In Eukaryotes: In this case, the inclusion of fungal β-lactam-yielding species, *lysine* gets biosynthesized *via* a distinct metabolic pathway wherein L-α-aminoadipic acid invariably appears as an exceptional intermediate; and subsequently, it may be removed carefully for the ensuing penicillin biosynthesis.

Precisely in fungi, the L-α-aminoadipic acid is made available *via* the prevailing **lysine biosynthetic pathway,** it may also be obtained alternatively *via* a **lysine catabolic pathway**, very much identical to the one frequently observed in the *actinomycetes;* and ultimately routed and channeled into the **penicillin biosynthesis.**

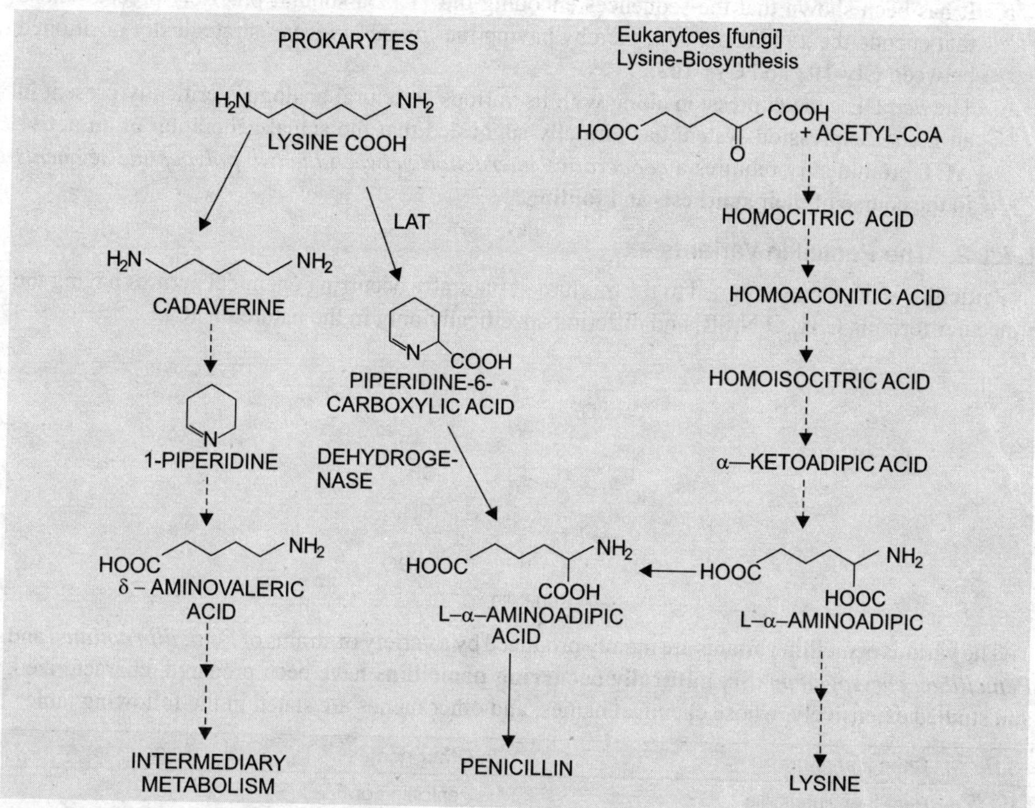

Fig.1.19 *Lysine Metabolism and Relationship to L-α-Aminoadipic Acid Production in Microorganism and Fungi*

B. Late Genes in the Biosynthesis of Hydrophobic Penicillins: Extensive research has amply proved and established that isopenicillin N (IPN) may be rightfully regarded as the most crucial **branch-point intermediate** in the penicillin pathway. Furthermore, its subsequent strategic conversion to a wide ranges of *hydrophobic penicillins,* such as: *Penicillins G* essentially designates the ultimate and final step particularly related to the **penicillin-producing segment of the pathway.**

Salient Features: The various salient features involving the late genes in the biosynthesis of the hydrophobic penicillins are as follows:

1. It has been observed that the L-α-aminoadipic acid moiety first gets dislodged by an enzyme, amidohydrolase, to give rise to the formation of 6-APA followed immediately by reaction with a CoA derivative to result into the formation of the targeted drug penicillin.
2. Enzyme actively engaged in catalyzing the reaction [in (1) above], **acyl-CoA-isopenicillin acyltrasferase** (ACT), normally occurs as a *heterodimer* usually comprising of two subunits of 29 and 11 kDa (*i.e.,* kilo dalton).
3. ACT represents a **'multifunctional enzyme'** which predominantly exhibits the characteristic features of *three* enzymes, namely: **acetyl-CoA-isopenicilin N acyltransferase (IAT), acyl-CoA-6-APA acyltransferase (AAT),** and **penicillin amidase.**
4. Interestingly, the aforesaid subunits [in (2) above] are articulately derived from a **40 kDa preprotein** by the aid of a **post translational processing mechanism;** and are legitimately encoded by a single gene, *pen* DE, that has been duly *cloned* as well as *sequenced* originating from two **fungal β-lactam producers.**
5. It has been shown that the sequences encoding the 11 kDa subunit precisely precede those that encode the 29 kDa subunit, thereby having the *'processing site'* strategically positioned between **Gly-102** and **Cys-103.**
6. The *pen* DE gene expression along with its various structural analogues critically present in an *E.coli.* expression system has virtually suggested that the actual generation of an **active ACT** prominently requires a *cooperative interaction between the two polypeptide segments* in the course of their **synthesis** and **folding.**

1.7.1.2 The Penicillin Variants

Penicillin is the name assigned to the mixture of naturally occurring chemical entities having the molecular formula $C_9H_{11}O_4N_2SR$, and differing specifically only in the nature of 'R':

Penicillin

The various penicillin variants are mainly produced by a variety of strains of *Penicillin notatum* and *Penicillium chrysogenum.* Six **naturally occurring penicillins** have been prepared, characterized, and studied extensively, whose chemical names, and other names are stated in the following table:

S.No	Chemical name	Other names
1.	Pent-2-enylpenicillin	Penicillin-I or F
2.	Benzylpenicillin	Penicillin-II or G
3.	*p*-Hydroxybenzyl penicillin	Penicillin-III or X
4.	*n*-Heptyl penicillin	Penicillin-IV or K
5.	*n*-Amylpenicillin	Dihydro-F Penicillin
6.	Phenoxymethyl penicillin	Penicillin-V

1.7.1.3 Production of Benzylpenicillins [Penicillin G]

Alexander Fleming's originally isolated strain of *Penicillium notatum* (Straub) afforded actually very low yield of **penicillin.** Vigorous search for improvement of strain revealed the isolation of

P. chrysogenum which distinctly gave much *higher yields of penicillin.* Importantly, the newer strains of *Penicillium* could even produce upto 180 folds higher yields in comparison to the original isolate that are solely based upon the novel phenomenon of **'mutation'** or the so-called **'genetic engineering'** methodologies.

In actual practice, **penicillin** is commercially produced in submerged vat cultures employing a highly purified and selected strain of *P. chrysogenum,* whereby the ultimate yield of the targeted product (**penicillin**) has been enhanced almost **three folds** *i.e.,* from 10 mcg.mL^{-1} to 30 mcg.mL^{-1}. Interestingly, these modified, researched, purified strains of **penicillium** do exhibit a number of marked and pronounced characteristic features, such as: high-titre values, improved growth, immense tolerance to the side-chain precursors, acetyltransferase activity, and ability to store intracellular requirement.

The various steps that are associated intimately with the production of **Benzylpenicillins [Penicillin G]** are stated as under:

1.7.1.3.1 Inoculum

Penicillium notatum (*i.e.,* Fleming's initial/original strain) together with other *'early isolates'* afforded exclusively low yields of **penicillin;** besides, they responded very sluggishly to the **submerged culture techniques** particularly. Contrary to this, an early strain of *P. chrysogenum* (**NRRL, 1951**), duly isolated from the moldy fruits, was observed to yield much higher yields of **penicillin.** Consequently, *the high-yield strain* was duly subjected to careful treatment with a broad-spectrum of time-tested **mutagenic agents**, for instance: UV-radiations, X-rays, and mechlorethamine (MBA)—a nitrogen mustard. Obviously, these mutagenic agents helped a long way in the appropriate selection of several **higher yielding mutants** in particular; and, in general, the judicious application of these ensuing mutagenic agents in sequence, along with certain repetitive treatments, ultimately grave rise to the newer strain **Q-176,** that essentially had the ability of producing maximum yields of penicillin.

Q-176 strain produced > 1000 Units. mL^{-1}
NRRL-1951 strain produced ~ 200 Units. mL^{-1}

Drawback: Both Q-176 and NRRL-1951 strains gave rise to the formation of a yellow water-soluble pigment known as **chrysogenin** that prominently introduced a distinct yellow tint to the final product of penicillin. Therefore, it was almost necessary to intensify the studies in the direction of **mutation** and **selection** to lay hand on such modified strains that failed to produce the undesired yellow pigment.

Developments in Better Penicillin-Producing Strains: It is worthwhile to observe at this point in time that a *major segment of strain-development programmes* ultimately culminated with the latest **high-yielding industrial strains** for the penicillin production. However, one may serenely take notice of the fact that all of these modified strains are truly the descendant variants of the mother strain Q-176.

Asexual Reproduction: Nevertheless, the penicillin-producing strains of *Penicillium* are found to be due to **asexual reproduction;** and, therefore, the scope of the 'conventional methods of genetic analysis' may not be applicable to them at all.

Parasexual Recombination: The incidence of a specific type of combination usually termed as **'parasexual recombination'** may take place by the help of **prevalent resultant-segregation** as well as **recombination of genes.**

Meticulous and intensive studies carried out by several researchers, namely: Roper (1952), Sermonti (1956), and Pontecorvo (1956) have evidently demonstrated that in the event when two genetically altogether different strains of *Penicillium* are allowed to grow simultaneously, the **hyphae** of the two strains in question will exhibit a tendency to fuse at a number of points. The formation of **diploid nucleus** shall come into being when the corresponding cells duly generated from the aforesaid *'union'* essentially comprise of nuclei from each of the respective fungal strains and invariably two nuclei strategically located in the close proximity within the cell ultimately get fused. In case, the ensuing *diploid nucleus* just per chance gets into a respective **conidium,** that happens to be uninucleate in nature, the eventual formation of an altogether **new strain** would be perpetuated.

Formation of Haploid Nuclei: Further effective division by diploid nuclei meiotically may give rise to the **formation of haploid nuclei** essentially having *distinct genetic combinations*. Interestingly, this very technique has a lot of potential and scope for future development of remarkably newer and useful industrial strains of penicillin-yielding fungi.

1.7.1.3.2 Production Media

Though the precise and exact compositions of the **penicillin-production media** really employed in any industry are more or less impossible to quote and determine, by virtue of the fact that such information(s) are regarded to be the **'trade secrets'** or **patented** by the actual users. Nevertheless, a large segment of these commonly used media invariably comprises of such ingredients as: corn steep liquor solids, lactose, glucose, calcium carbonate, potassium dihydrogen phosphate [KH_2PO_4], edible oil, and a penicillin precursor. Jackson (1958) promulgated a very useful and typical medium having essentially the following composition:

S.No	Ingredients	Quantity (%)	Remarks
1.	Fermentable carbohydrates		
	– Corn steep liquor solids	3.5	Organic
	– Lactose	3.5	Carbon
	– Glucose	1	Source
2.	Organic nitrogen source q.s.	q.s	
3.	Phenyl acetic acid	q.s	Penicillin precursor
4.	Potassium dihydrogen phosphate [KH2PO4]	0.4	
5.	Calcium carbonate	1	Acts as buffer
6.	Edible oil	0.25	
7.	Organic salts	q.s	Maintain salt-balance in medium

Note:

1. The pH after sterilization is carefully maintained between 5.5 to 6.0.
2. Higher lactose content ranging between 4 to 5% is desired with vigorously increased aeration and agitation environments maintained within the fermentor (*i.e.,* bioreactor).
3. The 'production media' contains both 'lactose' and 'precursor' which are not included in the inoculum media.

1.7.1.3.3 Biomass Production

It has been amply demonstrated that the ensuing production of penicillin exclusively depends upon the prevailing **biomass production;** and, therefore, it is absolutely desirable to achieve a relatively high biomass concentration in the fermentor (bioreactor). The very presence of carbon compounds (carbohydrates) besides other nutrients and additives is grossly responsible for the initial growth of the organism(s) almost achievable near the maximum specific growth rate. Importantly, the *rapid growth rate* prominently gives rise to an appreciable enhancement in the **initial O_2-uptake rate** as well as the **subsequent CO_2-evolution rate** accordingly. It is, however, pertinent to mention at this juncture that the ultimate *penicillin production* may be enhanced by suitably augmenting and greatly improving **mycelial biomass,** which could be accomplished appropriately by boosting up both the speed and rate of agitation.

1.7.1.3.4 Course of Typical Penicillin Fermentation

The actual course involved in typical penicillin fermentation on account of several undergoing chemical changes is represented explicity in Fig. 1.20.

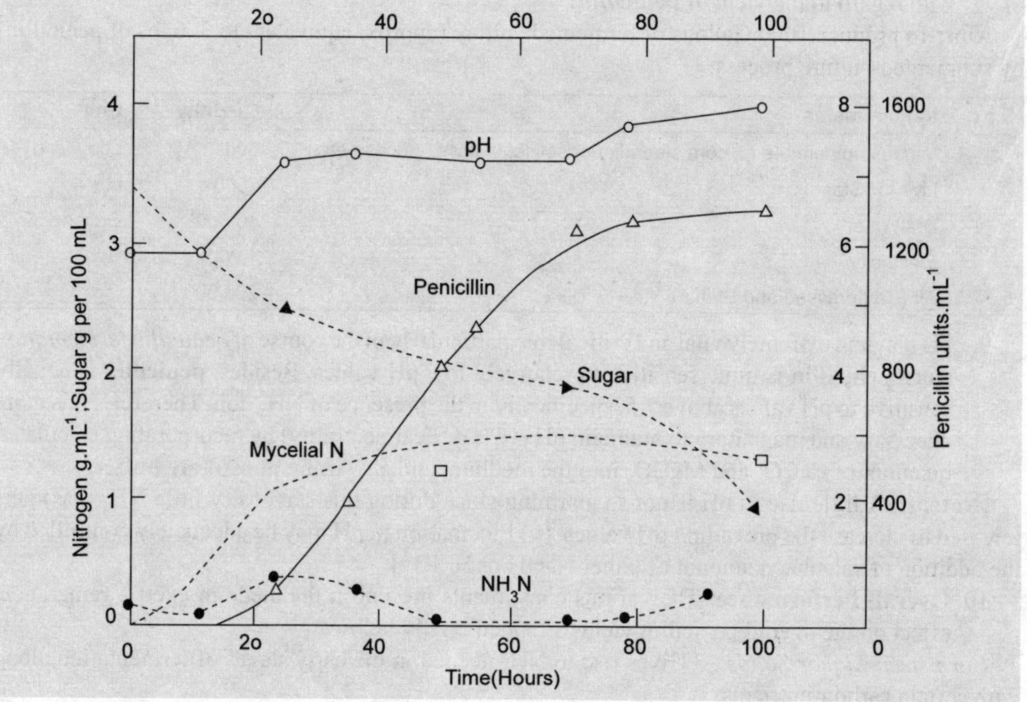

Fig. 1.20 *Various Chemical Changes Involved in a Typical Penicillin Fermentation with Added Phenyl acetic Acid Precursor.*

Salient Features: The various salient features intimately associated with the chemical changes incurred in Fig. 1.15 are enumerated below:

1. At the initial stage of fermentation pH remains rather constant, whereas the corn steep liquorcabon entities, glucose, and ammonia are being utilized simultaneously.
2. Optimum pH range for penicillin production rises maximum between 7 to 7.5 by a sequence of events, namely: carbon compounds (*i.e.,* carbohydrates) utilized and depleted — portion of lactic acid (from corn steep liquor) being consumed — ammonia (NH_3) released by deamination of aminoacids from corn steep liquor.
3. At this critical point in time pH remains virtually steady and constant as the method makes use of the lactose to form **penicillin,** further rise in pH arrested due to the fact that prevailing mold gets absolutely starved (of nutrients).
4. Completion of fermentation is indicated by pH rise to 8 or even higher by virtue of considerable depletion of **'lactose'** which smartly brings about *autolysis of the mycelium.*
   (**Note:** In usual practice, the penicillin fermentation is arrested and harvested before this specific and critical stage is achieved.)
5. **First 20 to 30 hours:** *i.e.,* during corn steep liquor solid and carbohydrate consumption the **fungal growth** turns out to be distinctly thick and heavy due to *three* possible reasons, namely: (*i*) disperse strands (of DNA); (*ii*) clusters of mycelium; and (*iii*) availability of definitive pellets of mycelium (ranging between 0.5 to 2 mm diameter).
6. Fig. 1.15 reveals vividly that the yields of penicillin are found to be **'linear** even at 22 hours, but in actual practice they range between 48 to 96 hours.

7. Ultimate yield of **penicillin** varies between 3 to 5% solely based upon *carbohydrate actually consumed,* and almost attains a level in excess of **1500 Units. mL^{-1}.**
8. Sylvester and Coghill (1954) have arrived at the following statistically averaged estimation with regard to the yield of **penicillin:**

Aim: To produce 1000 Gallons of fermented culture (approx. equivalent to 5–6 lbs of penicillin) by submerged-culture process.

S.No	Requirements	Quantity	Unit
1.	Various nutrients (*e.g.,* corn steep-liquor solids, lactose, glucose etc.)	500	Lbs
2.	Live LP-Steam	7500	Lbs
3.	DM-Water	10,000	Gallons
4.	Electricity	1,000	kwh
5.	Air (Compressed and Sterile)	250,000	

9. pH plays an extremely vital and critical role particularly in the course of *penicillin fermentation* since **penicillin** is quite sensitive to relatively low pH values. Besides, **penicillin** is equally sensitive to pH values above 7.5, specifically in the presence of NH_4^+ ion. Therefore, it is quite necessary and mandatory to maintain pH ~ 7 (*i.e.,* near neutrality) by incorporating calculated quantum of $CaCO_3$ and $MgCO_3$ into the medium, and also using **phosphate buffer.**

[**Note:** (*i*) A little rise in pH is not so alarming since during this stage very little NH_3 (gas) gets released to increase the prevailing pH values. (*ii*) Fluctuation in pH may be adequately controlled by the addition of calculated amount of either NaOH or H_2SO_4.]

10. **Overall Performance:** The various constituents present in the medium exert a remarkable effect on the overall penicillin yields as stated briefly below:

Corn steep-Liquor Solids — Gives rise to NH_3 needed in the early stages of fermentation along with certain carbon-nutrients.

Glucose — gets readily used-up to afford requisite mycelial growth but permits and restricts very little penicillin production.

Lactose — Gets only gradually degraded to *glucose* and *glactose:* and perhaps this rather not-so-rapid availability of glucose from lactose affords the much desired starvation environments urgently needed for penicillin production.

Liquid nutrients — Liquid nutrients (*i.e.,* fatty oils) are fully consumed by the respective fungus during penicillin production. However, some of the 'oil' is incorporated into the fermentation medium to serve as *'antifoaming agent'*. Most probably these oils (liquid nutrients) are duly subjected to degradation by the corresponding **'fungus'** either to the *2C-acetate* or similar compound level before being utilized in the actual formation of *mycelium* and **penicillin.**

1.7.1.3.5 Penicillin Nucleus: Two Amino Acids

One may observe the presence of *two specific amino acids* embedded into the **penicillin nucleus,** namely: **L-cysteine** and **D-valine** as depicted below:

It has been proved beyond any reasonable doubt that the adequate supplementation of **L-cysteine** and **L-cystine** *i.e.,* the two S-containing amino acids, predominantly enhanced the overall yields of **penicillin** to a much greater level and extent that occurred by the addition of all types of pure *'inorganic S-containing'* compounds.

Arnstein (1954) further substantiated and expanded the aforesaid findings by employing **isotopically labeled L-cysteine** (*viz.,* β–14_C, 35_S, and 15_N) to demonstrate precisely that the prevailing mold could induct this 'specific amino acid' directly right into the **'penicillin nucleus'.** Likewise, further researches carried out in this direction by Arnstein *et al.* using *isotopically labeled D- and L-valine* together with other *'inhibitor studies'*, invariably established the fact that the *C-skeleton* of **L-valine** gets duly incorporated very much into the **'penicillin nucleus'.**

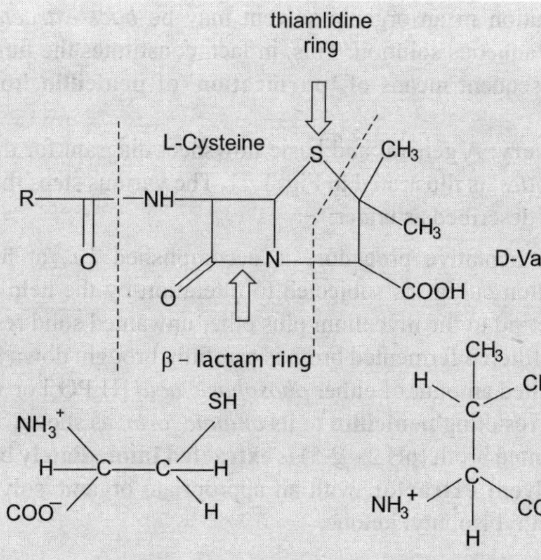

thiamlidine ring

L-Cysteine

R—C(=O)—NH— ; S ; CH_3 ; CH_3 ; N ; O ; COOH

D-Valine

β - lactam ring

NH_3^+ ; SH ; H—C—C—H ; H ; COO^-

L–Cysteine

CH_3 ; H ; CH_3 ; C ; C ; NH_3^+ ; COO^- ; H

D-Valine

1.7.1.3.6 Role of Enzyme Penicillinase

Penicillinase is an extra cellular hydrolysable enzyme adaptively generated by the specific members belonging to the *'coli form group of organism'*, in general, by most *Bacillus* species, and also certain strains of *staphylococcus.* **Penicillinase** actually hydrolyzes *penicillin* into *penicilloic acid* (a dicarboxylic acid) as given under:

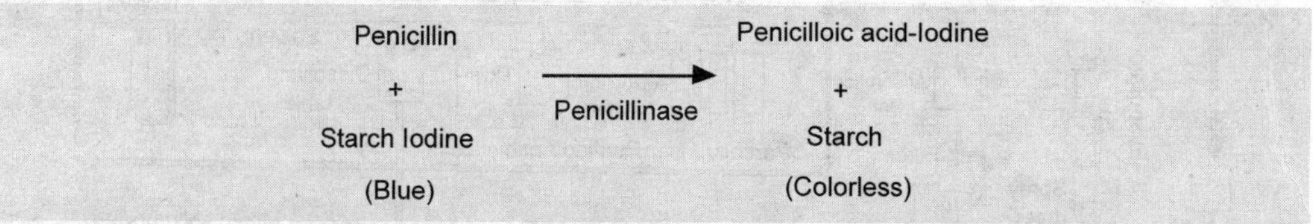

Characteristic Features: Penicillinase is vehemently present in a plethora of penicillin-resistant pathogenic strains of *Staphylococcus aureus*; and, therefore, is largely responsible for causing overwhelmingly **Penicillin-resistance** in the course of an infection. In addition to this the 'enzyme' aids in the rapid degradation of **penicillin** in the *penicillin-fermentation medium*, in the event of a possible contaminant which particularly produces the enzyme that not only has an easy access to, but also capable of growing in the fermentation broth.

1.7.1.3.7 Penicillin Production and Recovery

Principle: Penicillin in the *anionic (acid) form* is prove to extraction by solvent(s) as shown below:

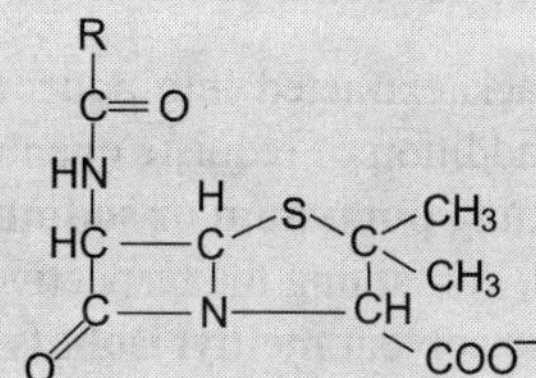

R ; C=O ; HN ; H ; S ; CH_3 ; HC—C ; C ; CH_3 ; C—N—CH ; O ; COO^-

Penicillin

Penicillin [Anionic (acidic) form]

The corresponding solution in an organic solvent may be *back-extracted* conveniently as its corresponding salt into an aqueous solution. This, in fact, constitutes the fundamental basis for the '**recovery**' as well as subsequent means of '**purification**' of **penicillin** from the respective duly harvested culture-broths.

Production and Recovery: A general and basic flowsheet diagram for the large-scale recovery and purification of '*antibiotics*' is illustrated in Fig. 1.21. The various steps that are usually followed in a sequential manner are described as under:

1. Once the entire fermentative procedure is accomplished *i.e.,* at harvest, the completed penicillin fermentation culture is subjected to filteration by the help of **heavy duty rotary vacuum filter** to get rid to the mycelium plus other unwanted solid residues.
2. The pH of the clear filtered fermented broth is carefully brought down between 2 to 2.5 by the addition of a calculated amount of either *phosphoric acid* [H_3PO_4] or *sulphuric acid* [H_2SO_4] so as to convert the resulting **penicillin** to its *anionic form,* as shown above.
3. The resulting fermented broth (pH 2 – 2.5) is **extracted immediately** by using a **Pod bielniak countercurrent solvent extractor,** with an appropriate organic solvent *e.g.,* amyl acetate, butyl acetate, or methyl isobutyl ketone.

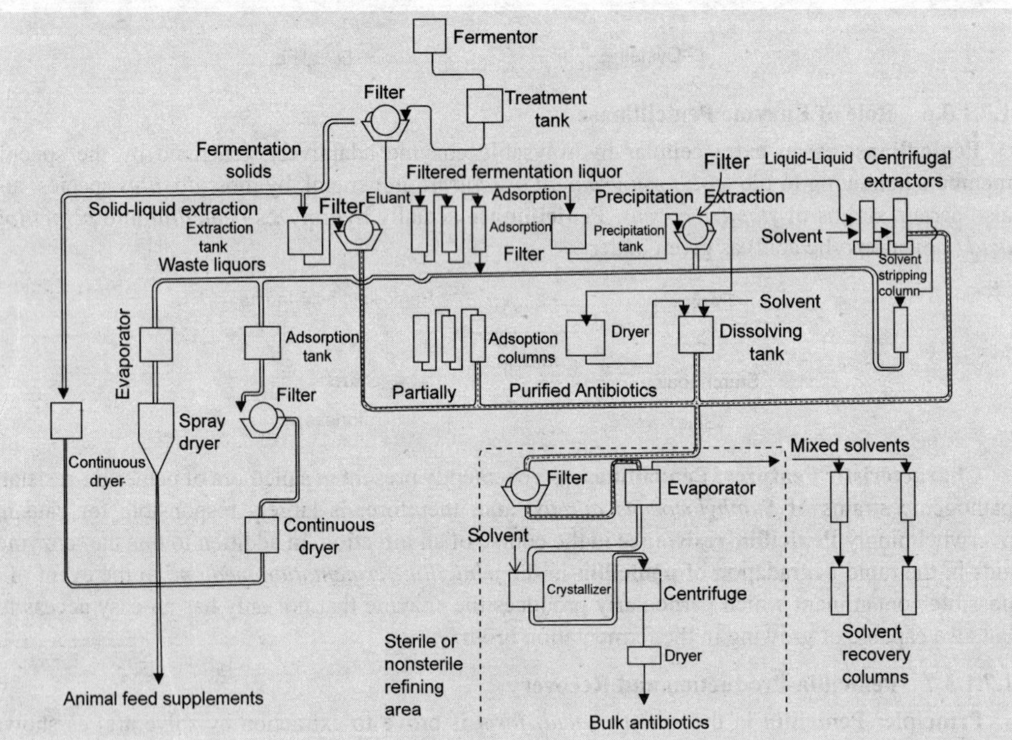

Fig. 1.21 *General and Basic Flow sheet Diagram for Large-scale Recovery and Purification of Antibiotics*

4. Penicillin, thus obtained, is back extracted into aqueous medium from the corresponding organic solvent by the careful addition of requiste quantum of KOH or NaOH to give rise to the formation of the corresponding **potassium or sodium salt of the penicillin.**
5. The resulting aqueous solution, containing the respective salt of penicillin, is again acidified and reextracted with the organic solvent **methyl isobutyl ketone**.
6. In fact, these shifts taking place between '**aqueous**' and '**solvent**' medium help in the ultimate *process of purification* of the **penicillin.**

7. The resulting solvent extract is finally subjected to a meticulous back-extraction with aqueous NaOH preferably, a number of times till extraction of penicillin is completed; and from this combine of aqueous extractions different established procedures are adopted to afford the penicillin to crystallize out either as **sodium or potassium penicillin.**
8. The crystalline penicillin thus obtained is washed, dried under vacuum, and the final product must conform to the requirements/specifications laid down by various **Official Compendia.**

Figure 1.22 illustratres a typical **'antibiotic'** fermentation plant. In actual practice, the *culture medium* could be conveniently batched as well as sterilized in the fermentor itself. Nevertheless, most of the fermentors are attached to a batching vessel and subsequently to the respective sterilizers as given in the above figure. The various feed vessels duly connected to the final-stage fermentor are invariably employed to supplement both *nutrients* and *precursors* during the on-going fermentative process. Importantly, the **seed** fermentor and the final-stage fermentor should be operable under stringent aseptic environments. The bioreactors are made of SS, having a capacity ranging between 30 and 300 m^3, agitation by 2/3 flat-peddled impellars, aeration done with compressed sterile air injection, generated heat dissipated by employing chilled-water cooling coils (maintained at 26 ± 2°C). Sterilization of the system done with live-steam injection ports adequately.

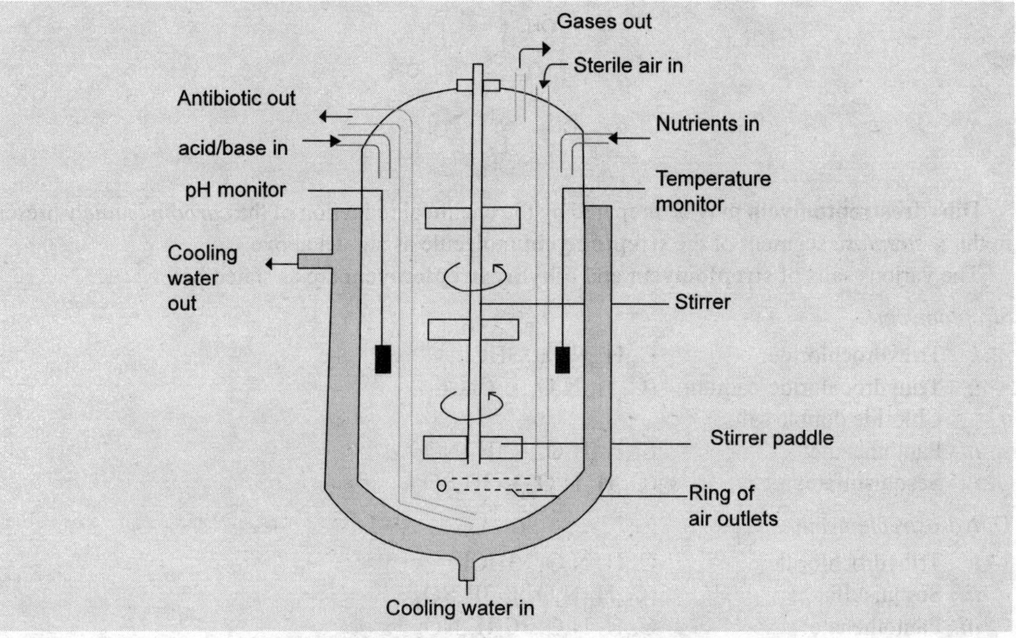

Fig. 1.22 *A Typical Antibiotic Fermentation Plant.*

1.7.2 Streptomycin

Streptomycin is produced by either of the two *Streptomyces* species, namely: *S. griseus* and *S. humidus*. The antibiotic is particularly active against Gram –ve bacteria *e.g., Mycobacterium tuberculosis*. Besides, it is also found to exert its activity against Gram +ve bacteria, and used therapeutically for curing infections inflicted by such organisms that distinctly show resistance to **penicillin.**

The wonderful epoch making discovery of **streptomycin** was meticulously carried out by three prominent researchers: Schatz, Bugie and Waksman (1944); and one of their first and foremost soil isolates (bearing No: 18-16) derived from *S. griseus* was, in fact, a *mother strain* still being employed largely as **industrial strains** across the globe even today. However, constant endeavour in selective mutation and purification of various strains articulately helped to enhance excellent practically achievable yields of today.

1.7.2.1 Chemical Structure

The chemical structures of two basic compounds, *viz.,* **streptomycin** and **dihydrostreptomycin** are as given below:

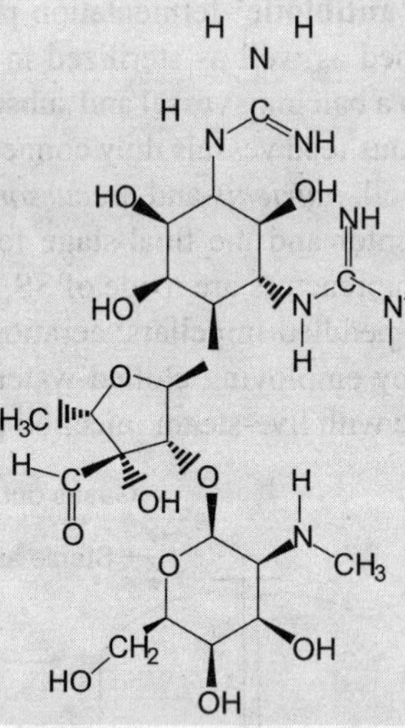

Dihydrostreptomycin may be prepared by the chemical reduction of the *carbonyl moiety* present in the *L-streptose* segment of the **streptomycin** molecule as shown above.

The various salts of **streptomycin** and **dihydrostreptomycin** are as stated below:

Streptomycin

i. Trihydrochloride: $C_{21}H_{39}N_7O_{12} \cdot 3HCl$

ii. Trihydrochloride-cadium: Chloride double salt $(C_{21}H_{39}N_7O_{12})_2 \cdot CaCl_2$

iii. Pantothenate: $C_{21}H_{39}N_7O_{12} \cdot C_9H_{17}NO_5$

iv. Sesquisulfate: $(C_{21}H_{39}N_7O_{12})_2 \cdot 3H_2SO_4$

Dihydrostreptomycin

i. Trihydrochloride: $C_{21}H_{41}N_7O_{12} \cdot 3HCl$

ii. Sesquisulfate: $(C_{21}H_{41}N_7O_{12})_2 \cdot 3H_2SO_4$

iii. Pantothenate: $C_{21}H_{41}N_7O_{12} \cdot C_9H_{17}NO_5$

Besides **streptomycin,** some other forms also exist as the ensuing fermentation products of *S. griseus* as given below:

S.No	Streptomycin Variants	Organism Used	Remarks
1.	Streptomycin	*S. griseus; S.humidus;*	Highly active
2.	Mannosidostreptomycin (Streptomycin B)	*S. reticuli*	Low antibiotic activity
3.	Hydroxystreptomycin (Reticulin)	*S. reticuli*	do
4.	Mannosidohydroxy streptomycin	*Streptomyces spps*	do

1.7.2.2 Choicest Medium

The choicest medium for the fermentative process of streptomycin production essentially comprise of:

a. **Carbon Source:** *e.g.,* dextrin, glycerol, glucose, starch, and similar economically viable substances.

b. **Nitrogen Source:** *e.g., naturally occurring processed agricultural products:* cotton seed meal, soyabean meal, corn steep liquor solids, casein-hydrolysate, yeast and its prepared extracts; and *pure inorganic salts:* ammonium sulphate [$(NH_4)_2$ SO_4], ammonium nitrate [NH_4NO_3].

c. **Vegetable/Animal Fat:** *e.g.* soyabean oil, linseed oil, fatty acids having more than 14Cchain lengths plus their corresponding esters, and lard oil.

Two research groups, almost over a gap of a decase suggested typical industrial medium best suited for the fermentation of streptomycin as given below:

S.No	Ingredients	Woodruff and McDaniel1	Hockenhull2
1.	Soyabean meal	1%	–
2.	Glucose	1%	2.5%
3.	Sodium chloride	0.5%	0.25%
4.	Extracted soyabean meal	–	4%
5.	Distiller's dried solubles	–	0.5%
6.	pH (Before Sterilization)	–	7.3–7.5

1.7.2.3 Inoculum

High-yeilding *Streptomyces griseus* spores accomplished through meticulous mutation procedures are stringently maintained either **soil stocks** or duly **lypholized** in an appropriate carrier, for instance: *sterile skimmed milk.* Consequently, the spores obtained from these **stock cultures** are carefully inoculated into a *'sporulation medium'* strictly under aseptic conditions. It has been observed that it duly caters for sufficient **'sporulated growth'** to gainfully initiate the much desired **liquid buildup of** mycelial inoculum in flasks or inoculum tanks respectively.

1.7.2.4 Streptomycin Production

Preamble: Streptomycin production outputs in **bioreactors** invariably respond overwhelmingly to relatively high degree of aeration as well as agitation. It has been duly established that the **'optimum production parameters'** for **streptomycin** are:

Fermentation temperature:	Varies between 25–30°C (~ 28°C)
pH:	Ranges between 7–8 (Max. between 7.6–8)
Duration:	Varies between 5–7 days
	(yield > 1200 mcg.mL^{-1})

Importantly, **streptomycin** is fairly *rough and tough,* and hence hardly gets destroyed by the presence of contaminating microorganisms as is the case with *penicillin.* Nevertheless, contaminants definitely minimize yields to a considerably extent.

Note: (1) The actinophage infections may prove to be harmful and serious in nature for both the inoculum and production vessels, because the *streptomycete* rapidly undergoes cleavage thereby reducing yields substantially.

(2) Development and application of *'tailor-made'* strains of *S. griseus,* specifically resistant to certain more common phages, are being used nowadays globally.

Production: The classical and widely promulgated commercial fermentation operation for the production of **streptomycin** essentially passes through *three* cardinal phases, namely:

Phase-1: It extends upto only *24 hours* wherein the rapid growth commences producing the large proportion of mycelium required for the fermentation. The highly *energised proteolytic* characteristic property of *S. griseus* predominantly sets free NH_3 right into the medium from the soyabean meal, and thus the carbon-enriched nutrients present in the soyabean meal are adequately consumed for the vigorous progressive growth. Nevertheless, the glucose up-take of the medium is rather on a very low ebb during this particular phase, and perhaps that could be the reason for reasonably lower (slight) streptomycin production. Interestingly, the ensuing pH of the medium rises from 6.7/6.8 to nearly 7.5 or so.

Phase-2: It is the most crucial and critical stage since during this phase streptomycin is eventually generated at a tremendously rapid rate that usually extends from 1 day to almost 6/7 days of incubation under perfect sterile environment. Because there is little growth of mycelium; and hence, the weight of mycelium almost remains constant. In fact, *three* events take place precisely in this specific phase, namely: (*a*) **NH_3** is fully consumed; (*b*) **glucose** also being used-up to the maximum extent; and (*c*) pH stands constant between 7.6 to 8.

Phase-3: With the virtually complete depletion of *'sugar'* from the fermentation medium the **streptomycin production** almost comes to a standstill situation. At this point in time, the ensuing fermentation is invariably harvested before the commencement of this phase of **senescense** *i.e., the 'period of old age'*.

Harvest-Recovery-Purification: Once the fermentation attains completion, the resulting **mycelium** is duly separated from the ensuing fermented broth by filtration; and thus, the **streptomycin** is finally recovered by one of the two methods described below based on the specific industrial concern.

Method-I: The **streptomycin** produced is adequately adsorbed from the fermented broth onto activated carbon particles, and subsequently subjected to elution from the carbon particles by means of diluted mineral acid till **streptomycin** gets eluted almost completely. The eluted product is precipitated by suitable solvents, filtered, and dried *under vacuum* before further purification.

Method-II: Fermentation broth is first acidified and subsequently filtered and neutralized. The resulting clear broth is forced *via* a packed column of **cation-exchange resin** to allow the adsorption of **streptomycin** on it completely. The column is washed with water (DM) soon after the completion of adsorption, and finally eluted with diluted HCl, and the liquid containing **streptomycin** is concentrated *under vacuo* almost to dryness. The crude antibiotic is dissolved in *methanol* and filtered, and *acetone* is now added so as to allow the complete precipitation of **streptomycin.** In the final treatment the ensuing precipitate is washed thoroughly with acetone and dried *in vacuo* before being solubilized in MeOH for the ultimate preparation of the desired **streptomycin-calcium chloride complex** in its purest form.

Note: *The final product obtained either from Method-I or II must rigidly conform to the standards of purity and assay as prescribed in the* ***Official Compendia.***

1.7.3 The Tetracyclines

The epoch-making discovery of chlortetracycline (aureomycin) in 1947 by Duggar paved the way for a number of structural analogues used as broad-spectrum antibiotic that belong to the tetracycline family. The tetracyclines which are found to be effective therapeutically are listed in the following table.

1.7.3.1 Salient Features of the Tetracyclines

Name of Compound	Official Status	Brand Name(s)	R_1	R_2	R_3	R_4	R_5
Tetracycline	BPC; (1973); USP;	Tetracyn(R) (Pfizer) SK-Tetracycline(R) (SK & F)	H	OH	CH_3	H	H
Oxytetracycline	USP;	Terramycin(R) (Pfizer)	OH	OH	CH_3	H	H
Chlortetracycline HCl	BP, USP; Eur.P. Int. P.; Ind. P.;	Aureomycin(R) (Lederle)	H	OH	CH_3	Cl	H
Demeclocycline HCl	BP. USP; Eur. P.;	Ledermycin(R) (Lederle, UK)	H	OH	H	Cl	H
Methacycline HCl	BP (1973); USP;	Rondomycin(R) (Wallace)	OH	=	CH_2	H	H
Doxycycline	USP;	Vibramycin(R) (Pfizer)	OH	H	CH_3	H	H
Rolitetracycline	USP;	Syntetrin(R) (Bristol)	H	OH	CH_3	H CH_2–N	

1.7.3.2 Nomenclatures

Based on the above conventional numbering of various carbon atoms and subsequent labeling of the **four** aromatic rings present in the tetracycline nucleus, oxytetracycline is chemically designated as:

"4-Dimethylamino-1, 4, 4*a*, 5, 5*a,* 6, 11, 12*a*-octahydro-3, 6, 10, 12, 12*a*-penta-hydroxy-6-methyl- 1, 11-dioxo-2 naphthacenecarboxamide".

Some other members of the tetracycline family may conveniently be named as follows:

Methacycline: 6-Methylene-5-oxytetracycline;

Doxycycline: α-6-Deoxy-5-oxytetracycline;

Rolitetracycline: N-(Pyrrolidinomethyl)-tetracycline.

1.7.3.3 General Characteristics of the Tetracyclines

Following are the *general characteristic features* of all the members of the tetracycline family:

a. The tetracycline is obtained by fermentation procedures from streptomyces species or by the chemical transformations of the natural products.

b. The important members of this family are essentially derivatives of an octahydronaphthacene, *i.e.,* a hydrocarbon made up of a system of four-fused rings.

c. The antibiotic spectra and the chemical properties of these compounds are quite similar but not identical.

d. The tetracyclines are amphoteric compounds, *i.e.,* forming salts with either acids or bases. In neutral solutions these substances exist mainly as zwitter ions.

e. The acid salts of the tetracyclines that are formed through protonation of the dimethylamino groupf of C-4, usually exist as crystalline compounds which are found to be very much soluble in water. However, these amphoteric antibiotics will crystallize out of aqueous solutions of their salts unless they are duly stabilized by an excess of acid.

f. The corresponding hydrochloride salts are used commonly for oral administration and are usually encapsulated owing to their bitter taste.

g. The water soluble salts are obtained either from bases such as sodium/potassium hydroxides or formed with divalent/polyvalent metals, *e.g.,* Ca^{++}. The former ones are not stable in aqueous solutions, while the latter ones, *e.g.,* calcium salt give tasteless products that may be employed to prepare suspensions for liquid oral dosage forms.

h. The unusual structural features present in the tetracyclines afford three acidity constants (pKa values) in aqueous solutions of the acid salds. The thermodynamic pKa values has been extensively studied by Lesson *et al.* and discussed in the chapter on 'Physical-chemical factors and biological activities'.

i. An interesting property of the tetracyclines is their ability to undergo epimerizaton at C-4 in solutions having intermediate pH range. These isomers are called epitetracyclines. The **four *epi-tetracyclines*** have been isolated and characterized. They exhibit much less, activity than the corresponding **'natural' isomers;** thus accounting for an apparent decrease in the therapeutic value of aged solution.

j. It has been observed that the strong acids and bases attack the tetracyclines having a hydroxyl moiety at C-6, thereby causing a considerable loss in activity through modification of the Cring.

Strong acids produce dehydration through a reduction involving the OH group at C-6 and the H atom at C-5*a*. The double bond thus generated between positions C-5*a* and C-6 induces a shift in the position of the double bond between the carbon atoms C-11 and C-11*a* thereby forming the relatively more energetically favoured resonant system of the naphthalene group found in the *inactive* anhydrotetracyclines.

The strong bases on the other hand promote a reaction between the hydroxyl group at C-6 and the carbonyl moiety at C-11, thereby causing the bond between C-11 and C-11*a* atoms to cleave and eventually form the lactone ring found in the *inactive* isotetracyclines.

k. The tetracyclines form stable chelate complexes with many metals, *e.g.*, Ca^{++}, Mg^{++}, Fe^{++}, etc.

A few typical examples for the tetracycline's shall be dealt with in the section that follows:

1.7.3.3.1 Tetracycline

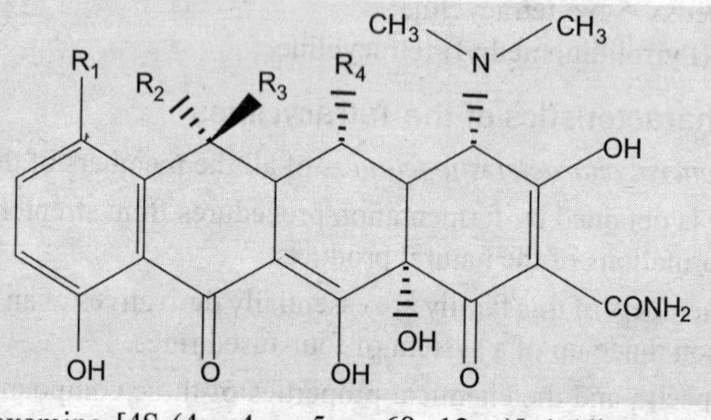

2-Naphthacenecarboxamine [4S-(4α, 4*a*α, 5*a*α, 6β, 12*a*α)]-4 (dimethylamino)-1, 4, 4*a*, 5, 5*a*, 6, 11, 12*a*-octahydro-3, 6, 10, 12, 12*a*-pentahydroxy-6-methyl-1-11-dioxo-; USP; Achromycin(R); Cyclopar(R); Panmycin(R); Tetracyn(R);

Tetracycline is the drug of choice in the treatment of chloera, relapsing fever, granuloma inguinale and infections produced by rickettsia, *Borrelia, Mycobacterium fortuitum* and *marinum,* and *Chlamydia psittaci* and *trachomatis* (except pneumonia and inclusion conjunctivitis).

It may be employed as an **'alternative drug'** in the following *two* situations, namely:

a. With silver nitrate in the prevention of neonatal ocular prophylaxis of chlamydial and gonococcal conjunctivitis, and

b. For treatment of actinomycosis, anthrax, chancroid, mellioidosis, plague, rat-bite fevers, syphilis and yaws.

It has also been reported to be beneficial in the treatment of *toxoplasmosis.*

Tetracycline Production

Tetracycline is produced on large-scale using the *submerged fermentation process* by *two* predominant strains employed across the globe, namely: (*a*) *Streptomyces aureofaciens* **[ATCC:**

13908–13911 and **NCL** B–9114]. In actual practice, the *stock cultures* are adequately maintained for reasonably long durations in the shape of **spores.** Importantly, the resulting spores are maintained strictly either under liquid N_2 (–70 to –80°C) or **lyphilized.** The **'bioreactor'** being employed is normally made up of stainless-steel along with SS connecting pipes, two-or three way SS gate-valves, SS-pumps (**Alpha Laval** - *Make*) provided with adequate agitation and compressed sterile air circulation. Besides, it must have all the necessary gadgets and recording devices meant for round-the-clock monitoring during the entire fermentative operation. Various *physical* and *physiological* parameters of the culture media in the **bioreactor** need to be controlled automatically, such as: pH regulation, supplementation with sterile nutrients during the fermentation run etc. In addition, a number of vital and critical tests are being carried out for the optimum growth of the antibiotic (**tetracycline**), for instance: strength of nutrients, morphology and growth of culture, antibiotic production, and sterility conditions.

Note: *Sterilization of the* **'liquid nutrient media'** *is normally carried out at 120°C for a period of 40 minutes.*

Culture Medium: It has been observed that the overall tetracycline production is solely governed by the ensuing C: N ratio of the nutrients (*i.e.,* sources) in the culture medium. However, in actual practice the various components that essentially provide **carbon sources** are, namely: *starch, sucrose* and *glycerol;* and **nitrogen sources** are, namely: *admixture of soyabean meal plus mineral salts, ammonium salts, amino acids, casein* (*milk*-protein), *meat-extract* (*animal*-protein) etc. Besides, the usable medium also comprises of **cotton-seed meal, peanut meal, corn steep liquor** etc. It is absolutely important as well as necessary to stringently maintain very **low concentration of Cl– ion** in the medium so as to accomplish **high production levels.** Deionized corn steep liquor and similar raw materials free from Cl^- ions may also be used gainfully. The optimum temperature should be 28°C and pH must vary between 5.5 to 6.5 (ideally 5.6 to 6.0).

Inoculum: The basic inherent characteristic features of the ensuing **inoculum** do play a major role for the biosynthetic production of **tetracycline,** such as: quality of vegetative inoculum or spores *i.e.,* its threshold age, genetic homogeneity, metabolic reative profile etc. Optimum tetracycline yield is duly accomplished from a medium that predominantly comprises of **inoculum** for 24 hours, and present within a range of 2–10% having an optimum pH value between 5.6 and 6.2.

Aeration: It is quite necessary and equally important to make available both vigorous and intensive **aeration** in the submerged cultures of *Streptomyces aureofaciens* right from the very initial stage of cultivation phenomenon. Any observed irregular aeration or interruption in aeration during the **firstfew hours** invariably gives rise to an appreciable extent of production of **tetracycline.**

Tetracycline Production: The tetracycline production is carried out in submerged aerated agitated bioreactor containing adequate virulent culture medium loaded with genetically homogenous and metabolically reactive inoculum. It essentially comprise of *three* distinct and vital stages, namely:

Stage-1: **Growth Phase:** It is mostly characterized by instant fast utilization of incorporated nutrients. There is a distinct enhancement of the **cell mass.** The phsophate (PO_4^{-3}) ion concentration has an enormous influence upon the prevailing culture medium. Interestingly, during the on-going production phase of the tetracycline fermentative procedure the **secondary mycelium** (*i.e.,* the *thin-hyphae*) is found to modulate the specific phosphate ions present in the culture medium. However, the *'production type of the mycelium'* is hardly generated particularly in the overwhelmingly presence of the PO_4^{-3} ions.

Stage-2: **Production Phase:** In this particularly phase the maximum quantum of the antibiotic is actually generated. Thus, the overall rate of growth of the concerned microorganism gets decreased substantially and almost ceases in due course.

State-3: Thus is, in fact, the last phase wherein the production of the tetracycline almost attains the lowest ebb. The mycelium undergoes due fragmentation and the process of cleavage commences apparently.

Isolation and Purification: Tetracycline is invariably obtained from the **clear filtrate** obtained from the acidic medium (*i.e.,* the fermented broth) by the help of sterilized SS-Plate Type Filter Press or Pdobielniak Counter Current Extractor (as mentioned under 'penicillin'). The clear filtrate is subjected to a process of adsorption upon an active substance *e.g.,* activated carbon, and elution subsequently. The eluted liquid is treated with a requisite amount of salts of alkaline earth metals to obtain the **precipitate of tetracycline** as its corresponding salts. The resulting salt is poorly water soluble, but fairly soluble in several organic solvents. Once the organic phase is separated, the **tetracycline** is adequately pushed into the aqueous phase (by the addition of diluted HCl). Finally, the **purified form of tetracycline** is salted out or crystallized carefully, and dried **under vacuum.**

1.7.4 Vitamin B_{12} (Cyanocobalamine; Cobamide)

Vitamin B_{12} is produced commercially by the aid of a **direct fermentation procedure** using *Streptomyces* species, for instance: *Streptomyces olivaceus.*

Rickes *et al.* (1948) first and foremost recovered the active crystalline **vitamin B_{12}**, as given below from a *S. griseus* culture (that also eventually produced the antibiotic **resein**).

Prolonged intensive and extensive researches have adequately proved and revealed that at least *'small quantum'* of vitamin B_{12} could be synthesized by a host of microorganism variants belonging specifically to *actinomycetes* and *bacteria;* and that relatively *'large quantum'* was prevalent particularly amongst the microorganisms pertaining to the *intestinal habitats.*

In general, cobamides (vitamin B_{12}) essentially comprise of a *'porphyrin nucleus'* to which the **ribose** and **phsphate** residues are attached strategically. Nevertheless, the cobamide variants do differ in their corresponding **purine, benzimidazole** on other base located in the **nucleotide-like segment of the molecule;** and besides, in the chemical functional moiety duly attached to the Co atom.

The various steps involved in the production of Vitamin B_{12} are enumerated sequentially as stated below:

1. *S. olivaceous* is allowed to grow with adequate constant aeration at 27°C preferably in a nutritionally rich crude-medium having **glucose** as a major source of **carbon.**
2. A potential source of cobalt (Co) between 2–10 ppm is duly incorporated into the above medium in the form of its salt cobalt chloride [$CoCl_2 . 6H_2O$] to serve as a **precursor.** Thus, the relevant organism meticulously scavenges low levels of cobalt from the prevailing medium, whereas the respective higher levels are proved to be toxic in nature.
3. Total duration of the fermentative process lasts between 3 to 4 days or until such time when **mycelium lysis** commences to take place. In this manner, a major segment of the vitamin B_{12} produced remains very much contained within the microbial cells until **autolysis*** comes into force; and, therefore, the recovery of the vitamin from the **'fermentation broth'** is tremendously simplified by actually initiating harvesting before autolysis has turned out to be adequately serious *i.e.,* a situation when **vitamin B_{12}** is still lodged within the mycelium securedly.
4. At harvesting stage, both the solids and the mycelium are duly *filtered* or *centrifuged* to separate them from the ensuing **'fermentation broth',** and dried subsequently for an appropriate usage in the form of either **vitamin B_{12} enriched** animal-or poultry-feed supplements.
5. **Alternative Method of Recovery:** In this specific instance, the **vitamin B_{12}** is predominantly released from the concerned cells by several tried and tested methodologies, namely: *alcohol treatment, heat, acidification* etc.

Example: The adequately completed **'fermentation broth'** is first acidified, treated with sodium sulphite so as to protect the vitamin, and finally the admixture of *culture* and *fermentation* broth is subjected to careful heating by employing steam-heated coils with agitation or passing low-pressure steam slowly with proper agitation.

6. The *'solid residues'* as well as *'spent mycelium'* are duly separated either by 'filtration' or *'centrifugation'*, and the resulting clear fluid thus obtained is meticulously evaporated strictly **under superb vacuum facilities.**

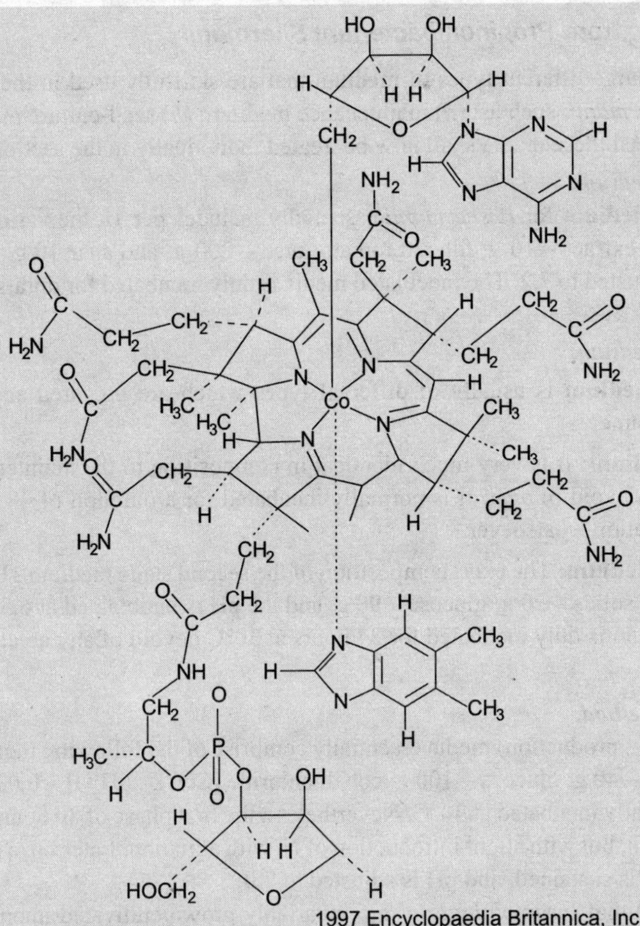

1997 Encyclopaedia Britannica, Inc.

Vitamin B_{12}

Note

1. Main bulk of vitamin B_{12} is used as such in solid dosage forms and liquid preparations.
2. Relatively small proportion of the vitamin B_{12} is further purified and crystallized for the exclusive treatment of pernicious anemia** and other vital medicinal usage *via* the IV route of administration.

Latest Method of Production

The latest method adopted for the present-day commercial production of **vitamin B_{12}** is usually carried out by adequately aerated submerged bacterial fermentations making use of strains of

Propionibacterium or *Pseudomonas* with a beet-molasses based culture medium and the adequate supplementation with requisite amount of the cobalt-salts.

Vitamin B_{12} may also be produced on a large-scale by using *Bacillus megaterium,* and the overall recovery from this fermentative procedure almost approaches quite similar to those obtained from the *Streptomyces* organisms.

The details of commercial production from *Propionibacterium shermanii* and *Pseudomonas denitrificans* are described as under:

1.7.4.1 Vitamin B_{12} from *Propinonibacterium Shermanii*

There are, in fact, *three* different types of medium that are skillfully used in the production of vitamin B_{12} from *P. shermanii,* such as: (*a*) maintenance medium; (*b*) seed-culture medium; and (*c*) main-culture medium. All these media shall now be treated individually in the section that follows:

(a) Maintenance Medium:

The **maintenance medium** for *P. shermanii* essentially includes per 1L the various ingredients as: tryptone 10g; yeast extract – 10 g; filtered tomato juice – 200 g; and agar 10 g. The pH of the prepared medium is adjusted to 7.2. The inoculated media is duly incubated for duration of 96 hours at 30°C.

(b) Seed-Culture Medium:

The **seed-culture medium** is usually of different types which are prepared according to the following *two* stages, namely:

1. **First-Stage Medium:** It is very much identical in composition to the maintenance medium and is precisely devoid of agar. It is normally incubated for a duration of 48 hours at 30°C without any agitation whatsoever.
2. **Second-Stage Medium:** The exert composition of the second stage medium 1L is as follows: corn steep liquor solids – 20 g; glucose – 90 g; and the pH is maintained at 6.5.

In general, the medium is duly incubated for 24 hours at 30°C devoid of any aeration, and pH is adjusted to 6.5

(c) Main-Culture Method:

The main-culture (*i.e.,* production) media essentially comprise of the following ingredients in 1L: corn steep liquor solids – 40 g; glucose – 100 g; cobalt chloride [$CoCl_2 . 6H_2O$] – 0.02g; and the pH adjusted to 7.0. It is usually incubated at 30°C. Nevertheless, the first phase of 80 hours is allowed to carry on without aeration, but with slight introduction of N_2 with agitation. Later on, a slight aeration to the tune of 0.1 v/v/m is sustained, and pH is adjusted to 7.0.

It has been observed that *'propionibateria'* are invariably grown/cultivated upon carbohydrate based media specifically and that too in an **unaerated environment.** However, the cobalt supplement is an absolute necessity for vitamin B12 production. Besides, it also solely depends upon either the internal generation or external supply of **5, 6-dimethyl benzimidazole** (or 5, 6-DBI). Importantly, the mutant strains of *P. shermanii* are capable of synthesizing their own 5, 6-DBI, which ultimately enhances the yield of vitamin B_{12} to an extent of 65 mg. L^{-1} in a pilot scale.

It is, however, pertinent to state here that the *'aeration'* definitely augments the formation of 5, 6-DBI, whereas it distinctly lowers the vitamin B_{12} biosynthesis at one of its various steps. Therefore, it is quite necessary and equally vital that the very *first stage* (80 hours) the fermentative process in the bioreactor must be carried out predominantly in an **anaerobic environment,** but a little agitation is still necessary until the main bulk of the carbohydrate present in the media is fully consumed for the growth and the ultimate formation of **cob amide.** Of course this kind of sequential steps will exert hardly any undue effect. The subsequent follow up stage (next 88 hours) is supplemented with *moderate agitation* and *slight aeration.* The *aeration* afforded at this stage essentially induces the biosynthetic pathway of 5, 6-DBI, whereby the resulting *cobinamide* gets converted ultimately to **cobalamin.**

1.7.4.2 Vitamin B12 from Pseudomonas Denitrificans

Quite recently a plethora of mutant strain variants have been duly developed that are prominently based upon the original wild-type of *P. denitrificans* used for the large-scale production of **vitamin B_{12}.**

Nevertheless, it essentially requires *three* different types of media, such as:

(a) Laboratory-Scale Medium:

Precisely the medium required essentially for the laboratoryscale fermentative process for producing vitamin B_{12} form *P. denitrificans* comprises in 1L the following constituents: beet molasses – 60 g; brewer's yeast – 1 g; N_2 amine – 1 g; ammonium phosphate $[(NH_4)_2HPO_4]$ – 2 g; magnesium sulphate $[MgSO_4.7H_2O]$ – 1 g; manganese sulphate $[MnSO_4.7H_2O]$ – 2 g; zinc sulphate $[ZnSO_2.7H_2O]$ – 0.02 g; sodium molybdate $[Na_2MoO_4.2H_2O]$ – 51.5 g; agar – 25 g; and pH adjusted to 7.4. The inoculated laboratory-scale medium is duly incubated at 28°C for 96 hours.

(b) Seed-Culture Medium:

It has almost the identical composition as stated in (*a*) above, but it is devoid of agar. It is incubated at 28°C on a *'rotary shaker'* for duration of 72 hours.

(c) Production-Culture Medium:

It consists of the following ingredients in 1L, namely: beet molasses – 1000 g; yeast – 2 g; ammonium hydrogen phosphate $[(NH_4)_2HPO4]$ – 5 g; magnesium sulphate $[MgSO_4.7H_2O]$ – 3 g; manganese sulphate $[MnSO_4.H_2O]$ – 0.2 g; cobalt nitrate $[Co(NO_3)_2.6H_2O]$ – 0.188 g; zinc sulphate $[ZnSO_4.7H_2O]$ – 0.02 g; sodium molybdate $[Na_2MoO_4.2H_2O]$ – 51.5 g; 5, 6-DBI – 0.025 g; and pH is adjusted to 7.4. The prepared media is duly incubated at 29°C for duration of 90 hours with constant agitation of 420 RPM and rate of aeration at 1v/v/m.

Source of Carbohydrate

In actual practice, the sugarbeet molasses loaded with 5 to 10% **betaine** (*i.e.,* trimethyl glycine) serves as an ideal source of carbohydrate. It also stimulates the production of **vitamin B_{12}** by promoting the synthesis of *α-synthetase.*

It has been duly observed that it specifically aids in the production of **δ-aminovulinic** acid *i.e.,* the very first and foremost intermediate in the **cobalamine biosynthesis.** It is pertinent to mention here that the aforementioned **cobalamin biosynthesis** by the organism

P. denitrificans essentially require the external supply of 5, 6-dimethyl-benzimidazole [*i.e.,* 5, 6-DBI] and cobalt salt.

Fermentation Phenomenon

The process of fermentation involving the growth of the *Pseudomonas* and the ensuing biosynthesis of the **vitamin B_{12}** particularly needs moderate aerated environment along with adequate agitation in the **'bioreactor'.**

1.8 Future Prospects

Biotechnological processes may be broadly viewed from *two* distinct and acceptable angles, namely: *first,* to a **small extent** which grossly need to be confined within a specifically well-defined area or system; and *secondly,* to a **large extent** wherein the ultimate eventful grand success of a plethora of the processes shall exclusively depend on the rationalized correct choice and meticulous operation of these systems. Most desirously in an industrial environment, the expected level and scale of operation will, certainly for realistic economic reasons, significantly, be substantially enormous; and, therefore, invariably in all instances the ultimate success will evidently requires the **closest cooperation** between the *process engineer* and the *bioscientist* thereby proving explicitely the most realistic interdisciplinary nature of the newer **biotechnological processes.**

The latest trend has just gained the momentum for the **overall improvement of various strains** *via* the spectacular application of **molecular genetics.** It is now possible to manipulate certain ear marked experimental parameters in stringently controlling *secondary metabolism;* and this glaring accomplishment has given rise to a very modest gains in the much-sought-after **production efficiency.** Many more future ambitious targets with specific reference to *molecular techniques* shall predominantly revolve around the identification of the prevailing **transcriptional** and **regulatory** mechanisms that would essentially either limit or restrict the expression of both foreign and native genes in producing viable strains. Besides, with advent of an ever-increasing knowledge of the wide-spectrum of biochemical and biophysical characteristic features of the *biosynthetic enzymes* shall ultimately allow their legitimate productive manipulation at the molecular level governed by X-ray crystallographic analysis of the prevailing active-site structures that would in turn ultimately permit the synthesis of a much wider range of **bioactive precursors** and **corresponding metabolites.**

Nevertheless, these **optimistic projections** are entirely supported by evidence upon a realistic consideration of the scientific merits of the application of recombinant DNA technology to the production of **antibiotics.** Off late an unfortunate situation has occurred unexpectedly due to the rapid spread of antibiotic-resistant organisms that necessitates the dire need for exploring new classes of antibiotics most pressing on one hand, and the economic cost of discovering and developing these newer breed of antibiotic on the other hand — is precisely discouraging such research endeavours globally.

In nutshell, perhaps once the problem of prevailing **'antibiotic resistance'** boils down to an even more acute situation, aggressive research into the development of *newer antibiotics* will, gain momentum out of necessity, come back into reasonable favour, and the full blast impact of **molecular genetics** shall be brought into force to bear on the problem.

Questions

1. Write an account on mutations and its applications. (JNTUA-May 2009)
2. Discuss isolation of pencillin by fermentation. (JNTUA-May 2009)
3. How do you design and optimize the parameters for the production of tetracyclins. (JNTUA-May 2009)
4. Antimicrobial spectrum and resistance. (JNTUA-May 2009)
5. Vitamin B12. (JNTUA-May 2009)
6. Explain about Isolation of mutants and factors influencing the rate of mutation. (JNTUA-Nov 2010)
7. Give detailed note on design of fermentation process. (JNTUA-Nov 2010)
8. Discuss screening of soil for organism producing antibiotics. (JNTUA-Nov 2010)
9. Describe the historical development of antibiotics. (JNTUA-Nov 2010)
10. Explain the historical development of antibiotics. (JNTUA-May 2009)
11. How the organism are screened from the soil for producing antibiotics. (JNTUA-May 2009)

12. Explain how a typical formulation process is designed. (JNTUA-May 2009)
13. Discuss isolation of fermentation products. (JNTUA-May 2009)
14. Vitamin B12. (JNTUA-May 2009)
15. Give a detailed account on historical development of antibiotics. (JNTUA-Nov 2010)
16. Write about primary and secondary screening of antibiotics. (JNTUA-Nov 2010)
17. Explain the protocol for the production of streptomycin by fermentation method. (JNTUA-Nov 2010)
18. Describe the methods for isolation of mutants. (JNTUA-Nov 2010)
19. What is a fermenter? (JNTUA-Dec 2009)
20. Describe the design of a fermenter with a neat sketch. (JNTUA-Dec 2009)
21. What are the factors that influence the rate of mutation? (JNTUA-Dec 2009)
22. Explain the procedure for isolation of tetracyclines. (JNTUA-Dec 2009)
23. Cultivation of virus. (RGUHS–Mar 2009)
24. Discuss different methods of evaluation of bacteriostatic and bactericidal substances. (RGUHS–Mar 2009)
25. With flow diagram discuss the production of vitamin B12 by fermentation processes. (RGUHS–Apr 2008)
26. Antifoaming agents used in fermentation. (RGUHS–Apr 2008)
27. Mutation. (RGUHS–Apr 2008)
28. Synchronous growth curves. (RGUHS–Oct 2007)
29. Organisms to produce streptomycin and penicillin. (RGUHS–Oct 2007)
30. Detail about evaluation of bacteriostatic and bacteriocidal disinfectant. (MGRU Apr-2004)
31. Write in detail about the maintenance of cell culture and its application. (MGRU Apr-2004)
32. Mention the application of official vaccine. (MGRU Apr-2004)
33. Type of culture media. (MGRU Apr-2004)
34. Bacterial counting method. (MGRU Apr-2004)
35. Basic principle of fermentation process. (MGRU Apr-2004)
36. Acid-fast staining. (MGRU Apr-2004)
37. Transcription. (MGRU Apr-2004)
38. What are the methods by which the micro organisms (bacteria) are differentiated. (MGRU 2003)
39. How penicillin is synthesized by germination technology. (MGRU 2003)
40. Differences between gram positive and gram negative bacteria. (MGRU 2003)
41. Differences between bacteria and virus. (MGRU 2003)
42. Microbiological assay of antibiotics. (MGRU 2004)
43. Methods for cultivation of virus. (MGRU 2004)
44. Composition of culture media for animal cell culture. (MGRU 2004)
45. Define the bacteriostatic. (MGRU 2004)
46. Define the bactericidal. (MGRU 2004)
47. Define the disinfectant. (MGRU 2004)
48. Define the antiseptic. (MGRU 2004)
49. Write in detail about the principle, operation and design of industrial horizontal jacketed autoclave. (MGRU 2004)
50. Explain the design and construction of fermentor. (MGRU 2003)
51. Briefly explain continuous culture. (MGRU 2003)
52. Write briefly on preparation of injection of penicillin. (MGRU 2003)

53. Give detailed structure of citric acid preparation by fermentation process. (MGRU 2002)
54. Bactericides used in disinfection process. (MGRU 2002)
55. Write any two differences between gram positive and gram negative cell wall in bacteria. (MGRU 2002)
56. Solid state fermentation. (MGRU 2002)
57. Draw a neat labelled diagram of "Steam Jacketed autoclave" and discuss its design and operation in detail. (MGRU 2001)
58. Draw the diagram of aerobic fermentor. Write a note on operation of fermentor. (MGRU 2004)
59. Write the principle and procedure involved in cup plate method for antibiotics. (MGRU 2004)

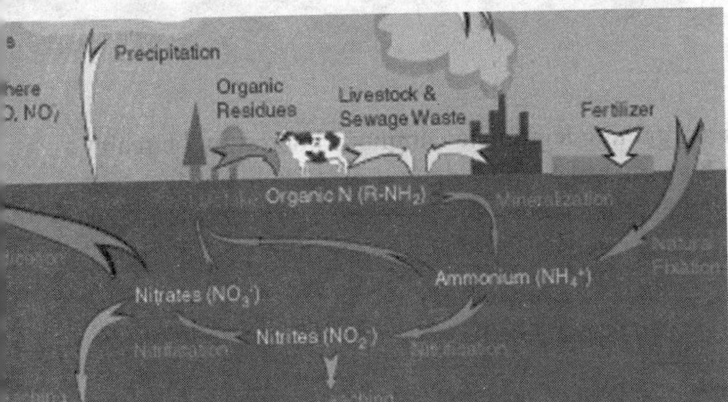

CHAPTER 2 Microbial Transformations

2.1 Introduction

Microorganisms do have the capability and accessibility for the conversion of one organic molecule into another precisely. Based upon the experimental evidences a good number of **complex bioconversions** which are usually accomplished by several specific microorganisms cannot be achieved by various normal chemical means. Interestingly, the **microbial transformations** of the molecules that are eventually found to be of immense industrial application invariably involve *oxidation, reduction, hydrolysis, condensation, isomerization* and the like.

Besides, it was adequately realized that microorganism articulately represent an exceptionally useful tool to have an in-depth knowledge with respect to the mechanism of **'heredity'** and **'genetic transfer'**; and, therefore, utilized progressively in elaborated **genetic investigations.**

It has been duly observed that all fermentations do not necessarily cause to participate **total microbial transformation** of carbon substrates *e.g.,* corn steep liquor solids, glucose etc. to rather smaller biosynthetic building blocks, for instance: acetate, and subsequent resynthesis to produce the *desired fermentative end product.* In this manner, therefore, certain microbial transformations essentially engage one, two, or a few step enzymatic transformations of the corresponding substrate to give rise to a fermentative product which is intimately related to the ensuing substrate chemically. At this critical juncture, it is quite evident that in case the microbial growth is closely linked with the transformation, a specific segment of this substrate or that of an alternate one, when present, should also get degraded partially so as to maintain a regular supply of **'carbon'** not only for the energy, but also for the growth of the cell.

Example: A typical example of a microbial transformation is explicitly represented by the *'second half'* of the dual fermentation of **α, ε-diaminopimelic acid: L-lysine,** because the *α, ε-diaminopimelic acid decarboxylase* enzyme obtained from *Acetobacter aerogenes* is predominantly used up in carrying out a single-step enzymatic decarboxylation of the α, β-diaminopimelic acid into L-lysine.

Nevertheless, **microbial transformations** are gaining legitimate enormous interest in the realm of the state-of -the-art fermentation industry by virtue of the glaring and overwhelming fact that **enzymatic reactions** may be gainfully employed to bring about some *chemical transformations* that are essentially:

- Quite expensive,
- Difficult to accomplish, and
- Next to impossible solely by chemical means.

Importantly, the **microbial transformations** of a host of specific *organic compounds* are duly accomplished by making use of such starting materials as: **growing cultures, resting cells, spores, enzymes, immobilized cells,** and **enzymes derived from microorganisms.** The commercial scale of the aforesaid **microbial transformations** is mostly performed under perfect sterile environments using **aerated and stirred bioreactors.** However, sterilization is absolutely necessary so as to avoid any possible contamination(s) that may give rise to either generation of *undesired products* or undue suppression of *desired reactions.* Obviously, the ultimate end products invariably get secreted very much *'outside the cell'*; and, hence, they either remain dissolved or found suspended in the final fermentation broth. The final product may be obtained from the above fermented broth by adopting the following steps in a sequential manner, namely:

- If filamentous fungus (*e.g., Penicillium notatum*) is the microorganism that has been used, it may be separated by simple filtration.
- Further recovery of the product from the filtered fermented broth may be obtained by any one of the following well-defined, time-tested procedures, such as:
  - adsorption to ion-exchangers
  - precipitation as their corresponding Ca^{2+} – salts
  - simple repeatative extractions with choicest solvents
  - Direct distillation from the medium (exclusively for **volatile products**).

2.2 Types of Reactions Mediated by Microorganisms

A plethora of microbial transformation reactions that are solely mediated by microorganisms are as stated under:

i. Vinegar (acetic acid) production,
ii. Gluconic acid production,
iii. Antibiotics production,
iv. Single-cell protein (SCP) from methanol,
v. Lactic acid production,
vi. Kojic acid, and
vii. Itaconic acid.

Of the five products stated above, (*iii*) has been discussed under Chapter-1; (*v*) shall be discussed separately under 4.4 in this chapter; and the remaining (*i*), (*ii*) and (*iv*) will be treated individually in the sections that follows:

2.2.1 Vinegar (Acetic Acid) Production

Vinegar fermentation enjoys the reputation of being one of the oldest known fermentative procedures to the mankind; and historically, it was obtained as an *unwanted spoilage of wine* as a natural event. In true sense, *vinegar* (acetic acid) is nothing but a **fermentation-derived food product** essentially comprising of not less than 4 g of acetic acid per 100 ml (*i.e.,* 4% *w/v*); and besides, it inherently possesses an **unique special flavour characteristic features,** which evidently protects and provides a clear-cut edge over the *artificial direct products* obtained *via* **pure synthetic routes** in flavour, mellow taste, and above all the competition.

The production of vinegar on commercial scale may be accomplished by several time-tested procedures as stated below, namely:

1. Traditional method,
2. Aerobic fermentation process,
3. Orleans process,
4. Packed-generator process,
5. Trickling generator, and
6. Submerged fermentor.

The aforementioned methods shall now be described individually in the section that follows:

2.2.1.1 Traditional Method

In this particular instance the production of vinegar essentially requires *two* different modes of fermentations, namely:

a. *Utilizing a specific yeast — i.e.,* to produce ethanol from cane-sugar (**sucrose** — obtained from *fruits, malt* etc.), and
b. *Utilizing Acetobacter species — i.e.,* to carry out the oxidation of ethanol *via* acetaldehyde to ultimately acetic acid.

In usual practice, the *substrate* for the **first-stage of fermentation** may be provided by almost a host of naturally occurring starting materials, such as: *ripe and sweet fruits e.g.,* apples, pears, plums, grapes, berries etc.; *honey; wine, malt* and the like. It is, however, pertinent to mention here that mostly the modern trends in the production of vinegar extensively make use of **apple-cider** and **wine,** in the presence of *two* predominantly employed fermentation organisms, namely:

1. *Saccharomyces cerevisiae;* and
2. *Saccharomyces cerevisiae* var. *ellipsoideus.*

The introduction of pressurized sulphur dioxide (SO_2) gas into the fermentative broth is an absolute necessity in order to control as well as monitor the bacterial growth effectively.

Caution: It is quite important to remove the inducted SO_2-the gas from the fermentative broth either by aeration or by other suitable means just prior to the oxidation of generated alcohol further to the desired vinegar (*i.e.,* acetic acid).

Once the alcohol-fermentation is fully accomplished, the resulting mass of yeast cells along with various other sedimented solid residues are permitted to settle down as completely as possible, and the *supernatant fermented alcoholic broth* is withdrawn carefully. Finally, the vinegar production is initiated from the above **'alcoholic broth'** by following the various steps detailed below sequentially:

1. Alcohol content adjusted between 10–13%,
2. Vinegar in small quantity added to enhance the acidity of the broth, and
3. Alternatively, *Acetobacter* cells may also be incorporated in such processes that would require *inoculation.*

2.2.1.2 Aerobic Fermentation Process

In general, the microbial oxidation of ethanol to acetic acid is nothing but an **aerobic fermentation process** which essentially demands an excessive oxygen (O_2) requirement.

Salient Features: The various salient features of an **aerobic** fermentation process are as given below:

1. *Acetobacter* cells are usually of a highly aerobic nature; and, therefore, any circumstantial development of an **'oxygen deficiency'** in the fermentation medium would directly affect their normal activities.
2. Oxidative conversion of *'ethanol'* to *'acetic acid' per se* needs an enormous quantum of oxygen which is evidenced by the following example: L of **Ethanol** when converted to **Acetic Acid** requires 552 g of **oxygen.**

3. *Evolution of Heat Energy*—Oxidation of ethanol to acetic acid evolves a considerable amount f heat energy that should ordinarily be dissipated from the fermentative broth in due course, example: 4.5 L (≡ 1 Gallon) of Ethanol when converted to **Acetic Acid** liberates proximately30, 250 BTUs (*i.e.,* **British Thermal Units**).
4. Interestingly, the latest developments in process design have adequately provided enough manipulative measure and controls with regard to the supply of *sufficient oxygen* to the fermentation broth and also sufficient arrangement for dissipation of heat either through circulation of chilled air or chilled water coils in the bioreactor.

In the age-old vinegar fermentation processes, besides those wherein a fortuitous souring of wine took place, were duly obtained by the introduction of an *'alcoholic liquid'*, either in the form of **fermented fruit juice** or **wine,** in shallow open vessel. The exposed air adequately caused due inoculation of the alcoholic solution by *Acetobacter* organism, whereas the ensuing large surface area catered for the much needed aeration. It has been duly observed that during an *extended incubation period,* the apparent growth of a **'bacterial scum'** essentially comprising of the **alcohol-oxidizing bacteria** got eventually developed on the surface of the liquid. In addition to the above, certain **nematodes** very specific to vinegar usually termed as **vinegar eels,** also found to have multiplied in these vessels both progressively and aggressively.

2.2.1.3 Orleans Process

Orleans, in France, first and foremost worked out gradually the **'production of vinegar'** from the original *vat fermentation* to the rather *more sophisticated* **'Orleans Process'** particularly for wine vinegars. Importantly, the said methodology is still being adopted in certain units in France to produce **fine and top quality table vinegars.**

In fact, the **Orleans process** essentially makes use of large fermentation vessels or barrels or casks placed either in *vertical* or in *horizontal* positions. A number of holes made in the walls of these fermentative vessels, strategically located above the **'level of liquid'**, allow the cross-sectional movement of air in them adequately. Consequently, the *Acetobacter* organism (bacteria) generate a substantial quantum of **'slime'** which eventually grow into a *layer* or *filu* or *vinegar mother,* right upon the surface of the alcoholic broth, carefully supported at the surface of the floating raft made up of wooden grating. It has been duly established that the culture cells in the slime layer are further placed together in position by the corresponding **cellulosic strands** caused by one of the *Acetobacter* species known as *Acetobacter xylinum.* However, in actual practice, a natural inoculum of *Acetobacter* cells is allowed to pile up either in the *casks,* or a portion of the *'vinegar mother'*, which is essentially transferred from the previous casks to boost and promote the process of **'acetification'.**

It is pertinent to state here that the phenomenon of oxidation responsible for the conversion of *ethanol* to *acetic acid via* this route is rather slow and sluggish. It usually demands an incubation span varying between 1 to 3 months at a stretch, and during this fermentative duration a plethora of other non- *Acetobacter* organisms are also rendered active, thereby giving rise to organic acids *viz., lactic acid, propionic acid* that eventually as their respective **'esters'** do impart/induce an exceptionally unique and pleasant fruity flavour and aroma to the ultimate **vinegar** thus produced.

Note: Nevertheless, long incubation period normally gives rise to a relatively higher loss of ethanol *via* evaporation and over oxidation.

2.2.1.4 Packed-Generator Process

Packed-generator process was developed initially by Schuzenbach, a German scientist, whereby the microbial oxidation of ethanol to acetic acid could be accomplished efficiently and adequately by a rather more rapid methodology. However, it is also known as the *'quick method'* and the *'trickle method'*.

In the **packed-generator process** the fermentation vessel *i.e.,* the **'vinegar generator'** usually consists of a large vertical tank that could be either open or closed at the top, and loosely packed with beech wood shavings, small twigs, evenly cut corn cobs, bamboo-stick bundles, or similar other packing substances. Consequently, a **bacterial film** made up of mixed *Acetobacter* species, other than those for the **Orleans Process** (section 4.2.1.3), eventually grows upon the exposed surface of the supporting agent. At this stage, the *alcoholic broth* (obtained separately by many known methods) is introduced in small lots at intervals from the top of the packed generator, which trickles down gradually *via* the packing medium (support) in order to make available sufficient contact of the alcohol with the bacterial cells; and this ultimately leads to the oxidation of **alcohol** into **acetic acid.** In usual practice, the **packed generators (vinegar generators)** are strategically provided with air-inlet devices positioned very much near the bottom to permit air to move-up through the generator, because the **'rise-of-air'** gets accelerated progressively by virtue of the **'heat'** being generated during the process of fermentation. Precisely, it is absolutely important and necessary to control and monitor the evolution of heat so as to allow the fermentative process to continue without any adverse/harmful effect; and it may be accomplished by any one of the following procedures, namely:

- **Rate of addition** of added *'alcoholic broths',*
- **Temperature** of the added *'alcoholic broths',*
- **Cooling-coils** provided in sophisticated generators, and
- **chilling** of incoming or recycled *'alcoholic broths'*

Salient Features

The salient features of **packed-generator process** are enumerated below:

1. **Alcoholic broth** is either adequately recycled through the same fermentor until the entire ethanol content gets *'oxidized'* completely, or it is passed through the several generators kept in series (*i.e.,* connected to one another) in order to oxidize the alcohol successively at each of the connected generators.
2. These generators (connected in series) invariably yield an appreciable concentration of **acetic acid** even up to 15% (v/v); and, therefore, are being employed extensively and specifically for the genuine production of **'white table vinegar'** across the globe.
3. Modern day **recalculating packed-generators** are duly stuffed with specially sized beech wood shavings (air-dried), 2 × 1.25 inches, and not-so-tightly rolled, and that may take up approximately 2000 cubic feet of the said material.
4. Satisfactory accumulation of **'bacterial film'** upon the supporting agent in the **'packed generator'** would render it operational effectively from several to many months at a stretch or until an unavoidable serious contamination caused due to the **slime-forming bacterium, Acetobacter xylinum** becomes prevalent.

a. Fermentor Designs:

The broad spectrum of **fermentor designs** involving the sustained performance of the *submerged fermentation approach* for **'vinegar fermentation'** has duly acclaimed a reasonably widely recognized development in process technology. In fact, the present day submerged fementations being utilized, extensively in the large-scale production of **'table vinegars'** and are entirely based upon the well-elaborated intensive aeration studies performed on *antibiotic fermentations* both during and after World War II.

Importantly, these submerged fermentations make use of *two* entirely different **'fermentor designs'** invariably termed as : (*a*) **acetator;** and (*b*) **cavitator.**

Acetator: Fig. 2.1 illustrates the schematic diagram of the Fring's submerged culture acetator.

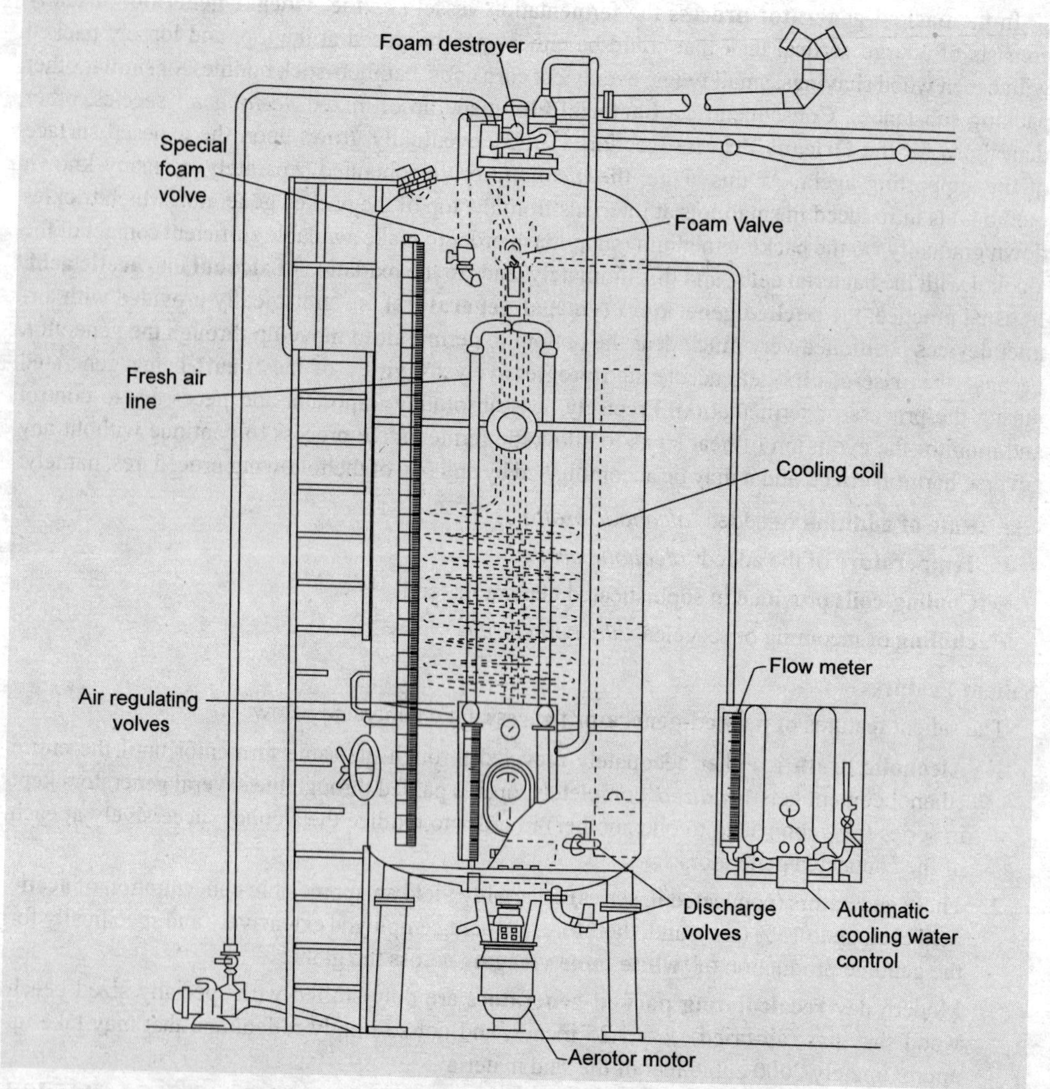

Fig. 2.1 *Schematic Diagram of Fring's Submerged Culture Acetator.*

Acetator normally operates as a *semi-batch-mode;* and, however, with certain modifications may now be utilized as a *continuous-flow-mode.* An effective **'aeration'** in the **Acetator** may be adequately accomplished with the aid of a fast-rotating ceramic disc strategically placed over an air nozzle to produce extremely fine dispersed air-bubbles, having consequent solution of O_2 in liquid-phase (*i.e.,* culture medium).

At the initial stage, the **Acetator** is fed with a mixture of fresh stock of *alcoholic solution* together with *actively oxidizing vinegar* obtained from a simultaneously operating fermentor. It is a common practice to determine the alcoholic and acid contents of the mixed alcohol stock with vinegar; and, if required, necessary adjustments are duly made to achieve adequate starting concentrations. Ideally, the acid content should vary between 1–1.5%, and an alcohol content between 4.5–10.8%. It is pertinent to mention here that start up alcohol concentration seems to be too high for sustaining the continuous operation; and, therefore, the fermentation broth is neither withdrawn for harvest, nor is fresh alcohol stock added, till such time when the fermentation has adequately gone through to accomplish an alcohol content nearly 0.5%. Fresh alcohol stock solution is further added automatically and the completed fermentation broth is withdrawn from the **Acetator** accordingly.

It is absolutely important to maintain the actual alcohol content of the **'harvested broths'** to stand nearly at 0.3% because of the following *two* reasons, namely:

1. Strength of alcohol content less than 0.3% shall cause harm to the organism, and
2. Alcohol content < 0.3% also gives rise to excessive foaming (which may be controlled by the addition of **silicones**).

Cavitator: Just like the **Acetator,** the **Cavitator** is also an *'automated device'* that essentially caters for both charging with alcoholic solution and discharging of completed fermentation broth. Because this fermentator *i.e.,* **Cavitator** is rated as highly efficient and capable of producing acetic acid at a much faster speed and pace, it is appreciably smaller in size and dimension in comparison to the corresponding *packed vinegar generators* (see section 2.1.4).

Advantages: The various distinct advantages of the **Cavitator** are as enumerated under:

1. It neither forms *'slime'* nor the *'vinegar eel'*.
2. Since, the rate of O_2-removal from the culture medium by the *Acetobactor* cells is so large and predominant that neither the **'oxidative browning'** of the *'apple cider'* nor of *'wine mash'* ever occurs.
3. A small quantum of **'residual alcohol'** is invariably left behind in the vinegar as it is recovered from the fermentor; and, therefore, in this particular process the vinegar is usually stored to permit broth **'aging'** and subsequent *'microbial depletion'* of this residual alcohol.
4. **Superior Vinegar.** In actual practice, the vinegar removed from the **Cavitator** prominently contains a host of *'suspended microorganisms'*, quite unlike the *'packed vinegar generators'* (wherein the microorganisms are intimately attached to the beech wood shavings), and during storage of the vinegar these microorganisms specifically oxidize the residual alcohol and simultaneously attribute splendid additional *'pleasing alterations'* both in the overall aroma and taste to yield a **'superior vinegar'.**

Methodology: The various steps involved are as follows:

1. It is a complete continuous fermentation process.
2. It essentially comprises of *five* vital stages, namely:

Stage-1: The cavitation force developed by the rotor at the time air bubbles are formed.

Stage-2: The air-diffusion takes place during the passage of the bubbles to the surface.

Stage-3: An advanced stage whereby the air-diffusion at the point at which the bubbles usually burst at the surface.

Stage-4: At this stage, the surface-aeration caused by the atmospheric pressure on account of the constant change of surface exposed to atmosphere both by the agitation and circulation of the liquid very much within the tank.

Stage-5: This is the final stage whereby the air induced into the liquid by a **vortex action** as the liquid flows over the cone and through the draft tube. All the aforesaid five distinct and critical stages have been duly shown in the following Fig. 2.2.

3. Diammonium hydrogen phosphate $[(NH_4)_2\ HPO_4]$, as an additional nutrient supplement is judiciously incorporated both at start-up and in the course of continuous operation. Eventually, the progress acquired in, fermentation is estimated periodically by finding the *'acid'* and *'alcohol'* contents of the broths. However, it is quite important to induct fresh-air into the fermentors, during this period, along with the recirculated air of the fermentor so as to afford just sufficient O_2 to fulfill the combined demands of the prevailing **microbial respiration** as well as **alcohol oxidation.** Besides, adequate care needs to be taken with respect to the feed-rate of the **fresh alcohol stock** to maintain the *required and stipulated low-alcohol content* in the finished vinegar *i.e.,* the fermented broth.

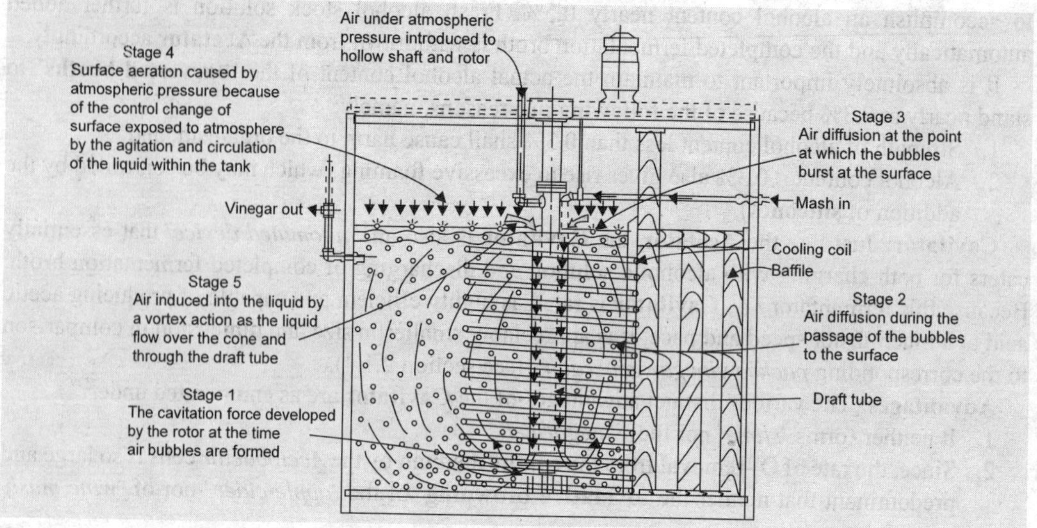

Fig. 2.2 *Schematic Diagram of the Cavitator.*

2.2.1.5 Trickling Generator

The **trickling generator** still holds a coveted position and extensively employed in vinegar production, as depicted in Fig. 2.3.

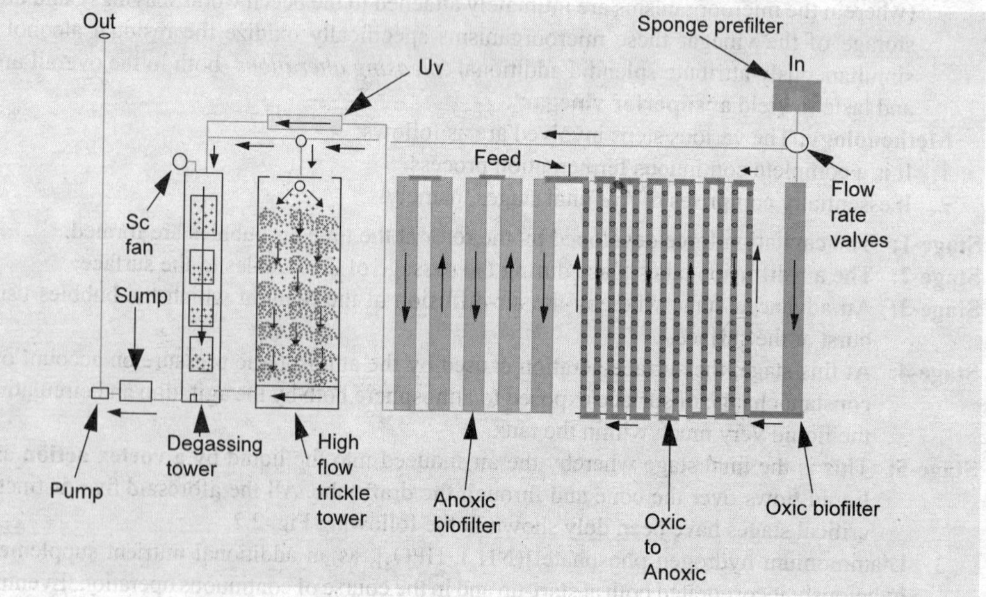

Fig. 2.3 *Diagram of a Trickling Generator for Acetic Acid.*

In actual practice, the starting material is adequately sprayed over the surface and trickles gradually through the shavings containing organisms into a basin located in the bottom, where the partially converted solution (*i.e.,* alcohol converted to acetic acid), as shown below, is duly chilled and pumped again to the top of the generator.

It has been duly observed that the **'trickling generator'** process is capable of converting between 88–90% of total ethanol added into acetic acid; whereas, the rest of ethanol (10–12%) gets either used up for the primary metabolism or released along with the waste air. Interestingly, the prevailing temperature in the upper portion of the **trickling generator** stands at about 29°C; whereas, in the lower segment it remains at 35°C (hence, it is partially cooled and recirculated from the top).

In nutshell, it takes almost 72 hours to yield 12% acetic acid by this methodology.

2.2.1.6 Submerged Fermentor

The **submerged fermentor** first and foremost makes use of either *fruit wines* or *special mashes* having reasonably rather low concentrations of ethanol. Indeed with such a low-yielding methodology/ technique the aeration was not absolutely critical and important. However, as on date the emergence and recognition of high-yielding methodologies that essentially yield 13% acetic acid in amounts ranging up to 50 m^3, predominantly demands highly controlled and regulated means of **aeration.**

Interestingly, the fermentors very much look alike other bioreactors (see chapter 1). The fermentation tanks are usually made up of stainless steel that has an arrangement of stirring at the bottom. The aeration assembly comprises of a suction rotor having the incoming air flowing down *via* a SS pipe located at the top of the fermentor. In order to dissipate the elevated temperature during fermentation process **efficient heat-exchangers** are engaged (through which cold water is passed constantly) to control the temperature around 25 ± 2°C; besides, **mechanical foam eliminators** should be pressed into service to arrest the nuisance caused due to foaming.

Methodology: The various steps involved in the production of acetic acid (**household vinegar**) by the **submerged fermentor process** are as stated under:

1. Household vinegar (13% acetic acid) is usually produced in a semicontinuous, absolutely automatic process, in an environment (atmosphere) of adequate aeration and constant mechanical stirring together with a start-up material which essentially composed of approximately 7–10% acetic acid plus 5% ethanol.
2. The concentration of **ethanol** is determined continuously by suitable method during the fermentative process; and when the concentration dips down to a level varying between 0.05 and 0.3% achievable within a span of 36 hours. At this particular juncture, about 50–60% of the fermented solution is removed and duly replaced with a new lot of **'mash'** containing 0 to 2% acetic acid and 10–15% ethanol so as to recharge the fermentor accordingly.

It has been duly established by researchers that one may obtain upto 98% yields at 40°C *via* fully continuous processes, as shown in Fig. 2.4.

Advantages over Trickling Generator

The advantages score of the **submerged process** upon the **trickling generator** are as described below:

1. The **production rate** with the **submerged process** per m^3 is almost 5 folds greater than the corresponding **trickling generator process** and 10 folds higher than the **surface fermentation process.**
2. Submerged process require much lesser capital investment per production amount, merely 1/5th of the total plant area is required for its due installation, vulnerability of faster conversion to different mash variants in a much shorter duration, and above all reasonably lower manpower cost involved on account of highly automatic controls and measures.

Recovery: The end-product acetic acid (household vinegar) obtained by the sub-merged process is invariably **turbid** in appearance by virtue of the presence of microorganisms (mostly in suspended form); and, therefore, the product must be clarified by adequate filtration. One may make use of plate-type filters along with appropriate filter-aids are mostly recommended and used gainfully. The coloured filtrate (acetic acid) may be decolourized by the help of **potassium ferrocyanide** [$K_4Fe(CN)_6$], if necessary.

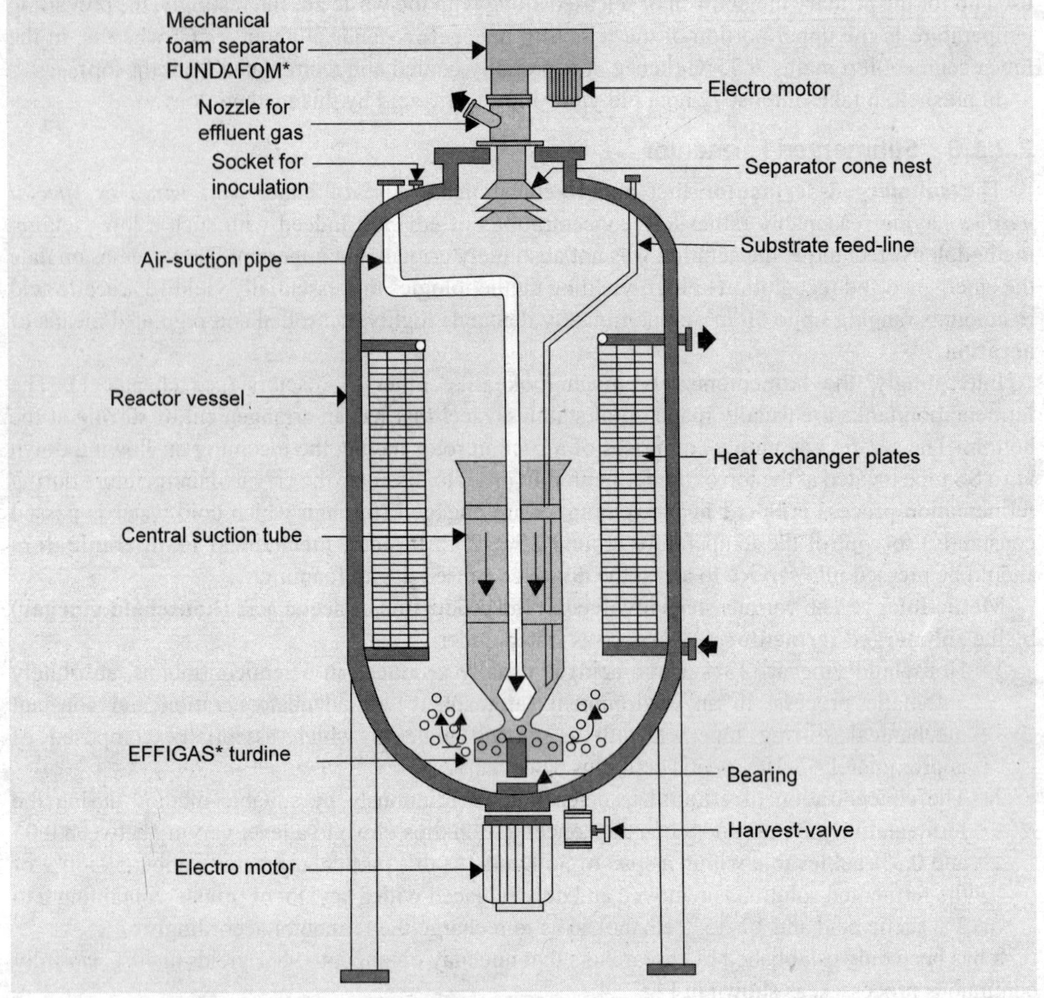

Fig. 2.4 *Diagrammatic Sketch of Submerged Fermentor for Acetic-Acid Production.*

2.2.2 Gluconic Acid Production

Gluconic acid possesses enormous commercial applications in a variety of product and product utilities in pharmaceuticals as well, namely:

- Manufacture of metal, leather and food.
- **Calcium gluconate** to provide and supplement Ca^{2+} to pregnant mothers.
- **Na^{+} and Ca^{2+} salts** in alkaline serve as effective metal sequestering agents for Fe^{3+}, Al^{3+}, Cu^{2+}.
- **Ferrous gluconate** caters for Fe for the treatment of anemia in humans.
- **Sodium gluconate** finds its use as a sequestering agent in detergents.
- **δ-gluconolactone** functions as a baking powder additive.

In the domain of **'industrial microbiology'** *gluconic acid* enjoys a creditable long historical evidence. Alsberg (1911) first and foremost reported the production of *gluconic acid* commencing with the *Pseudomonas.* In 1928, the first ever commercial surface process by making use of a **'fungus'**, *Penicillium leuteum-purpurogenum,* saw the light of the day gracefully which remarkably gave a yield ranging between 80–87% of its theoretical values.

Interestingly, as to date the **submerged processes** have gained a world-wide acceptance and recognition by employing either the **fungus**—*Aspergillus niger* or the *bacterium—Acetobactor suboxydans,* which ultimately gave rise to a range of value-added products, such as: gluconic acid; glucose oxidase; and sodium — and calcium-gluconates.

Note: There are several organisms that have been duly optimized *via* research to yield *'gluconic acid'*, but unfortunately have not been exploited commercially, prominently include the following: **fungi:** *Endomycopsis, Gonatobotrys, Penicillinum, Pullularia, Scopulariopsis;* **bacteria:** *Vibrio, Pseudomonas.*

Fermentation Production. The production of **gluconic acid** from *glucose* is predominantly carried out by a *flavoprotein* which is termed as **glucose-oxidase*,** or more precisely **glucoseaerodehydrogenase** that essentially serves as an enzyme mediating this oxidation. The overall reaction takes place in two steps as illustrated below:

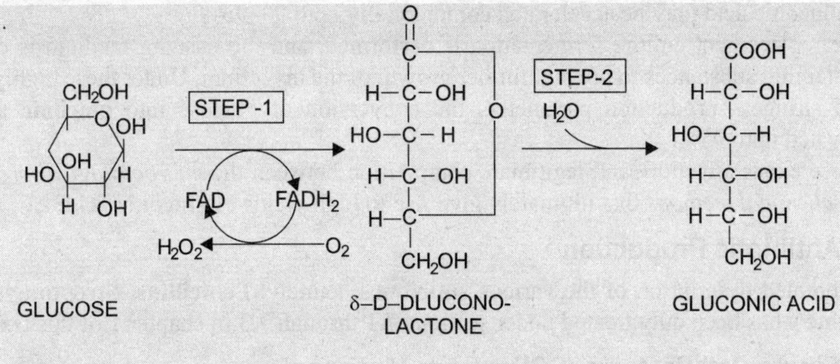

STEP -1   FAD → $FADH_2$ O_2 → H_2O_2 STEP-2 H_2O

GLUCOSE   δ–D–DLUCONO-LACTONE   GLUCONIC ACID

FAD = Flavin Adenine Dinucleo

$FADH_2$= Flavin Adenine Dinucleotide Dihydrate

Step-1: The dehydrogenation of a mole of D-glucose in the presence of FAD gives rise to the formation of δ-D-gluconolactone. Besides, the transference of 2 H-atoms from $FADH_2$ to oxygen (O_2) yields a mole of hydrogen peroxide (H_2O_2) that gets instantly split up into a mole of water (H_2O) by the help of the enzyme catalase.

Step-2: The resulting product obtained from **Step-1** *i.e.,* δ-D-gluconolactone takes up the water from the previous step and legitimately yields a mole of **gluconic acid.**

Methodology: The various sequential steps involved in the production of **gluconic acid** are as stated under:

1. The *Aspergillus niger* (fungus) — gluconic acid fermentation may be preferably accomplished by submerged culture process usually at pH ranging between 4.5 to 6.5, predominantly needs a growth culture medium wherein both P and N are limiting.
2. The *A. niger* mycelium, once formed in an initial gluconic acid-growth fermentation adequately, is judiciously reutilized in the ensuing successive **'replacement culture'** fermentations, of course, as long as the prevailing **glucose-oxidase activity** of the mycelium remains highly virile and active.
3. Soon after the initial fermentation process yields the mycelium, the consequent successive fermentations are nothing but **exclusively enzymatic transformations** specifically brought about by the ensuing *glucose-oxidase* of the mycelium. In usual practice, the entire fermentative run lasts for 20 hours at 28–30°C having a high aeration rate ranging between 1-15 vvm.
4. Recycling of the mycelium evidently gives rise to lowering of the requirement for inoculum built-up. However, as and when the system is in dire need of inoculum, it is introduced as *spores* or *pregerminated spores* directly to the **production fermentor.**

5. Growth culture medium for **gluconic acid production** essentially comprises of glucose (25%) together with various salts, $CaCO_3$, a boron compound, and sometimes even corn steep liquor is added. The overall fermentation is invariably carried out at 28 ± 2°C supported by adequate agitation, aeration, and control of heat generation either using water-jacketed fermentors or employing cooling-coils.
6. Once the fermentation is completed, the **gluconic acid** is recovered by neutralization of the *fermented broth* with calculated amount of $Ca(OH)_2$ in order to permit the crystallization of calcium gluconate. Finally, **gluconic acid** is recovered from the calcium gluconate (salt) by the addition of a measured and calculated quantity of concentrated H_2SO_4.

Important Highlights: Following are some of the important highlights of **gluconic acid production:**

1. Simply by enhancing the pressure in the system, the solubility of O_2, and hence the production of gluconic acid may be accelerated commercially upto 90–95%.
2. The replacement culture fermentation is performed, and the ensuing medium is devoid of containing substances to prevent further growth of the mycelium. Under these highly specific and stringent production parameters the conversion of glucose into **gluconic acid** gets elevated upto 95%.
3. These exists a healthy and legitimate competition between the *microbiological process* and the *chemical methods* that ultimately give rise to high yields of **gluconic acid.**

2.2.3 Antibiotic Production

An elaborated description of the various antibiotics, namely: **Penicillins, Streptomycins,** and **Tetracycline's** has been duly treated under sections 7.1 through 7.3 in chapter 1 of this text book.

2.2.4 Single-Cell Proteins (SCPs) from Methanol

The terminology **single-cell protein (SCP)** was first and foremost coined by some researchers at the famous MIT-Massachusetts Institute of Technology (USA) in the year 1966. As to date, SCP, covers a rather broad spectrum coverage not only confined to isolated cell protein but also to the ensuing microbial biomass derived from either uni-and multicellular organism, yeasts, filamentous fungi or algae that may be employed extensively both as *'food'* or *'feed additives'*. It has been duly established that the usual protein content (average) in the **microbial biomass** varies between 45-55%, but in certain specific organism it may be as high as 80%. Because of the presence several essential nutrients *'biomass'* has gainfully been exploited as an *'ideal'* supplement to conventional food products across the globe.

Interestingly, in overall comparison with the traditional means and ways of generating proteins both for food or feed, commercial production of microbial biomass affords the following cardinal advantages, such as:

a. Generally the microorganisms exhibit an exceptionally high rate of multiplication,
b. Microbes possess high-protein content,
c. Capable of using a plethora of different C-sources, a few of them could even be waste products,
d. Strains with predominantly high yield and markedly excellent composition may be either selected or produced quite easily and conveniently, and
e. Production of *microbial biomass* is absolutely independent of either seasonal or climatic variation.

The Central Food Technology Research Institute (CFTRI) at Mysore (India) carried out an intensive and extensive research on the utilization of **blue-green-algae** obtained from the marine sources, **Spurulina,** as a prominent supplement to diet in elderly and convalescent subjects. The marine-algae is duly cultured, and carefully dried, powdered and used either as **tablet** (1g) or **capsule** (1g). It essentially comprises of protein (upto 60%), essential vitamins and certain unsaturated fatty acids. **Spurulina** is being used largely as a supplement to the diet of humans both in India and abroad as well.

Disadvantages of Microbial Biomass. The *three* most vital disadvantages of microbial biomass are as stated below:

1. A good number of microorganisms give rise to *serious toxic products;* and, therefore, one has to ascertain that the **biomass** is absolutely devoid of such substances.
2. Microorganisms invariably present in the **biomass** may give rise to unavoidable indigestion and allergic reaction(s) after consumption.
3. The excessive high level of nucleic acids (DNA and RNA) present in the **microbial biomass products** is extremely undesirable.

The SCP Phenomenon. In actual practice, the production of SCP exclusively involves the following *four* major steps that are precisely independent either upon the specific kind of substrate or type of microorganism being employed, namely:

1. Preparation of an appropriate medium by making use of various suitable carbon sources *e.g.,* carbohydrates, starch, corsteep liquor, glucose etc.,
2. Very stringent and effective control, management and prevention of contamination of *medium* and also the entire *plant system,*
3. Meticulous production of the desired microorganism essentially required for the fermentative procedure, and
4. Recovery of the generated *microbial biomass* and its subsequent processing stages involved.

Salient Features: The various salient features with regard to the production of SCPs are described as given below :

1. Medium for SCP Production. Importantly, the medium for SCP production varies as per the type of microorganisms being used.

Examples

a. **Green Algae** (*Chlorella, Scenedesmus, Spirulina*) — may be cultivated autographically without making use of a dissolved carbon source.

b. **Heterotrophic organisms** (*humans*) — may be grown heterophically using C-sources derived from two distinct categories, namely:

   i. **Fossil:** *viz.,* n-alkanes, methanol, ethanol, gaseous hydrocarbons and the like; and

   ii. **Renewable:** *via.,* molasses, CO_2, whey, solid substrates polysaccharide hydrolysates, and effluents of various industries like — distilleries, breweries, potato and canning industries, confectionary industries, and wood-pulp industries.

***n*-Alkanes:** Serve as the most preferred C-source for a wide spectrum of industrial requirements.

Source of N: Ammonia gas (NH_3) for *Saccharomycopsis lipolytica salts: e.g.,* Fe^{2+}, Mn^{2+}, Mg^{2+}, PO_4^{3-} etc.

Fungus and Higher Fungi: Mushrooms *i.e.,* fruiting bodies of higher fungi, has proved to be an excellent delicacy for foods meant for human consumption in a host of countries across the globe which has almost touched the mark of 106 MT each year.

Example: *Chaetomium cellulyticum* (a **fungus**) has been gainfully and successfully cultured on a variety of solid substrates *e.g.,* sawdust, straw, wood chips, composted straw, agricultural wastes, and forestry wastes.

Precautionary Measures: It is, however, pertinent to state here that specifically in the **biomass production** the following precautionary measures must be taken religiously, such as:

- Culture medium and the entire plant (fermentor etc.) should be free from any possible contamination.
- Gaseous components of the culture medium *viz.,* CO_2, NH_3 etc, and the circulating compressed air must be sterilized by allowing it to pass through filters.

- Various other components in several instances are duly sterilized by live-steam.

2. Microorganism: The microorganism being used is suitably cultured in the respective culture medium in perfect clean and hygenic environmental conditions. However, the **microorganisms** which is meant to be cultured in the medium should essentially possess the under mentioned basic characteristic features, for instance:

a. Must be **non-pathogenic** in nature to humans, animals, and plants,
b. Essentially possess excellent nutritional value,
c. Must be devoid of any *'toxic'* component whatsoever,
d. Should be largely exploitable as food or feed, and
e. Overall **'production cost'** must be reasonably low to render it commercially viable.

3. Choice of Fermentor: In actual practice, **the choice of fermentor** *i.e.,* the *cultivation vessel* or *bioreactor* solely depends upon the exact microorganisms to be employed for the operation. Generally, aeration is regarded to be a vital and important functional operation the entire cultivation phenomenon. Heat is invariably produced during cultivation due to the evolution of CO_2; and, therefore, it has got to be dissipated by using a cooling device effectively (cooling coils or heat exchangers).

Figure 2.5 illustrates the outline of an industrial fermentor employed by Imperial Chemical Industry (ICI) to commercially produce SCP starting from *Pseudomonas methylotrophus* grown carefully upon **methanol.** By the help of the aforesaid fermentor it may be quite feasible to produce a definite quantum of **microbial biomass** ranging between 4 to 30 g. L^{-1} at 38–40°C and at pH 6.8. Importantly, the production is invariably allowed to continue for an indefinite duration to accomplish the maximum achievable targeted economy.

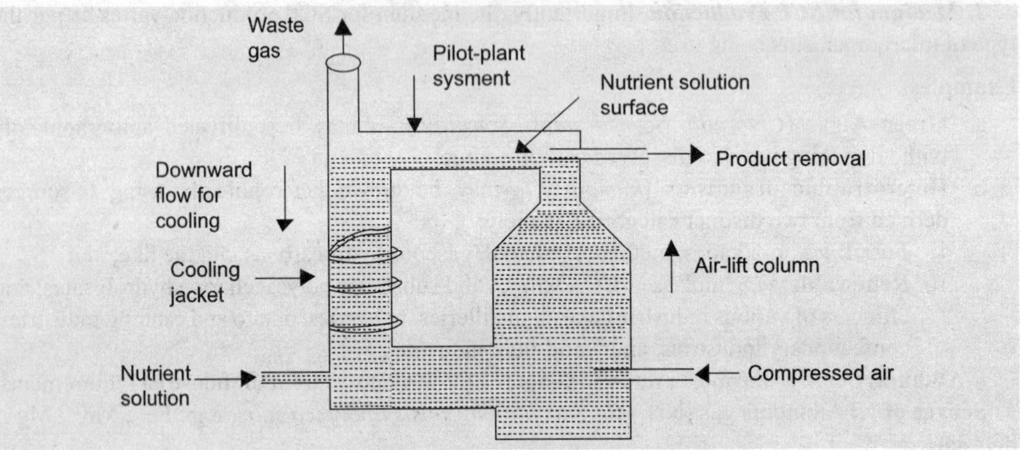

Fig. 2.5 *ICI-Fermentor to Produce SCP from Methanol.*

4. Harvesting of Microbial Biomass: The various steps that are usually followed for the harvesting of microbial biomass are as described below in a sequential manner:

i. **Bacteria** and **yeast** *i.e.,* single-cell organisms are invariably recovered by adopting one of these methods, namely: **flocculation, floatation** and **centrifugation.**
ii. **Filamentous bacteria** *e.g., Penicillium notatum* are mostly recovered by simple filtration;
iii. Maximum amount of **'water'** needs to be discarded before proceeding to the final stage of drying.
iv. Adequate precautionary measures are absolutely mandatory to perform the entire operation under utmost clean, hygenic and sterilized conditions to maintain the product and the broth which eventually gets transferred from the plant absolutely free of bacterial contamination.

v. The **final dried products** are found to be fairly stable bacteriologically only if they are treated and handled as per the stringent operational directives.

vi. **Microbial biomass,** in certain instances only, essentially requires an elaborated and well-defined after-treatment either in order to minimize drastically the unwanted components in the said product or to isolate the respective protein(s).

vii. Reduction of **nucleic acids** (DNA and RNA) are required to be accomplished on top priority because they may prove to be quite hazardous to health, *viz.,* **fungi** (2.5 to 6%); **microorganisms** (10 to 16%); **algae** (4 to 6%); and **yeasts** (6 to 10%). However, the various means and ways that are usually engaged in the removal of nucleic acids from the microbial biomass normally include: **activation of endogenous nucleases during the last-stage of microbial biomass production; chemical extraction procedures; and ultimately the alkaline hydrolysis.**

2.2.5 Lactic Acid Production

Preamble: Scheele (1780) first discovered the presence of **lactic acid** [$CH_3CH(OH)COOH$)] in the *sour milk.* Pasteur (1857) *i.e.,* almost a gap of 77 years after Scheele's epoch making discovery proved and established that the souring of milk was due to microbiological fermentation by a causative organism. As on date, there are indeed several evidences to show that a plethora of microorganisms are capable of producing at least small amounts of **lactic acid** which is present in several fermented foods and beverages.

Subsequently, the first ever microbial production of an **'organic acid'** was that of **lactic acid** carried out in the year 1880 *i.e.,* almost after 23 years from Pasteur's observation. Nowadays, both the **chemical procedures** and the **biological processes** are not only *extremely competitive* but also *appreciably cost-effective.*

Organisms for Lactic Acid Production: In fact, there are *two* different types of lactic acid organisms that have been duly recognized, namely: (*a*) Heterofermentative; and (*b*) Homofermentative, which would be explained as under:

A. Heterofermentative Organisms: These organisms usually yield certain quantum of **lactic acid,** but simultaneously and most probably by virtue of the ensuing **pentose-phosphate metabolic pathway** they may give rise to the production of several chemical substances, such as : ethanol, acetic acid (vinegar), CO_2, and traces of a few other products.

Example: *Leuconostoc mesenteroides* — it is of no utility for the commercial lactic acid fermentative procedures due to the fact that a substantial quantum of the **'substrate carbon'** is consumed in yielding products other than **lactic acid.**

B. Homofermentative Organisms: These strains of lactic acid producing bacteria invariably yield maximum quantum of **lactic acid** and only trace amount of other products. In fact, these organisms make use of the specific metabolic pathway to yield **pyruvic acid** which gets subsequently reduced by the corresponding enzyme, **lactic dehydrogenase,** to produce **lactic acid.** It has been observed that the overall percent conversion of hexose-sugar to **lactic acid** is almost equivalent to two moles of lactic acid for every mole of hexose-sugar (theoretical yield) consumed by the respective organism.

Examples:

1. *Lactobacillus delbrueckii* — it is used for the commercial production of lactic acid in fermentative procedures using *corn-dextrose media.*
2. *Lactobacillus bulgaricus* — it makes use of **'lactose'** as a source of carbon and finds usage in lactic acid production starting from **whey media.**
3. *Lactobacillus pentosus* — it specifically utilizes the **'pentoses'** obtained from the **'sulphitewaste liquor'** for **lactic acid** production on a large-scale.

Other Potential Homofermentative Species: There are some other species which belong to the class of **homofermentative organisms,** such as: *Lactobacillus casei; Lactobacillus leichmannii;*

and *streptococcus lactis* — all do possess potential industrial importance and recognition. These organisms are essentially anaerobes; however, they may withstand certain extent of O_2. Interestingly, *S. lactis* is found to be relatively much less sensitive to O_2; and, hence, may be regarded as a **facultative aerobes** rather than **obligate anaerobes;** and, therefore, the bioreactors should be used in an absolutely O_2-free atmosphere.

Theoretical Aspects: The biosynthetic pathway of **lactic acid** starting from glucose essentially takes the route via glyceraldehyde-3-P, 1, 3-di-P-glycerate, and pyruvate as given in Fig. 2.6. It may be further expatiated by the reducing power generated effectively during the oxidation of **glyceraldehydes phosphate** is eventually transferred with an NAD-dependent enzyme **lactate dehydrogenase** to the corresponding pyruvate, and this ultimately gets *reduced stereospecifically* to give rise to the *two* optical isomers **L(+) or D(–) lactic acid.**

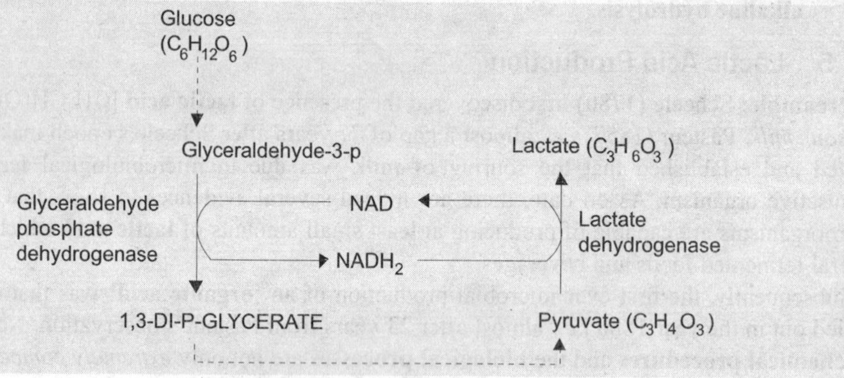

Fig. 2.6 *Lactic Acid Production from Glucose Using Lactobacillus delbrueckii.*

Fermentation Medium: In USA, the C-source used commercially for the production of **lactic acid** from a variety of available media, such as: molasses, whey, and partially refined corn-sugar (containing dextrose); whereas, several other countries extensively employ either previously hydrolyzed potato starch or other suitable C-substrates *i.e.,* semi refined sugars, maltose, lactose, sucrose, and dextrose.

Ideally, the **fermentation medium** must comprise of glucose (12–13%), diammonium acid phosphate [$(NH_4)_2HPO_4$] (0.25%), and small amount of B-vitamins. The fermentative operation is usually initiated in huge fermentors (capacity: 25–120 m^3) at a temperature ranging between 45 to 50°C plus an excess of $CaCO_3$ (solid) supplemented to maintain the pH varying between 5.5 to 6.5 strictly. The entire fermentation usually takes almost 3 days (72 hours) under the aforesaid experimental parameters. Because, **lactic acid** is found to be toxic to the organism, *two* specific procedures have been successfully tried and tested so as to remove the product (*i.e.,* lactic acid) both simultaneously and continuously from the **'fermented broth',** namely:

a. **Electrodialysis:** A method of separating electrolytes from colloids by passing a current through a solution containing both.

b. **Continuous Culture:** A continuous culture was duly carried out in a **membrane reactor** that ultimately led to the production of **lactic acid** to the extent of 80 g/l.h.

Extraction and Recovery: There are *four* distinct procedures that may be adopted for the **extraction and recovery** of *lactic acid* from the fermented broth as described under:

Method 1: At harvest, a calculated amount of $CaCO_3$ is added to the fermented medium, pH adjusted to 10, and the contents are heated and filtered subsequently. By doing so a host of desirable goals are accomplished, such as:

1. All of **lactic acid** gets converted to calcium lactate,
2. Most organisms are killed and eliminated,

3. Help in the complete coagulation of protein present in the medium,
4. Removes excess of $CaCO_3$, if any, and
5. Decomposes any residual sugar(s) present in the medium.

Lactic acid is now recrystallized as **calcium lactate** and decolourized by adding activated carbon. The latter step may be accomplished alternatively by preparing the zinc salt of lactic acid which happens to be comparatively less soluble.

Method 2: In this particular instance the **'free lactic acid'** is subjected to extraction with isopropyl ether (solvent) successively from the pre-heated and filtered fermentation broth. This phenomenon is based upon the principle of **counter-current continuous extraction.** In fact, the desired **'lactic acid'** is finally recovered from the medium of *isopropyl ether* by further affecting **counter-current extraction** with water, in which the former is soluble because both are polar in nature.

Method 3: The *'lactic acid'* thus obtained is converted into its corresponding **methyl ester** which is separated from the fermentation broth by distillation followed by hydrolysis of the corresponding ester by simply boiling in dilute aqueous medium.* Subsequently, the **lactic acid** is recovered from the aqueous medium by evaporation of the water, and the liberated methanol may be collected by distillation.

Method 4: In this specific procedure, the lactic acid is obtained as its corresponding **secondary and tertiary alkylamine salts** which are subsequently extracted from the aqueous medium with appropriate organic solvents completely. The solvent is removed usually by distillation and the residual 'salt' is then decomposed carefully to obtain **lactic acid.**

Note: In general, it is quite important and necessary that the 'recovery processing equipment' must be quite resistant to the corrosive action of the high concentration of lactic acid being accumulated. Hence, invariably one should make use of stainless-steel equipment for the recovery of lactic acid in its purest form and quality.

Grades of Lactic Acid: Depending upon the actual usage and application one may come across different **'grades of lactic acid'** available commercially in trade, namely:

1. 'Crude' or 'Technical' Grade: It is a coloured product solely meant for commercial application at various concentrations ranging between 20–80%. It may be prepared by using H_2SO_4 to eliminate Ca^{2+} from the calcium lactate salt obtained from the heated and filtered fermentation broth by adopting these steps sequentially *viz.,* filtration, concentration, refiltration to remove additional $CaSO_4$. Hence, the **crude** or technical grade lactic acid comprises of several impurities and may be used where **purity** of the product is not so critical and essential, such as: deliming of hides in leather industry.

2. "Edible" Grade: It is usually having a straw-coloured appearance and mostly available at strengths ranging between 50–80%. It is mostly used in food and beverage industries to maintain optimum pH for better storage and shelf-life of products.

3. 'Plastic' Grade: It is more or less colourless and available in strengths varying between 50–80%. Invariably prepared from technical grade lactic acid *via* adequate refining processes.

4. 'USP' Grade: It is a pharmaceutical grade lactic acid having strength of 85% and mostly used in pharmaceutical formulations.

2.2.6 Kojic Acid

Kojic acid (5-hydroxymethyl-4-pyrone) though does not possess a free carboxyl moiety but still named as an **'acid'** by virtue of the fact that it gets ionized to liberate H^+ ions as shown below:

It is usually produced by **fungi** belonging to the groups *Aspergillus flavus, A. oryzae* and *Aspergillus tamaril* preferably in surface culture. However, high yields of **kojic acid** by the direct fermentation of glucose as indicated below:

However, it may also be obtained from pyruvic acid, acetic acid, glycerol, and ethanol. It find its application as *flavour-enhancing additives,* also as food additives to *inhibit tyrosinase.*

Glucose —(Aspergillus flavus ; A. oryzae ;)→ kojic Acid

2.2.7 Itaconic Acid

In 1931, **itaconic acid** was first ever demonstrated to be a metabolic product of *Aspergillus itaconicus.* Within a span of next decade it was duly observed that certain strains of *Aspergillus terreus* also give rise to the formation of **itaconic acid.** In actual practice, the mutants of both strains are profusely employed even today for its large-scale production.

Theory: Itaconic acid is produced by way of the **tricarboxylic acid cycle** (TCA-cycle), whereby D-isocitric acid in the presence of the enzyme aconitic-acid hydrolase loses a mole of water to yield *cis*aconitic acid. The resulting product undergoes decarboxylation (*i.e.,* loses a mole of CO_2) in the presence of the enzyme aconitic-acid decarboxylase to produce the desired product itaconic acid. The aforesaid two steps may be summarized as stated under:

HO — CH — COOH
|
CH — COOH
|
CH_2— COOH

D-Isocitric acid

↓ Step-1 : Aconitic acid hydrolase (Hydrolysis) (H_2O lost)

CH — COOH
||
C — COOH
|
CH_2— COOH

cis - Aconitic acid

↓ Step-II : Aconitic acid decarboxylase (Decarboxylation) (CO_2 lost)

CH_2
||
C — COOH
|
CH_2— COOH

Itaconic acid

The above is the biosynthetic pathway of itaconic acid *via* the TCA-Cycle.

Alternatively, the destruction of *itaconic acid* by the help of **itaconic acid oxidase** yields *two* undesirable products, namely: **succinic acid** and **itatartaric acid.**

Importantly, Ca^{2+} ions specifically inhibit the enzyme **itaconic acid oxidase;** and, therefore, Ca^{2+} ion additions predominantly enhance the overall yield of the desired product **itaconic acid.**

It has been duly observed that the appropriate usage of the **immobilized cells,** the actual production of **itaconic acid** has been adequately increased upto 0.73 g/l.h.

Interestingly, the present day practice is to make use of the strain *Aspergillus terreus* exclusively in the batch-wise submerged fermentation process. In this process a 15% (w/v) solution of sucrose is employed that leads to its conversion into the **itaconic acid** to the extent of 78% of the theoretical yield. It is, however, pertinent to mention here that the effective and progressive fermentation of **itaconic acid** occurs only at pH values less than 2.6. At higher pH values either the desired acid undergoes degradation or ceases to produce any product.

Cautions: There are two important 'cautions' that have to be observed strictly, namely:

1. Fermentor liners should be fabricated with acid-resistant material, and
2. Accumulation of itaconic acid is found to be sensitive to the presence of 'trace metals' in the fermentation medium.

Applications of Itaconic Acid: The various applications of itaconic acid are enumerated under:

1. It is used largely in the plastic industry.
2. **Copolymers** with its corresponding *esters* and other *monomers* find their utilities in the paper industry for wall paper and other paper products.
3. **Copolymers** are also used in the manufacture of adhesives.
4. An **itaconic acid acronitrile copolymer** is observed to be more readily dyed in comparison to certain other polymers.

2.3 Design of Biotransformation Processes

It has been adequately observed that the most crucial and pivotal biotransformation processes are designed and based upon a variety of chemical reactions which may be classified under several categories, such as: (*a*) oxidation; (*b*) reduction; (*c*) hydrolysis; (*d*) condensation; (*e*) isomerization; (*f*) formation of newer C–C bonds; and (*h*) introduction of hetero functional moieties.

In general, the various kinds of biotransformation processes involving typical chemical reactions along with certain specific examples and the percentage efficiency of conversion are summarized in the following Table: 2.1. A possible explanation of the reaction(s) involved has been included in order to have a better understanding of these chemical pathways.

Table 2.1 Biotransformation Reactions of Different Types

S. No	Type of Reaction	Typical Example(s)	Efficiency of Bio-transformation %	Explanation
I	**Oxidation Reactions**			
	1. **Hydroxylation**	*B. subtilis* Tryptophan → 5-Hydroxytryptophan	100	The hydroxylation at C-5 occurs by the presence of *B. subtilis*
	2. **Oxidation** of aliphatic side chains with the formation of carboxyl, aldehyde, or ketone functions.	n-Dodecylbenzene *Nocardia* → sp. Phenyl acetic acid	80	The 12 C-side chain gets oxidized to methane carboxylic acid in the presence of *Nocardia Sp.*
	3. **Epoxidation**	1,7 -Octadiene *Pseudomonas oleovorans* → 7 -8 -Epoxy-1-octene	–25	*P. oleovorans* helps in the epoxidation at C-7 and C-8 ; positions of 1, 7-octadiene.
	4. **Oxidative** cleavage of aromatic rings	Naphthalene *Corynebacterium nov. sp.*→ Salicylic acid [ATCC 15570]	70	One aromatic ring of naphthalene undergoes cleavage to form salicylic acid in the presence of *C. nov. sp.*

	5. **Oxidation** of *heterofunctional* oxida*moieties e.g.,* amino functions to nitro function.	2 -Amino -4 - alkyl imidazole *Streptomyces* → *s.p* 2 -Nitro -4 alkyl imidazole	50 ; 25 ; 36	*Streptomyces sp.* helps in the oxidation of amino (–NH_2) function into the nitro (–NH_2) function.
II	**Reduction Reactions**			
	1. Reduction of an aldehydic carbonyl presence of function.	Benzaldehyde *Saccharomyces* → *cerevisiae* Benzyl alcohol	50	Reduction of an aldehydic function takes place in the presence of *S. cerevisiae*
	2. Reduction of a heterofunction *e.g.,* **Nitro group.**	Nitropentachloro benzene *S. aureofaciens* → Pentachlor aniline	—	The presence of *S. aureofaciens* helps in the reduction of nitro moiety into the amino group.
III	**Hydrolytic Reactions (Hydrolysis):**			
	1. Hydrolysis of CN (nitrile) function.	Analkyl nitrile *Brevibacterium* → At pH9.0 An alkylamide	—	*Brevibacterium* helps in the conversion of an alkyl nitrile to either an **'amide'** at pH 9.0 or a corresponding carboxylic acid.
	2. Hydrolysis of esters of carboxylic acids	*d*,1 –Menthyl laureate *Mycobacterium phlei* → 1 -Menthol	—	*Mycobacterium* esters of *phlei* aids in the hydrolysis of *d*,1-menthyl laureate into 1- menthol.
	3. Hydrolysis of C = C bonds.	Anhydrotetracycline *Streptomyces aureofaciens* → Tetracycline	—	*S. aureofaciens* helps in the hydrolysis of anhydrotetracycline so that the carbon-carbon double bond between C-6 and C-5*a* is abolished to obtain **tetracycline** by undergoing hydration.
IV	**Condensations**			
	1. N-Glycosidation	6 -Azauracil *E.coli.* [ATCC 10798] → 6-Azauracil-riboside	16	*E. coli* causes the N-glycosidation of 6-azauracil into 6- azauracil riboside due to the condensation reaction.
	2. O-Glycosidation	Cyclofenil *Beauveria Sulfurescens* [ATCC 7159] → Methylyglucopyranoide structural analog	60	*Beauveria sulfurescens* helps in the condensation of cyclofenil into the corresponding methylglucopyranosie derivative.
	3. N-Acetylation	6–APS + D-Phenylglycine methylester *Kluyvera citrophila* → Ampicillin	63	*K. citrophila* causes the N-acetylation of 6-APS and D-phenylglycine, methyl ester to yield the desired antibiotic ampicillin *via.* biotransformation.

Summararily, biotransformation designs have been accomplished with tremendous success for a plethora of compounds, namely: cardiac glycoside 'digoxin', acetyltropine, benzylisoquinoline etc. So far, the various typical examples that have been cited are exclusively related to a variety of chemical reactions in the presence of microorganisms.

In addition to the above remarkable explicite examples it has been amply demonstrated and adequately substantiated scientifically that **'plant cells'** are also capable of transforming a wide range of substrates; and, therefore, carry out a large number of reaction(s), for instance: oxidation, hydroxylation, reduction, methylation, glucosylation, acetylation, aminoacylation and the like. Interestingly, the **plant cells** may reasonably tolerate a variety of compounds, namely: steroids, phenolics, alkaloids etc., when incorporated exogenously *via* the growth medium.

Examples: A few glaring examples are given below:

1. Transformation of Steviol (aglucon) into Stevioside (glucoside): The transformation of **Steviol** (i.e., hydroxydehydrostevic acid) by the cells of *Stevia rebaudiana* (Bert.) Hemsl. (*Eupatorium rebaudianum Bert.*) *Compositae,* also called *yerba dulce* (*Habitat* : Paraguay), into a glucoside known as **stevioside** which is proved to be 300 times sweeter than *sucrose,* and hence used as a sweetener.

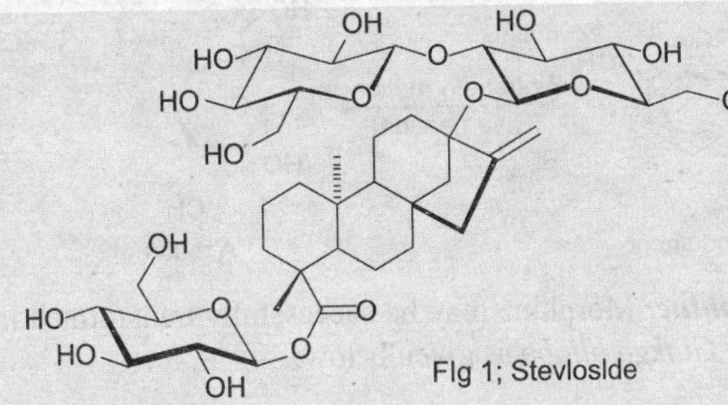

Fig 1; Stevioside

2. **Glycosylation of salicylic acid** by the cultures of *Mallotus japonica* yields a product that possesses an appreciable high analgesic activity, and also exhibits excellent better tolerance in the stomach in comparison to acetylsalicylic acid (*i.e.,* aspirin).

3. Hydroxylation of β-Methyl digitoxin to Digoxin: It has been observed that the most significant biotransformation process of pharmaceutical importance is the **12-hydroxylation of** β**-methyl digitoxin** to **digoxin** by the aid of cell cultures of *Digitalis lanata.* In fact, the two cardiotonic compounds *digitoxin* and *digoxin* are duly isolated from the leaves of **Digitalis.** It is a well-known fact that the cardiotonic substance **digoxin** cannot be produced either by microbial biotransformation (bioconversion) or chemically.

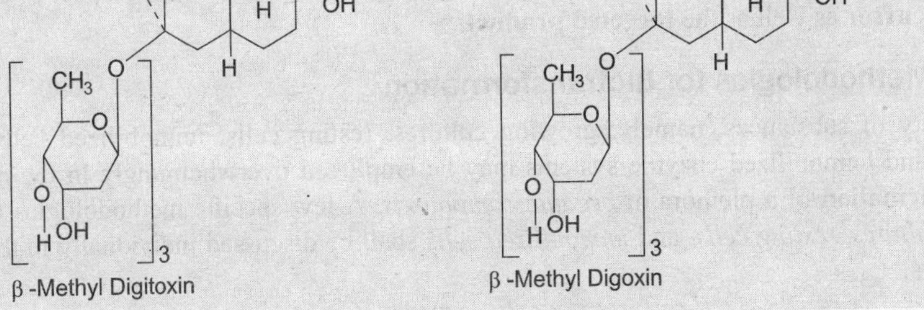

β -Methyl Digitoxin β -Methyl Digoxin

It is worthwhile to mention here that the biotransformation (*hydroxylation*) of β-methyl digitoxin into the more desirable and substantially less toxic drug, **β-methyl digoxin** by the cell cultures of *Digitalis lanata* is significant remarkably.

4. Arbutin from Hydroquinone: It has been observed that **arbutin,** a naturally occurring β-D-glucoside, usually found in the leaves of *Pyrus communis, Pyrus serotina, Bergina crassifolia,* and *Arctostaphylos uvaursi.* In fact, the biotransformation procedures involving the conversion of hydroquinone into its β-D-glucoside, **arbutin,** by the help of different cell systems, such as: *Rauwolfia serpentina, Datura innoxia,* and *C. roseus.* In actual practice, one may obtain upto even 18 $g.L^{-1}$ of **arbutin** from the cell suspension cultures of *R. serpentina* after a continuous feeding of *hydroquinone* into the culture medium for a duration of 7 days at a stretch. However, the aforesaid technique has a major disadvantage due to the fact the *'cells'* invariably accumulate not only **arbutin,** but also another by product known as ***para*-hydroxy-phenyl-O-β-D-primveroside** upto 6 $g.L^{-1}$, which is rather difficult to separate from the desired substance **arbutin.**

Biotransformation
[R.serpentina]

Hydroquinone → A rbutin

5. Codeine from Morphine: Morphine may be successfully transformed into **codeine** by using the suspension cultures of *Ginkgo biloba* as given below:

a. *G. biloba*

ii. Morphine → Codeine

b. Biotransformation

6. Scopolamine from Hyoscyamine: Hyoscyamine may be conveniently transformed into **scopolamine** by making use of the suspension cultures of *Anisodus tanuticus* as shown under.

A. tanuticus

Hyoscyamine → Scopolamine

Biotransformation

Importantly, the concentration of **scopolamine** may be enhanced reasonably by augmenting the initial concentration of hyoscyamine to a certain extent.

One may summarize the *three* cardinal absolute preconditions or requirements for a successful biotransformation of a *'precursor'* into a targeted product as stated under:

a. The culture medium should have adequate **enzymes** very urgent and quite necessary for the ensuing transformation of a precursor to the desired product,
b. The **'targeted product'** should be generated at a rate predominantly **faster** than its rate of metabolism, and
c. The *'culture medium'* must be having enough limit of tolerance with respect to the **added precursor** as well as the **targeted product.**

2.3.1 Methodologies for Biotransformation

A variety of substances, namely: growing cultures, resting cells, immobilized cells, spores, enzymes, and immobilized enzyme systems may be employed overwhelmingly in the **microbial biotransformation** of a plethora of *organic compounds.* A few specific methodologies involving *growing cultures, resting cells,* and *immobilized cells* shall be discussed individually in the section that follows:

2.3.1.1 Growing Cultures

The methodologies that are intimately associated with **growing cultures** essentially involve the strains that are cultivated in an appropriate culture medium, and subsequently a concentrated substrated solution is usually incorporated after an appreciable growth of the culture after a lapse of 6 to 24 hours.

A few noteworthy variants of this particular procedure are as stated below:

a. Usage of a relatively very large inoculum,
b. Incorporating the concentrated substrate immediately without permitting, a growth phase to commence,
c. Usage of **'emulsifiers'** *e.g.*, Tweens (*i.e.*, Tween-20, 40, 60, 80—synthetic surfectants) or **water-miscible solvents** *e.g.*, acetone, ethanol, dimethyl formamide (DMF), dimethyl sulphoxide (DMSO) may be employed to aid the dissolution of rather sparingly soluble substances quite conveniently.

Salient Features: A few distinct salient features of this **growing culture** process are as enumerated below:

1. In certain instances where the solubility limits are at a low ebb *e.g.*, **steroid biotransformations,** the quantum of substrate that may be incorporated are usually performed at **substrate concentrations** ranging between 0.1 to 10 $g.L^{-1}$ of the medium; whereas, in certain cases even upto 30 $g.L^{-1}$ may be converted successfully.
2. **Solvent Concentrations** varying between 5 to 15 $mL.L^{-1}$ of the culture medium may be employed in certain specific cases of *steroid biotransformation,* and the substrate is incorporated and subsequently converted into the desired fine crystalline form. However, it is pertinent to state here that these so-called **pseudo-crystalline fermentation procedures** may be performed by using comparatively high concentrations of the substrate *e.g.*, 15 to 50 $g.L^{-1}$ with progesterone—a female sex-hormone.
3. ***Lipophilic Substrate:*** The **lipophilic substances** may be subject to biotransformation significantly by employing a **polyphase system.**

   Example: An *aqueous phase* comprising the cell material or the enzyme is overplayed with a *water-immiscible fluid phase* wherein the **'substrate'** has been duly dissolved. Consequently, the ensuing **'substrate'** gets across gradually into the prevailing *aqueous phase;* and as the biotransformation phenomenon gains momentum, the desired product passes right into the solvent phase ultimately. Interestingly, in certain very specific instances, the actual prevailing biotransformation takes place almost exclusively at the ensuing interface of the aqueous and solvent phases.
4. ***Ideal Optimal Biotransformation Reaction Parameters:*** Ideally the biotransformation reaction parameters as applicable to large-scale plant equipments and accessories are invariably performed in an environment under perfect sterile conditions preferentially in **adequately aerated and stirred bioreactors,** wherein *bioconversions* taking place being controlled and monitored meticulously by **spectroscopically** or **chromatographically** (HPLC, HPTLC, GC). However, the on-going process is normally terminated (arrested) on accomplishing a **maximal titer value.** Sterility is an absolute must throughout the entire operation because any type of uncalled for contamination would give rise to several happenings, such as:

   a. Suppress the desired reaction;
   b. result into several faulty conversion products; and
   c. Cause total substrate breakdown.

2.3.1.2 Resting Cells

In such critical situations when the enzyme induction afforded by the added substrate is not quite necessary and urgent, **resting cells** may be employed profusely and effectively. However, the **resting cells** do offer a tremendous advantage whereby the *growth inhibition by the substrate* is eliminated completely. Besides, the presence of high-cell densities that essentially promote an enhanced level of productivity may be employed; simultaneously, the very *risk* of any possible scope of contamination is minimized appreciably. Interestingly, there are several biotransformation reactions that exclusively and predominantly take place in the **'buffer solution'** and this eventually renders the ultimate recovery of the **'desired product'** relatively easy and convenient.

2.3.1.3 Immobilized Cells

In more recent times, a host of biotransformation methodologies do make use of the **immobilized cells** thus affording the biggest even advantageous plus point that the process could be carried out simultaneously; besides, the *cells* might be employed over and over again.

Applications: In actual practice, the immobilized bacterial cells that invariably catalyze either **single-stage reaction** or **multi-stage reaction,** are presently exploited in the large-scale production of **L-alanine, aspartic acid,** and **malic acid.**

2.4 Selection of Organisms

The **selection of strains** either from its *natural sources* or from the various *available cultures* which are solely responsible for catalyzing the desired biotransformation reaction(s) is not only vital and critical but also of great importance. It has been observed that there are quite a few microorganisms that usually carry out the desired bioconversions with the help of a related chemical entity. In steroid one may encounter a rather difficult problem due to the lack of selective methods so as to identify the colonies precisely which usually perform the ear-marked specific activity.

Example: The **'plate assay'** may be successfully employed to select such organisms which may aromatize several steroidal entities, for instance: 19-nor steroids; 19-substituted steroids; and sterols (*e.g.*, β-sitosterol, ergosterol etc.) into **equilin** and **related oestrogen.**

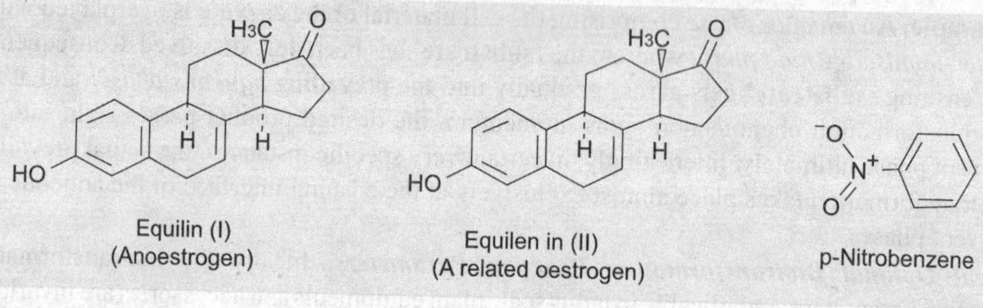

Equilin (I)
(Anoestrogen)

Equilen in (II)
(A related oestrogen)

p-Nitrobenzene

These ring A aromatic oestrogenic products I and II above usually react particularly with the reagent ***para*-nitrobenzene diazonium fluoborate** to give rise to the production of an *intense red colouration.* Therefore, the development of such colonies in a solid medium containing an appropriate steroidal substrate, are duly replicated before the reagent is sprayed; and thus, a red-ring gets developed all around the *active colonies.*

Modified Enrichment Method

The **modified enrichment method** is invariably used for the isolation of mutants blocked in the substrate dissimilation mechanism. In this specific instance, a steroid substrate is normally incorporated as the sole C-source exclusively in a **'minimal medium'** seeded adequately with the soil dilutions. The cells that cause the degradation of the substrate will ultimately grow; and are, therefore, subsequently transferred to the same medium but particularly enriched with another C-source, for instance: **glucose.** However, the mutants may be present which are strategically blocked at different stages in the process of degradation of the steroid substrate, but may consume glucose as the C-source.

Besides, the *resulting intermediates* may get **accumulated**, whereas the *lesion-bearing mutants* can be **isolated** conveniently. Furthermore, mutants may also be isolated which are incapable of accumulating an **'undesirable compound'.**

Example: An *'undesirable reaction'* initiated by *Aspergillus ochraceus* which eventually blocked the ensuing transformation of **11α-hydroxyprogesterone** into **6β-11α-dihydroxyprogesterone** was duly prepared that could only yield the derivative **11α-hydroxy-progesterone.**

It has been profusely established and reported that a fairly large number of microbial strains *viz.,* **eubacteria, yeasts, molds,** and **streptomycetes** may be stored and maintained strictly as per the recommended **'standard methods',** such as : **agar slant, soil culture, frozen culture,** and **lypholized culture** preserved at temperatures ranging between –20°C to –170°C.

Filtration Enrichment Method: In this case, after mutagenesis the **spores of filamentous organisms** *e.g.,* actinomycetes, fungi, are made to develop in a *liquid minimal medium.* The ensuing microcolonies of **prototroph** thus developed are meticulously separated by **filtration,** whereby the spores of **auxotroph** that were unable to grow left behind in the filtrate. The filtrate obtained in this manner in subsequently plated and the resulting colonies are adequately checked for *auxotrophic characteristics.*

Penicillin-Selection Procedure: In **penicillin-selection procedure** the prevailing growing cells are killed selectively by the *'antibiotic'* treatment, thereby enriching the *auxotrophs* that are incapable of growing upon the *'minimal medium'*. Thus, exclusively based upon their mode of action a plethora of 'inhibitors' other than penicillin may also be employed effectively in this procedure, namely: **dihydrostreptomycin** for *Pseudomonas aeruginosa;* **nystalin** for *Hansenula polymorpha, Penicillium chrysogenum, Aspergillus nidulans,* and *Saccharomyces cerevisiae;* **nalidix acid** for *Salmonella typhimurium;* **colistin** for the penicillin-resistant *Hydrogenomonas* strain H16.

Sodium Pentachlorophenolate: The salt **sodium pentachlorophenolate** also affords enrichment procedure by virtue of its **greater toxicity** particularly against the *'germinating spores'* in comparison to the *'vegetative cells'*.

Example: The above method has been successfully applied with several organisms, such as: *Penicillium chrysogenum; Streptomyces aureofaciens; Streptomyces olivaceus;* and *Bacillus subtilis.*

It is, however, pertinent to state at this juncture that the applications of the aforesaid enrichment methods may cause an enhancement of *'auxotrophs'* between 10 to 100 times, thus increasing considerably the probability of obtaining mutants. Importantly, one may observe that the variants of mutants present in the initial original population may get shifted to an appreciable extent, such as : an enhanced proportion of **proline auxotrophs** may be accomplished in *E. coli* after the due *auxotroph enrichment.*

Spraying with Reagents (or Incorporating Indicator Dyes)

One may observe either the presence or absence of *specific enzyme activities* almost directly in the colonies that are allowed to grown on plates by employing either of the *two* available common procedures, namely: (*a*) spraying with appropriate reagents; and (*b*) incorporating indicator-dyes right into the culture medium.

Inhibition of Assay Organisms: In this specific instance the *antibiotically-active compounds* may be detected quite easily and conveniently by measuring the **inhibition of sensitive assay organisms.**

This procedure allows the precise determination (assay) of the *'antibiotic content'* of an unknown solution using a reference standard simultaneously.

Agar Plug Method: The **agar plug method** is regarded to be one of the most reliable and precise techniques wherein the **agar cylinders** having *'single-colonies'* are transferred to test plates after due incubation preferably in a moist chamber as depicted in Fig. 2.7 given below:

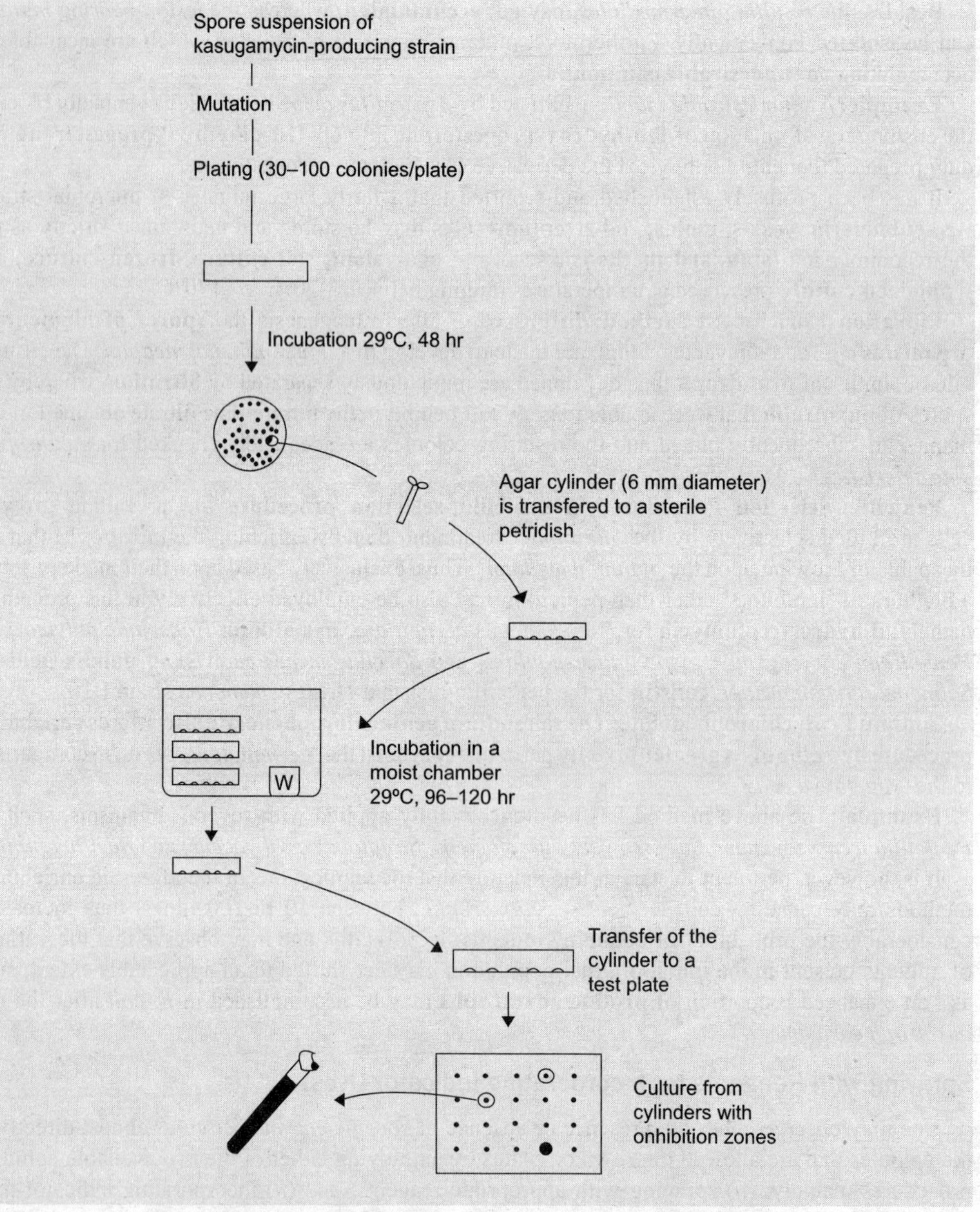

Fig. 2.7 *'Agar plug' Method in Kasugamycin Strain Development*

In fact, the actual observed diameter of the resulting *'zones of inhibition'* invariably caters for a definite measure of the capability of *'antibiotic production'* of each strain under investigation.

Suitability of Agar Plug Method: The method is fairly suitable for such processes where only a differentiation between productivity and non-productivity is sufficient *e.g.,* detecting the production of **specific constitutive enzymes.**

Drawbacks: This method has several drawbacks which may be summarized as given under:

1. There exists only a slight correlation between antibiotic formations in the *'plate culture' Vis-a- Vis* antibiotic production is submerged fermentation.

2. Strains that produce at high yields on being grown on plates may yield at only low yields or even almost nil in the prevailing liquid culture.
3. When screening is adopted and initiated employing *high-yielding strains,* further enhancements in yield invariably cannot be detected by the help of this procedure.

2.5 Biotransformation Process and its Improvements with Special Reference to Steroids

In true sense, the **'biotransformation process'** *i.e.,* the ensuing **regiospecific and stereospecific bioconversions,** is nothing but a pure **biological process.** Nevertheless, these processes are not only simple but also chemically well-defined; and, therefore, invariably the various organic substances are duly modified into the corresponding *reversible products.* Beyond any reasonable doubt these reactions are suitably catalyzed by the help of certain highly specific enzymes usually present abundantly in microbial, plant, and animal cells; which in turn do catalyze a host of transformation reaction processes.

Microbial Cells: Bertrand (1986) first and foremost initiated a methodical, scientific approach to microbial transformation whereby the **'microbial cells'** definitely produced better results in comparison to the **plant** and **animal cells.** In fact, the microbial cells do possess substantially **greater surface volume ratio** due to which they have a tendency to *grow faster* and afford reasonably *higher rate of metabolism.* In other words, these essential characteristic features predominantly help in accomplishing highly specific as well as efficient transformation of the prevailing substrate in which they normally grow. Perhaps this could be the reason why various phenomenons, such as: growing, resting or adding of the dried microbial cells or enzymes duly isolated from these cells into the substrate to cause transformation effectively. Importantly, the particular agents undergoing transformation usually remain suspended into a medium for proper usage either in agitated/aerated bioreactor or in packed columns for continuous operations. Lastly, **'microbial cells'** may be carefully immobilized on the solid support both for prolonged operation and enhanced desired stability.

Plant Cells: Plant cells have been profusely exploited in bringing about superb *biotransformation processes* towards the ultimate objective for the successful production of a large spectrum of exclusive novel drug molecules, namely : **Cardiac glycoside** — digoxin; **Sweetening agent** — stevioside; **skin lightening agent** — arbutin; **CNS-depressant** — codeine etc. It has been observed that the **'plant cells'** have the enormous built in tolerance for a variety of chemical substances, for instance: steroids, alkaloids glycosides, phenolics, antibiotics and the like. Interestingly, these cells markedly behave and perform in a much better manner in comparison to the **'microbial cells',** particularly in such an event when highly specific **enzymatic biosynthetic pathways** are required as a top priority.

Animal Cells: The application of **animal cells** *viz.,* organ perfusion preparation, cell culture preparation, are employed mostly in carrying out the biotransformation process involving organic compounds, preferentially at the laboratory scale only.

In a nut-shell, amongst all the *three* above cited cells the application of **microbial cells** for *biotransformation process* is the most preferred one by virtue of the fact they largely replace the involvement of a good number of **chemical steps** and their subsequent purification and recovery.

2.5.1 Biotransformation of Steroids

A large cross section of naturally occurring **steroids** belonging to the *animal* and *plant* kingdom significantly exhibit remarkable **hormonal characteristic features,** for instance : **animal source** — corticosteroids, oestrogens, sex-hormones, cholesterol *etc.;* plant source — ergosterol, cardiac glycosides, β-sitosterol etc., In general, **all steroids** essentially possess the same basic structure *i.e.,* a *cyclopentanoperhydrophenanthrene.*

Examples: Various examples of **steroids** are as given below:
Glucocorticoids: Cortical; Cortisone; Corticosterone; Dexamethasone;
Mineralocorticoids: Aldosterone; Fludrocortisone;
Androgens: Testosterone; Oxandrolone;
Oestrogens: Estrone; Estriol; Estradiol;
Gestogens: Progesterone:
The structures of several naturally occurring steroidal hormones are as given below:

Glucocorticoids

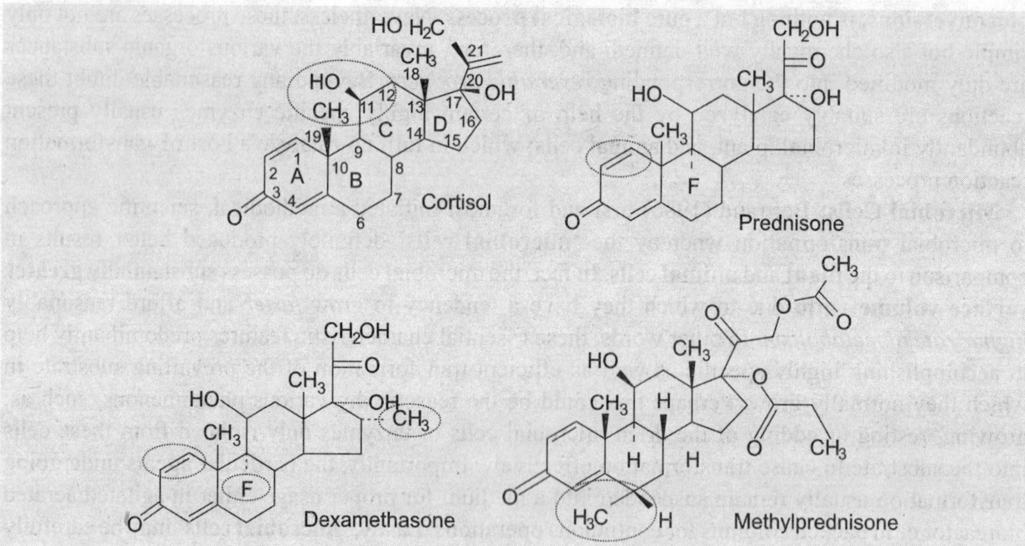

Figure *Chemical structure of cortisol and of main synthetic glucocorticoids, such as prednisone, methylprednisolone and dexamethasone*

Mineralocorticoids

Androgens

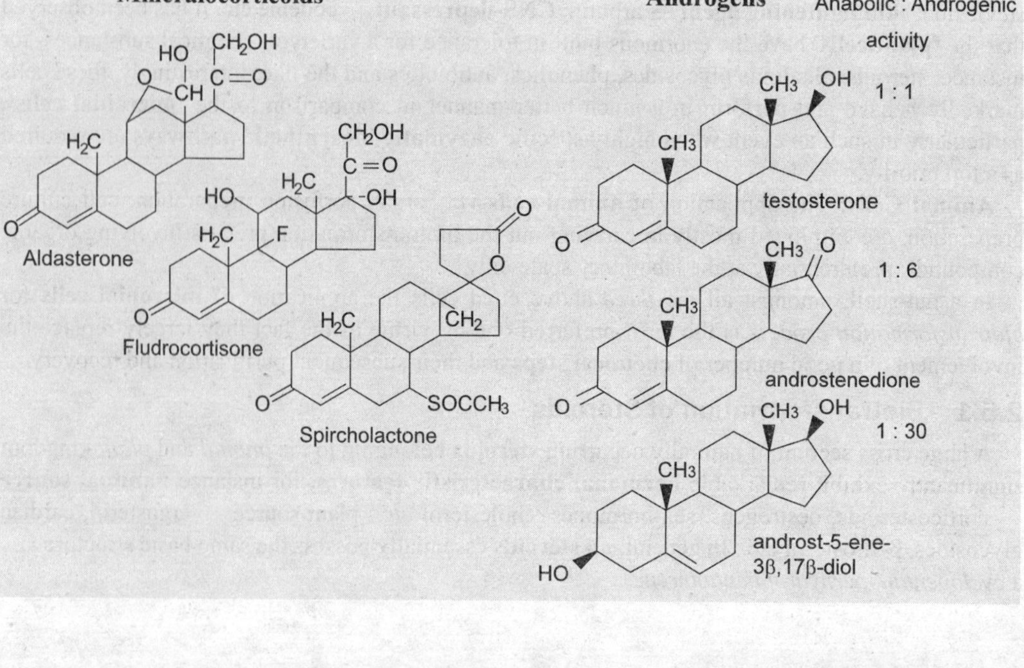

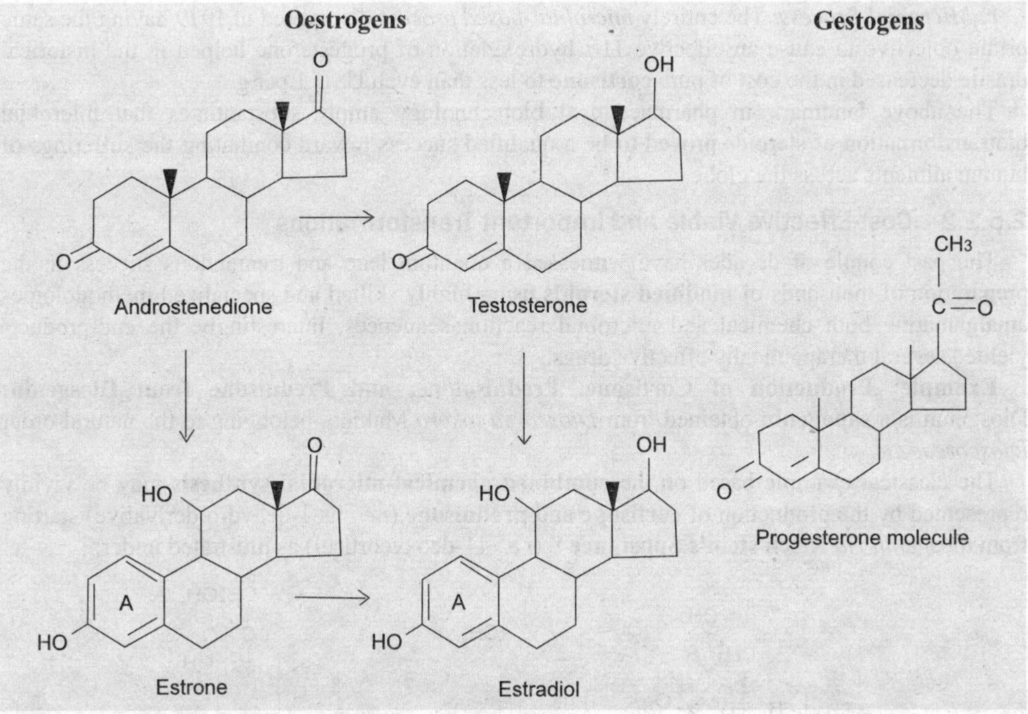

Oestrogens

Gestogens

Androstenedione

Testosterone

Progesterone molecule

Estrone

Estradiol

It is, however, pertinent to state at this point in time that the **steroids** known till date invariably take care of a variety of human diseases so satisfactory that the dire need for further development of certain newer steroid biotransformation processes is more or less restricted. Nevertheless, the research is, at present, geared toward the **optimization** of the prevailing available procedures, such as:

a. Utilization of *immobilized cells* or *enzymes,*

b. Augmentation of *existing reaction system e.g.,* by the help of **polyphase systems,**

c. Finding improved and efficient starting materials, and

d. Minimizing degradative side reactions.

Future Developments: There are, in fact, *two* predominant aspects on which the future developments in **steroid biotransformation** are based, namely:

i. Application of **plant-cell cultures,** and

ii. **Genetic engineering research** upon the microorganisms.

2.5.1.1 Types of Transformations/Biotransformations

The various types of transformations/biotransformations that are of particular interest with respect to the **steroids** are as described under:

a. Total Synthesis: The **'total synthesis'** of *cortisone* (yield = 1g) obtained from *deoxycholic acid* (615 g) *via* the original chemical process essentially involved as many as 31 different individual reaction steps which eventually held the cost of the product abnormally high. Hence, this kind of research is only limited to *academic interest* and very little *commercial interest.*

b. Site-specific and Stereospecific Manipulation: Intensive and extensive research with regard to microbial introduction of an O-atom strategically into the steroid nucleus particularly in a **site-specific and sterospecific fashion** encouraged the *11α-hydroxylation of progesterone,* and that too without any prior activation whatsoever. Interestingly, these biochemical processes proceeded quite effectively and efficiently, which ultimately paved the way for a viable, feasible and cost-effective production of cortisone. Cost of 1g of cortinsone stood at USD 200 per g in 1949.

c. Microbial Process: The entirely *microbial-based process* discovered in 1979 having the same prime objective to cause an effective 11α hydroxylation of progesterone helped in the historical drastic decreased in the cost of pure **cortisone** to less than even USD 1 per g.

The above landmark in pharmaceutical biotechnology amply substantiates that microbial biotransformation of steroids proved to be a qualified success toward combating the sufferings of human ailments across the globe.

2.5.1.2 Cost-Effective Viable and Important Transformations

The past couple of decades have witnessed a quantum leap and tremendous success in the preparation of thousands of **modified steroids** using highly skilled and specialized methodologies amalgamating both chemical and microbial reaction sequences. Interestingly, the end-products yielded several therapeutically effective drugs.

Example: Production of Cortisone, Prednisolone, and Prednisone from Diosgenin: Diosgenin is a **sapogenin** obtained from *Dioscorea tokoro* Makino, belonging to the natural order *Dioscoreaceae.*

The classical example based on the **combined chemical-microbial synthesis** may be vividly represented by the production of **cortisone** and **prednisone** (*i.e.,* its 1-dehydro derivative) starting from *diosgenin via* **Reich stein's Substance S** (*i.e.,* 11-deoxycortisol) as illustrated under:

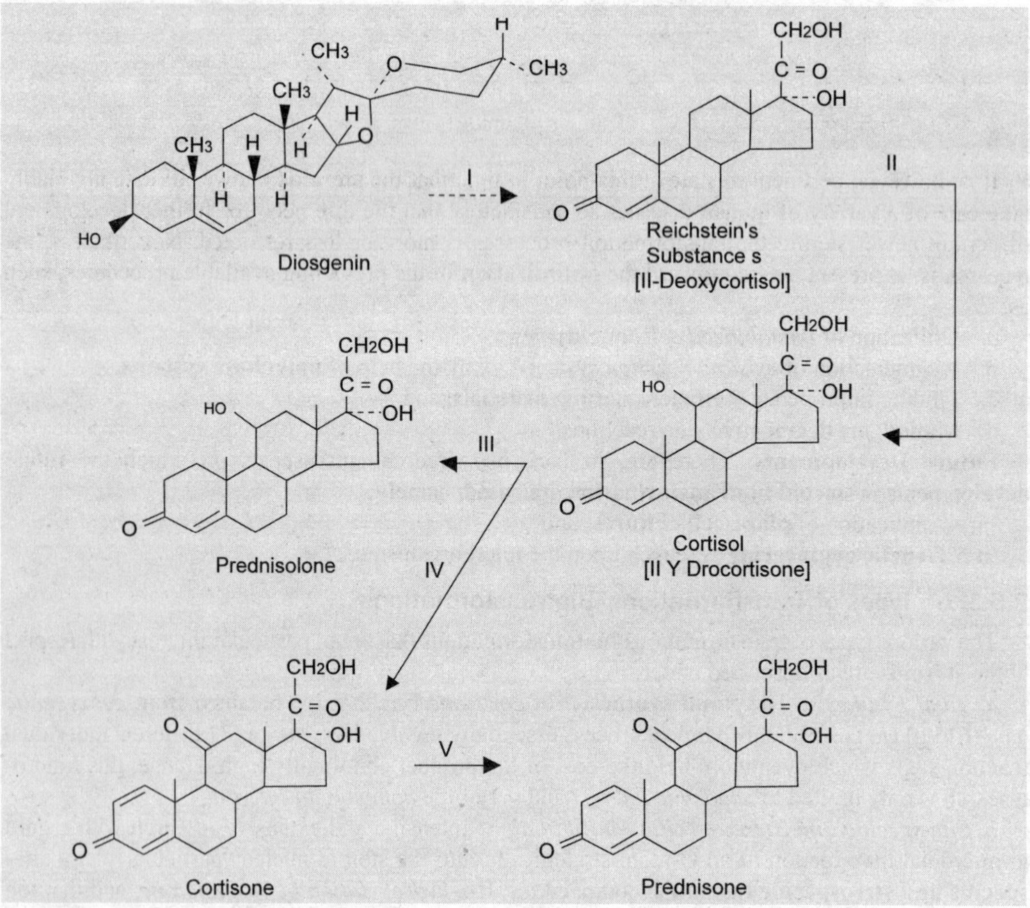

The explanations of the aforesaid reactions are as stated below:

Step-1: Diosgenin undergoes several chemical-microbial transformations to give rise to the formation of **Reich stein's Substance S** which may also be called as 11-deoxycortisol.

Step-2: The resulting Reich stein's Substance S undergoes 11β-hydroxylation in the presence of the microorganism *Curvularia lunata* to yield **cortisol** *i.e.,* hydrocortisone.

Step-3: Cortisol obtained from the previous step-III affords dehydration at C-1 position in the presence of the organism *Corynebacterium simplex* to produce **prednisolone.**

Step-4: It is essentially a non-microbial step and gives rise to **cortisone** *via* chemical oxidation whereby the 11-hydroxy moiety is converted to a 11-ketonic function conveniently.

Step-5: Once again the organism *Corynebacterium Simplex* (see step III) has been successfully utilized to cause dehydration at C-1 to yield the desired product prednisone.

The concerted efforts of various researchers across the globe exclusively based upon *a host of microbial reaction sequences* have left a lasting impression upon its great **economic significance** and **immense values.**

Examples: There are *two* typical examples that evidently expatiate the above observations, namely:

a. Progesterone transformation to the corresponding C-19 steroid has been adequately exploited on a commercial scale in the feasible production of **testosterone** and **oestrogen,** and
b. **Oestrogen** production may also be accomplished by the **meticulous microbial dehydration** of ring A present in the steroidal nucleus.

Summararily, the various experimental parameters invariably adopted for carrying out the innumerable **bioconversion reaction sequences** of this specific nature are given in Table 2.2.

Table 2.2 *Typical Examples of Certain Commercial Steroid Processes*

S.No	Product	Substrate	Reaction	Microorganism Used	Manufacturer
1.	11α-Hydroxy-progesterone	Progesterone	11α-Hydroxylation	*Rhizopus nigricans*	Upjohn Co., (USA)
2.	Cortisol	11-Deoxycortisol (Reichstein's substance S)	11β-Hydroxylation	*Curvularia lunata*	Pfizer Inc., (USA).
3.	9α-Fluoro-16α-hydroxycortisol tisol	9α-Fluorocortisol	16α-Hydroxylation	*Streptomyces Roseochromogenes*	Lederle Labs.
4.	Prednisolone	Cortisol	1-Dehydrogenation	*Arthrobacter simplex*	Schering Corp. (USA)
5.	1-Dehydro-testololactone	Progesterone	1-Dehydration side-chain cleavage	*Cylindrocarpon radiciola*	Squibb % Sons
6.	Androstadiendione	β-Sitosterol	Side-chain cleavage	*Mycobacterium fortuitum mutants*	Upjohn Co. (USA), Searle and Co. (USA)
7.	Triendiol1	Diendiol2	1-Dehydrogenation	*Septomyxa affinis*	Upjohn Co. (USA)

1. Triendiol: 11β, 21-Dihydroxy-1, 4, 17 (20)-pregnatriene-3-ones (i.e., precursors employed in the production of 6α-methylprednisolone).

2. Diendiol: 11β, 21-Dihydroxy-4, 17 (20)-pregnadiene-3-ones.

It has been established beyond any reasonable doubt that the commercial production of **testosterone** and **oestrogen** may be accomplished by the transformation of *progesterone* into a corresponding **C-19 steroid** specifically. Besides, the strategic microbial dehydration of ring A is successfully exploited resulting into the oestrogen production. In fact, the wisdom and precise manoeuvre of certain specific experimental parameters a host of **'bioconversion reactions'** of this particular pattern may be accomplished legitimately, and *six* of them have been duly provided in the following Table: 4.3 expatiately.

In fact, **batch fermentative procedures** have since been able to cause several *steroidal transformations;* however, considerable progress has also been accomplished by the skilful usage of both *enzymes* and *immobilized cells.* Interestingly the latter procedures invariably offer a large number of **advantages,** such as:

- Minimized risk of possible contamination,
- Easier mode of product recovery,
- Significantly shorter conversion times, and Enhanced substrate concentrations

Table 2.3 *Operational Parameters of Several Steroid Transformations.*

S. No	Product	Substrate	Yield (%)	Medium	Microorganism	Experimental parameters employed
1.	1-Dehydrotestololactone	Progesterone	50	I	*Cylindrocarpon radiciola*	25°C; 72 hr.
2.	1, 4-Androstadiene-3, 17-dione	Progesterone	85	II	*Fusarium solani*	25°C; 96 hr.
3.	15α-Hydroxy-4-pregnene-3, 20-dione	Progesterone	11	III	*Streptomyces aureus*	25°C; 72 hr.
4.	11α-Hydroxy-4- androstene-3, 17-dione	Androstene-3, 17-dione	25	IV	*Rhizopus arrhizus*	28°C; 96 hr.
5.	11α-Hydroxy progesterone	Progesterone	91	V	*Aspergillus ochraceus*	28°C; 120 hr.
6.	Prednisolone	Hydrocortisone	93	VI	*Arthrobacter simplex*	28°C; 120 hr. Pseudo crystal Fermentation.

Media Composition as per Table 4.3.

1. Corn-steep liquor (dry wt. basis) 3g; Dihydrogen ammonium phosphate ($NH_4H_2PO_4$) 3g; Calcium carbonate ($CaCO_3$) 2.5 g; Soyabean oil 2.2 g; Progesterone 0.5 g; DW q.s. to 1L; pH 7.0;
2. Peptone 15 g; Corn-steep liquor 6 ml; Glucose 50 g; DW q.s. to 1 L; pH 6.0; Progesterone 0.25 g should be incorporated only after 48 hr.;
3. Soyabean oil 2.2 g; Soymeal 15 g; Glucose 10 g; Calcium carbonate ($CaCO_3$) 2.5 g; Progesterone 0.25 g; DW q.s. to 1 L;
4. Peptone 20 g; Corn-steep liquor 5 ml; Glucose 50 g; DW q.s. to 1 L; pH 5.5 to 5.9; Androstendione 0.25 g to be incorporated only after 27 hr;
5. Peptone 10 g; Yeast extract 5 g; Sucrose 30 g; DM water q.s. to 1 L; pH 6.5; Progesterone 40 g carefully dissolved in acetone and added to the ensuing growing culture after 24 hr.;
6. Peptone 5 g; Corn-steep Liquor 5 g; Glucose 5 g; DW q.s. to 1 L; pH 7.0; Finely powdered hydrocortisone, 1–50%, duly suspended in ethanol; incorporated carefully into a 24 hr. old culture medium.

In actual practice, it has been duly observed that even more than one essential biochemical step may be carefully combined together and engaged in order to achieve several such **steroid transformations** both gainfully and efficaciously.

Examples: There are at least well recognized, tested and tried instances that explicitly exemplify the aforesaid **steroid transformations,** such as:

1. Application of Immobilized Mycelium: The **immobilized mycelium** of *Curvularia lunata* or the immobilized cells to *Arthrobacter simplex* have been intensively and extensively exploited to effectively perform the **two-step reaction** as evidenced in the conversion to **prednisolone** from the Reich stein's substance S (*i.e.,* 11-deoxycortisol).

2. Application of Fungal Spores: The utility of a number of **fungal spores** *e.g., Penicillium notatum,* are being employed directly to augment the catalytic transformation(s) of a plethora of such bioconversion processes.

3. Application of Solvent System: Based on the universal fact that since most *steroidal substrates* are immiscible in aqueous medium, the ensuing transformation parameters have been meticulously developed for certain selected and specific steroids in a particular **solvent system** that happens to be invariably water-immiscible *e.g.,* transformation of **'testosterone'** with the immobilized cells of *Nocardia rhodochrous.*

4. Application of Two-Phase System: In general, the organic solvent is most frequently found to be toxic to the cells as well as enzyme; therefore, one may alternatively make use of an aqueous **two-phase system.**

Example: Prednisolone may be obtained by the 1-dehydration of *cortisol* by the aid of cells of *Arthrobacter simplex* precisely in a **two-phase system** comprising essentially of the following *two* substances, namely:

a. Polyethylene glycol (PEG) 8000 : 25% (*w/w*), and
b. Dextran T40 : 6% (*w/w*)

2.5.1.3 Microbial Cleavage of Sterol-Side Chains (at C-17)

Since 1970s, the world experienced an ever growing demand for a large cross-section of **steroidal drugs** that eventually caused an appreciable shortage of various available *steroid precursors* for carrying out various bioconversion reaction *e.g.,* **diosgenin**. In fact, **diosgenin** — a sapogenin is obtained from a variety of plant sources, such as: *Dioscorea rokoro* Makino, *Dioscorea composita Dioscorreaceae;* and the South African Plant *Testudinaria sylvatica.*

An aggressive and highly intensified researches were aimed at for the exploitation and feasibility attempts on the broad-based utilization of low-cost sterols derived from either *animal sources* **(zoosterol)** *e.g.,* **Cholesterol** or *plant sources* **(phytosterol)** *e.g.,* **β-sitosterol, stigmasterol,** and **campesterol.**

Objectives: The major **objective** of all such elaborated investigations was the highly selective removal (elimination) of an array of aliphatic side-chain moieties, thereby resulting into the formation of propionic acid and acetic acid, without further cleavage of the **basic steroid nucleus** at all.

It has been duly established and proved that the ensuing 8-carbon side-chain undergoes appropriate Cleavage to give rise to the formation of a **C-17 keto compounds** ultimately as depicted under:

HO Cholesterol + CH_2-OOCR' / $R''COO-CH$ / $CH_2-O-P(=O)(O^-)-O-CH_2CH_2\overset{+}{N}(CH_3)_3$ Phosphatidylcholine

↓ lecithin cholesterol acyltransferase(LCAT)

R''COO Cholesterol ester + CH_2-OOCR' / $HO-CH$ / $CH_2-O-P(=O)(O^-)-O-CH_2CH_2\overset{+}{N}(CH_3)_3$ lysophosphatidylcholine

Side-Chain Cleavage of Cholesterol

2.5.1.4 Mycobacterial Cleavage of Steroid Nucleus (Ring 'B')

The degradative product 3-hydroxy-9, 10-secoandrosta-1, 3, 5(10) triene-9, 17-dione is produced redominantly starting from **cholesterol** (a *zoosterol*) *via* a strategically cleavage of the ring 'B' in the teroid nucleus, besides the generation of *two* extremely useful intermediate products, namely: **ndrostendione** and **androstadiendione** as described below:

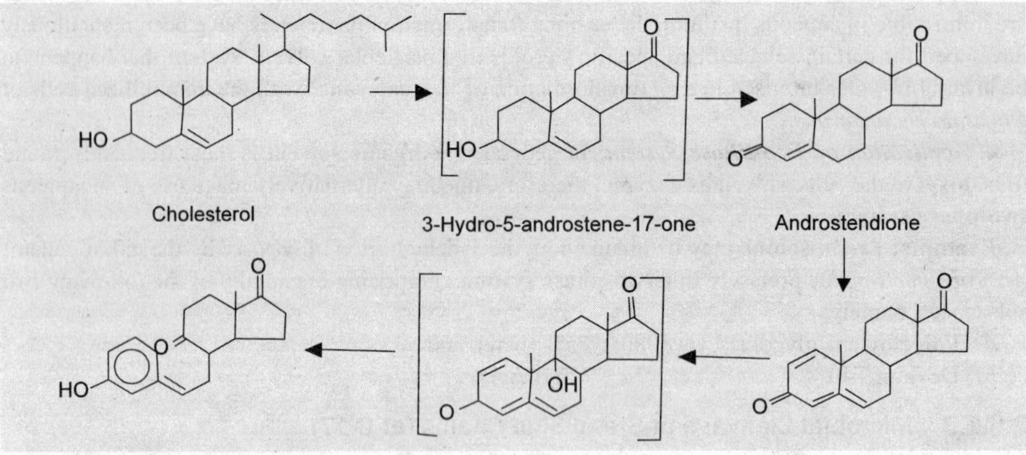

Cholesterol

3-Hydro-5-androstene-17-one

Androstendione

A plethora of highly sophisticated techniques are duly available to block selectively and precisely he cleavage of the steroidal nucleus:

- Cleavage reaction may be entirely blocked by appropriate chemical modification of the substrate.
- Conversion may take place largely in the presence of certain inhibitors that specifically check either C-1(2)-dehydration or 9α-hydroxylation, for instance:
  a. bivalent ions that critically replace Fe^{2+} ion,
  b. chemical entities which chelate Fe^{2+} or Cu^{2+} ions,
  c. compounds that specifically block *sulphhydryl moieties e.g.,* Pb^{2+}, Co^{2+} and Ni^{2+}.
- Mutants having *inactive enzymes,* such as: C-1(2)-dehydrogenase or 9α-hydroxylase may be employed. It is, however, worthwhile to state here that *Mycobacterium* mutants that are solely responsible for the transformation of various sterols, namely: **cholesterol, stigmasterol,** and **sitosterol** into the corresponding main products, such as: **androstenedione** and **androstadiendione** have been isolated duly. It has been observed that these mutants are incapable of causing further cleavage of the said two main products.

Specific example: The product 9α-hydroxy-4-androstene-3, 17-dione may be obtained from the various substrates *e.g.,* β-sitosterol, stigmasterol, campesterol and cholesterol in the presence of the organism *Mycobacterium fortuitum* using a specific medium* at 30°C for a period of 336 hrs at a stretch.

2.5.2 Steroid Bioconversion via Fermentative Procedures

Steroids *i.e.,* the highly biologically active compounds are usually produced by a host of vital organs in the human body, namely: testies, ovaries, placenta and the adrenal cortex. The nature of the **steroids** are exclusively dependent upon the various functional moieties attached on the steroid nucleus plus the side chains at C-17 which in turn attribute classical and extremely specific spectrum of biological activities *e.g.,* anti-inflammatory agents, antifertility agents, contraceptives, oestrogenic agents, sterility profile and the like.

Microorganisms invariably do play a vital and pivotal role in the steroid bioconversions as enumerated below in a sequential order:

a. *Corynebacterium simplex* aids in the dehydrogenation of **cortisone** to yield **prednisone**
b. *Rhizopus arrhizus* (a *fungal* sp.) helps in the hydroxylation of **progesterone** therapy giving rise to the corresponding steroid **11α-hydroxyprogesterone** by introducing an O-atom at C-11 position.
c. *Rhizopus nigricans* (a *fungal* sp.) is also able to hydroxylate progesterone to give rise to the formation of 11α-hydroxyprogesterone.
d. *Corynebacterium* simplex may cause the effective dehydrogenation of either **cortisol** or **hydrocortisone** to yield **prednisolone.**
e. *Nocardia restrictus* affords the biotransformation of **δ4–cholestene-19-hydroxy-3-one** into the desired **oestrone.**
f. *Cunninghamella blakesleeana* (a *fungus* sp.) aids the hydroxylation of **cortexolone** to form **11-hydroxy cortisone** by the introduction of an O-atom at C-11 position strategically.
g. **Yeast strains** also cause conversion of **androstendione** into the corresponding male-sexhormone **testosterone.**

Interestingly, in the typical steroid bioconversion *via* fermentative procedures the desired microorganism, *Rhizopus nigricans,* is allowed to grow in a fermentation tank charged with an appropriate growth culture medium along with optimized incubation parameters to **accomplish biomass** upto the maximum possible extent. It is, however, pertinent to mention here that the ensuing fermentation procedures essentially require both **aeration** and **agitation** to accomplish rapid growth. Hence, it is always preferred to incorporate **steroid** (*e.g., progesterone*) right into the **bioreactor** loaded with *Rhizopus nigricans.* The end-product is subsequently recovered with **methylene chloride,** adequately purified by chromatography, and ultimately obtained in its purest form by recrystallization.

Generally, the **bioconversion of steroids** is invariably accomplished by employing exclusively the *submerged aeration technique* carried out in SS-tanks (fermentors) charged with *minimal nutritional quantities* so as to permit the maximum ease and conversion with regard to the extraction and purification of the ultimate desired transformation substance.

In usual practice, the fermentative procedure is adopted efficiently by either of the *two* following phases, namely:

Phase-I: It represents predominantly the **'growth phase'** whereby the maximum extent of the *culture-growth* is accomplished. And for the culture-growth one may require both optimized temperature and aeration parameters. However, the duration of incubation solely depends upon the type of culture being employed, such as: **bacteria:** 12–24 hrs; **fungi:** 24–72 hours. Besides, one must adhere to strict environmental conditions as per the laid-out norms.

Phase-II: When the **'growth-phase'** almost comes to an end, the careful addition of the respectively steroid commences. In certain instances, one may carry out the addition of steroid very much along with the inoculation procedure. Importantly, the quantum of steroid need to be added solely depends upon *three* vital components, namely:

(*a*) Transforming capacity of culture; (*b*) potential toxicity of substrate; and (*c*) nature of product. It has been duly observed that **deoxycorticosterone** possesses an appreciable antifungal activity. It is absolutely essential to contain the **'problem of toxicity'** in the *culture medium* by subjecting to either continuous or periodic incorporation of substrate into the fermentation vessel. The organic solvents that are utilized profusely may include: **acetone, ethanol,** and **methanol,** which essentially contribute *two* main advantageous factors, such as: (*a*) afford relatively low toxicity for the conversion enzymes; and (*b*) cause appreciable solubility of steroids. Importantly, **dimethylformamide** (DMF) does possess an exceptional solubility characteristic feature for **steroids;** whereas it's non-toxic level stands at below 2% concentration in the culture medium.

It is, however, pertinent to state here that the **'bioconversion capacity'** actually based upon the *load of the prevailing substrate,* and the ability of the *microorganism.*Questions

Questions

1. Discuss applications of biotransformation process in steroids. (JNTUA-May 2009)
2. Add short note on selection of organism for biotransformation process. (JNTUA-Nov 2010)
3. How the design of biotransformation process is performed? Explain. (JNTUA-May 2009)
4. Explain the biotransformation of steroids in detail. (JNTUA-May 2009)
5. What is Biotransformation? Give detailed account on the design of biotransformation sses. (JNTUA-Nov 2010)
6. Write in detail about recombinant DNA technology. Write about the production of Insulin by recombinant DNA technology. (MGRU 2004)
7. Define and classify sterilization. (MGRU 2004)
8. Define microbial biotransformation. Explain the type of reaction. (MGRU Apr-2004)
9. Outline the biotransformation of steroids. (MGRU Apr-2004)
10. Single cell protein. (MGRU Apr-2004)
11. Give in detail about preparation of any one antibiotic by fermentation process. (MGRU 2002)
12. Define microbial transformation? How to synthesis steroid from sterol using microbes. (MGRU 2004)

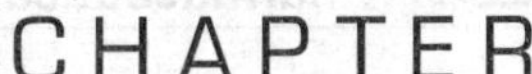

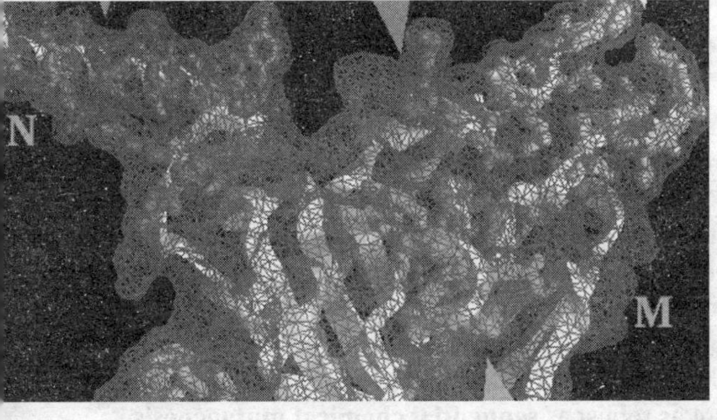

CHAPTER

3

Genetic Recombination

3.1 Introduction

Kark Ereky, the famous Hungarian agricultural economist, was the first to have coined the terminology—**'biotechnology'** in the year 1919; and since then, it has now become more or less a *'buzword'* in the enormous development of medicines, wines, enzymes, agricultural production, animal production, gene-therapy, cloning and the like. With the advent of sea-change in the armamentarium of biotechnological progress in the past several decades based on the glaring fact that there could be a tremendous potential to produce altogether newer range of **'products'** from raw materials with the help of the **'living organisms'** exclusively*.

The past 25 years have witnessed an astronomical progress amalgamated with immense and intense *'practical realization'* of **'biotechnology'** which has paved the way to enable the present day medical scientists to detect, isolate, generate as well as characterize the various proteins which are intimately associated with the appropriate and desired coordination of the innumerable essential functionalities related to perfect human life and health. It has been adequately observed and demonstrated that numerous *in vivo* phenomena which are ascertained to be significantly causative in pathophysiological imbalance may not only be judiciously identified, but also be reasonably rectified/ manipulated so as to regain the much desired normal functionalities in humans.

It is, however, pertinent to mention here that this comparatively latest new methodology and technology essentially involves the marked and pronounced synergism of discoveries in recombinant DNA methodology, DNA alteration, gene-splicing, genetic engineering, immunology, and immunopharmacology, with progressive and remarkable advances in the area of *'automation'* and *'data-analysis'* to evolve not only a cogent but also a 'high-tech' industry in the near future.

In a broader perspective the **'genetic recombination'** means—*'the joining of gene combinations in the offspring that were not present in the parents'*.

Hopwood, between 1977–1979, has thoroughly discussed the potential applications and utilities of genetic **'recombination'** in industrial streptomycetes. Subsequently, within a span of 10 year *i.e.,* between 1977–1986 several researchers* have put forward articulated efficient methodologies for the genetic recombination by means of **protoplast-fusion.** Ironically, enormous valuable information's available with regard to *protoplast fusion,* an appreciable volume of specific examples of applications of recombination to **strain-improvement** are lacking significantly.

The *two* cardinal possibilities in support of this lack of information's are:

a. Most successful applications/utilities have been reserved as **'proprietary information'** and

b. Prevailing recombination perhaps is not as robust as **sequential chemical mutagenesis.**

Therefore, one may infer judiciously that even if the prevailing recombination is not as robust as the random mutagenesis in the ensuing process of strain development, it is certainly and gainfully beneficial for the construction of recombinant entities having specific useful traits which may not be readily generated by mutagenesis. It is pertinent to mention here that under such a situation, it is invariably useful to make use of recombination as a **'complementary method'** to further augment **random mutagenesis exclusively for the strain development.**

Interestingly, the *'mother nature'* since 3.5 billion years has been both actively and passively, covertly and overtly engaged in carrying out what we may most legitimately term as the **'natural genetic experiments'** in this Universe. These accomplishments could only be materialized by the aid of the following intricate and complicated biological processes taking place *in vivo,* such as:

- *Mutation: i.e.,* random heredity alteration;
- **Crossing-over:** *i.e.,* breakage and exchange of corresponding segments of the homologous chromosomes;
- *Recombination at meiosis: i.e.,* fertilization.

In downright reality, these aforesaid biological phenomena have immensely participated and positively contributed to the current diversity of life in this world. Besides, there exists plethora of historical and scientific evidences that stand to prove that humans have been also actively engaged in manipulating genetic characteristic features of various species since more than 10,000 years *via* extensive and intensive experiments related to the *two* vital and pivotal aspects, namely; (*a*) **inbreeding;** and (*b*) **cross-breeding.**

The various glorious accomplishments of the human endeavors may be summarized as stated below:

- Modern robust strains of wheat, corn, high-yielding rice which are a far cry from their primitive and puny ancestors.
- Varied breeds of cows, sheep, poultry, dogs, cats etc.,
- Development of larger and sweeter oranges, grapes, seedless, watermelons, papaya, vegetables, and also the flamboyant ornamental decorative plants.
- Hybridizations: *e.g.,* **tangelo** *i.e.,* crossing the tangerine and the grapefruit; **mule** *i.e.,* crossing a donkey and a horse; *alsatian dog i.e.,* crossing a German Shephard dog and a wild wolf (often used for police work).
- **Hybrid Antibiotics:** Hopwood *et al.** in 1985 were pioneer in producing *hybrid antibiotics*—the ones produced by a genetic hybrid. A **hybrid antibiotic** may be regarded as an entity that may essentially and predominantly embody the structural features invariably found in two altogether different metabolites and thereby represent the formation of a newer 'natural product'.

It is, however, pertinent to state here at this point in time that the latter specific feature does not necessarily draw a line of distinction of the *hybrid antibiotics* from relatively older techniques adopted for the production of newer antibiotics, for instance:

- Precursor-directed biosynthesis
- Mutasynthesis

- Hybrid biosynthesis
- Protoplast fusion
- Intraspecific mating
- Biotransformation methods

Another school of thought believes the **'hybrid antibiotics'** simply as a bunch of *'new metabolites'* that may crop up from the novel and unique combinations of genes, accomplished by the introduction of genes from one microorganisms into another or due to the *targeted mutation* of the **secondary metabolism genes** very much within the same microorganism.

Sadee 1987 in his rather most compelling article postulated a **'third revolution in modern medicine'** in which he has revealed critically that practically most of the gross structures and physical characteristics of every organism owes its origin exclusively and primarily to the *'genetic code'* inherited and strategically located within the nucleus of each cell. Importantly, the main building blocks of the cellular structure *vis-à-vis* architecture rest upon the carbohydrates, proteins, lipids and the nucleic acid. **Enzymes** that predominantly represent a special class of proteins invariably build and utilize these prevailing molecules all along the various stages of cell transformations, namely: maturation, maintenance, and finally reproduction.

3.2 Transformation [Synonym: Metamorphosis]

Transformation (or **metamorphosis**) refers to a specific type of mutation occurring in bacteria. It results from DNA of a bacterial cell penetrating the host cell and finally becoming incorporated into the genotype of the host.

In a generalized expression one may regard the uptake of **'foreign DNA'** (or **transgenes**) by the aid of the plant cells as a marked and pronounced biological phenomenon termed as **transformation.** In actual practice, a plethora of well-defined processes and techniques have been developed, tried and tested so as to introduce meticulously the *'transgenes'* into the plant cells. However, one may categorize the **foreign DNA** (or **transgenes**) into the following *two* major groups, namely:

a. Agrobacterium Mediated Gene Transfer, and
b. Direct Gene Transfer.

Nevertheless, the aims and objectives of the study shall normally determine largely the nature and type of plant cells essentially used for the ensuing **'transformation'.**

Example: Gene regulation studies must meet the following *vital cell criteria* as enumerated under:

i. Cells should be competent enough to take up DNA and thereafter initiate the expression of transgene,
ii. Production of transgenic tissues the cells should also be meristematic, and
iii. Transgenic plants may be produced only when the cells do possess the ability to regenerate complete plants.

Interestingly, in plants the **'stable transformation'** are of *two types*, namely: (*a*) **Non-integrative stable transformation*** *i.e.,* when the transgene is maintained in quite stable status in an extra chromosomal state, such as: **virus vectors;** and (*b*) **Integrative stable transformation** *i.e.,* when the transgene becomes integrated into the plant genome and are heritable in nature.

3.2.1 Agrobacterium-Mediated Gene Transfer

It has been duly established that gene transfer through *Agrobacterium* is invariably accomplished in the following *two* methods:

3.2.1.1 Co-culture with Tissue Explants

In actual practice, the *'suitable gene construct'* is strategically inserted carefully very much within the T-region of a disarmed Ti plasmid; and for this one may use either a *'cointegrate'* or a *'binary vector'*. Consequently, the **'recombinant vector'** is placed carefully in the *Agrobacterium* that is invariably co-cultured with the plant cells or tissues' to be transformed for about 48 hours.

Importantly, in the instance of several plant species, normally *'small leaf-discs'* (having a few mm diameter) are cut carefully from the surface of pre-sterilized leaves the subsequently employed for co-cultivation, such as: *tobacco, tomato, petunia* etc. Consequently, the **'transgene'** thus accomplished essentially comprises of a *specific selectable reporter gene e.g.,* the 'bacterial *neo* genene'. The resulting *neo* gene is strategically hooked on the *appropriate regulatory sequences* which are found to be functional in plant cells. In actual practice, such a *'gene'* is invariably termed as **chimaceric gene** because it predominantly consists sequences derived from several different genes.

It has been duly observed that in the course of **leaf disc agrobacterium co-culture,** a chemical entity known as **acetosyringone** duly released by plant cells thereby causing specific induction of the **vir genes** that particularly afford the plausible transfer of **recombinant T-DNA** into a plethora of the prevailing plant cells. In doing so the resulting T-DNA would eventually get integrated into the *plant genome;* and hence, the **transgene** would be expressed. Consequently, the *transformed plant cells* will become resistant to **kanamycin** (an antibiotic) on account of the expression of **neo gene.** After a gap of 48 hours, the treated leaf-discs are meticulously transferred onto a generation medium containing suitable concentrations of both *kanamycin* and *carbenicillin* as shown in Fig. 3.1. The two *'antibodies'* do play specific roles, namely:

a. **Kanamycin**—permits exclusively the *'transformed plant cells'* to undergo division and regeneration of **'shoots'** in 3–4 weeks duration; and *b.* **Carbenicillin**—helps in killing *Agrobacterium* cells only. At this stage, the shoots are adequately separated, rooted, and ultimately transferred into the prepared soil-bed.

Salient Features: The prevalent salient features of co-culture with tissue explants are as enumerated under:

1. The agro *bacterium* does infect certain specific **monocot** plant species and ultimately gives rise to the formation of **crowngall cells,** such as: *Asparagus* or causes apparent swellings, for instance: *Allium cepa, Dioscorea bulbifera,* besides *Chlorophytum* and *Narcissus.* In most of these instances, the critical production of the **opines** by the corresponding crown gall cells and swelling tissues was noticed evidently.
2. Besides, the integration of T-DNA into the genomes of at least two plant species, namely: *Dioscorea bulbifera* and *Orzyza sativa* has been well established and amply demonstrated. Nevertheless, the efficiency of transformation is observed to be at low ebb.
3. Importantly, an appreciably efficient degree of transformation of the *monocot cells* may be accomplished by the induction of **acetosyringone** in the course of co-culture of plant cells with the aid of *Agrobacterium.*
4. A few plant species are found to secrete such chemical entities that essentially and precisely inhibit the usual induction of the *vir operons* by **acetosyringone.** *Example:* Secretion of 2, 4-dihydroxy-7-methoxy-1, 4-benzoxazin 3-one (DIMBOA) that specifically inhibits **vir gene induction;** and this problem may be circumvented by adding an excess of acetosyringone. However, this technique help in the successful transformation in several cereal species *e.g., barley, maize, rice* and *wheat.*

3.2.1.2 In Planta Transformation

It has been observed that inhibition of *Arabidopsis* seeds in the freshly prepared cultures of *Agrobacterium* ultimately gives rise to the stable integration of T-DNA strategically present in the *Arabidopsis* genome. It seems that the prevailing *Agrobacterium* cells eventually gain entry into the corresponding seedlings in the course of the germination process, are adequately held up within the plants; and subsequently, when flowers undergo the process of development (*i.e.,* blooming) they ultimately transform either the ensuing **'zygotes'** or the **'cells'** which yield zygote.

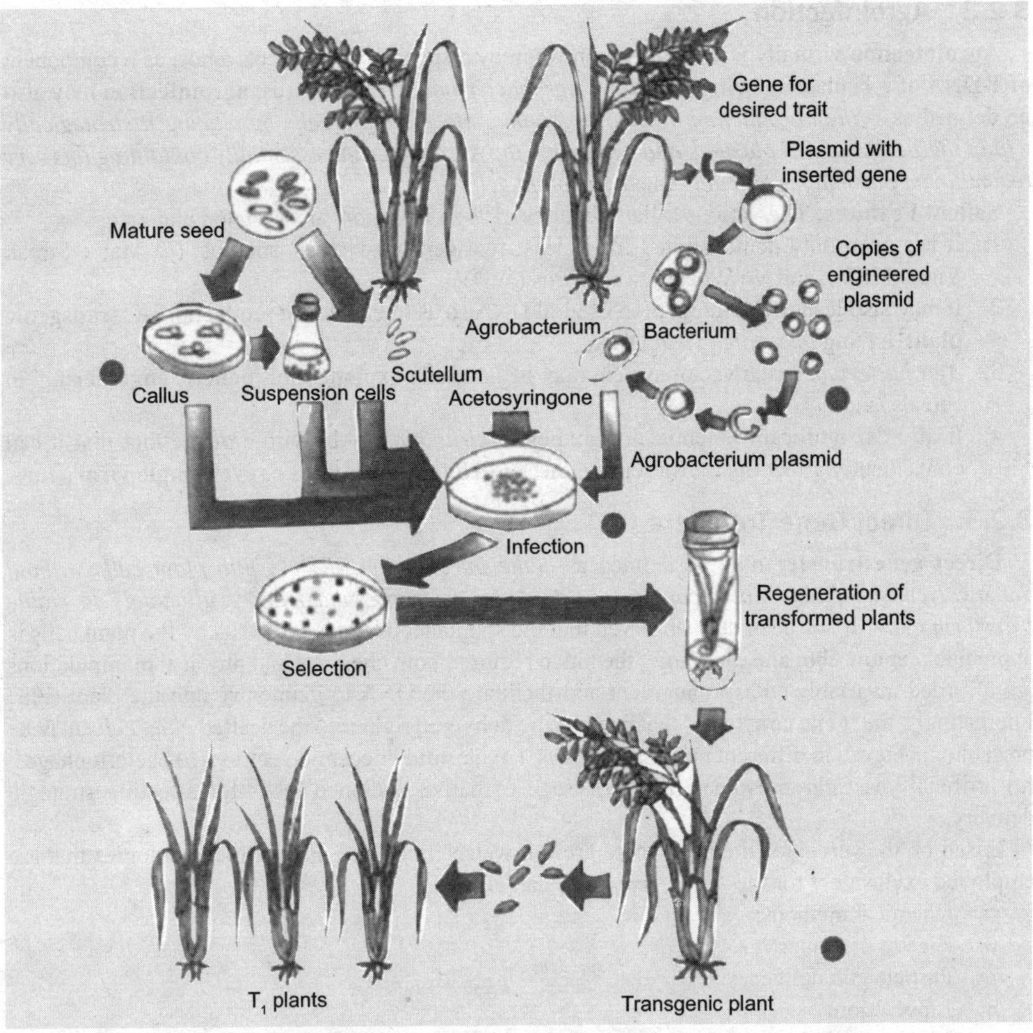

Fig. 3.1 *A Sequential Diagrammatic Representation of the Methodology for Agrobacterium-Mediated Gene Transfer.*

Another viable and feasible approach is invariably accomplished when the *'just budding flowers'* of the *Arabidopsis* plants are duly dipped into a freshly prepared culture of *Agrobacterium,* and subsequently a partial vacuum is generated so as to augment and facilitate entry of the corresponding **bacterial cells** right into the body of the exposed plants. Consequently, the plants are allowed to grow, selfed, and the *'progeny'* thus obtained are subjected to vigorous methodical screening for the identification of the **generated transformants.**

Advantages: The various glaring advantages of the *two* aforesaid approaches of *Agrobacterium* transformation methodologies are as given below:

a. Absolute elimination of the need for regeneration from the **tissue explants,**

b. Methodologies involved are relatively not so cumbersome and easy; and, therefore, may be adapted with other plant species with an equally **high successful rate,**

c. possess little risk of **'somaclonal variation',** although the probability for the mutations independent of stable T-DNA integrations do prevaily by virtue of the incidence of the abortive T-DNA insertions.

3.2.2 Agroinfection

Agroinfection virtually is a phenomenon whereby a specific virus infects a host as a component of T-DNA of a Ti plasmid being carried by *Agrobacterium.* In other words, **agroinfection** may also be defined as—*'the introduction of a viral genome into the plant cells by placing it strategically within the T-DNA of a Ti plasmid, and employing the Agrobacterium essentially containing this very recombinant plasmid for co-culture with the plant cells'.*

Salient Features: The various salient features of *'agroinfection'* are as stated under:

1. It has been duly demonstrated for at least two germini-viruses, such as: (*a*) Maize Streak Virus (MSV); and (*b*) Wheat Dwarf Virus (WDV),
2. It may also lead to the integration of viral DNA so as to enable the production of **'transgenic plant'** having *integrated viral* DNA.
3. *Agrobacterium* based vector system may be gainfully exploited for **'genetic engineering'** in cereals, and
4. It affords significant potential for studies in *virus biology* by virtue of the fact that it can conveniently affect the transference either of **deletion mutations** or even **single viral genes.**

3.2.3 Direct Gene Transfers

Direct gene transfer may be defined as—*'the introduction of DNA into plant cells without the involvement of any biological agent e.g., Agrobacterium, and leading ultimately to stable transformation'.* It has been duly observed that the spontaneous uptake of DNA by the plant cells is appreciably at low ebb; and, therefore, the much required both chemical and physical manipulations are afforded invariably so as to augment and facilitate the DNA to gain entry into the plant cells. Interestingly, the **'gene construct'** that needs to be delivered right into the desired *plant cells* may be present or achieved in different manners, such as: (*a*) plasmid or cosmid vectors; (*b*) bacteriophages; (*c*) artificial yeast chromosomes; and (*d*) usage of native uncloned DNA for affecting strategic delivery.

Based on the survey of literature there are **ten** well-defined and distinct methodologies that are employed exclusively for the *'direct transfer'*, namely:

i. Chemical methods;
ii. Electro oration;
iii. Particle gun delivery;
iv. Lipofection;
v. Microinjection;
vi. Macroinjection;
vii. Pollen transformation;
viii. DNA Delivery *via* growing pollen tubes;
ix. Laser-induced gene transfer;
x. Fiber-mediated gene transfer; and
xi. Transformation by ultrasonication.

Each of the aforesaid method shall be treated individually in the section that follows:

3.2.3.1 Chemical Methods

It has been duly established that there are certain chemical substances, such as: polyethylene glycol (PEG), polyvinyl alcohol (PVA), and calcium phosphate [$Ca_3(PO_4)_2$] predominantly increase the uptake of DNA by the plant protoplasts exclusively and squarely.

PEG-Mediated DNA Delivery. The various sequential generalized steps adopted for the PEG mediated DNA delivery are as stated under:

1. The plant protoplasts are suitably suspended in a *transformation medium* enriched with Mg^{2+} ions instead of the Ca^{2+} ions.

2. Linearized plasmid DNA essentially having the *'gene construct'* is carefully added into the protoplast suspension obtained in (1) above.
3. To the resulting solution PEG (20% concentration) is added and pH adjusted to 8.0
4. The *'protoplasts'* thus obtained is subjected to a five-minute **thermal-shock treatment** at 45°C followed by an immediate transfer to **ice** just prior to the addition of DNA, because it significantly enhances the frequency of transformation by **several orders of magnitude.**

[**Note:** Carrier DNA incorporation at this specific stage does promote transformation; however, in actual practice it is neither desirable nor necessary at all.]

5. After a certain stipulated duration of *'incubation'*, the prevailing concentration of PEG is reduced adequately while that of CA^{2+} ion is increased appreciably in order to accomplish an **enhanced transformation frequency.**

Example: Transformation of tobacco protoplasts **(Necotiana):**

It has been observed that when the **'synchronized tobacco protoplasts'** subjected to transformation either in the course of *mitotic phase* or *S-phase* give rise to the formation of **3% transformed colonies;** whereas, the corresponding **'non synchronized tobacco protoplasts'** yielded only 1.5% effective transformation.

In actual practice, the treated protoplasts are ultimately cultured so as to regenerate adequately **cell wall** and thereby produce **callus colonies** from which the desired plants regenerated subsequently. It is, however, pertinent to state here that the proper use of a **'selectable marker'** would certainly go a long way for the judicious selection of the transformed protoplasts in an appreciable extent.

3.2.3.2 Electroporation

Electroporation may be defined as—*'the legitimate introduction of DNA into the cells by exposing them critically for specific very short durations directly to the electrical pulses of high-voltage field strength which perhaps induced transient pores in the plasma lemma'.*

Importantly, these generated/applied electrical pulses invariably enhance the permeability of protoplast membrane and evidently facilitates the logical entry of DNA molecules right into the cells, provided the DNA is in direct contact with the membrane desirably. In general, there are basically **two** marked and pronounced systems of electroporation, namely: (*a*) low-voltage long-pulses method; and (*b*) high-voltage short-pulses method.

Example: Tobacco mesophyll protoplasts: The actual *realistic* values are as given below:

First instance:

Low-voltage long-pulses method: 300–400 V cm^{-1} for 10–15 ms
(milliseconds; exponential decay);

Second instance:

High-voltage short-pulses method: 1000–1500 V cm^{-1} for 10 μs.
(Microseconds; square-wave pulse generators);

Fig. 3.2(*a*) illustrates the details of the output characteristic featurs of the two principal types of electroporation methods in actual usage *viz.*, high-voltage short pulse machine, and low voltage exponential decay machine; wherein pulse duration (mS) is plotted along the X-axis and voltage (V) along the Y-axis.

Fig. 3.2(*b*) depicts the **'circuit-diagram'** of a low voltage, exponential decay machine.

Salient Features of Electroporation

The various salient features of *'electroporation'* are as enumerated under:

1. In a broader perspective, low-voltage long-pulses technique give rise to relatively high rates of transient **transformation;** whereas, high-voltage short-pulses method produce usually high rates of **stable transformation.**

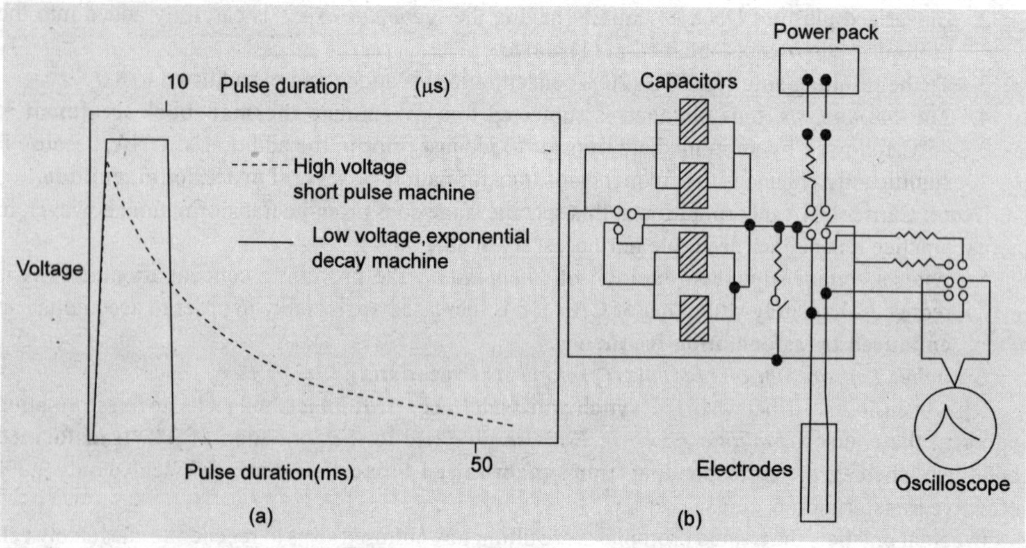

Fig. 3.2 *(a) Output Characteristic Features of Two Major Type of Electriporation Devices; and (b) Circuit Diagram of Low Voltage Decay Machine.*

2. In several extensive and intensive studies in electroporation experimental parameters yielding almost 50% protoplast viable survival may invariably give the highest rates of **stable transformation.**
3. The *transformation frequencies* may be critically enhanced by several-fold by means of the following *two* manners, namely:
   a. Sudden thermal-shock treatment (45ºC) to the ensuing protoplasts just before electroporation, and
   b. Presence of low concentration (~ 8%) of PEG in the course of electroporation.
4. Certain plant species are found to be appreciably sensitive to PEG; and hence, *electroporation* may be adopted as the *'method of choice'*.
5. A plethora of plant species are amenable to PEG-induced gene transfer (see section 2.3.1); and, therefore, is regarded to be much more efficient, dependable and reliable in comparison to *electroporation.*
6. *Electroporation* has been successfully and gainfully expoited to afford the production of fairly **stable transformed cell-lines** and/or **plants in several plant species,** such as; maize, petunia, rice, tobacco, wheat, sorghum, etc.

   Example: **For Tobacco:** The frequency of transformation was quite high and ranged between 2–8% (in the presence of 7% PEG).
7. *Electroporation* has been employed fruitfully to deliver strategically DNA into the intact plant cells.
8. In accomplishing *electroporation* the corresponding transformation frequencies may be adequately improved upon by adopting any one of the following *four* means, namely:
   a. Employing field strength of 1.25 kV cm^{-1},
   b. Incorporating PEG after addition of DNA,
   c. thermal-shock treatment of protoplasts at 45ºC for 5 minutes prior to the addition of DNA, and
   d. Specifically employing **'linear DNA'** instead of **'circular DNA'.**

3.2.3.3 Particle Gun Delivery [Synonyms: Biolistic or Ballistic Method of DNA Delivery]

In early 1990s, the **particle gun delivery** method was conceived and put into practice which essentially made use of 1–2 μm **tungsten** or **gold** particles, precoated with the DNA to be employed exclusively for transformation, are adequately accelerated to such a degree of velocities that gainfully enable their entry right into either the plant cells or the nuclei. In reality the actual **'particle acceleration'** is accomplished by employing an appropriate and specific device that precisely varies both in design as well as function. There are *two* most effective and equally successful devices that usually aid in causing acceleration of the particles, namely:

a. Utilization of pressurized helium gas, and

b. Utilization of the released electrostatic energy by a droplet of water after exposure to a very high voltage.

Interestingly, the relatively earlier devices actually employed **blank cartridges** *via* a sophisticated and modified firing mechanism to afford the needed energy for the particle acceleration; and this perhaps originated the nomenclature **particle gun** to this type of approach.

Helium pressurized device: The *helium pressurized device* mainly comprise of the following essential components, such as:

i. Gas-acceleration tube;

ii. Rupture disc;

iii. Stopping screen;

iv. Macro carrier carrying particles precoated with DNA; and

v. Target cells as shown in Fig. 3.3.

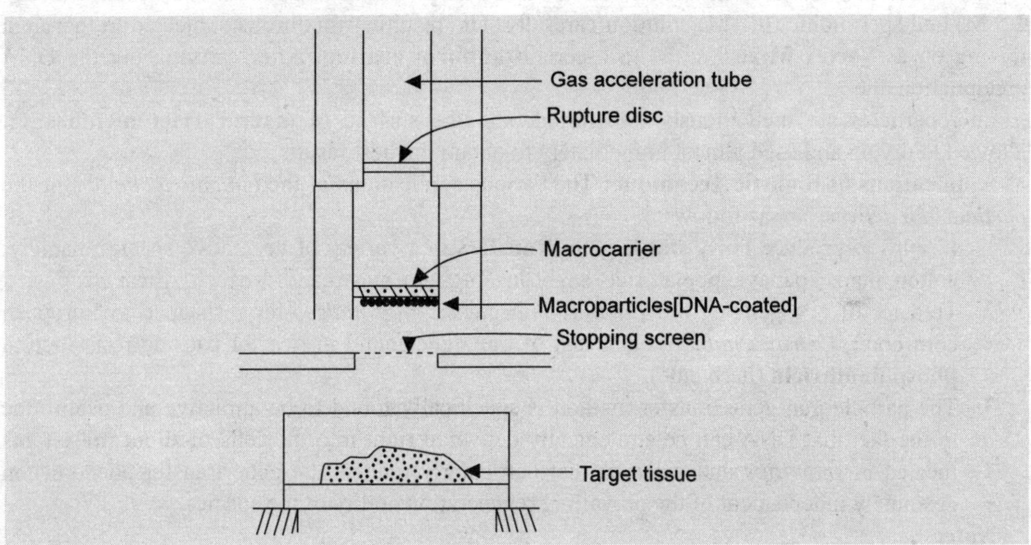

Fig. 3.3 *A Helium Pressurized Device Particle Gun Involved in DNA Delivery Showing Macroparticles Coated with DNA being conveyed in the Target Tissue.*

The aforesaid components (*i*) through (*v*) are sequentially enclosed in a **chamber** so as to enable creation of partial vacuum that precisely facilitates particle acceleration and thereby causes reduction in damage to plant cells. Once the partial vacuum is affected in the *gas acceleration tube,* adequately pressurized helium gas is made to release in the said tube in order to break the strategically positioned rupture disc. In this manner the **helium shock waves** are generated that *specifically accelerates the macroprojectile to which the DNA-coated microprojectiles are attached duly.* Thus, the **macroprojectile** is adequately retained by a stopping screen, while the **microprojectiles** pass *via* this screen and ultimately get embedded right into the **target tissue** cells meticulously positioned 10 mm below the stopping screen.

Notes:

1. Helium is invariably preferable to air by virtue of the fact it is not only lighter but also offers several advantages options.
2. In actual practice a 1000 psi (pounds per square inch) of pressurized helium gas is employed for causing acceleration.

Macrocarrier (Macroprojectile): It is a 2.5 cm diameter having 0.06 mm thickness plastic membrane that is usually employed once only. Its light mass usually affords rapid advantageous acceleration.

Microparticles (Microprojectiles or Microcarriers): They normally vary in diameter from 0.5 to 0.2 μm. However, the average size of 1.0 μm is employed commonly.

a. **Tungsten Particles:** These are relatively cheaper, with usual irregular shape and size, found to be toxic to some specific cell types, and exhibit **surface oxidation** that may ultimately lead to precipitation of DNA. Besides, they have a tendency to form aggregates after the addition of DNA and this gives rise to the reduction of **expected particle dispersion.**

b. **Gold Particles:** These are found to be comparatively more uniform in size (1–3 μm) and shape. They usually exhibit *lower toxicity, variable degree of coating with DNA,* and hence are much **more expensive.**

DNA-Coating: The most critical factor with regard to the coating of microparticles with DNA is normally achieved through precipitation. In actual practice, it may be accomplished by mixing together 1.25–18 mg microparticles and 0.5–70 μg of the plasmid DNA in a calcium chloride (0.25–2.5 M) and spermidine (0.1 M) solution carefully. The resulting mixture is subjected to thorough mixing on a **'Vortex Mixer'** so as to ascertain **uniform coating.** After carrying out the DNA precipitation, the

microparticles are meticulously transferred onto the surface of **macrocarrier membranes,** allowed to dry up and used almost immediately to obtain the best results,

Applications of Biolistic Technique: The various applications of the *biolistic technique* or the *particle gun delivery* are as follows:

1. It helps to produce fairly **stable gene transfers** in a variety of vegetative species, namely; cotton, maize, papaya, poplar, rice, soybean, sorghum, sugarcane, tobacco, wheat etc.
2. Transfer of **cry gene*** from *Bacillus thurigiensis into maize;* for resistance to European corn-borer, *Ostrinia nubialis;* and that of **bar gene** found in rice for causing resistance to **phosphinothricin** (herbicide).
3. The particle gun gene transfer method is specifically found to be attractive and useful due to the fact that DNA can be strategically delivered right into the cells of **shoot meristems** located in *short tips* and *embryos* that particularly renders the gene transfer phenomenon absolutely independent of the prevailing regeneration ability of the species.

Note:

a. Biolistic technique is virtually applicable to all plants species and may even be extended to the animal cells as well.

b. Its only major constrain/limitation being the rather expensive specialized acceleration device (*i.e.,* the particle gun).

3.2.3.4 Lipofection

Lipofection may be defined as—*'the introduction of DNA into cells via liposomes'*. It is considered to be the ultimate method of choice for DNA delivery into the animal cells particularly when being cultured *in vitro.*

Lipofection also enjoys the reputation of being one of the initial few methods of delivering DNA into the plant protoplasts. However, the transformation frequencies of the order of 4×10^{-5} have been observed. The *integrated DNA* evidently does not undergo rearrangements; however, multiple copies may obviously get integrated in *tandem*.

Special Features: Following are the *two* special characteristic features of *'lipofection'* namely:

1. Invariably, plasmid DNAs 9 kb, and of even larger dimensions have been adequately integrated quite intact.
2. Higher *transformation frequencies* with PEG and *electroporation* render them even more attractive.

3.2.3.5 Microinjection

In the event of **microinjection,** the DNA solution is injected almost directly right inside the cell by the help of *capillary glass micropipettes* using *micromanipulators* of a microinjection set of apparatus.

It has been demonstrated amply via actual experimental procedures that it is much more convenient and efficacious to make use of *'protoplasts'* instead of the *'cells'* because the cell-wall specifically gives rise to serious interference with the process of microinjection.

Salient Features: Following are some of the most important salient features of microinjection, such as:

1. Process of microinjection is technically not only demanding but also time-consuming *i.e.*, one may microinject upto 50 protoplasts in a span of 60 minutes.
2. Quite successful transformation by microinjection of cells and protoplasts has been accomplished in *Brassica* sp., alfalfa, tobacco etc., with achievable **transformation frequencies** ranging from 14 to 66%. However, the corresponding results with cereals are rather not so encouraging.
3. In order to achieve high transformation rates, it is a must to incorporate the DNA right into the nucleus or the cytoplasm of the specific cell. Hence, the success rate is found to be the highest with particularly the non-vacuolated embryonic cells and the densely cytoplasmic ones. A logical and plausible explanation with respect to the extremely low transformation rates amongst large vacuolated cells is due to the DNA being delivered into the vacuole directly which gets degraded consequently.

3.2.3.6 Macroinjection

Macroinjection may be defined as—*'injection of plasmid DNA (or uncloned native DNA) right into the lumen of developing inflorescence* using a hypodermic syringe.'*

It has been adequately advocated that the DNA is usually taken up by *microspores* in the course of certain particular state of their development. In 1987, an attempt was made to inject DNA specifically in the developing inflorescene of rye; and eventually a rather much lower frequency (0.07%) of the *transformed plants* was recovered in the progeny. In reality, the concept of macroinjection is quite easy and simple; however, the *two* glaring problems encountered are, namely: (*a*) poor attainable **frequency;** and (*b*) inconsistency in achievable **stable transformants.**

Table 3.1 summarize the characteristic features with respect to the vital and pivotal **DNA delivery techniques** for the **plant cells** exclusively.

Table 3.1 *Comparison of Certain Vital and Pivotal DNA Delivery Techniques for the Plant Cells*

S.No	Characteristic Features	DNA Delivery	Techniques		
		Agrobacterium Mediated	Chemical and Electrical	Microinjection	Particle Gun
1.	1. DNA construct (Max. size)	< 50 kb	5–20 kb	16 kb	–

S.No	Characteristic Features	DNA Delivery Techniques			
		Agrobacterium Mediated	Chemical and Electrical	Microinjection	Particle Gun
2.	Plant Range(s)	Restricted	All plants	All plants	All plants
3.	Obtainable efficiency	Relatively	Relatively	—	–
4.	Integrity of DNA insert.	Not affected by rearrangements	High degree of rearrangements	—	High degree of rearrangements
5.	Number of copies integrated.	Invariably single or a few copies	High frequency of multicopy insertions.	1 to 5	High frequency of multicopy insertions.
6.	Special equipment required	No	No (chemical) Yes (Electrical)	Yes	Yes
7.	Regeneration protocol	Needed	Needed	Needed quite often	Not necessary (use of embryos and shoot tips)
8.	Protoplasts culture	Not required	Necessary	May be required	Not needed
9.	Applicable to organized meristems	No	No	Yes	Yes
10.	Applicability to cereals	Applicable	Used frequently	Possible	Applicability high
11.	Chimeric plants	No	No	Quite often (in case of meristems employed)	Quite often (in case meri stems bomarded)

3.2.3.7 Pollen Transformation

It has been duly reported by some researchers that **'gene transfer'** could be accomplished by simply allowing DNA to soak in *pollen grains* just prior to their actual usage for **pollination.** It is, however, pertinent to state here that these studies failed to be substantiated by other researchers who specifically made use of **'cloned genes'**. Though apparently the proposed methodology seems to be quite attractive bearing in mind its overall applicability and superb simplicity, yet till date there exists little definitive evidence and ample proof for a **transgene** being actually transferred by the air of pollen soaked in the DNA solution.

3.2.3.8 DNA Delivery via Growing Pollen Tubes

In this specific technique, first of all the **stigma** of a flower is carefully incised sometime after its *pollination;* and *secondly* the **DNA solution** is duly smeared onto the incised surface painstakingly. In actual practice the accurate and precise **'time of stigma excision'** shall virtually depend upon the *rate of pollen-tube growth* that may vary from 5–20 minutes to 2–3 hours.

Examples:

i. **Rice:** In this particular instance the plasmid DNA containing *nptil* **gene** was duly applied onto the incised surface of the stigma. Consequently, 20% of the seeds thus obtained actually showed the presence of *nptil* **gene** in copy numbers varying from 1-300.

ii. **Barley:** In this case, the following observations were made, namely:
- transformation frequency ranged between 10^{-3} to 10^{-4} of the seedlings thus accomplished
- expression level of *nptil* **gene** was rather low
- both mature plants and their corresponding progeny failed to show any *nptil* **expression.**

Special Notes: Following are some of the *'special notes'* with respct to the DNA delivery *via* growing pollen tubes:

1. Methodology may be promising, easy and simple but its integrity with respect to its *consistency in results* and *stable transformations* are yet questionable, and
2. Two vital aspects, such as: mechanism of DNA transfer into the zygotes, and supporting factors affecting it must be studied more intensively and aggressively.

3.2.3.9 Laser-Induced Gene Transfer

The application of laser has been employed effectively and successfully for high frequency (10^{-3}) **transfection** of animal cells. In reality, the lasers puncture transient holes in the cell membrane specifically *via* which DNA would gain entry into the cell cytoplasm. In fact, the usage of lasers to afford delivery of DNA into the plant cells was a pretty long practice; however, there is little available information(s) with regard to its **transient expression** or **stable integration.**

3.2.3.10 Fibre-Mediated Gene Transfer

In this specific and articulated approach the DNA is strategically delivered into the *cell cytoplasm* and *nucleus* by means of the **silicon-carbide fibres** having 0.6 µm diameter and 10 µm length.

The methodology essentially involves the intermixing of **suspension culture cells** and **plasmid DNA** having *gus* **gene** along with the silicon-carbide fibres, all of which are adequately suspended in the culture medium with utmost precautions. The ultimate mixture was thoroughly mixed in a vortex mixer, and the resulting cells were quantitatively estimated for their **transient *gus* gene expression.** The frequency of gus positive cells was observed to be 10^{-4}. It has been observed that the silicon-carbide fibres meticulously mediated the exact delivery of DNA right into the cytoplasm as well as the nuclei of cells in a manner very much akin to **microinjection**.

Applicability of this particular technique was successfully extended to both maize and tobacco suspension culture cells. Unfortunately, it has not yet been well substantiated and established whether the transformation(s) thus accomplished give rise to **fairly stable integrations of the transgene.**

3.2.3.11 Transformation by Ultrasonication

In several vegetative species wheat, tobacco and sugar beet **explants** after being cultured for certain duration were adequately sonicated with plasmid DNA that essentially carried *marker genes,* e.g., cat, nptil and gus. It has been observed that when the **sonicated calli** were carefully transferred to selective medium-it gave rise to adequate shoots; whereas all such **controlled calli** (not sonicated with plasmid DNA) proved to be 100% fatal.

Example: Tobacco: In this specific instance the transgenic plants were duly obtained at an approximate frequently of 22 per cent.

3.3 Conjugation

In biology, the union of two unicellular organisms accompanied by an interchange of nuclear material (as in *Paramecium*) is termed as **conjugation.**

In another version, one may explain *conjugation* as a sexual process of DNA transfer which may essentially take place either between individuals of the same or different biological species. However, it is pertinent to mention here that during the process of conjugation, a part or whole of the bacterial chromosome may be transferred into the recipient cell; even large plasmids are invariably exchanged. In actual practice, however, the segments of the transferred chromosome get strategically integrated into the chromosome of the recipient cell by a known process of recombination.

It has been well-established that the *natural processes* that are essentially involved for the specific **'gene transfer'**, in actual practice, vary significantly in their *range* and *specificity.* In fact, these are of *two* distinct types, namely:

a. ***Imprecise nature:*** In a broader perspective the natural processes involved are rather imprecise in nature that predominantly renders the recovery of the **'desired gene'** combination solely dependent not only on efficient *screening* but also on *selection,* and
b. ***Restricted range:*** Besides, the *'natural processes'* encountered do possess a restricted range with regard to the various species that are involved depending on *two* vital phenomena, namely: (*i*) **sexual compatibility** *i.e.,* sexual reproduction; and (*ii*) **transduction** *i.e.,* the prevailing *virus-host range.*

Importantly, the two aforesaid **natural processes** (*a*) and (*b*) invariably put forward a highly serious limitation upon the particular movement of genes across the *taxonomic*** borders.*

In general, the **classifical genetics** until recently, represented the only *modus operandi* whereby heredity*** could be studied and manipulated logically and effectively. Interestingly, in the recent past, the emergence and development of newer techniques have more or less allowed unprecedented logical changes in the genetic make-up of organisms, even permitting to the extent of exchange of DNA between dissmilar organisms (species). However, the manipulation of the genetic material in organisms may now be accomplished clearly in *three* well-defined manners, such as; (*a*) *organismal;* (*b*) *cellular;* and (*c*) *molecular.* These *three* ways shall now be treated individually in the section that follows:

3.3.1 Organismal

In true sense, the **'genetic manipulation'** of whole organisms has been taking its usual natural phenomenon by *sexual reproducion* since the very beginning of *'time'* on this earth. The remarkable evolutionary progress in practically all living creatures in this planet (earth) has invariably involved both *viable* and *active* interactions between the genomes and the environment. The wisdom and knowledge in human beings have been practised and exploited both profusely and abundantly in the specific field of **'agriculture'** for decades even centuries in causing **active control of sexual reproduction.** Importantly, in the recent past the **'genetic manipulation'** has been effectively and progressively employed with quite many **industrial microorganisms,** *e.g.,* yeasts, in the production of industrial alcohol from *molasses** and *'malt wort';* baking industry; and production of **'streptokinase'** to name a few. It essentially involves several important stages in a sequential manner, such as: *selection, mutation, sexual crosses, hybridization,* etc. Nevertheless, it is considered to be a very random process and may normally take a long-span of time to accomplish the desired results-if at all in certain specific instances. Undoubtely, it has exhibited an enormous and immense broad-spectrum of benefits having much improved species of **animals** and **plants.** But in the biotechnological-based industries there have been an astronomical improvement in the growth of productivities, for instance: **enzymes** and **antibiotics.**

3.3.2 Cellular

Cellular manipulations of DNA have been practised since more than four decades. These invariably involve either *cell fusion* or the *culture of cells* and the *subsequent regeneration of whole plants from these cells.* Therefore, it may be regarded either as a **semi-random** or a **directed process,** evidently in contrast to the aforesaid *organismal manipulations;* and the ensuing alterations can be recognized and identified more rapidly. A few most typical and glaring successful biotechnological examples of such specific methodologies generally include **monoclonal antibodies (MABs)** and the meticulous **cloning of a plethora of important plant species.**

3.3.3 Molecular

In reality, the spectacular **molecular manipulations** of DNA and RNA took place for the very first time almost four decades ago; and since then opened the flood-gates of an altogether new era of **genetic manipulation** thereby enabling a much desired and directed control of the targetted changes. It is otherwise baptized as **genetic engineering** or **recombinant DNA technology that** is now bringing forth not only the sea changes but also the dramatic advancements to **'biotechnology'** in the specific fields of life-saving medicines, food-products, beverages, agricultural products etc. Importantly, in these techniques the personnel's, intimately associated with the molecular manipulations, are able to predict and know a lot more with regard to the **genetic alterations** being affected. Indeed it is now quite feasible and practicable to either add or delete parts of the DNA molecule with a reasonably high extent of accuracy and precision and the resulting product may be identified and hence recognized conveniently. The latest trend in research activities have been geared towards **current industrial ventures** for altogether newer types of organism, and numerous chemical entities varying from viable commercial chemicals and pharmaceutical substances.

One of the most wonderful achievements of **'conjugation'** is the glorious and superb success in ***in vitro*** **fertilization** and **embryo transfer techniques,** whereby childless couples, invariably suffering from serious sterility problems, to have their own babies, otherwise widely known as **test tube babies.** Predominantly, the above mentioned techniques involving either **embryo-splitting coupled with embryo transfer** and/or **hormone-induced superovulation** may be exploited for the fast and rapid multiplication of farm animals, such as: sheep, pig, cattle, horse etc. The excellent art of **'genetic engineering'** has been gainfully extended to develop **transgenic* animals** that are particularly resistant to some ailments, with a distinct capability of rapid-growth rates, efficient feed-conversion, and having an appreciable enhanced ability to generate certain important and valuable **biochemical's** that may be amply and suitably excreted through **milk, urine** or blood from which they may be adequately *isolated* and *purified* consequently. In short, the latter aspects are collectively known as **'animal biotechnology'**; whereas, the last instance is termed as **molecular farming.**

Table 3.2 records some of the typically selected contributions of **'biotechnology'** to human welfare embracing the various aspects, namely:

- Medical biotechnology
- Industrial biotechnology
- Animal biotechnology
- Environment biotechnology
- Plant biotechnology.

Table 3.2 *Typically Selected Contributions of Biotechnology to Human Welfare.*

S. No.	Biotechnological Aspects	Researched Products in Use	Comments
1.	**Medical Biotechnology**	• Monoclonal antibodies (MABs) employed for diagnosis of human diseases *e.g.*, Hepatitis B plus other viral diseases; cancer; sexually transmitted vinereal diseases etc.	*Accomplished by Hybridoma Technology*
		• Indispensable drug substances *e.g.*, Human insulin; human interferon; human and bovine growth hormones etc.	Accomplished by genetically engineered bacteria.
		• *Gene therapy* to cure genetic ailments *e.g., cystic* fibrosis; Huntington's chorea.	Such highly sophisticated techniques are almost in their final stages of development.
		• DNA probes employed for the diagnosis of human ailments *e.g.*, kala-azar; malaria; sleeping-sickness etc.	Obtained by genetically engineered microorganisms.
		• Exact identification of real parents/ criminals using DNA or Autoantibody Finger-Printing.	Extremely precise and reliable based on human blood stains, semen strains, and hair roots.

S. No.	Biotechnological Aspects	Researched Products in Use	Comments
		• Infants with specified sex by artificial insemination with X of Y carrying sperms prepared by sperm separation techniques.	It is believed that uncontrolled activities may alter the natural sex-ratio in the races of the universe.
2.	**Industrial Biotechnology**	• Specific production of life-saving **antibiotics**' *e.g., erythromycin;* metabolites as: actinomycetes; *mitomycin; penicillin; streptomycin etc.*	Obtained by such secondary metabolites as: actinomycetes; fungi; and microorganisms.
		• Commercial production of viable and useful chemical entities *e.g.*, acetone; citric acid; gluconic acid; glycerine; lactic acid etc.	Obtained by microorganisms (mainly bacteria) from relatively less useful substrates
		• Production of useful enzymes *e.g.*, α-amylase; proteases; lipases etc.	Produced from bacteria, fungi for use in such industries as: dairy; detergent; leather; textile; and also in **medicines.**
		• Conversion (transformation) of cheaper and less useful compounds into more useful and important ones *e.g.*, **sorbose** from *sorbitol;* and **steroidal hormones** from *sterols*.	Using either **immobilized enzymes** or **microorganisms** in aerobic *fermentors*.
		• Fuel (*viz.* **biogas, ethanol**) from rather less useful, cheaper and abundantly available substrates *e.g.*, Bagasse; Sugarcane; Wood *etc.*,	Obtained via. fermentation by Microorganisms [Cowdung based Biogas being immensely popularized in rural environments in India].
		• Production of **immunotoxins** by linking together and *a natural toxin.*	Help in the destruction of *specific antibody* specific-cell types and thus may afford a potent treatment of cancer.
3.	**Animal Biotechnology**	• Evolution of **'transgenic-animals'** to yield enhanced milk output, growth resistance to certain diseases, and production of some vital **proteins** in blood/milk/urine.	A host of transgenic cattle, chicken, fish, mice, pigs, rate, and rabbits have been produced.
		• **Test-tube babies** in humans, essentially involves *in vitro* fertilization and suitable embryo transfer.	Infertile couples may have babies.
		• Both **embryo-splitting** and/or **hormone-induced super ovulation** involving embryo-transfer together with *in vitro*.fertilization.	Gives rise to rapid multiplication of a host of animal variants with *superior genotype.*
4.	**Environmental Biotechnology**	• Biocontrol and management of plant borne diseases and insect pests by employing amoeba, bacteria, fungi, viruses etc.	Environment-friendly techniques; and specifically avoids the use of pesticides that may cause undue pollution.
		• **Detoxification** of industrial effluents and wastes *e.g.*, spent-wash in distilleries.	By the help of genetically engineered microbes.
		• Bio-degradation of petroleum and Management of crude-oil spills.	By the aid of a strain of *Pseudomonas putida.*
		• Efficacious treatment of sewage wastes and deodourization of human excreta.	Strains of microorganisms to deal with such problems developed

S. No.	Biotechnological Aspects	Researched Products in Use	Comments
5.	**Plant Biotechnology**	• Conservation of **germplasm** via storage in liquid-N_2 (at – 196°C, termed as *cryo-preservation*) or *via* slow growth.	Specifically beneficial in *clonal crops e.g.,* producing tubers, storage roots etc.
		• **Gene transfers** (genetic engineering) for affording storage protein improvement, insect resistance, herbicide resistance, protection against plant viruses etc.	A **revolutionary development** in crop modification and improvement. Mostly using *Ti-plasmid* of *Agrobacterium* and *via* **particle gun** and DNA uptake
		• *Embryo culture* to preserve and rescue **inviable hybrids** and to recover *haploid plants** for interspecific hybrids.	Most widely practiced and recognized applications.
		• Fast and rapid clonal multiplication via meristem culture, *e.g.,* several forest and fruit trees like **'teak'**.	Extraordinarily high rates of multiplication in comparison to the very low conventional procedures.
		• Molecular markers e.g., RFLPs and RAPDs-for exclusive linkage mapping and mapping of the **quantitative trait loci.**	A **recognized powerful tool** for indirect selection of quantitative traits.

3.4 Transduction

Transduction may be defined as—'*a phenomenon causing genetic recombination in bacteria in which DNA is carried from one bacterium to another by a bacteriophage*'.

In other words, the genetic make-up of the cell may be altered by **transduction,** besides several other biological processes *viz., mutation, sexual recombination, transformation, phage conversion* and the like. It is, however, pertinent to mention here that in the specific incidence of *transduction* the DNA is especially transferred from one cell into another by a virus that may be either **generalized** or **specialized.**

Recombinant DNA Technology

In the articulated phenomenon of **gene transmission** *via* natural processes one may encounter *two* major and serious drawbacks, namely:

a. Accomplishment of imprecise gene transmission that essentially renders the recovery of the *'desired gene combination'* solely dependent on absolutely efficient screening and selection, and
b. Corresponding range of gene transmission with respect to the species involved is invariably restricted based entirely upon the *sexual compatibility* (*i.e.,* **sexual reproduction**) and also the virus host range (*i.e.,* **transduction**).

In short, these two aforesaid drawbacks give rise to a serious degree of limitation upon the specific movement of the genes involved across the **taxonomic boundaries.**

Boyer and Cohen (1973) established through their spectacular practical demonstration *i.e.,* by introducing a *small segment* of *DNA* (usually of **foreign origin**) into a *bacterial plasmid** that eventually paved the way towards rapid and remarkable advances in **recombinant DNA technology.** The resulting **hybrid plasmid** obtained in this manner was subjected to further growth in the environment of the most common as well as fast producing bacterium E. coli. Importantly, this altogether unique and splendid technique ultimately caused the evolution of **recombinant DNA** (*i.e.,* **hybrid DNA** is generated by piecing together the various segments of DNA obtained from a variety of sources; also invariably known as rDNA) **technology.**

In actual practice, the **recombinant DNA molecules** are invariably obtained by adopting one of the following *three* **cardinal objectives,** namely:

a. To obtain a large quantum of **copies** (or *replicas*) **of particular DNA fragments,**
b. To recover huge amounts of the **'protein generated solely by the concerned gene,** and

c. To integrate specifically the **'gene' in question** into the *corresponding chromosome* of a **'target organism'** where it **express itself strategically.**

It is pertinent to mention here that to accomplish the above cardinal objectives (*a*) through (*c*)—**'it is absolutely essential and prerogative to first obtain a large number of copies (or replicas) of the concerned genes'**. In order to achieve this objective, the **particular DNA segments** are integrated meticulously into a self-replicating DNA molecule usually termed as **vector.** It is worthwhile to state here that the most commonly used *vectors* are either *DNA viruses or bacterial plasmids.*

Summararily, the various steps articulately concerned with piecing together the **DNA segments** of divergent origin and causing them into an **appropriate vector** together give rise to **recombinant DNA technology.**

Thus, the tremendous growth and advancement for the rapid isolation of *rate and unique proteins,* and their subsequent *commercial production* by the aid of fast-growing microorganisms. Nevertheless, newer breeds of microorganisms were engineered and researched with especially inserted and tailor-made characteristic features for various qualified applications in the fields of medical, agricultural and ecological domain.

Figure 3.4 vividly depicts the basic concepts and processes that are intimately associated with **genesplicing** and **recombinant DNA technology.**

There is another extremely vital and prodominant aspect of **recombinant DNA technology** is the specific and critical use of **antibodies** in biotechnology, diagnosis, and therapy.

Salient Features of Antibodies: The different salient features of **antibodies** are as enumerated below:

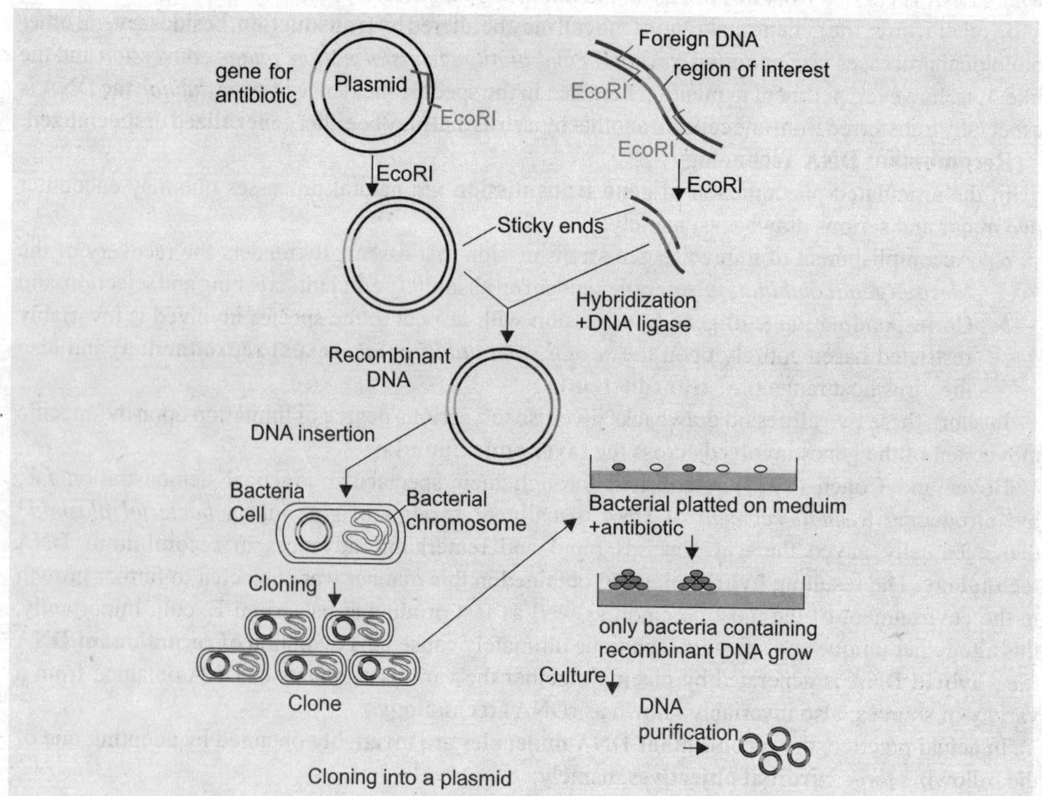

Fig. 3.4 *Various Stages of Gene Splicing and Recombinant DNA Technology*

1. These are exclusively produced by the *plasma cells* (*i.e., β-lymphocytes* or *B-cells*); and are essentially comprised of **four protein-chains** inter-linked by **disulphide-bonds.**
2. The exterior surface of the **'antibody'** essentially has a very **specific indentation,** or **lock** which would critically show cognizance of the **specific foreign** entity or **key** which helps its due *binding* or *complexation.*
3. They are solely produced in each individual for executing their **specific immunological experience** with **antigens.**
4. Fusion of B-cell and mycloma cancer cell led to the formation of **hybridoma** that essentially retained the two main characteristic features belonging to its two parent cell. A hybridoma has the ability to grow **indefinitely** very much akin to the cancer cell; and, in fact, it constitutes the **major discovery** that ultimately leads to the well-known **hybridoma technology.**

3.5 Protoplast Fusion

In bacteriology, a **protoplast** may be defined as—*'the sphere remaining after Gram-positive bacteria have had their cell contents lysed; and the bacterial cell wall constitutes are absent'*.

However, in the Gram-negative organisms these spheres do retain an outer wall layer and are usually termed as *spheroplasts*.

Interestingly, the **protoplast fusion** (or **somatic hybridization**) is one of the most vital and important applications of **protoplasts culture.**

Significance of Protoplasts Fusion: The various cardinal significance of protoplast fusion is, namely:

1. for hybridization between *genera'* or *species* that are incapable to cross by the normal and conventional *modus operandi* of **sexual hybridization,** and
2. Significance fully realized in **plant kingdom** by virtue of the fact that the *hybrid cells* are capable of being inducted to regenerate into **whole plants consequently.**

Evidence from literature amply reveals that Cocking (1960) first produced large quantum of *protoplasts* by specifically making use of *cell-wall degrading enzymes.* As to date the actual techniques of *protoplasts production* have undergone a tremendous extent of **articulated refinement**. It is, however, pertinent to state at this juncture that it is now quite convenient and possible to **regenerate whole plants** from the **protoplasts,** and also to **fuse protoplasts** of variant plant species.

Example: Carlson *et al.* (1972) were pioneer in producing legitimately a **somatic hybrid plant** by meticulously fusing the protoplasts of *Nicotiana langsdorfii* and *Nicotiana glauca.*

Soon after their wonderful break through and achievement a host of **divergent somatic hybrids** have been produced successfully.

Techniques of Protoplast Fusion: There are *two* recognized techniques invariably employed for the protoplast fusion.

3.5.1 Spontaneous Fusion

It has been duly observed that in the process of isolation of protoplasts for culture i.e., the situation when the enzymatic degradation of cell walls gets normally affected, certain protoplasts strategically located in its vicinity may undergo fusion to yield **homokaryons** or **homokaryocytes** each having 20 to 40 nuclei in all. Importantly, the incidence of actual occurrence of **specific multinucleate fusion bodies** is invariably abundant and frequent, when the **protoplasts** are derived from **actively dividing cells.** In fact, the prevailing spontaneous fusion is found to be highly **intraspecific** in nature.

Alternatively, the **spontaneous fusion** of protoplasts may also be accomplished by bringing them into close contact *via* **micromanipulators** or **micropipettes**. It has been duly established that the relatively younger leaves are quite prone to experience this type of fusion. Besides, there exists a definite co relationship between the actual age of the leaf employed for the isolation of *protoplasts* and the corresponding percentage of protoplasts experiencing the spontaneous fusion.

3.5.2 Induced Fusion

In actual practice, however, the **somatic hybridization** is invariably exploited for the *fusion of protoplasts* by following *two* distinct routes adopted quite often, namely: (*a*) *interspecific fusion*—using two different species; and (*b*) employing two *diverse sources within the same species*. Therefore, to accomplish this cardinal objective one needs to adopt **induced fusion** having an appropriate agent (**fusogen**); whereas the *spontaneous fusion* may not prove to be effective and useful.

Examples:

a. **In animals:** *Sendai virus* (**inactivated**)—is required to intiate the process of **induced fusion,** and

b. **In plants:** PEG treatment; $NaNO_3$ (at high pH) + Ca^{2+} (high concentration); and electrical impulse—are needed to achieve the phenomenon of **induced fusion.**

It has been duly observed that in the plant kingdom the respective inducing agent, as stated above; exert its action in two stages, namely:

a. Bringing together the protoplasts, and

b. Causing them to adhere to one another for affording fusion ultimately.

Figure 3.5 vividly illustrates the various means to accomplish successfully the fusion of plant protoplasts spread over to almost three decades (1970 to 2000).

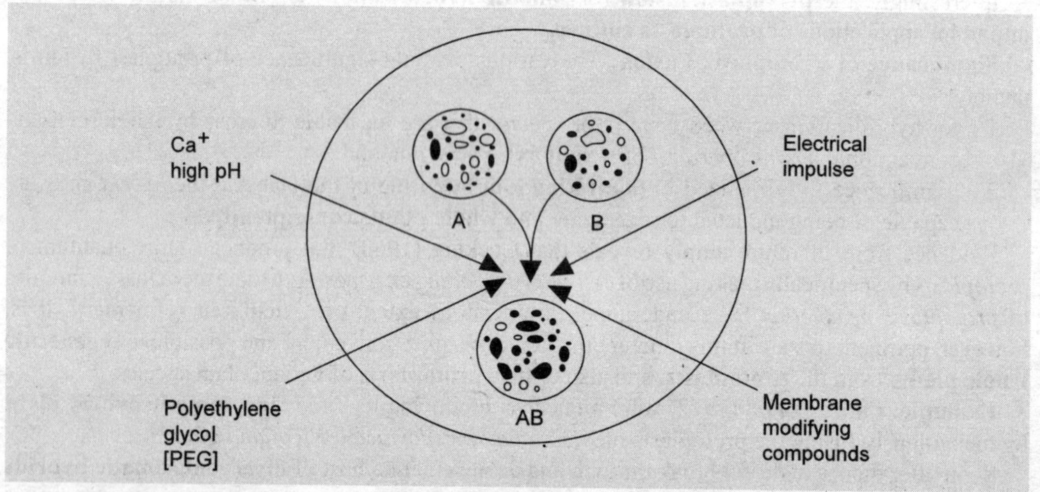

Fig. 3.5 *Various Experimental Parameters Employed for Induction of Protoplasts Fusion.*

The following *four* modes of treatment essentially associated with the production of *induced fusion* shall be treated individually as under:

i. Sodium Nitrate ($NaNO_3$) Treatment

ii. Calcium Ions (Ca^{2+}) Treatment at High pH,

iii. Polyethylene Glycol (PEG) Treatment, and

iv. Electrical Impulse (Fusion).

3.5.2.1 Sodium Nitrate ($NaNO_3$) Treatment

The $NaNO_3$-treatment method was employed gainfully for the fusion of protoplasts obtained from the root tips of **maize** and **coat** seedlings; however, the method is not preferred so abundantly on account of its rather low frequency of fusion, specifically when **extremely vacuolated mesophyll protoplasts** are employed. The various steps that are being adopted sequentially are illustrated in Fig. 3.6.

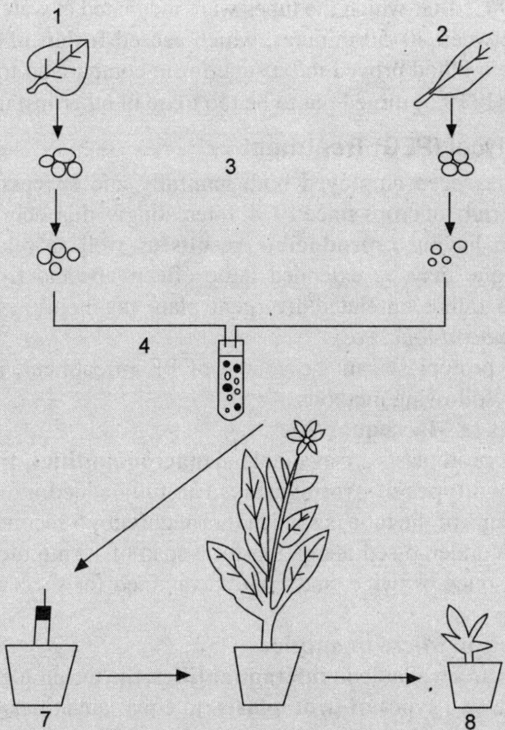

(1) Nicotiana longsdorfii (2) Nicotiana glauca (3) Leaf meosphyll cells treated with enzymes to digest away the cell walls (4) Protoplasts are mixed and suspended in NaNO to cause cell fusion (7) Shoots grafted onto a parent plant; the hybrid scion matures to produce fertile flowers and seeds (8) Seeds germinate to produce seedlings similar to sexually produced amphidiplold

Fig. 3.6 *Various steps Involved in Sodium Nitrate Treatment for Production of Interspecific Somatic Hybrids in the genus Nicotiana.*

Step 1: An **'aggregation mixture'** comprising of sodium nitrate (5.5% w/v) in sucrose solution (10% w/v) is first prepared into which the isolated protoplasts are duly suspended.

The aforesaid mixture significally serves as a **fusion-inducing mixture,** and affords **fusion** upon adequate incubation in a water bath maintained at 35 ± 2ºC. However, one may accomplish **higher frequency of fused protoplasts** by subjecting the resulting mixture to centrifugation and the **'pellet'** resuspended and reincubated for at least one or more additional cycles.

Step 2: The **fusion-inducing mixture** obtained in step 1 is promptly replaced by a **liquid culture medium;** and the protoplasts contained in this mixture are reincubated (35 ± 2ºC). If so required the aforesaid cycle may be repeated at least one or two times before **plating the protoplasts** on a solid medium. Thus, the fusion of protoplasts may be monitored adequately at various stages *via* intensive examination under an **inverted microscope.**

1. Nicotiana longsdorfii 2. Nicotiana glauca 3. Leaf meosphyll cells treated with enzymes to digest away the cell walls 4. Protoplasts are mixed and suspended in NaNO to cause cell fusion 7. Shoots grafted onto a parent plant; the hybrid scion matures to produce fertile flowers and seeds 8. Seeds germinate to produce seedlings similar to sexually produced amphidiplold

3.5.2.2 Calcium Ions (Ca^{2+}) Treatment at High pH

Bhojwani and Razdan (1983) devised a method involving centrifugation (spinning) of the *protoplasts* taken up in a **fusion-inducing solution** (0.05 M $CaCl_2 \cdot 2H_2O$ in 0.4 M mannitol at pH

10.5) for 30 minutes at 50ºC, after which the tubes were incubated at water-bath maintained at 37ºC for a duration ranging between 40–50 minutes, which caused **fusion of protoplasts** to the extent of 20–50%. However, the method proved to be superior in comparison to other methods in certain cases, whereas the high pH (10.5) turned out to be too toxic in other instances.

3.5.2.3 Propylene Glycol (PEG) Treatment

PEG, as a **fusogen,** has been employed both gainfully and successfully in carrying out the **protoplasts fusion** in a variety of crops since 1974. Interestingly, this technique essentially attributes high frequency of fusion having **reproducible results** as well as relatively **lower cytotoxity.** Nevertheless, this technique may be extended quite effectively and fruitfully for the **fusion of protoplasts** belonging to rather unrelated/divergent plant taxonomy, such as: *suyabean-barley; soyabean-maize;* and *soyabean-tobacco.*

The **agglutination** of protoplasts, in the course of PEG-treatment, may be accomplished by adopting either of the *two* following methods:

Method-1: Protoplasts in Macroquantities

In a situation, when the protoplasts are available in **macroquantities,** 1 ml of the prepared culture medium along with the **two types of protoplasts** is carefully added into 1 ml of 56% solution of PEG, and finally the contents of the tube is shaken thoroughly for 5 seconds only. Consequently, the protoplasts are allowed to undergo sedimentation for a span of 10 minutes, washed with the liquid growth (culture) medium once or twice, and finally examined for successful achievement of both **agglutination** and **fusion.**

Method-II: Protoplasts in Micro quantities

In case, the protoplasts are available in **microquantities,** the technique of **drop cultures** may be employed effectively. The **two types of protoplasts,** in equal quantities [*i.e.,* 100 μL each or 4 to 6 drops] are mixed and placed carefully in a *Petri-dish,* and allowed to settle at room temperature (20 ± 2ºC) for a duration of 5 to 10 minutes. Now 50 μL PEG (2–3 drops) are carefully added from the periphery in each Petri-dish, that are subjected to incubation for 30 minutes at room temperature (24ºC), which ultimately leads to agglutination of the **protoplasts**. Subsequent to the PEG treatment the resulting protoplasts are washed meticulously during which the **protoplasts fusion** takes place largely. At this stage the PEG is replaced by the culture medium to permit the *ultimate growth of the fused protoplasts.*

3.5.2.4 Electrical Impulse (Fusion)

It has been observed that when the protoplasts are duly placed into a small culture vessel having *electrodes,* and an *adequate potential difference is applied,* the ensuing protoplasts would get accumulated in between the electrodes. At this critical juncture if one applies an extremely short electrical impulse (shock), it will afford the induction of **protoplasts fusion** as depicted in Fig. 3.7 including the various stages involved from (*a*) through (*d*).

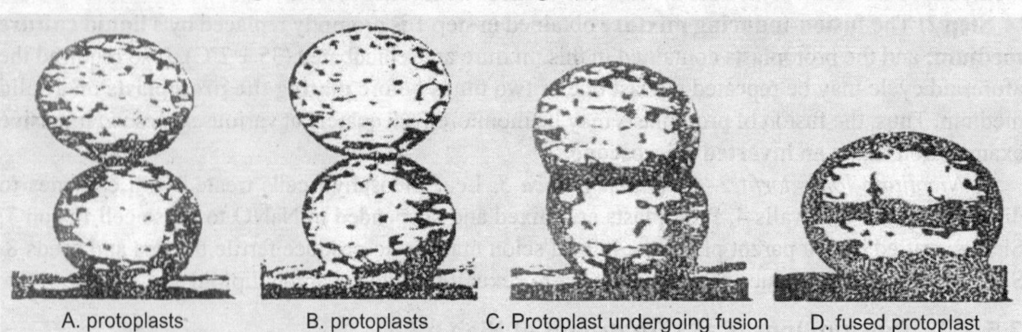

Fig. 3.7 *Various Stages from (a) to (d) Depicting Protoplast Fusion Induced by Application of Electrical Impulse (Shock)*

3.6 Gene Cloning

The word **'clone'** has been derived from the Greek, *klon*-meaning a *cutting* used for propogation. A real extension of the terminology using **'gene'** exclusively for the propogation of animals (including humans) may be regarded as **'gene cloning'**.

Ever since the British scientists*, in 1997, carried out the successful cloning of **sheep** (named **DOLLY**) by meticulously transferring the *nucleus* from an udder-cell of an adult sheep right into the cytoplasm of an **eunucleated fertilized egg.** Subsequently, the resulting **'egg'** was neatly transplanted into the uterus of a *surrogate mother* wherein it eventually developed just like a normal *zygote* ultimately into a **'normal lamb'** that has now grown into a **normal adult sheep.** Therefore, one may rightly conclude and infer, based on the above actual realistic experimental evidences, that—**'when complete animals are duly accomplished from the somatic cells of an animal'**—it is usually termed as **'animal cloning'.**

Soon after the American researchers gained a qualified success in accomplishing the cloning of **Rheus Monkey** by employing meticulously the unique **embryo-splitting technique,** which is well recognized across the globe to be the *nearest* and the *closest* species to the **humans specifically** wherein embryo-splitting has been enormously successful.

Interestingly, the terminology **'clone'** legitimately conveys different meanings in various disciplines of **'biological sciences'**, such as;

a. **Microbiology:** the asexual progeny of a single cell,

b. **Botany:** a group of plants propogated from one seedling or stock. Members of the group are absolutely *identical* but **do not reproduce from seed,**

c. **Tissue Cultures:** a group of cells descended from a single cell. The term commonly (or In the Body) refers to the multiple offspring of single T or B lymphocytes that essentially have identical **surface receptors** or **immunoglobulin** (IgS), and to the offspring of malignant WBCs, and

d. **Immunology:** a group of lymphocytes that develop from a sensitized lymphocyte; they are all capable of responding to a **specific foreign antigen.**

Advantages of Cloning

Following are the cardinal advantages of **'cloning'** in the modern revolutionary biotechnological era, namely:

1. A highly sought after biotechnologically researched device because it permits the **indefinite multiplication** of an elite **desirable genotype** having the least risk of *segregation* and *recombination* during the course of **meiosis,** that should predominantly and critically **precede sexual reproduction,** and
2. The ensuing technique of **'cloning'** affords an enormous and tremendous promise in the field of **'genetic research',** particularly in the better understanding and in-depth knowledge with respect to the ever complicated and difficult phenomena intimately associated with the **'aging'** and **'curing'** of innumerable **genetic diseases.**

It is, however, pertinent to state at this point in time that the **'Cloning Process'** and its various pivotal and vital aspects with respect to the *'gene cloning'* constitute a major area, and hence, need to be explored at length in the sections that follows:

3.6.1 Cloning Process

Literally it refers to—*'a cutting used for propagation'.* In the present context cloning means, to make identical copies. The recent advances accomplished in the field of *"Biotechnology"* the cloning process has been exploited in the following *seven* aspects, namely:

i. DNA – cloning,

ii. Cloning larger DNA fragments in specified cloning vectors,

iii. Cloning Eukaryotic DNAs in bacterial plasmids,
iv. Cloning Eukaryotic DNAs in phage genomes,
v. Cloning cDNAs,
vi. Expression cloning.
vii. Amplifying DNA: The Polymerase Chain Reaction (PCR)

The above diversified cloning processes shall be dealt briefly as under:

3.6.1.1 DNA-Cloning

The DNA cloning is nothing but a broad based technique whereby large quantum of a particularly DNA-segment are produced. Usually, the resulting DNA segment which is to be cloned is first linked to a vector DNA that serves as a vehicle for carrying foreign DNA into a suitable host cell, such as the bacterium *Escherichia coli.* The vector (*i.e., E. coli*) essentially contains sequences which in turn permit to be replicated within the host cell. In order to clone DNAs within bacterial hosts *two types* of vectors are commonly *employed, namely:*

a. The DNA segment to be cloned in introduced into the bacterial cell by **first** joining it to a plasmid and **secondly,** causing the bacterial cells to take up the plasmid from the medium, and
b. The DNA segment is joined to a portion of the genome of the bacterial virus lambda (λ) which is subsequently allowed to infect a culture of bacterial cells. Thus, a huge quantum of viral progeny are produced, each of which contains the foreign DNA segment.

It is, however, pertinent to mention here that by following either of the two methods stated above—the DNA segment once gets inside a bacterium, it will undergo the replication process with the bacterial (or viral) DNA and partitioned to the daughter cells (or progeny viral particles). In this manner, the actual number of bacterial cells which are actually formed.

Besides, cloning may also be employed as a versatile method to **isolate in a pure form any specific DNA fragment** amongst a relatively large heterogeneous population of DNA molecules.

3.6.1.2 Cloning Larger DNA Fragments in Specified Cloning Vectors

It has been observed that neither plasmid nor lambda phage (λ) vectors are adequately suitable for cloning DNAs whose length is more than 20-25 kb. This specific lacuna has revitalized the interest of researchers to look into the development of several other vectors which might facilitate to clone much larger segments of DNA. However, the most important to these vectors are termed as **yeast artificial chromosomes (YACs).**

YACs are nothing but artificial versions of a normal yeast chromosome. They normally comprise of all the elements of a yeast chromosome which are absolutely necessary for the specific structure to be replicated during S-phase and subsequently segregated to daughter cells during mitosis, including:

- One of more origins of replication,
- Having telomeres at the ends of the chromosomes, and
- A centromere to which the spindle fibers may get attached during chromosome separation.

Invariably, the YACs are designed in such a fashion so as to provide essentially:

a. A gene whose encoded product permits those particular cells having the YAC to be selected from those that lack the element, and
b. The DNA fragment to be cloned like other cells, subsequently the yeast cells shall pick up DNA from their respective medium that caters for the path whereby YACs are introduced directly into the cells.

It has been observed that DNA fragments cloned in YACs range typically from 100kb to 1,000 kb in length. Example:

'The restriction enzyme usually recognizes the eight-nucleotide sequence GCGGCCGC, which in turn specifically cleaves mammalian DNA into fragments approximately one million base pairs long'.

Fragments of this length can now be introduced conveniently into YACs and subsequently cloned within host yeast cells.

3.6.1.3 Cloning Eukaryotic* DNAs in Bacterial Plasmids

A foreign DNA intended to be cloned is strategically inserted into the plasmid to give birth to a recombinant DNA molecule. However, the plasmids used for DNA cloning are exclusively the modified versions of those occurring in the bacterial cells. Consequently, the bacterial cells are able to take up DNA from their medium. This particular phenomenon is termed as *'transformation'* and forms the basis for cloning plasmid in bacterial cells.

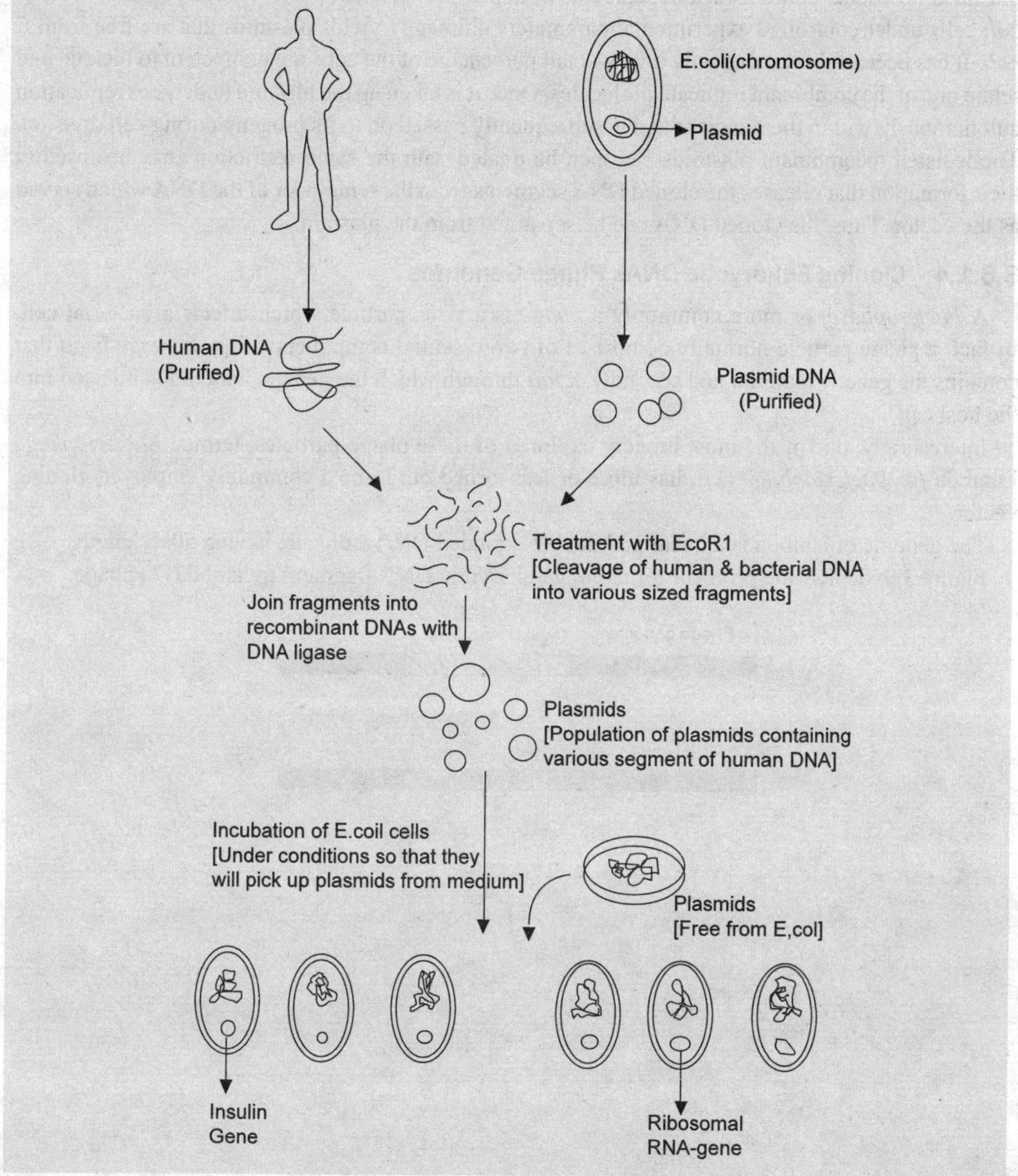

Fig. 3.8 *DNA Cloning Using Bacterial Plasmids.*

Figure 3.8 represents the DNA cloning using bacterial plasmid. First of all the recombinant plasmids each containing a different foreign DNA insert are added to a bacterial culture (*E. coli*) which has been previously treated with Ca^{2+} ions. These bacteria are gainfully stimulated to take up DNA from their respective surrounding medium upon exposure to a brief thermal-shock treatment yielding plasmid DNA (purified). Secondly, human DNA is also obtained in the purified form. Subsequent treatment of human DNA and plasmid DNA with EcoR1 result into the cleavage of human and bacterial DNA into various sized fragments. Now, these small fragments join together to yield recombinant DNAs with DNA ligase and thus give rise to the *plasmids.* These populations of plasmids invariably contain various segments of human DNA. Incubation of these plasmids with *E. coli* cells under controlled experimental parameters ultimately yields plasmids that are free from *E coli.* It has been observed that only a very small percentage of the cells are competent to pick up and retain one of the combinant replicate molecules. Once it is taken up the plasmid undergoes replication autonomously within the recipient and is subsequently passed on to its progeny during cell division. The isolated recombinant plasmids can then be treated with the same restriction enzymes used in their formation that releases the cloned DNA segments from the remainder of the DNA which served as the vector. Thus, the cloned DNA can be separated from the plasmid.

3.6.1.4 Cloning Eukaryotic DNAs Phage Genomes

A *bacterophase*, or more commonly a *phage* is a virus particle which infects a bacterial cell. In fact, a phage particle normally comprises of two essential components; first, a *phage head* that contains the genetic material and secondly, *a tail* through which the genetic material is injected into the host cell.

Interestingly, one of the most broadly explored of these phage particles, termed *Bacteriophage* Lambda *[or bacteriophage* (λ)], has more or less turned out to be a commonly employed cloning vector.

The genome of lambda is a linear and double-stranded DNA molecule having 50kb length.

Figure 3.9. depicts the protocol for cloning eukaryotic DNA fragment in lambda (λ) phage.

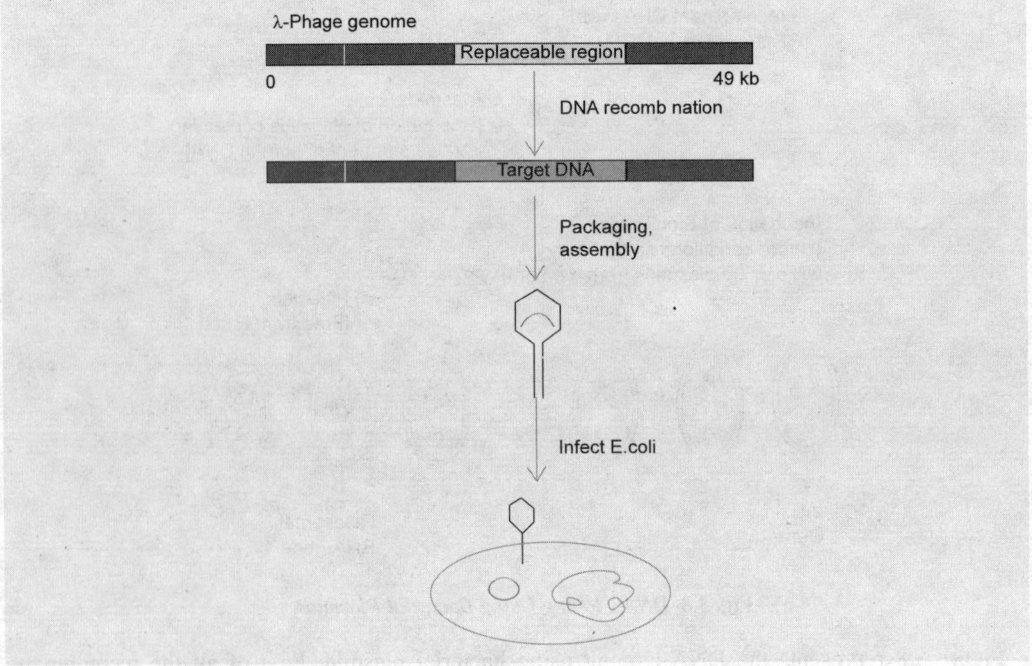

Fig. 3.9 *Sequence for Cloning DNA Fragments in Lambda (l) Phage*

In usual practice, the modified strain (mutant) employed in most cloning experiments contains two cleavage sites for the enzymes EcoR1 that ultimately fragments the genome into *three* large segments. However, the two outer segments essentially contain all information's required for the infectious growth, whereas the middle fragment could be rejected conveniently and replaced suitably by a piece of DNA upto 25kb in length.

It has been observed that the genes of eukaryotes are often split, with non-coding intervening sequences—known as *introns,* thereby separating the coding regions—termed as *exons*. The two outer segments undergo *splicin* with eukaryotic fragment to result into the formation of recombinant DNA. Consequently, the recombinant DNA molecules can be packaged into phage heads *in vitro* and in turn these genetically engineered phage particle may be employed to infect host bacteria. Once gaining entry into the bacteria, the eukaryotic DNA segment is adequately amplified along with the viral DNA and subsequently packaged into an altogether new generation of virus particle that are released when the cell undergoes *lysis.* The released particles thus obtained infect new cells, and without any loss of time either a *plaque* or a clear spot in the *'bacterial lawn'* is visible distinctly at the site of infection. Each plaque, which is nothing but a zone of lysis, possesses millions of phage particle, each carrying a single copy of the same eukaryotic DNA segment. Interestingly, a single pertridish may accommodate more than 10,000 different plaques.

3.6.1.5 Cloning cDNAs

It is pertinent to mention that the explanation of cloning cDNAs has been specifically restricted to cloning DNA fragment isolated from extracted DNA *i.e.,* genomic fragments. In other words, the isolation of a genomic DNA means the eventual isolation of a particular gene or a family of genes out of a pool of hundreds of thousands of unrelated sequences. Besides, it becomes more or less necessary to study the following different aspects during the course of isolation of genomic fragment, namely:

- Non-coding intervening sequences,
- Regulatory sequences flanking on either sides the coding portion of a gene,
- Different members of a multigene family that invariably lie very close in the genome,
- Evolution of DNA sequences, such as duplication and DNA of various species *vis-à-vis* their rearrangement, and
- Interspersion of transposable 'genetic elements'.

There are **two** aspects which are very important with cloning cDNAs, namely:

a. Analysis of gene structure, and
b. Analysis of gene expression.

Figure 3.10. Illustrates the manner by which cDNAs are synthesized for cloning in a plasmid.

In order to clone cDNAs, *first* of all a sizable population of mRNA is isolated; *secondly,* it is employed as a template to provide a single stranded DNA complement; *thirdly,* the resulting product (single stranded) is duly converted to a double stranded population with the help of a DNA polymerase; and *fourthly,* they are finally combined with the desired vector. It is quite evident that essentially mRNA populations typically consists thousands of altogether different species, and as with experiments employing genomic DNA fragments, the clones should be invariably screened to isolate only one particular sequence from a heterogeneous population of recombinant molecule.

From Fig. 3.3, it may be observed that when polypeptide (A) and mRNA are annealed, it provides a small segment of primer attached to poly (A) to the tail of mRNA. Now, with the help of reserve transcriptase the primer to poly (A) gets fully developed. Alkali helps in the separation of DNA and RNA strands to give rise to fully developed primer alone, which on treatment with RNA polymerase 1 yields the combined product. The resulting product when digested with S1 nuclease two separate strands of the primer and poly (A) are obtained. Lastly, integrate cDNA into the plasmid vector that will produce a bacterium wherein DNA can be cloned.

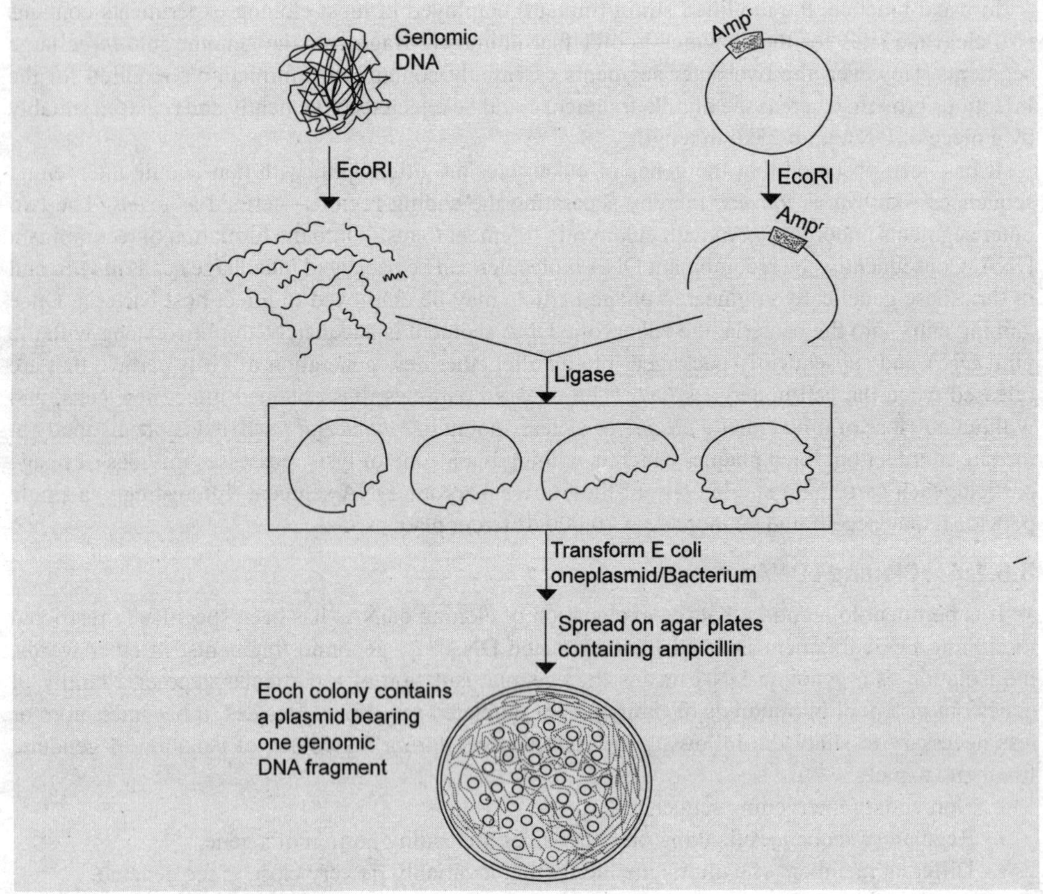

Fig. 3.10 *Synthesis whereby cDNAs get Cloned in a Plasmid.*

3.6.1.6 Expression Cloning

For practical applications it is quite important that such systems must be available wherein the cloned genes may be expressed. In other words, **expression cloning** is an alternative method for identifying a phage plaque which essentially contains a particular cDNA. In this specific method the cDNA being cloned is inserted directly in the downstream region from a strong bacterial promoter, which adequately ensures that the foreign DNA is not only transcribed but also translated in the course of the infections process. Interestingly, those phage which has originally incorporated the gene being sought must form plaques that essentially possess the protein encoded by the gene. Further identification of the plaque is performed on replica plates of employing a labeled probe which binds particularly to the encoded protein. The antibodies serve invariably as the most commonly used probe to identify the desired cloned genes which have been critically located on the replica plate whereas the genes may be subsequently isolated from the viruses on the original plate.

3.6.1.7 Amplifying DNA: The Polymerase Chain Reaction (PCR)

The conventional molecular cloning techniques may be considered *in vitro* DNA—amplifying tools. Interestingly, the latest development in the field of synthetic DNA has evolved an altogether new method for the rapid amplification of DNA *in vitro,* broadly termed as the *Polymerase Chain Reaction* (PCR). In reality, PCR is capable of multiplying DNA molecules to the extent of a billion fold *in vitro,* thereby giving rise to huge amounts of very specific genes employed for various purposes, such as: cloning, sequencing or mutagenesis. In short, PCR utilizes the enzyme DNA polymerase, which eventually copies DNA molecules.

The polymerase chain reaction (PCR) for amplifying specific DNA sequences has been shown in Fig. 3.11. [*Stage – A through Stage – F*]. These six stages have been duly explained here under:

Stage A: The target genes (DNA—combinant form) if first heated to affect the separation of the strands of DNA; secondly, a reasonably excess amount of two oligonucleotide primers, of which one is complementary strand, is added along with DNA-polymerase;

Stage B: As the resulting mixture attains the ambient temperature, the excess of primers relative to the target DNA makes sure that most target strands anneal to a primer exclusively and not to each other. In this way, the primer extension ultimately gives rise to a copy of the original double stranded DNA.

Stage C: Further follow up of three above mentioned steps sequentially *viz;* heating, primer annealing and primer extensions results into the formation of a copy of the original double-stranded DNA. In other words, DNA polymerase extends the primers employing the target strands as a template.

Stage D: Another prime extension of the resulting product yields the second double-stranded DNA.

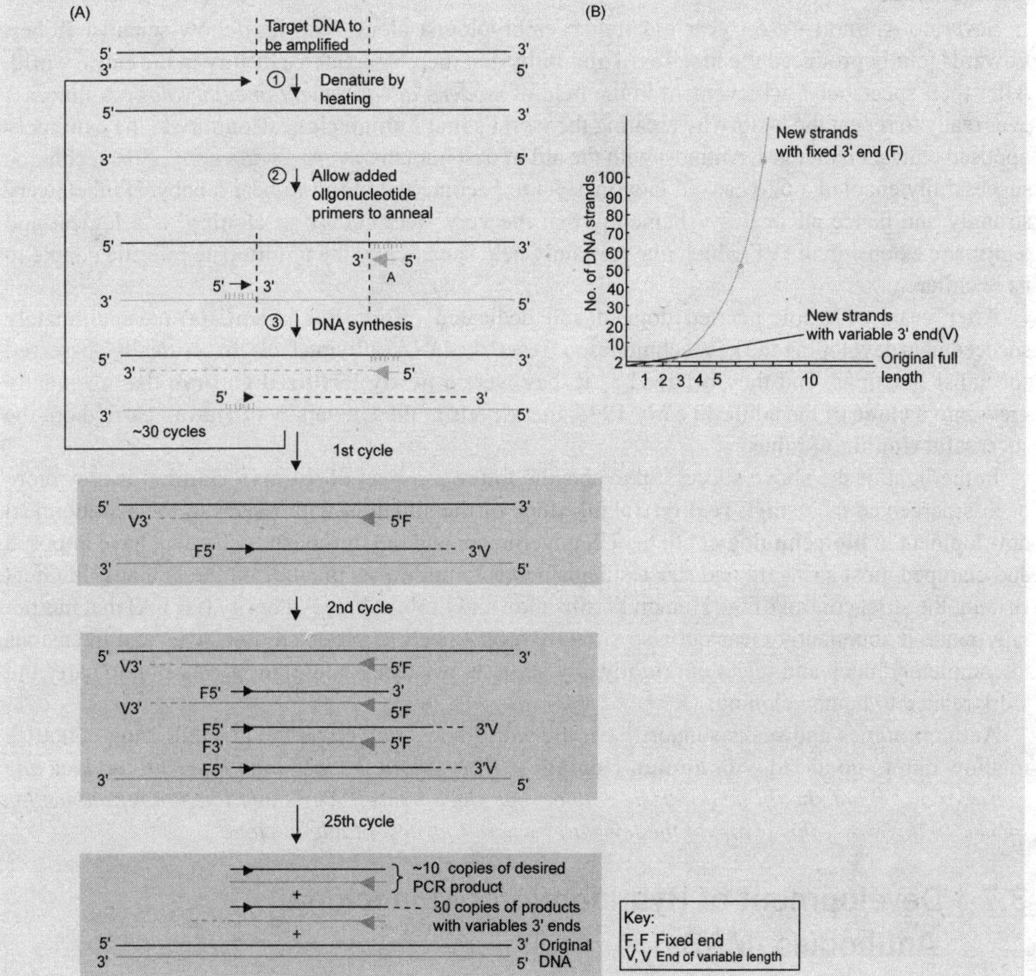

Fig. 3.11 *PCR for Amplifying Specific DNA Sequences*

Stage E: The end product obtained from the previous step is subjected to incubation for a suitable duration; and the resulting mixture is heated once again so as to separate the strands. Subsequently, the mixture is brought to the room temperature whereby the primers aptly get hybridized with the complementary regions of newly synthesized DNA. Thus, the whole process is repeated. In this particular instance, the two additional PCR-cycles give rise to 8 to 16 copies, respectively, of the original DNA sequence.

Stage F: It represents a plot between the number of PCR cycles (along the X-axis) and the copies of the target gene (along the Y-axis). The graphical illustration depicts the effect of carrying out 20 PCR cycles on a DNA preparation initially having only 10 copies of a target gene. The resulting graph is **semi logarithmic** in nature.

Advantages of PCR-Technique

PCR-technique has **two** cardinal advantages, namely:

a. Each and every cycle virtually doubles the content of the original target DNA, and

b. A 106 to 108 fold increase in the target sequence is actually achieved after a 20–30 PCR cycle run.

Human Clone

Severino Antinori—a 53 year old Italian embryologist along with his fellow scientist Robert Edwards jointly produced the first **Test Tube Baby** and thereby created a history in the entire world. After their spectacular achievement in the field of *modern advancement in embryology* Antinori is ever ready to repeat the history by creating the world's first **human clone.** Contrary to the extremely opposed ethical challenges, Antinori with the aid of first human *in vitro fertilization* (IVF) technique successfully enabled a 62 year old lady in 1994 to become the oldest to bear a baby. He feels very strongly and hence advocates vehemently that the very **'technology of cloning'** is a logical and legitimate extension of IVF which may certainly help specifically the unfortunate infertile couple to have children.

After years of whole-hearted dogged and dedicated efforts the **'scientists'** have ultimately succeeded in developing the key techniques to **'reset'** the DNA of living cells that critically possessed specialist functions; and they behaved as if they were a **newly fertilized embryo** that eventually grew into a **clone** of the adult. In early 1998, the experts at the University of Hawaii carried out the successful **cloning of mice**.

In the light of the above successful events the future prospect of **'human cloning'** is now more or less perceived as a **stark reality.** Taking stock of the situation with regard to the astronomical development in **biotechnology** both the US government and the European Parliament have imposed and clamped most stringent and strictest legislations to outlaw its practice on the humans. In Great Britain, the strict control of the Human Fertilization and Embryology Authority (HFEA) that has not only made it abundantly clear but also strongly pronounced its clear cut objectives and intensions to completely block and reject out rightly any requests whatsoever to grant permission to carry out work related to human cloning.

Antinori argues and seeks support from the world body as well as the law enforcing countries to allow him to go ahead with **human cloning**—*"What about the man who does not produce any sperm at all? What should he do? If he cannot reproduce himself why should he not reproduce his 'genes' in this way—this is one of the few cases where it is acceptable to clone".*

3.7 Development of Hybridoma for Monoclonal Antibodies (MABs)

Hybridoma may be defined as—*'the cell produced by the fusion of an antibody-producing cell and a multiple mycloma cell'.*

Importantly, the **'hybrid cell'** is capable of producing a *continuous supply of identical antibodies'*.b

Another school of thought explains **hybridoma** as—'a hybrid cell obtained by fusing a B lymphocyte with usually a tumour cell of the antibody forming system or of B-lymphocytes (*i.e.,* B-cells), that are invariably known as **myclomas.**

The **hybridoma** thus produced essentially possesses the inherent capability to produce antibodies by virtue of two cardinal facts, namely: (*a*) on account of the **B-lymphocyte genome;** and (*b*) due to its capacity for indefinite growth *in vitro* caused by the tumour (mycloma) cell involved in the fusion. Hence, specific hybridomas are either cultured *in vitro* or made to pass *via* the **mouse peritoneal cavity** to obtain the desired *monoclonal antibodies* (MABs); and this sequential procedures encountered is usually termed as **hybridoma technology.** It is, however, pertinent to mention here that the development of the hybridoma technology helped to solve insurmountable technical problem(s) intimately associated with the generation of antibodies which are duly recognized to be *monospecific in nature* because they are **monoclonal**. In 1984, the **Nobel Prize** for *Physiology and Medicine* was bagged by Georges Köhler and Cesar Milstein for their remarkable discovery. The said prize was duly shared with Niels Jerne, who introduced the concept of clonality of the immune response *i.e.,* the theoretical basic foundation upon which the entire methodology is solely based.

3.7.1 The Principle of Monoclonal Antibody Production

The principle of monoclonal antibody production is not only graceful but also stylish. Interestingly, one may *'capture the particular synthesis'* of a single antibody-forming cell and **'immortalize'** it in the very *tissue culture*. Nevertheless, the normal antibody-forming cells cannot be grown and preserved indefinitely (perpetuated) in culture, tumours of the antibody-forming system *i.e.,* **myclomas,** may be grown indefinitely in culture. Therefore, it is earnestly required to have a method for bringing together in one single cell the two cardinal functionalities, namely: (*a*) *altogether different abilities for the synthesis of a specific antibody;* and (*b*) *ability to grow indefinitely in culture.* However, the efforts of Köhler and Milstein succeeded in accomplishing this wonderful aim and objective by allowing to fuse an antibody-forming cell with a mycloma cell, resulting into the formation of a hybrid cell commonly known as a **hybridoma.**

The crucial problem of **selecting** the antibody-forming cell of the desired specificity is articulately resolved by fusing relatively huge numbers of the **antibody-forming** cells on one hand and the **mycloma cells** on the other. The resulting hybridomas are then meticulously examined (or selected) specifically for those which are exclusively engaged in the synthesis of the **'antibody'** having the desired (or anticipated) specificity.

3.7.2 Cell Fusion

Figure 3.12 vividly illustrates the underlying principle of generating **monoclonal antibodies,** which are duly accomplished by the fusion of an *antibody forming cell* (invariably a spleen cell) with a *myeloma cell particularly* in the presence of one of a variety of **fusing agents** *e.g.,* polyethylene glycol (PEG).

[Cells from an immunized mouse are fused with myeloma cells and undergo HAT medium selection. The fused cells, called hybridomas, are then screened for their ability to react to the antigen of interest. The clones of interest are then sub cloned and expanded.]

This ultimately results into the formation of **'hybridoma'. Separation of fused hybridoma cells from normal spleen cell population:**

The separation of fused hybridoma cells from the normal spleen cell population is achieved most conveniently by virtue of the glaring fact that the spleen cells normal die off in culture after a short period of time. Interestingly, the **unfused myeloma cells** and the **hybridoma cells** are absolutely 'immortal'; and, therefore, the dire need of an efficacious and specific method is of prime necessity to get rid of the *unfused myeloma cells.* It is achieved by employing myeloma cells which are killed in the presence of the drug **aminopterin.**

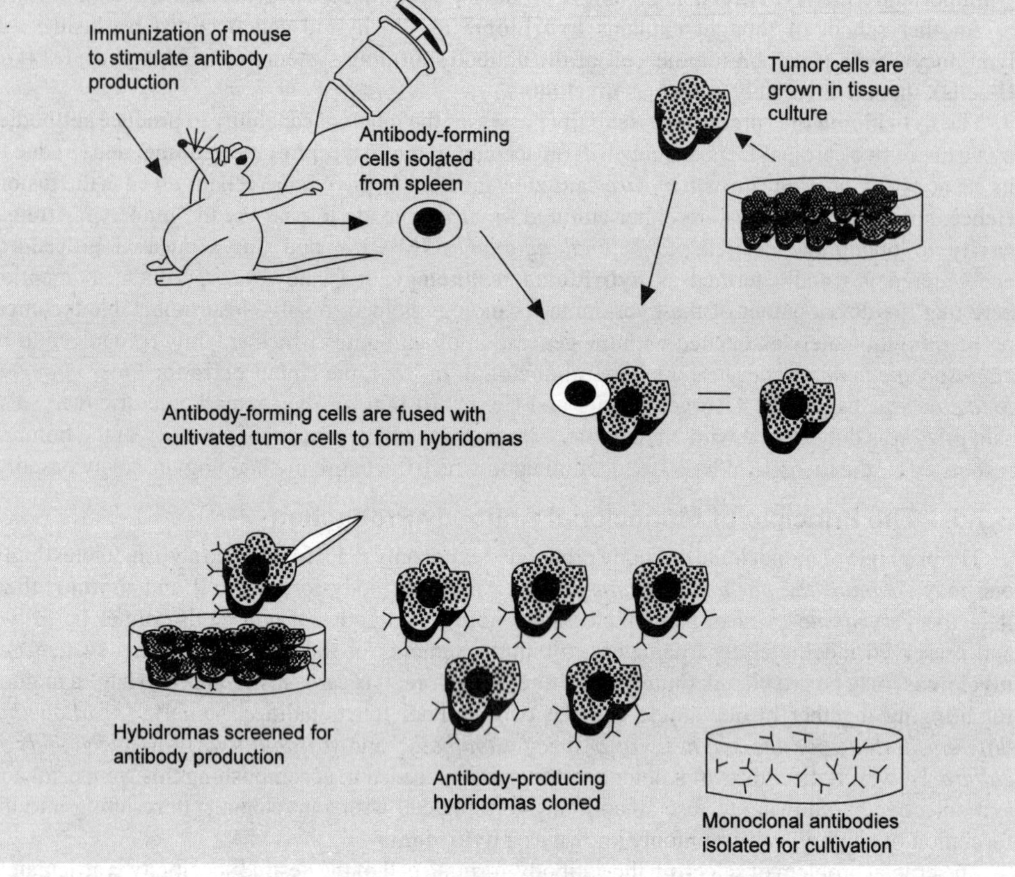

Fig. 3.12 *Production of Monoclonal Antibodies (MABs).*

Aminopterin

8-Azaguanine (8 AzG)

Just like a plethora of cells, myeloma cells, predominantly make use of *two* altogether **distinct pathways for the nucleotide synthesis,** namely: (*a*) synthetic pathway (major one); and (*b*) *salvage pathway* (minor one)—as depicted in Fig. 3.13.

Salient Features: The various salient features of Fig. 3.13 are as stated below:

1. Normal cells invariably synthesize nucleotides by employing both pathways.
2. The very incorporation of the drug **8-azaguanine** to the normal cells, enables it to penetrate right into the DNA through a reaction catalyzed by a specific enzyme HGPRT* *via* the salvage pathway. Such cells eventually prove to be fatal as they simply cannot function with an **altered base.**
3. Evidently, a variant cell that cannot get along with the **salvage pathway** by virtue of the fact that it specifically lacks HGPRT should be **8 AzG resistant;** and, therefore, would not be killed by the said drug substance (*i.e.,* 8 AzG).

4. Therefore, **such HGPRT–** mutants may be selected particularly with this drug; and these are the actual myeloma cells generally employed for the desired fusion.

Explanation: *In pyrimidine biosynthesis $CoFH_4$ is oxidized to FH_2, thereby using up FH_4. In* ***purine biosynthesis*** *$CoFH_4$ is converted to FH_4 non enzymatically so that FH_4 can be reconstituted to $CoFH_4$.* ***Aminopterin*** *blocks the conversion of FH_2 to FH_4 so that no more FH_4 can be generated. As soon as it has depleted the existing FH_4, the cell can no longer function. As a consequence of the* ***pyrimidine pathway*** *now using up virtually all of the FH_4, the purine pathway also stops; however, the cell still carries out DNA synthesis via the* ***salvage pathway.***

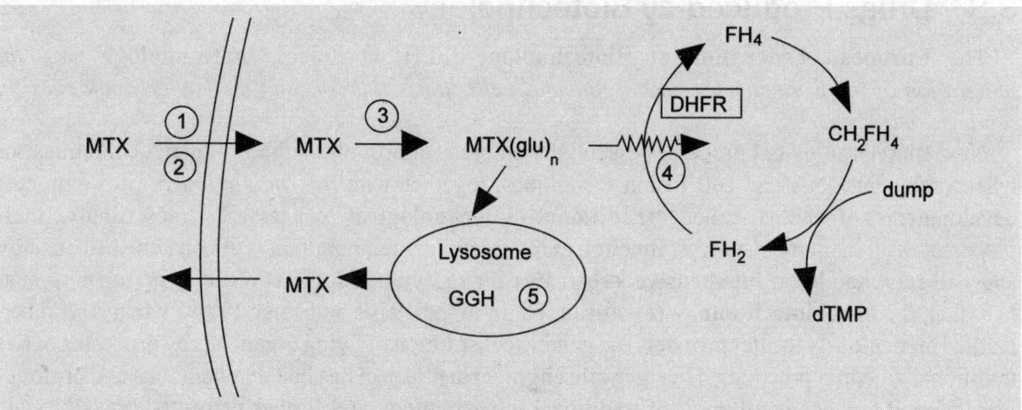

Fig. 3.13 *Aminopterin Works by Blocking the Reduction of Dihydrofolate (FH_2) to Tetrahydrofolate (FH_4).*

5. **Aminopterin** acts on the major *synthetic pathway* (or **De Novo Biosynthesis**) by interfering directly with the conversion of dihydrofolate (FH_2) to tetrahydrofolate (FH_4) and also preventing a series of **one-carbon transfers** particularly. Hence, in the very presence of aminopterin the cell cannot synthesize nucleotides via the **main synthetic pathway;** and, therefore, should take the **salvage pathway** instead.
6. A normal cell can still grow in the presence of aminopterin, whereas a HGPRT– cell cannot, perhaps due to the fact that the prevailing **HGPRT– mutants** cannot carry out the salvage pathway; and the net effect would be the fatal fate of the ensuing HGPRT– cells in the presence of aminopterin.
7. In a situation, when **HGPRT– myeloma cells** get fused with the normal B lymphocytes (or B cells), it has been duly observed that the resulting hybridomas are capable of growing in the presence of *aminopterin* because the normal cell profusely contributes functional HGPRT.
8. In another situation, when two chemical entities *e.g.,* **hypoxanthine** and **thymidine,** which are recognized as the precursor molecules employed by the enzyme HGPRT in the **salvage pathway,** are duly incorporated into the medium, evidently the ensuing hybridoma is capable of using the alternate pathway in the synthesis of DNA.
9. Importantly, the **unused normal spleen cells** usually **die** as they are not capable of growing for longer span in the **tissue culture,** and the **unfused myeloma cells** get killed by the *aminopterin.*
10. As a result the only **fused hybridomas** are able to grow adequately. This particular phenomena is known as the **HAT selection** (*i.e.,* hypoxanthine, aminopterin, thymidine selection).

Four Important Principles of HAT-Selection:

The *four* most important principles of HAT selection are as enumerated under:

a. When the **major synthetic pathways** are blocked by the folic acid analogue **aminopterin,** the cell should employ the **salvage pathway.** This pathway essentially contains the enzyme HGPRT.

b. **HGPRT– myeloma cells** may be selected particularly because they can grow in the presence of 8-azaguanine (*i.e.,* 8-AzG). **HGPRT+ cells** incorporate 8-AzG into DNA. HGPRT– cells do not incorporate the toxic molecule. Hence, HGPRT– cells can grow in its presence.
c. HGPRT– cells die in the presence of HAT because both the **major synthetic pathway** and the **salvage pathway** are blocked virtually.
d. Fusion of the **HGPRT– myeloma cells** with the **HGPRT+ spleen cells** allows growth in HAT by incorporating the missing enzyme for the **salvage pathway.**

3.8 Drugs Produced by Biotechnology

The **European Federation of Biotechnology** (FEB) considers **'biotechnology'** as—*'the integration of natural sciences and organisms, cells, parts thereof, and molecular analogues for products and services.'*

New Biotechnological processes essentially embrace almost all methods of genetic modification by recombinant DNA and cell fusion techniques, together with the *'magic touch'* of the modern developments of the so-called **'traditional-biotechnological processes'.** Interestingly, these processes will, in many instances, function at relatively low temperature, will consume little energy, and will rely mainly on **inexpensive substrates** for biosynthesis. However, it is pertinent to state here that, the **new biotechnology revolution** begin in the 1970s and early 1980s, when researchers learned meticulously to alter precisely the genetic constitution of living organisms by processes outwit traditional breeding practices. This **'genetic engineering'** aspect has had a tremendous and profound impact upon practically all areas of traditional biotechnology and further permitted breakthroughs in **medicine** and agriculture, specifically in those that would be rather difficult and impossible by traditional breeding approaches. In fact, some of the most spectacular and exciting advances, will be in the newer **pharmaceutical drugs** and *'gene therapies'* to treat previously incurable diseases, with a view to produce much healthier foods, safer pesticides, latest and innovative environmental technologies, and above all the **new energy** sources.

Although there are a large number of **'drugs'** that have been evolved *via* the biotechnological processes, but the following typical examples shall be treated at large in the sections that follows:

i. Altepase [Activase(R)],
ii. Human Insulin [Humulin(R)],
iii. Humatrope: Growth Hormone, and
iv. Hepatitis B [Recombinant HB (Merck)—a Hepatitis B vaccine]

3.8.1 Alteplase (BAN, USAN, INN); Activase(R)

Recombinant Tissue-type Plasminogen Activator; rt PA;

Form	Molecular Formula	Molecular Weight
Non-glycosylated	$C_{2736}H_{4174}N_{914}O_{824}S_{45}$	64, 497.9
Glycosylated	$C_{2569}H_{3894}N_{746}O_{781}S_{40}$	59, 008.4

USP;

Description: Alteplase (activate) in a glycosylated protein of 527 residues having the amino acid sequence of human tissue plasminogen activator (τ-PA) and produced by the recombinant DNA technology.

Note: The name may be elaborated on the label by sets of initials mentioned in parentheses so as to indicate the specific method of production, *example:* (rch): indicates the production from the genetically-engineered Chinese hamster ovary cells.

Storage: Alteplase need to be stored preferably at –20ºC or even below in perfectly sealed containers.

In fact, various elaborated studies meticulously carried out by researchers revealed vital and important observations with regard to the *'stability conditions'* of **alteplase** as detailed below:

Lee *et. al. 1990*: concluded that **'alteplase'** must not be mixed in the same container with medicinal compounds such as: *dobutamine, dopamine, heparin* or *glyceryl trinitrate*, because there was indeed ample available **evidence of incompatibility;**

Frazin (1990): observed that dilution of a proprietory preparation of **alteplase** (Activase) to 0.09 and 0.16 mg . mL^{-1} with 5% (w/v) glucose injection distinctly resulted in the precipitation of the drug. Frazin made the following *two* observations:

a. **Alteplase** is formulated with arginine as a solubilizing agent, and dilution with 5% (w/v) glucose to concentration below 0.5 mg of **alteplase** per mL usually makes precipitation possible, and

b. Dilution with 0.9% (w/v) NaCl (*i.e.,* **Normal Saline Solution**) is possible to concentrations as low as 0.2 mg. mL^{-1} before the precipitation becomes a risk.

Units: The **activity** of *alteplase* may be measured in terms of **International Units (IU)** by employing the **2nd** International Standard for the *Tissue Plasminogen Activator* established in 1987, although it is an usual practice to express the doses by **weight.** The **Specific Activity** of *alteplase* is 580 000 IUs. mg^{-1}.

Pharmacokinetics: It has been duly observed that **alteplase** gets cleared from the plsma, chiefly *via* metabolism in the liver.

Uses and Mechanism of Action: The various applications and possible mechanism of action of **'alteplase'** are as follows:

1. It is a **thrombolytic agent,** which is a predominant representative of a *single-chain form of the endogenous enzyme tissue plasminogen activator* meticulously produced by the **recombinant DNA technology.** Very much similar to the **endogenous tissue plasminogen activator,** it converts *fibrin-bound plasminogen* to the corresponding **active form of plasmin**, thereby causing in marked and pronounced **fibrinolysis** and **dissolution of clots.**
2. **Alteplase** has almost negligible effect upon the circulating, unbound plasminogen; and hence, may be termed as a **fibrin-specific agent.** It was perhaps thought that **fibrin specificity** could be an absolute necessity for minimising the prevailing risk of ensuing haemorrhage intimately associated with the application of **thrombolytics;** although the latest **fibrinspecific drugs** usually give rise to appreciable bleeding in comparison to the non-specific thrombolytics.
3. Alteplase is employed very much akin to **steptokinase** both in the management and treatment of **thrombo-embolic disorders,** specifically the **myocardial infarction** and **venous thrombo-embolism.**

3.8.2 Humulin: Humulin(R)

Humulin: Humulin(R) is the branded product of the famous pharmaceutical manufacturer, Lilly, containing **human-insulin** and **its host of variants,** being produced by it in different countries across the globe.

Description of Insulin: Insulin is a **pancreatic-hormone** essentially involved in the *regulation of blood-glucose concentrations* and also having a specific role in the protein and lipid metabolism. In usual practice, the **human,** porcine, **bovine** or **mixed porcine-bovine insulin** is administered to such patients having **insulin-dependent diabetes** mellitus in the management and control of their blood-glucose concentrations. It may also be used necessarily in certain **non-insulin-dependent diabetics.** Insulin is also an essential component of the emergency management and control of **diabetic ketoacidosis.**

Drawbacks: The two most predominant drawbacks of insulin are as stated below:

1. **Hypersensitivity reactions** may take place.
2. **Hypoglycaemia** occurs most abundantly giving rise to serious complications of insulin therapy.

Importantly, it has been established beyond any reasonable doubt that **insulin** is—*'a hormone produced by the* β-cells *of the islets of Langerthans of the pancreas and essentially comprise of two separate chains of amino acids, the A and B chains, joined together by two disulphide bridges'*.

It is, however, pertinent to mention here that the **insulin** produced by a variety of species specifically conforms to the **same basic structure** but has **different sequences** of amino acids in the chains.

Porcine, Human, and Bovine Insulin's: The difference(s) in the *three* insulin variants are as stated under:

Type of Insulin	Molecular Formula (Molecular Weight)	Comments
Porcine Insulin	$C_{256}H_{381}N_{65}O_{76}S_6$ [5777.6]	Differs from human insulin in only one amino acid in the B-chain.
Human Insulin	$C_{257}H_{383}N_{65}O_{77}S_6$ [5807.7]	–
Bovine Insulin	$C_{254}H_{377}N_{65}O_{75}S_6$ [5733.6]	Differs from human insulin not only in this same amino acid in the B-chain, but also in two other amino acids in the A-chain.

Proinsulin: Proinsulin has been recognized as the **precursor of insulin** which happens to be a single polypeptide chain incorporating the A as well as B chains of insulin usually connected by a peptide known as the **C-peptide** (also called the *connecting peptide*). It has been adequately observed and established that the **insulins of various species** may have more or less the **identical composition;** whereas, the composition of the **proinsulins** are not so, in that the *number and sequence of amino acids* present in the **C-peptide may vary significantly.**

Steiner *et al.** (1969) reported that **insulin** gets synthesized by the islet β-cells from a single chain, 86-amino acid polypeptide precursor and **proinsulin**. The latter is eventually synthesized in the polyribosomes of the prevailing rough endoplasmic reticulum of the β-cells obtained subsequently from an even larger polypeptide precursor termed as **preproinsulin.** Besides, the B chain of preproinsulin is extended at the NH_2 – terminus by at least a cluster of 23 amino acids. Subsequently, proinsulin passes through the Golgi apparatus and rightly enters the storage granules, where ultimately the actual conversion to insulin takes place.

Importantly the actions of such proteolytic enzymes as: *endopeptidase* and *thiol-activated carboxypeptidase's*, eventually upon **proinsulin** finally give rise to the formation of equimolar quantum of **insulin** along with the connecting C-peptide. It has been observed that the resulting insulin molecule essentially comprises of chains A and B, having 21 and 31 amino acid residues, respectively. The aforesaid two chains are in turn connected by two disulfide linkages, with an extra disulfide linkage strategically positioned within chain A as illustrated in Fig. 3.14.

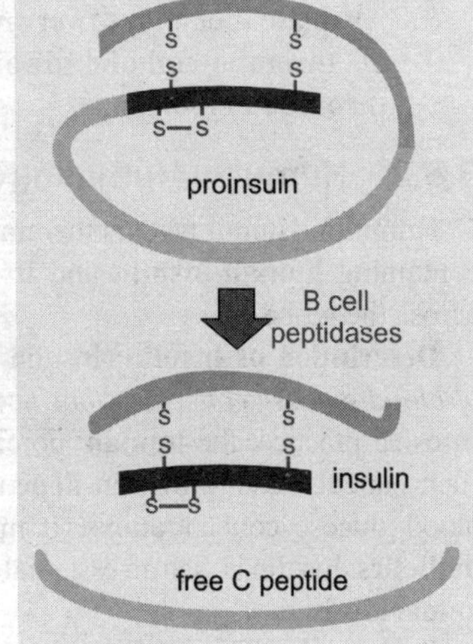

Fig. 3.14 *Conversion of Proinsulin to Insulin.*

There are, in fact, *five* different types of **insulins** as stated below:

i. Conventional insulins,
ii. Single-peak insulins,
iii. Highly purified insulins,
iv. Monocomponent insulins, and
v. Purified insulins.

These **five variants** of insulins shall now be treated individually in the section that follows:

A. Conventional Insulin's:

The earlier commercial insulins were actually derived by extraction from **bovine** or **porcine** or mixed **bovine** and **porcine pancreases,** and were subjected to subsequent purification by recrystallization only. The **insulins** produced by such well specified methods were invariably termed as: **'conventional insulins'** simply to distinguish them from insulins that have been further purified by several techniques.

Fractionation of Extracts: An extract of *'insulin'* that has been recrystallized only once may be separated into *three* distinct fractions or components usually termed as the '*a*', '*b*', and '*c*' fractions. The composition of each separated component is as given below: **Component '*a*':** It consists of largely high molecular weight substances. It is only usually observed in *very impure preparations* because repeated recrystallization will help to discard most of it. **Component 'b':** It consists mostly of **proinsulin** and **insulin dimers. Component '*c*':** It consists of **insulin, insulin esters, arginine insulin,** and **desamido insulin** respectively.

Note: A number of pancreatic peptides *e.g.,* glucagon, pancreatic polypeptide, somatostatin, and vasoactive intestinal peptide are also invariably found in products that have not undergone any additional purification.

B. Single-peak Insulins:

The sophisticated analytical technique, **gel filtration,** shall afford a significant reduction in the content of *pancreatic peptides* or *insulin derivatives.* Hence, the products purified by gel filtration are generally called as *single-peak insulins.*

Note: Gel permeation and size-exclusion chromatography (SEC) are the other nomenclatures of the gel filtration process.

C. Highly Purified Insulins:

In addition to gel filtration the crude product may be further purified by **ion-exchange chromatography** (IEC) that will further lower the **proinsulin** content, and may also reduce the contamination caused by **insulin derivatives** and **pancreatic peptides.** An insulin product, specifically in Great-Britain, that has been duly purified by gel-filtration and ion-exchange chromatography is termed as **highly purified insulins.**

D. Monocomponent Insulins:

In UK, the **insulin product** obtained by the purification of gel filtration and ion-exchange chromatography is commonly known as **monocomponent insulins.**

E. Purified Insulins:

Food and Drugs Administration (FDA) in USA has designated the terminology 'purified insulins' for such preparations prepared in the same manner; and **containing essentially less than 10 ppm of proinsulin.**

These days much of the **insulin** produced has the **amino-acid sequence** very much similar to that of the **human insulin**. In actual usage there are several human-insulin variants, such as:

Human insulin (emp): produced by the **enzymatic modification** of insulin obtained from the **porcine pancreas.** It is also known as **semisynthetic human insulin.**

Human insulin (crb): produced by the **chemical combination** of A and B chains that have been duly obtained from bacteria genetically modified by *recombinant DNA technology*.

Human insulin (prb): produced by **proinsulin** obtained from bacteria genetically modified by recombinant *DNA technology.**

Human insulin (pyr): produced from a **precursor obtained from a yeast** genetically modified by recombinant DNA technology.*

Structurally Modified Insulins

The **structurally modified insulins** are invariably produced *via* **chemical modification** of the **insulin molecule.** A *few typical examples are* cited as under:

a. **Dalanated Insulins:** It is prepared by the careful removal of the C-terminal alanine from the prevailing B-chain of insulin.

b. **Insulin Defalan:** It is prepared by the critical removal of the **terminal phenylalanine.**

c. **Sulphated Insulin:** The introduction of sulphated moieties at strategical locations of the amino acid chain.

Note: None of these insulins (*a*) through (*c*) have received any recognition and wide usages.

Insulin Argine and **Insulin Lispro** have been developed quite recently. Based upon the **recombinant DNA technology** several insulin analogues have been developed with **altered pharmacokinetic profiles** in the recent past; some of which are under progressive clinical trials and evaluations.

Table 3.3 summarize the various versions of Humulin, name of manufacturers, composition; and therapeutic usage.

Table 3.3 *Summary of Humulin(R) Variants*

S. No	Humulin(R) Variants	Manufactured By	Composition	Usage
1.	**Humulin 70/30**	Lilly, USA	Mixture of isophane insulin suspension (**human, crb**) 70% and insulin injection (**human, crb**) 30%.	*Diabetes mellitus*
2.	**Humulin 20/80, 30/70, and 40/60**	Lilly, South Africa	Mixtures of insulin injection (**human**) and isophane insulin injection (**human**) respectively in the proportions indicated.	–do–
3.	**Humulin 10/90, 20/80, 30/70, 40/60, 50/50**	Lilly, Canada	Mixtures of insulin injection (**human, prb**) and isophane insulin injection (**human, prb**) respectively in the proportions indicated.	–do–
4.	**Humulin BR**	Lilly, USA	Buffered regular **human insulin (crb)**	–do–
5.	**Humulin I**	Lilly, Italy	Isophane insulin injection (human)	–do–
6.	**Humulin L**	Lilly, Australia	Insulin zinc suspension (**human, prb**)	*Diabetes mellitus*
7.	**Humulin Lente**	Lilly, UK	Insulin zinc suspension (30% amorphous, 70%, crystalline) (**human prb**)	–do–
8.	**Humulin M1, M2, M3, M4, M5**	Lilly, UK	Mixtures of insulin injection (**human, prb**) 10%, 20%, 30%, 40% and 50% and isophane insulin injection (**human, prb**) 90%, 80%,70%, 60% and 50% respectively.	–do–
9.	**Humulin U**	Lilly, USA	Insulin zinc suspension (crystalline **Ultralenta (human, prb)**	–do–
10.	**Humulins NPH**	Lilly, Belgium	Insulin suspension (human, biosynthetic)	–do–
11.	**Humutard**	Lilly, Sweden	Insulin zinc suspension (human) (amorphous 30%, crystalline 70%)	–do–

3.8.3 Humatrope(R); Growth Hormone

Growth hormone is an *anabolic hormone* secreted by the anterior pituitary which stimulates tissue growth and **anabolism.** It is found to affect fat, **carbohydrate** and **mineral metabolism.**

3.8.3.1 Somatropin BAN, USAN, INN Humatrope(R); Umatrope(R); B.P.; Eur. P.,

Description: It is a **synthetic human-growth hormone** essentially possessing the normal structure of the major (22K) component of natural human pituitary growth hormone. It comprises of a single polypeptide chain of 191 amino acids having disulphide linkages between positions 53 and 165, and between 182 and 189.

The actual *'method of production'* of the growth hormone is clearly indicated on the **'label',** for instance:

epr: indicates production by enzymatic conversion of a specific **precursor** produced by a bacterium genetically modified by *recombinant DNA technology*.

rbe: indicates production from bacteria genetically modified by *recombinant DNA technology*.

rmc: indicates production from genetically engineered and transferred mammalian (mouse) cells.

Storage: Samotropin needs to be stored at 2–8°C in perfect airtight containers particularly in dosage forms of not less than 2.5 units. mg^{-1}. However, the bulk solution must be stored at –20°C in airtight, containers.

***Units:* One Ampoule of the First International Standard (1987):** 4.4 units of the human growth hormone (somatropin) are contained in 1.75 mg of freeze-dried purified human growth hormone, with 20 mg of glycine, 2 mg of mannitol, 2 mg of lactose, and 2 mg of sodium bicarbonate.

International Reference Reagent for Somatropin (1993)

1 mg of the first International Reference Reagent for **Somatropin (1993)** can be assumed, for the purpose of formulation of *therapeutic* as well as diagnostic products to possess the equivalent of **3IU of growth hormone activity.** Very much in line with the above statement of facts the European Pharmacopoea states categorically that—**'1 mg of anhydrous somatropin is equivalent to 3IU of biological activity.**

Pharmacokinetics: Somatropin is well-absorbed after subcutaneous or IM injection. After IV injection it has a half-life of about 20–30 minutes; however, after subcutaneous or IM administration the prevailing serum concentrations usually decline having a half-life of 3–5 hours, on account of the relatively more prolonged release from the site of injection. It is found to be metabolized in the liver and excreted in bile.

Uses and Mechanism of Action: Somatropin is a synthetic human growth hormone; and **Somatrem** is its corresponding **methionyl analogue.** The *'drug'* promotes the growth of muscular, skeletal, and other tissues, stimulates protein anabolism; and also affects fat and mineral metabolism. The hormone exhibits a **diabetogenic action** upon the *carbohydrate metabolism specifically*.

The secretion is observed to be **pulsatile** and solely depends upon the **neural and hormonal influences,** such as: (*a*) *hypothalamic release-inhibiting hormone e.g., somatostatin, and* (*b*) *hypothalamic releasing hormone e.g.,* **somatorelin.** In fact, there are certain physical and physiological factors that largely influence an enhanced secretion of the growth hormone, such as: *sleep, emotional stress,* and *hypoglycaemia.*

3.8.4 Hepatitis B [Recombivax HM (Merck)—A Hepatitis B Vaccine]

The **Recombivax HB *(Merck),*** a *hepatitis B vaccine,* is one of the most recent and significant developments in the field of **recombinant DNA technology,** that essentially comprise of highly specific antibodies which act like **magic bullets.**

It has been duly observed that **hepatitis** tends to cause a severe *acute infection* and may ultimately lead to *chronic infection* and **permanent liver damage.** It is essentially caused by **hepatitis B virus (HBV);** and recognized as an enveloped and double-stranded DNA virus. It has been adequately revealed through meticulous studies that individuals who are at the most vulnerable and greatest risk for infection include: IV-drug abusers (*e.g.,* morphine/heroin addicts); homosexual men; HBV-infected mothers; and above all the health care workers. It is now almost mandatory under stringent law-enforcing authorities that **'Blood Banks'** must now routinely screen for the **HBV-antigens,** which practice has substantially minimized the obvious exposure and risk for infection in persons requiring **multiple transfusions.** Previously called **serum hepatitis.** Importantly, the hepatitis B infection may be prevented through a vaccine created using **recombinant DNA technology.** However, complete protection can be accomplished *via* two vaccinations 1 month apart and a third dose 4 months later; an increased **anti-HBs antibody titer value** evidently shows **successful vaccination.** The following categories of person(s) must be vaccinated:

- All health care staff members
- Patients with renal disease requiring hemodialysis
- Police personnel's and other public safety workers
- Family members and sexual partners of those infected with HBV
- Persons who travel frequently and extensively abroad.

Note: The Centers for Disease Control and Prevention (CDCP) recommends that pregnant women should be meticulously tested for HBs Ag so that the newborns can be vaccinated.

Caution: *Individuals who have not been vaccinated against HBV and receive a needle stick or mucous membrane contact either with blood or with other body secretions should immediately contact their* ***occupational health department.***

Figure 3.15 evidently illustrates the various steps being followed in a sequential manner with regard to the production of a **genetically engineered vaccine** *e.g., Hepatitis B Vaccine.*

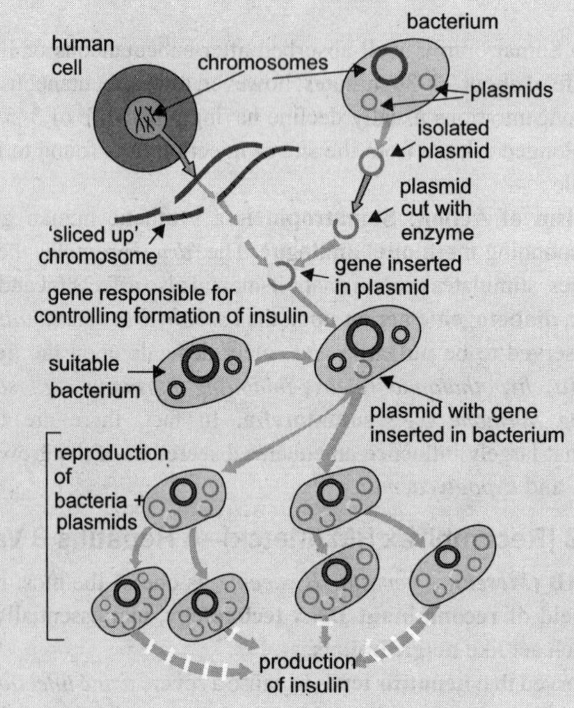

Fig. 3.15 *A Schematic Diagram Illustrating a Genetically Engineered Vaccine.*

Step 1: Genetic material (DNA) is dul extracted from the ensuing *hepatitis virus.* At this stage the *'surface proteins'* essentially provoke an *immune response.*

Step 2: The 'individual genes' are adequately analyzed and identified.

Step 3: The **'specific gene'** which categorically directs production of *surface protein* is located carefully.

Step 4: In this most critical steps the **gene** is removed from the viral DNA and inserted into the **plasmid** carefully.

Step 5: The **plasmids** are meticulously inserted into the corresponding yeast cells.

Step 6: Yeast is allowed to grow *via* fermentation. In this manner the cells reproduce and generate more quantum of surface protein.

Step 7: After a duration of 48 hours the corresponding yeast cells are ruptured to free the ensuing *'surface protein'*. The resulting mixture is duly processed so as to extract the purify the *surface protein.*

Step 8: A large amount of **surface protein particles,** in its purest form, are obtained which ultimately provoke an **immune response** effectively.

Step 9: The resulting **surface proteins** are adequately mixed with appropriate preservations together with other ingredients to obtain the **vaccine.**

Antigenic Markers for HBV-Infection

In fact, there are *three* **antigenic markers** that have been duly identified **for the HBV infection,** namely:

a. HBsAg: A surface antigen located on the viral envelope that represents one of the earliest markes and appearing in the blood during incubation,

b. HBeAg: Obtained from the protein capsid surrounding the DNA, and also is a marker for causing active infection, and

c. HBc: A core antigen that does not circulate in the blood, and helps in the stimulation of the production of the primary antibodies against HBV. These antibodies are not protective and, hence, provide no immunity.

Questions

1. What do you understand by recombinant DNA technology and write the principle and procedure involved in the production of monoclonal antibodies. (JNTUA-May 2009)
2. Give biotechnological approach on activase and humulin. (JNTUA-May 2009)
3. Humatrope. (JNTUA-Nov 2010)
4. Describe about the development of hybridoma for monoclonal antibodies in detail. (JNTUA-May 2009)
5. Explain in detail about Hybridoma technology for production of monoclonal antibodies. (JNTUA-Nov 2010)
6. Write the applications of monoclonal antibodies. (JNTUA-Nov 2010)
7. What is cloning? Explain. (JNTUA-Dec 2009)
8. Describe the drugs like monoclate. (JNTUA-Dec 2009)
9. What is hybridoma technology? (JNTUA-Dec 2009)
10. Describe humanized monoclonal antibodies. (JNTUA-Dec 2009)
11. PVP. (JNTUA-Dec 2009)
12. Humatrope. (JNTUA-Dec 2009)
13. Hybridoma techniques. (RGUHS–Mar 2009)
14. Discuss transformation and transduction. (RGUHS–Mar 2009)
15. What is hybridoma technology? Discuss the production and applications of monoclonal antibodies. (RGUHS–Apr 2008)

16. Conjugation. (RGUHS–Apr 2008)
17. Describe the process of genetic engineering. Explain the role of different enzymes used in the process. Listout the applications. (RGUHS–Oct 2007)
18. Describe hybridoma technology. (MGRU Apr-2004)
19. Write a note on recombinant DNA technology. (MGRU 2003)
20. How insulin is prepared by genetic engineering method. (MGRU 2003)
21. Write in detail about recombinant DNA technology. Write about the production of Insulin by recombinant DNA technology. (MGRU 2004)
22. Gene transfer by conjugation. (MGRU 2004)
23. Write the procedure for the western blotting technique. (MGRU 2003)
24. Recombinant DNA technique. (MGRU 2002)
25. Recombinant DNA techniques. (MGRU 2002)
26. Write down the advantages of genetic engineering. (MGRU 2001)
27. Define hybridoma technology? Write the stages involved in the production of monoclonal antibodies. (MGRU 2004)
28. Define Plasmid. (MGRU 2004)

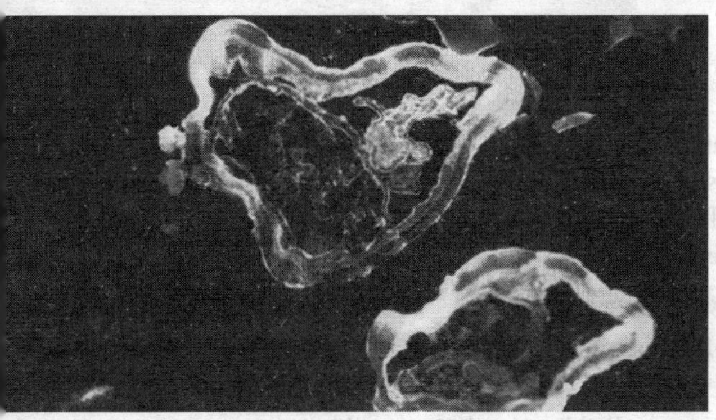

CHAPTER 4

Immunology and Immunological Preparations

4.1 Introduction

The **'science of immunology'** virtually saw the light of the day through the earnest efforts of Edward Jenner in 1798 who assumed to be true on the basis of reasoning that the value of '*vaccination*' as a probable means of protection against the cowpox (vaccinia) ailment. In fact, it was Jenner who first and foremost suggested the protective means of '*vaccination*' with non-virulent cowpox against smallpox infection. It is, however, pertinent to mention here that the science of *immunology* ultimately got its legitimate recognition as a branch of knowledge requiring systematic study and method only in 1881 when the entire universe witnessed an epoch making spate of progress put forward by two eminent scientists Louis Pasteur and Robert Koch. In reality, Pasteur's development of a vaccine for **anthrax** *i.e.,* an acute infectious disease caused by Bacillus *anthracis*, using attenuated organisms was enormously hailed by many scientists across the globe.

Elie Metchnikoff (1833), a noted Russian scientist spotted the pivoted role of *phagocytes* in causing immunity in the course of an extensive and intensive research due to infection of the popular waterflea, *Daphnia*, by a specific fungus. Metchinkoff's observations and findings put forward the well-known **phagocytic theory,** which essentially postulated that the prevailing '*inflammatory responses*' in the human body were, in fact, the very outcome of numerous on-going *cellular reactions* instead of the *vasculogenic reactions* as suggested earlier by Julius Cohnhein. In short, the preliminary as well as the pioneering work of Metchinkoff not only proved adequately but also established the justified role of the cellular substances present in the blood in accomplishing pathogenic microorganisms to a significant extent.

Interestingly, Metchinkoff's articulated concept and belief that '*inflammation produced*' happen to be a **'protective'** rather than a **'destructive'** phenomenon. As on date, it has been recognized beyond any reasonable doubt that the phagocytic activity of human WBC designates the *primary line of defense* against invasion on the body by a host of pathogenic organisms. Virchow and Pfeiffer vehemently opposed *Metchinkoff's phagocytic theory* based on their claim that the entire process caused solely due to the action of **antibodies,** which they ultimately laid as the fundamental foundation of the very understanding of the ensuing **immume bacteriolysis.**

Salient Features of Metchnikoff's Doctrine

The various salient features of Metchnikoff's doctrine are, namely:

a. Importance of *activated microphage,*

b. Latest concept that certain diseases are controlled by *circulating antibodies,*

c. '*Phagocytes*' (specialized cells) active participation in causing protection against other prevalent diseases,

d. *'Humoral antibodies'* responsible for the *pathogenesis of autoimmune* plus other *immunogenic ailments,* and

e. Certain diseases are also produced by *cell-mediated reactions.*

Later on in 1890 Vohn Behring, duly recognized **'antibodies'** present in serum to diphtheria toxin. Denys and Leclef (1895) observed that phagocytosis invariably get enhanced by immunization to a substantial extent. Bordet in 1899 observed that the lysis of cells by antibody essentially requires the earnest cooperation of various serum factors that are now collectively known as **'complement'.** Landsteiner in 1900, discovered the ABO antigens, a magnificent invention that eventually laid the foundation stone of the **'science of serology'**. Richet and Portier (1902) introduced the terminology '*anaphylaxis*' *i.e.,* opposite of *prophylaxis*. In 1903, Almorth Wright based on the clue derived from the *'humoral theory'* propounded another theory termed as the **'theory of opsonization'** in relation to opsonic activity to phagocytosis. In other words, it explains that *antibodies* as well as *phagocytes* are equally important and necessary to cause infectious diseases, and supplement each other in the **complete eradication of pathogenic organisms.** His remarkable research outputs conferred on him the Noble Prize in 1908. Almost after a lapse of 22 long years, Zinsser (1925) put forward a well-defined and explicite contrast between *immediate* and *delayed-type hypersensitivity.* Lastly, Heidelberger and Kendall (1930-35) carried out an elaborated **'precipitin studies'** an antigen-antibody interactions.

4.2 Principles

The *'science of immunology'* categorically deals with the specific mechanisms by which the *living tissues* invariably react to the so called *foreign biological materials,* such as: *invading pathogenic microorganisms*, so that ultimately either immunity or resistance gets developed in vivo to combat the dreadful diseases in the humans and animals. The credibility as well as the integrity of the defense mechanism system of the host, and in turn its ability to undergo critical and specific reaction(s) thereby counteract the possible invasion by microorganisms seems to be of prime and vital importance for the ultimate survival of the individual.

Obviously, the *'foreign biological materials'* quite often gain entry into a living body through such barriers as: hair, skin or ruptured spaces. Consequently, the *innate immune mechanisms* of the body triggers its action to offer adequate protection required spontaneously, which is actually carried out by WBC or leucocytes. It has been duly observed that this particular mechanism is absolutely insufficient to afford full protection in most of the instances commonly encountered; and, therefore, the body does respond through an *immune system.*

In fact, the entire prevailing *'immune system'* is essentially made up of cells and macromolecules that usually give rise to a rather complex network of cellular and molecular interactions so designed to negate the adverse effect caused by microorganisms and parasites. In other words, one may explain this intricate immune response as a mechanism explicitely exhibited either by humans or higher organisms, whereby a very critical as well as specific response is invariably drawn out against the probable invasion of well-defined pathogenic microorganisms and other foreign substances. Besides, it may also be regarded as a *'specific physiological response'* which protects human beings against a plethora of dreadful diseases. Interestingly, the ensuing immune response is appreciably signified by memory, specificity and above all the capability to differentiate between *'self'* from *'non-self'* at the molecular level even.

4.3 Antigens and Haptens

The two terminologies *viz.,* **antigens** and **haptens** are intimately associated with *immunology;* and, hence one may understand and have a clear concept about them as far as possible.

4.3.1 Antigens

An **antigen** is either a cell or molecule which will bind with preexiting antibody but will not definitely cause induction of antibody production.

Antigen may also be defined as – *'a macromolecular entity that essentially elicits an immune response via the formation of specific antibodies in the body of the host'.*

In a broader perspective the antigen (or **immunogen**) is invariably regarded as the afferent branch of the prevailing immune system, as illustrated in Fig. 4.1 below, and is any cell or molecule which would provoke an *immune response* very much in an immunological viable and competent individual. Generally, immunogens (antigens) must fulfill the following two cardinal characteristic features, namely:

a. Should be larger than 2000 in molecular weight, *e.g.,* protein, glycoprotein and carbohydrates, and

b. Must be absolutely foreign to the individual into whom they have been introduced appropriately.

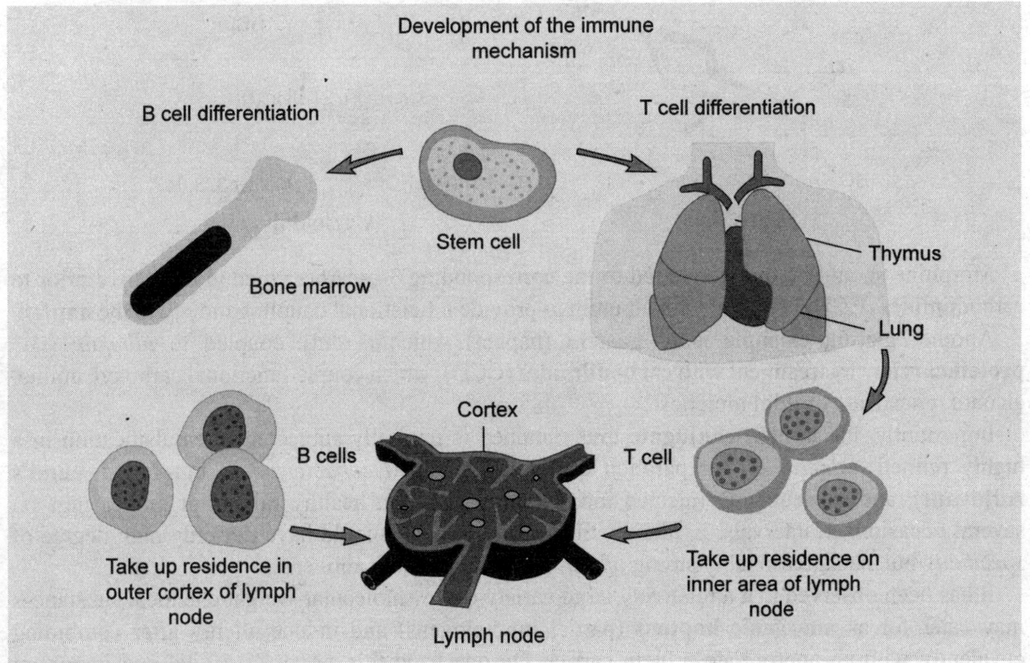

Fig. 4.1 *Immune Mechanism*

Example: The most befitting example of an *'antigen'* is ones own erythrocytes (WBC). Because, they will not induce antibody formation in oneself but will definitely react with an antibody essentially contained in an improperly matched blood transfusion.

It is, however, pertinent to state here that quite often an antigen is a protein, but it could also be a polysaccharide or nucleic acid or any other substance. Importantly, it may also be possible that a foreign substance (*e.g.,* **protein**)-not necessarily belonging to a pathogenic microorganism, may act as an *antigen* so that on being injected into a host, it may induce antibody formation. Besides, they may turn out to be antigenic and thereby cause stimulation of antibody production, incase they are intimately and lightly get bound to certain macromolecules, for instance: proteins, carbohydrates and nucleic acids.

4.3.2 Haptens

In usual practice, the relatively smaller, less rigid or rather less complex molecules usually are not immunogenetic in their purest form, but may be made so by simply linking them strategically to either larger or more complex structures. Consequently, the smaller molecules are invariably termed as **haptens;** whereas, the larger molecules or cells are known as *carriers.*

Hapten may also be defined– *'as a substance that normally does not act as an antigen or stimulate an immune response but that can be combined with an antigen and, at a later time, initiate a specific antibody response on its own'.*

Furthermore, small molecules (micromolecular), such as: drug substances, that may serve as *'haptens'* and can normally be made antigenic by coupling them chemically to a macromolecular substance *e.g.,* protein, polysaccharide, carbohydrate etc. The *hapten* is obtained from a non-antigenic compound (micromolecule) e.g., **morphine, carteolol** etc., which is ultimately conjugated*, covalently to a **carrier** macromolecule to render it antigenic.

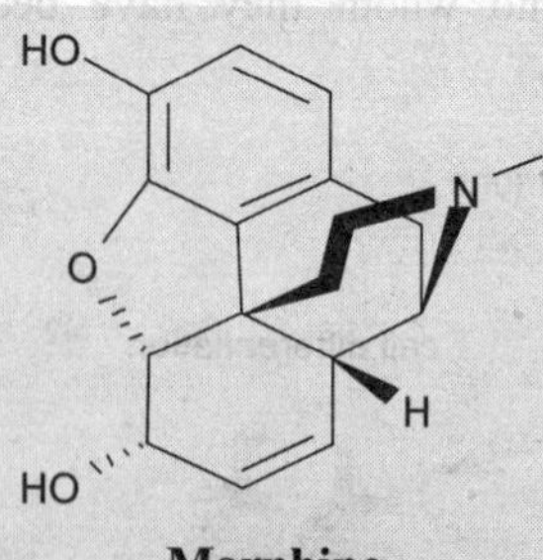

$C_{16}H_{24}N_2O_3.HCl$ Mol.wt.328.84

Morphine 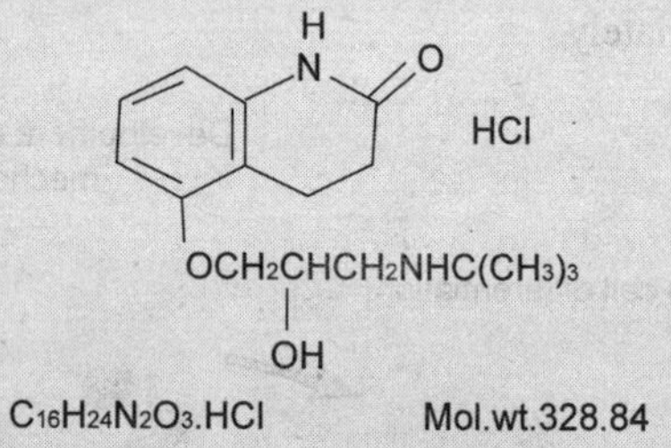 **Carteolol**

Morphine should be first converted to the corresponding 3-o-carboxymethyl derivative prior to carbodiimides (CCD) coupling with albumin to provide a functional coupling moiety in the **hapten.**

Another glaring example is of **gastrin** (hapten) which is duly coupled to *albumin* (*i.e.,* **proteincarrier**) by treatment with **carbodiimides** (CCD), which couple functional carboxyl, amino, alcohol, phosphate or thiol moieties.

Importantly, the **hapten-conjugate** thus obtained is normally subjected to emulsification in a highly refined *'mineral oil'* preparation containing-killed *Mycobacterium* (**Complete Freund's Adjuvant**), and subsequently injected intradermally either in healthy rabbits or guinea pigs on several occasions at intervals. Evidently, the serum antibody should have not only high degree of *specificity* but also a reasonably strong *affinity* for the prevailing antigens.

It has been observed that a relatively large variety of low molecular-weight chemical substances may cater for as **allergenic haptens** (partial immunogens) and induce allergy after combining covalently with an appropriate protein carrier. On one hand this serves as a vital and important phenomenon specifically in drug allergy; however, the most widely found **'environmental**

allergens'. Perhaps the most notable exception in the instance of common allergic contact dermatitis produced by a variety of plants, drugs, clothing additives and other similar substances.

Examples:

a. **Urshiols:** The *allergenic constituents i.e.,* the *oleoresin fraction,* derivatives of *pentadecycatechol* or *heptadecylcatechol,* that are solely responsible for causing **contact dermatitis** in North America usually belong to the natural order *Anacardiaceae,* the genus *Toxicodendron* (Rhus), and quite often include **oak, sumac** and **poison ivy.**

b. Several plants which essentially belong to the natural order *compositae viz.,* **ragweeds,** also responsible for causing *contact dermatitis,* and the *allergens* have been duly isolated and characterized as **sesquiterpinoid lactones.**

4.4 Immune Systems

Immunology, the generation of an *immune response* or the *defence mechanism exclusively* depends upon the interaction of the *three* most vital components of the **immune mechanism,** namely: (*a*) Immunogen stimulation; (*b*) humoral immune system; and (*c*) cellular immune system. Since 1901 and 1984 an enormous and substantial research inputs, were made by various scientists across the globe which have enabled the inhabitants of the world to lead a better and safer quality of life through the evolution of **'immunotechnology'** *i.e.,* conglomeration of various immune systems. During the said long period (1901-1984) the wonderful findings of scientists and researchers not only brought them wide recognition through most coveted Noble Prizes but also paved the way towards the introduction of remarkable and most trustworthy remedies for complicated not-so-easy diseases of the present day.

It would be worthwhile to make a brief and comprehensive illustration of some of these meaningful contributions in a chronological manner as stated below:

• ***Emil von Behring (1901):*** Awarded with Noble Prize for his interesting discovery that quite a few diseases are caused due to the *expression of toxins,* which he demonstrated by inoculating healthy animals with **diphtheria tetanus toxins** to generate **antitoxins.**

• ***Jules Bordet (1919):*** Bagged the Nobel Prize for proving that erythrocytes may be haemolyzed with particular antibody and complement accordingly. His work further demonstrated quite successfully the strategical involvement of certain biological processes taking place *in vivo,* namely: **bacterial agglutination, neutralization of the precipitin reaction,** and **complementary mediated immune haemolysis.**

• ***Karl Landsteiner (1930):*** Became the Nobel Laureate for his epoch making findings for a deeper and vivid immunological concepts with regard to the discovery of **blood group antigens** *i.e.,* AB- O blood groups, that was eventually used for successful transfusions in humans.

• ***Ehrlich's Selection Theory:*** It is directly associated with antibody production, and it was amply revealed that during the intricate phenomenon of acquiring *'immunity'*, the critical substances that are exclusively responsible for the **fine specificity of recognition** were revealed to be the **globular proteins** that are strategically located in the *γ-fraction of blood serum.* Subsequently, Landsteiner experimentally demonstrated the aforesaid theory to be **'false',** based on blood transfusions. In other words, Ehrlich failed to substantiate his assumption that traces of each individual kind of antibody are carried out in the organism specifically ; whereas, Landsteiner adequately proved that antibodies may only be generated under the influence of foreign substances, *i.e., via* an **instructive process.**

• ***Linus Pauling's Instructive Theory (1940s):*** Pauling was pioneer in assigning a *'helical structure'* to the protein molecules; and, soon after proposed the **instructive theory.** He even went a step ahead and postulated a **'template theory'** particularly for the *synthesis of antibody molecules* that could have a relatively broad range of diversity in shapes. However, at a later stage a renowned immunologist Sir Macfarlane Burnet heavily criticized the *'template theory'* on logical grounds.

• ***Natural Selection Theory (1955):*** Niels Kaj Jerne put forward the 'natural selection theory' for the production of **antibody.** In fact, his proposed theorization revolves round his logical explanation that – *'the antigen neither serves as a template nor as an enzyme modifier'*. In other words, the antigen is exclusively a **highly selection carrier** closely associated with a spontaneously circulating antibody to a *'system of cells'* that is capable of reproducing this antibody. It has been duly observed that **globulins** are being synthesized in a large variant of different configuration. At this juncture the introduction of an antigen into the blood stream essentially gives rise to the selective attachment onto the *surface of the antigen* only such *globulin molecules* that should exhibit a complementary configuration. In short, Niels Kaj Jarne brought back a new lease of life to the **'Ehrlich's Selection Theory'** almost after a long gap of *six decades*.

• ***Clonal Selection Theory:*** Burnet in 1957, put forward **clonal selection theory** with regard to **'antibody formation'** that vehemently offered a positive clue that each *cell* following an usual contact with an *antigen* yields a **clone**** of cells that would be exclusively engaged in the production of antibody of a particular kind. Importantly, Burnet's theory suggests *two responses* taking place, namely: **primary** and **secondary,** of which the latter one seems to be more powerful by virtue of the fact that **'antigenic memory** ultimately gives rise to **colossal clonal expansion** in an extraordinarily rapid manner in the course of subsequent exposure to antigen. Hence, the said theory has not only been accepted across the globe but also attracted enormous glory, fame and recognition which enabled Burnet to bag the Nobel Prize in 1960 (also shared by Sir Peter Medawar).

It is, however, pertinent to mention here that Niel's Kaj Jerne also overwhelmingly was honoured with the Nobel Prize in 1984 i.e., almost after a gap of 24 long years for his ever enlightening and wonderful discovery of the following two aspects in the immunological concepts, namely:

a. Clonal expansion concept, and
b. Evaluation of **idiotype network** in regulatory mechanism of immune responses.

• ***Rodney R Porter and Gerald M Edelman (1972):*** The pioneering discovery made by Porter and Edelman with regard to the *elucidation of the structure of antibody molecule,* which is extremely vital and important in the elaborated study of **antigen-antibody interactions,** helped them to be honoured with the most coveted and prestigious Nobel Prize in 1972. Importantly, their findings not only proved but also established the most glaring fact that the **four polypeptide chains comprising of each immunoglobulin molecule may be enzytmetically cleaved** into *three distinct segments,* such as: *two* **antibody fragments (Fab);** and *one* **crystalline fragment (Fc).**

• ***Wu and Kabat's Observations:*** In 1970, these researchers adequately demonstrated the presence of specific **'hypervariable regions'** strategically located on the **'antibody molecule'.** These critical observations, in fact, virtually paved the way towards the rapid and tremendous progress in the field of **immunology;** and, therefore, legitimately caused a geometrical development equally stretched over the two most virulent segments of *medicine* as well as *modern biology*, for instance: organ and tissue transplantation, vaccinology, and molecular biology.

• ***Identification of HLA-Complex:*** The structure and eventually the specialized role and functions of the *human leucocyte antigens* (HLA) complex were scientifically revealed by Snell, Dausset and Benacerraf in late seventies earned them the Nobel Prize in 1980.

• ***Somatic Hybridization:*** The ever sensational production of **immunologically homogeneous monoclonal antibodies** was accomplished through a wonderful major historical breakthrough by two

Immunologists: George Kohler and Ceasar Milstein in the year 1975, which bagged them the Nobel Prize in 1982.

• ***S. Tonegawa's Immunoglobulin Gene Rearrangement:*** The evolution of *somatic recombination theory* logistically suggesting the individual coding in fragments of the ensuing variable and constant regions that are ultimately resembled to generate an **enormous quantum of binding sites ;** and, therefore, various binding sites may be adequately obtained due to the different *combinations and* *permutations* of relatively lighter and heavier chains. At this material time Tonegawa's remarkable epoch making discovery of the most plausible *mechanism of shuffling of several gene segments* in the plasma cells (*i.e.,* antibody secreting cells) producing a huge variety of **antibody molecules.** In short, Tonegawa's spectacular and superb scientific observations on the *immunoglobulin gene rearrangement* made an appreciable contribution both in the fields of **immunology** and **molecular biology.** Tonegawa was rightfully awarded with the prestigious Nobel Prize in the year 1987.

In a nut-shell, one may interestingly observe and access the tremendous sea-change in the most scientific and logistic progress and development during the period 1901-1987 and even after that in the fields of **immunology** and **molecular biology** which, of course, have enormously improved upon the quality of life of humans across the globe irrespective of their caste and creed.

However, the **'immune systems'** may be viewed from the following two aspects critically, such as:

a. Manipulation of immune system, and
b. Types of immunity.

4.4.1 Manipulation of Immune Systems

The *'immune system'* or the *'immune defense mechanism'* in an individual person may be subjected to a wide spectrum of articulated well-planned manipulation against a host of dreadful and even fatal infectious diseases, caused by highly dangerous and most pathogenic microorganisms, such as: cholera, polio, chicken-pox, small-pox, diphtheria, measles, whooping cough, Hongkong Flu, anthrax, jaundice, hepatitis A, B and C and the like by immunization squarely and effectively. The underlying principle of immunization is solely based on injecting an individual subject with an appropriate dosage with a sterilized and pre-tested/evaluated preparation of a **pathogenic microorganism** (disease-causing microorganism) that has been rendered harmless absolutely.

It has been duly proved and established beyond any reasonable doubt that **immune system** predominantly and essentially possess two extremely special characteristic features which not only enable the body in preventing the individual from the dreadful infection but also ensure that he must not suffer from the same infection once again *i.e.,* one normally suffers from certain infectious ailments only once in one's life-time (*small-pox, measles* etc.,). Interestingly, the said *two* special characteristic features are, namely: (*a*) **Memory**: and (*b*) **adaptability.**

More explicitely one may understand that the very first encounter of an infections agent, the body starts to learn whether it is either a *foreign entity* or a *nonself entity:* and subsequently gets adapted to fight back the caused infection (MEMORY). But, the same individual on being exposed to the infecting agent, the body in turn exhibits a substantially increased agent; the body in turn exhibits a substantially increased immune response that is actually dependent on the earlier encounter. In the science of immunology these are invariably termed as **primary and secondary immune responses.** Consequently, as a fundamental characteristic features one may proclaim that the immune system has acquired adequate **adaptability.**

4.4.2 Types of Immunity

The various types of immunity that are commonly identified, characterized and studied at length are as stated below:

i. Humoral Immunity
ii. Cell-mediated Immunity,
iii. Innate (or Natural Immunity),
iv. Acquired Immunity, and
v. Non-specific Immunity.

These different types of immunities shall now be treated individually in the section that follows:

4.4.2.1 Humoral Immunity

Antibodies are *immunoglobulin* (Ig) *molecules* (*e.g., serum proteins*) and they are usually comprised of several categories designated as IgA, IgD, IgE, IgG, and IgM respectively. However, it is pertinent to state here that each category essentially possesses certain specific characteristic features, such as: size, carbohydrate content, *electrophoretic-migration velocity, quantum of antigen-combining sites, immunological response, and immunological objective.*

Examples:

a. ***IgM:*** Almost always enjoys the reputation of being the first class of antibody generated invariably in most *humoral responses* but normally gets switched over to the corresponding IgA, IgE, or IgG at the very early stage in the immune response.

b. ***IgG:*** Most versatile important and abundantly available class of antibodies taking part in largest **humoral immune reactions.** Besides, it happens to cross the placenta thereby providing a newly born baby absolute temporary immunity against whatever immunogens the mother has earlier against IgG.

c. ***IgA:*** Antibodies are invariably found in a plethora of such secretions as: tears, saliva and mucous membranes. These are quite frequently termed as our **first-line-of-defense mechanism** by virtue of the fact that most **bacteria, viruses** and **fungi** that eventually gain entry into the body do cross a mucous membrane.

d. ***IgE:*** Antibodies are equally important in our body's defense against the **parasitic worm infections** specifically. Prominently and predominantly several allergic manifestations give rise to the release of **histamines** *e.g.,* allergy due to pollens, house dust, dust mite, human hair, food allergens etc., which in turn afford the apparent discomforts resulting into extrinsic asthma, hay fever, or hives, or excessive sneezing (during changes of season due to pollens in the air).

e. Antibodies normally serve as **surface receptors** strategically located on certain *immunologically active cells* so as to enable them to bind immunogen.

Importantly, the different types of cells or entities that are held responsible for contributing immensely to the **humoral immunity** are as follows:

i. B Lymphocytes (or B Cells),
ii. Immunodominant peptides (IDPs),
iii. Antigen-presenting cell (APC),
iv. T Cell subsets
v. Class II MHC (major histocompatibility complex) proteins.

It would be worthwhile to have a closer and detailed description and functionalities of each of the cell or entity cited above in the selections that follows:

4.4.2.1.1 B Lymphocytes [or B cells]

The **B lymphocytes** or **B cells** are so named because they were first and foremost found in the *Bursa* of Fabricius of birds.* It has been observed that in 'birds' the multipotent stem cells actually originate in the bone marrow usually migrate to the *bursa*, and here they virtually get differentiated into specific antibody synthesizing cells. In fact, **antibody molecules** are normally generated by the plasma cells which are vividly differentiated from B cells. It has been found that B cells are concentrated in various parts of the body, such as: spleen, mucous-associated lymphoid tissue, and regional lymph nodes, where they actually await contact by the foreign *epitopes* which promptly initiate the process of conversion into the plasma cells.

Interestingly, the characteristic features of B cells may be enumerated as stated below:

1. B cells possess essentially surface immunoglobulin (sIgs) plus a number of receptors.
2. The sIg form an integral part of B cells; and, therefore, act as receptor for antigens.

3. B cells may also have immunoglobulin (Ig) in their cytoplasm.
4. Initially, when B cells are *'immature'*, sIg molecules which are exhibited specially belong to IgM category that do not cross link with other IgMs.
5. IgD molecules appear prominently on the surface showing extremely high levels with B cell marching ahead to its developmental pathway.
6. Activation of B cell initiates loss of IgDs together with other receptors appearing in the membrane that eventually enhance the phenomenon of activation.
7. B cells may undergo activation by the aid of lipopolysaccharide preparations from Gram-negative organisms *e.g., E. coli, Salmonella.* Besides, activation may be followed by the appearance of a plethora of surface receptors for Igs, ocystalline fragment (Fc) component of heavy Ig chain, and also for **Epstein-Barr virus.**
8. Antigen critically triggers selection of an appropriate antibody-producing cell and this selection is exclusively based upon the *surface receptors.*
9. *Receptors* which are found to be absolutely specific for an **antigenic determinant** not only provoke but also interact with B cells to initiate strategic proliferation and generate a clone of **blast cells,** most of which are capable of giving rise to the **same antibody.**
10. A portion of the prevailing *blast cells* get segregated and pass into the *plasma cells* (*i.e.,* **antibody secreting cells**), while others do remain behind in *lymphoid tissue* in the form of **memory cells.**
11. B cell is characterized by a **genetic composition** which enables it to produce only *one specificity* of antibody; and this is accomplished *via* **random rearrangement of genes** which essentially control and monitor both gross and minute antibody structure.
12. B cells are produced continuously *in vivo* throughout life since the life-span of a mature B cell is only a few days unless contacted by the immunogen for that it remains specific.

4.4.2.1.2 Immunodominant Peptides (IDPs)

It is, however, a universal truth that **'antibody production'** invariably takes place through the earnest cooperation and interaction of various types of cells. It has been duly observed that either *macrophages* or other cells having *identical lineage* encounter predominantly the extra cellular foreign immunogen present in the blood or lymph, undergoes phagocytocis, and ultimately meets complete destruction. Importantly, in the course of the *'phagocytic phenomenon'* the ensuing **macrophage** critically identifies and recognizes **epitope structures** present on the immunogen, and notably protects them in the shape of short peptide chains having 10-18 amino acid lengths that are usually referred to as immunodominant peptides (IDPs).

4.4.2.1.3 Antigen-Presenting Cell (APC)

The antigen has to be presented correctly and precisely onto the surface of an **antigen-presenting cell** (APC) which is normally a **macrophage,** or similar cell. Most commonly the antigen is presented in association with self Ia molecules duly coded by MHC-genes.

4.4.2.1.4 T Cell Subsets

T Cells or **thymus-derived T lymphocytes** do play extremely vital and equally important roles in the domain of **immune response mechanism,** particularly in the cell-mediated immunity (CMI). In true sense, the different types of immunological functionalities mediated by them usually fall under *two* distinct categories, namely: *(a) effector responses;* and *(b) regulatory responses.*

Examples of Effector Functions (Responses): The various types of effector functions are as stated under:

i. Tuberculin reaction (or delayed hypersensitivity response),
ii. Destruction of tissue grafts, and

iii. **Lymphokines** *vis-à-vis* their ability to perform *'killer functions'* of other cells due to the secretion of soluble chemical mediators,

Example of Regulatory Function (Response): The essential kind of regulatory function involves their close cooperation with B cells to give rise to the formation of **antibodies.** Explicitely and precisely but for their excellent mutual cooperation, a good number of antigens would have **not** succeeded in the induction of *antibody formation* in animals.

T cells, in general, possess a host of **'subpopulations'** that essentially contribute remarkable, explicit and above all an excellent array of immune responses, for instance: **cytotoxicity, killer properties** and **significant suppression.**

Emergence: The **'thymus'** is the focal point wherein the actual emergence of pre-T cells invariably commence and undergo **massive proliferation** and **differentiation** to get converted into **immunocomplement T cells.** Consequently, the resulting cells undergo migration right into the blood stream and along with B cells help to populate the prevailing secondary lymphoid organs. T cells get matured in **thymus,** migrate to the **peripheral regions of thymus**, and ultimately to **spleen** where they are subjected to further stage of maturation thereby yielding a variety of **T cell subsets.**

Kinds of T cell Subjects: There are in all **four** kinds of T cell subsets that have been duly identified based on their surface markers, namely:

a. T helper cells (TH cells or CD_4 cell): An appropriate TH cell is one that essentially possesses a good number of surface receptors arranged in a series and is capable of interacting with the class II major histocompatibility complex [or class II MHC] of the APC, and also specific for the epitopes present on the IDP. Besides, the T cell receptor series prominently comprises of T cell receptors (TcRs) that are found to be quite specific for:

- the prevailing foreign epitopes on the IDP,
- CD_4 (T_4) receptors that essentially interact with class II MHC structures,
- CD_{28}– which being a co stimulatory structure, and
- CD_3– surface molecules that predominantly cater for a possible communication linkage between T_CR, CD_4, and the cytoplasm of the T_H cell.

Interestingly, the prevailing interaction between the APC and TH cells gives rise to the secretion APC yielding a *cytokine* termed as interleukin-1 (IL-1), which prominently aids to activate the T_H cell.

Furthermore, the activated T_H cell subsequently gives rise to another cytokine known as interleukin-2 (IL-2) that eventually acts as an **autocrine** there by raising the T_H cell to a relatively *higher peak of metabolic activity* and also inducing T_H cell proliferation. In actual reality, the ensuing **activated** and **duplicated** T_H cells adequately generate more IL-2 and do help in the production of IL-4, IL-6, and IL-13 in addition to quite a few other molecules, including CD_4OL, which activate suitable B cells in a concerted manner.

Two subsets of T helper cells (T_H) [CF_{4+}] (Th1 and Th2):

The **T helper cells** (TH) are of *two* types, namely: (*a*) Th1 cells; and (*b*) Th 2 cells which would be discussed separately at length as under:

1. **Th 1 cells:** It is, however, pertinent to state here that since the remarkable discovery of subsets of T helper cells *i.e.,* Th 1 and Th 2, gained wide recognition and acceptance for the first time in 1986, a tremendous and copious volume of work has been duly accomplished and concepts with newer ideas conceived.

Salient features of Th 1 cells: The various salient features of these cells are as follows:

i. They activate macrophages,

ii. Their **clones** specifically give rise to interleukin (IL-2), interferon (IFN γ), and tumour necrosis factor (TNF-β),

iii. They produce strong delayed-type hypersensitivity reaction (DTH-reaction), *iv.* They invariably generate cytokines for its own proliferation *e.g.,* **autocrine growth factor** IL-2 for Th 1, and

v. They produce cytokines which cross-regulates each other's development and activity *viz.,* IL-4 and IL-10 suppressing Th 1.

2. Th 2 cells: The **salient features** of Th 2 cells are as enumerated below:

i. Their clones give rise to IL-3, IL-4, IL-5, IL-10 and IL-13. However, it was earlier believed that IL-10 to be the product of Th 2, and later on it was demonstrated to be the product of both Th 1 and Th 2.

ii. They generate weak DTH reaction involving relatively higher level of **'antibody production'.**

iii. They product cytokines for its own proliferation *viz.,* **autocrine growth factor** IL-4 for Th 2.

iv. They also produce cytokines, which essentially cross-regulate each other's development and activity *e.g.,* IFN-γ suppressing Th 2.

In general, **leishmaniasis,** is found to be a *'model'* for the functional dichotomy of helper T-cells, whereby Th 1 associated with resistance and Th 2 with susceptibility of this ailment.

b. Cytotoxic T cells [CTLs or Tc]: These represent a subset of T cells that essentially act as **'killer cells'** and are strategically located in the human peripheral blood. In fact, they kill the cells which are invariably infected either with a virus or any other pathogenic (*i.e.,* disease producing) microorganisms. CTLs are also termed as **effector T cells,** or **CD8 cells**. Since the Tc cells are recruited to an area **infested** with viral infection, growing tumour, or foreign organ (*i.e.,* transplanted organ like kidney); and those with T_CR_s specific for the epitopes of the target shall eventually get bound to the **'target cell'** which specifically exhibits either the *foreign tumour* or *virus epitopes* in perfect harmony with its class I MHC surface structures. Interestingly, this usually affords an activation of the IL-2 receptors upon the *recruited* as well as *attached* **Tc cells.** As a result the ensuing IL-2 generated by the TH cells **activates, proliferates,** and also **differentiates** TC cells, thereby enabling their conversion to the corresponding CTL cells ; and, therefore, causing an effective initiation of the **'effector phase'** of the prevailing **immune response mechanism** to a considerable extent.

c. Suppressor-inducer T cells [Ts]: These cells are believed to serve as suppressor of helper T cells (T_H) on one hand and in turn cause inhibition of the B cells to generate antibodies significantly. They are essentially found to bear CV8 markers.

d. Delayed Hypersensitivity T cells [TDH]: It has been recently demonstrated and advocated that the delayed hypersensitivity cells (TDH) essentially form an integral part of a subset of T cells that have been shown to take part actively in **delayed hypersensitivity reactions.**

The following two Figs. 4.2 and 4.3 evidently illustrate the development of T cells before they are actually exposed to the antigen, and the subsets of T cells that actively participate in the regulatory immune response mechanism respectively.

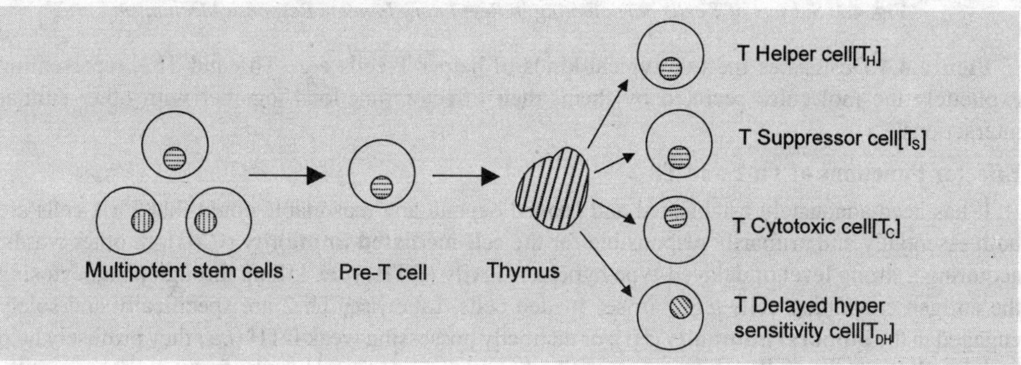

Fig. 4.2 *Development of T cells prior to their Exposure to Antigen*

Explanation of Fig. 4.2: A situation when the T cells are under the process of **'differentiation'** and **'proliferation'** in the *thymus,* these are invariably termed as **thymocytes.** Subsequently, these thermocytes eventually emerge as completely differentiated and fully distinguishable T cells that essentially undergo clonal expansion on being subjected to interaction with the ensuing antigen, such as: T_H ; T_S ; T_C ; and T_{DH}.

Explanation of Fig. 4.3: It vividly illustrates the various emerging subsets of T cells that actually take part in the regulatory immune response mechanism thereby giving rise to T_S (suppressor T cell), B lymphocyte (B cell), T_C (cytotoxic T cell), and macrophage respectively. The *'arrows'* indicated here designate the activating signals explicitely and squarely.

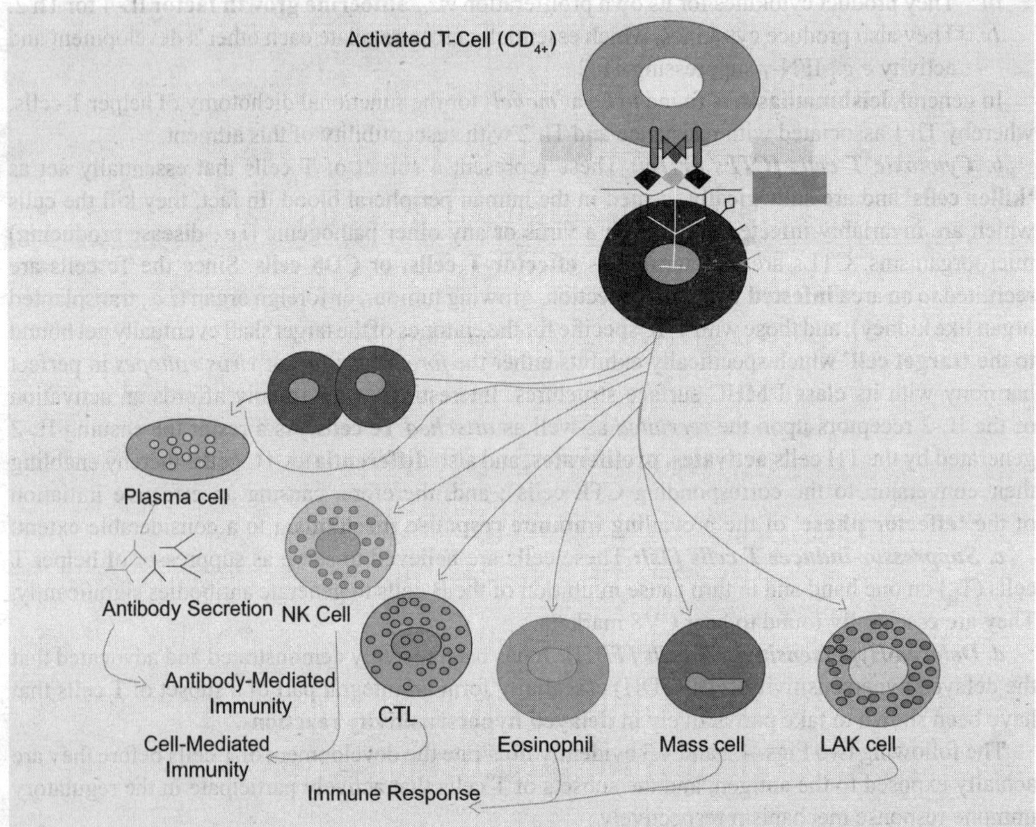

Fig. 4.3 *Subsets of T cells participating in Regulatory Immune Response Mechanism*

Figure 4.4 Designates the two typical kinds of helper T cells e.g., Th1 and Th2, representing explicitely the molecules secreted by them, their effector functions together with other similar interactions.

Effector Functions of Th 1 and Th 2

It has been adequately established and proved beyond any reasonable doubt that **Th 1 cells** are both essentially and primarily responsible for the **cell-mediated immunity** (CMI). In other words, acquiring a strong level of delayed-type hypersensitivity (DTH) (*i.e.,* killing through phagocytosing the antigen containing cells *e.g.,* viruses loaded cells. Likewise, Th 2 are specifically and solely engaged in the **humoral immunity** (HI); or distinctly possessing weak DTH (*i.e.,* they profusely help both B cells and other cells in generating antibodies adequately. Based on the fact that IFN-γ, usually released by Th 1 cells, causes *induction* and subsequent *conversion* of B cells to a good number of

IgG isotypes have undoubtedly raised doubt upon the integrity of the aforesaid classification linked to their *effector functions*. In order to get rid of such an ambiguity the *effector functions* of Th 1 and Th 2 logically may be classified exclusively based on the observed *'biological activities'* of the cytokines produced by them.

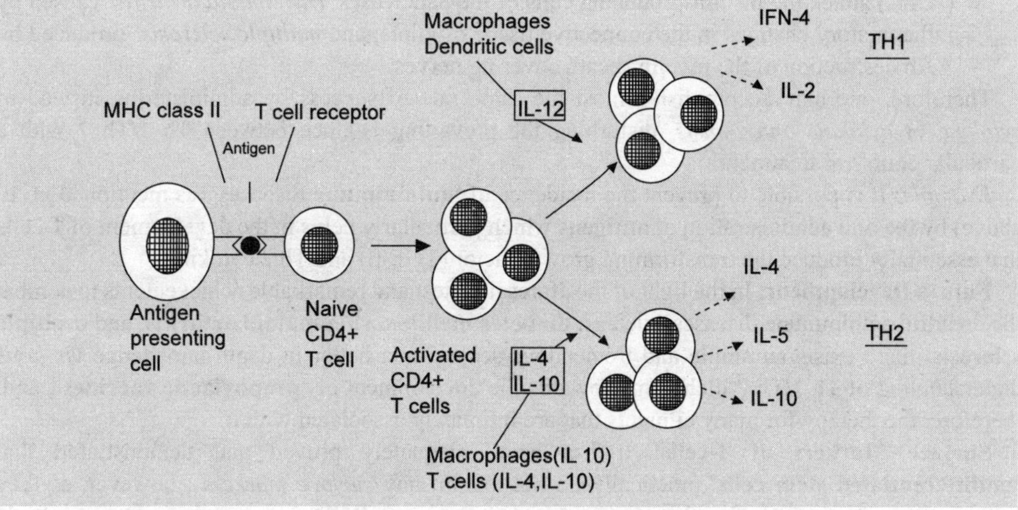

Fig. 4.4 *Molecules Secreted by Th 1 and Th 2 cells; Effector Functions and Interactions*

Examples:

Principal cytokine of Th 1 being IFN-γ: It plays *two* vital roles:

a. Activation of microphages for microbicidal action, and
b. Stimulation for the production of IgG antibodies.

Principal cytokines of Th 2 being IL-4 and IL-5:

a. *IL-4:* causes induction of B-cell switching to IgE production, and
b. *IL-5:* causes activation of eosinophils; and both IgE and eosinophil mediated defense is very vital for eliminating certain, but not all *helminths.*

Th1 and Th 2 [Subsets of CD_{4+} helper T-cells] and Diseases

The Th 1 and Th 2 helper cells have been observed to be intimately linked with several dreadful ailments. Evidently, it is on account of the critical indulgence by each separate cytokines that are associated with the management and control of **serious pathological immune responses.** A few such infectious diseases are, namely: (*a*) leischmaniasis; (*b*) allergic disease conditions (which involves **mast cells** and IgE; and also **autoimmune diseases.**

Importantly, one is loaded with so much solid evidences to suggest that modulation of Th1/Th2 equilibration by the adequate and timely administration of either **recombinant cytokines** or **cytokine antagonists** helps to change the flare up and intensity of the disease.

Examples:

a. ***IL-12:*** When given at the time of infection usually increases significant resistance to a host of several **intracellular pathogens,** such as: protozoa, viruses, fungi, and microorganisms.
b. ***IL-12:*** May also be indicated for the effective treatment of cancer, and allergic symptoms, and is also under active investigation in certain antineoplastic vaccine protocols.
c. ***IL-12:*** Invariably finds its usage as **vaccine adjuvant** along with specific sensitizing dosage resimens of **'antigen',** which not only helps in the genuine conversion of Th 2 pattern into Th 1 pattern, but also augment resistance to ensuing infection and thereby suppressing the prevailing Th 2 dëpendent pathological conditions appreciably.

d. ***IL-10:*** Can reasonably suppress **lipopolysaccharide-induced** endotoxemia and also inflammatory bowel disease in experimental animals.

e. ***Th 2 cells:*** On being subjected to *'selective induction'* may be used for the treatment and cure of tissue **autoimmune diseases** *e.g., diabetes mellitus:* in which the autoantibodies (AAbs) attack the insulin-producing cells of the pancreases; *rheumatoid arthritis:* caused by inflammatory changes in the connective tissue of joints; and *multiple sclerosis:* produced by AAb destruction of the myclin sheath covering nerves.

Therefore, one may accomplish almost the same rate of success by administering instead of *cytokine* or *cytokine antagonists,* disturbing the prevailing balance between Th 1/Th 2 with a particular course of treatment.

Example: It is possible to prevent the incidence of **'autoimmune diseases'** (as mentioned in *'e'* above) by the oral administration of **antigens** which particularly helps in the development of T-cells that essentially produce the transforming growth factor (TGF-β) and Th 2 cytokines.

Future Development: In the light of the aforesaid latest and remarkable achievements to combat the dreadful autoimmune diseases, such as: **diabetes mellitus, rheumatoid arthritis,** and **multiple sclerosis,** there exists an ample and tremendous scope for a better in depth knowledge *vis-à-vis* understanding of Th 1/Th 2 dichotomy towards the development of **'prophylactic vaccines'**; and, therefore, the therapy for many ailments that are intimately associated with it.

Surface Markers of T-cells: It has been adequately proved and demonstrated that **'undifferentiated stem cells'** practically do not exhibit any *surface markers* ; however, as they happen to travel through the **thymus cortex** and **the medulla**, they are subjected to multiple divisions and thereby accomplish maturity to a significant extent. Consequently, **thymus** helps to programme T-cells which pass through it to follow meticulously the prevailing T-cell differentiation into the various subsets; and, hence, it essentially encompasses its legitimate development to perform various immune functions as illustrated in Fig. 4.5 below.

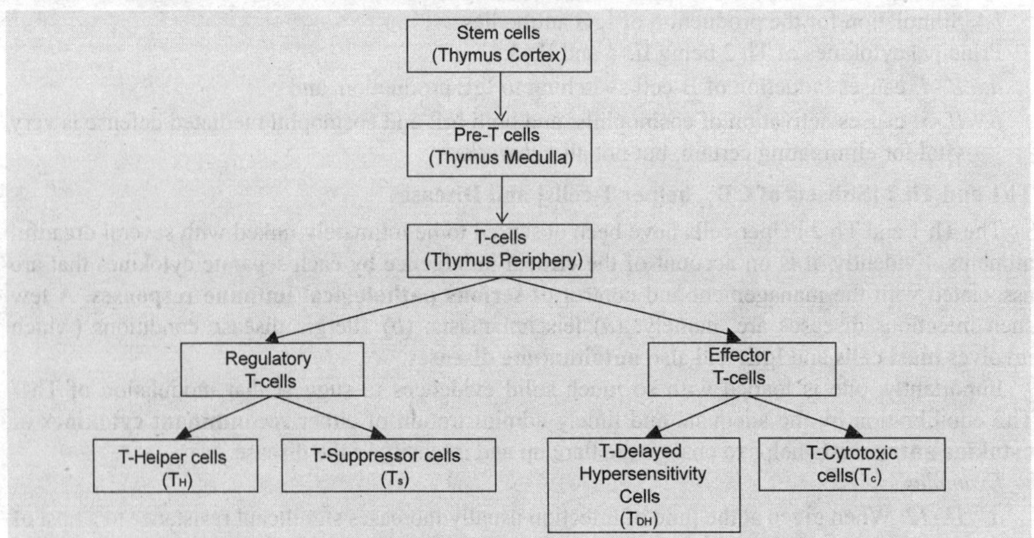

Fig. 4.5 *Block Diagram of Thymus Programme T-cells Passing through it to follow T-cell Differentiation in Subset Variants*

Interestingly, in the **life-span** within the *thymus*, lasting for nearly three days, the T cells start showing typical and specific **surface markers.** Besides, these surface markers are nothing but macromolecules (*e.g.*, **glycoprotein's**) that have a well-defined clear cut distinction from the **glycoprotein's that are strategically coded for by the major histocompatibility complex (MHC)**

genes shared equally by all T-cells. However, a good part of these markers have been duly well defined both in human T cells as well as in mouse T cells.

In actual practice, however, there are several other surface markers that are critically and exclusively exhibited on a population of T cells; and, therefore, these are invariably employed to identify the T cell subsets and their individual prevailing functions as depicted in Table 1 below:

Table 4.1 *Surface Markers of T-cells and Their Corresponding Subsets.*

T-Cells	Surface Markers	T-Cell Subsets	Individual Functions
T-Cells	CD_{4+}	T-helper cell (T_H)	– Regulator cells ; – Inducers of T_C cells that are CD_8; – Stimulate B cell to generate antibodies;
	CD_{8+}	T-cytotoxic cell (T_C)	– Kill (lyse) antigen-loaded target cells (i.e., effector cells)
	CD_{2+}; CD_{8+}; CD_3-cell receptor	T-suppressor cells (T_S)	– Prevent production of antibody by B cells; – Exert action on CD_4 and TH cells.
	Unknown (?)	T-delayed hypersensitivity cell (T_{DH})	– Rejection of **'grafts'**; – Aggravation of inflammatory response by effector cells; – Induction of IDH to cause secretion of **lymphokines** to affect phagocytes;
K-cells	CD_{2+} ; CD_{3+} ; CD_{8+} ; CD_{16} ;	–	– Surveillance of tumours; – Affect Fc receptors for Fe regions of IgG – Exhibit distinct antibody-dependent killer activity ;
NK-cells	CD_{2+}; CD_{56+}; CD_{4-}; C_{8-};		– Surveillance of tumours ;
	CD_{3-};		– Exhibit both anti-microbial and antiviral profile.

Differentiation between T-cells and B-cells in Immune System

The cardinal points of differentiation between T-cells and B-cells in the prevailing human immune system are *three*, which are enumerated as under in Table 2.

Table 4.2 *Differentiation between T-cells and B-cells in Immune System.*

S.No	T-Cells	S.No	B-Cells
1.	Usually act at short range, thereby causing cidal action on the **'target cells'**.	1.	Secrete antibodies that may exert its action strategically located at far away distances.
	Fail to secrete antibodies, but secrete ILs.		Antibodies positioned on the surface of B-cells are normally termed as B-cell receptors.
	Retain on their surface T-cell receptors showing **homology** with antibodies.		
2.	T-cells do recognize: (a) *antigens* solely located on cell surface, and that too in presence of MHC; and (b) Foreign extracellular antigens and microorganisms by the cell.	2.	B-cells do recognize free antigens in the circulating system of body that essentially includes: blood and lymphatic system.
3.	T-cells predominantly recognize the 3. *'Peptide fragments of antigens'* which 'are found to undergo partial degradation inside the cell; and carried to the cell surface subsequently.	3.	B-cells are known to recognize the *intact antigens'* and certainly **not** their corresponding **'fragments'**.

T-cell Receptors: It is quite well known that **'surface receptors'** in particular are fit to recognize the **'free-antigens'.** In fact, the receptors for B-cells have already been identified fully as **IgM monomer molecular entities** that have been strategically anchored onto the cell surface *via* the crystallizable fraction (Fc) region in such a fashion that fragment antibody binding (Fab) region are more or less absolutely '*free*' to interact with the antigen. It is, however, pertinent to state here that the T-cells do possess '*receptors*' that are prominently **antigen-specific**. In one of the recent studies it has been established duly that the T-cell receptors is nothing but a **heterodimer** comprised of two distinct chains, namely; α-chain, and β-chain, duly hooked on by several disulphide bonds [– S– S–]. Besides, each chain is strategically folded into two separate domains that are analogous to not only constant but also to the *variable regions* of an **immunoglobulin molecule.** Intensive and extensive studies with regard to the **genetic organization** of the *α-chain* and *β-chain* have duly revealed that each individual chain is adequately and specifically coded by an altogether separate set of genes. Evidently, the **α-chain genes** are located on the 14*th chromosome*, and the corresponding **β-chain genes** are present on the *7th chromosome*. More recently, two further chains, namely: *γ-chain* and *δ-chain* have been discovered, identified and hence recognized that are also found to be encoded by corresponding individual set of genes.

Figure 4.6 illustrate below a T-cell heterodimer, comprising of α- and β-polypeptide chains that are duly linked by several disulphide (– S– S--) bonds

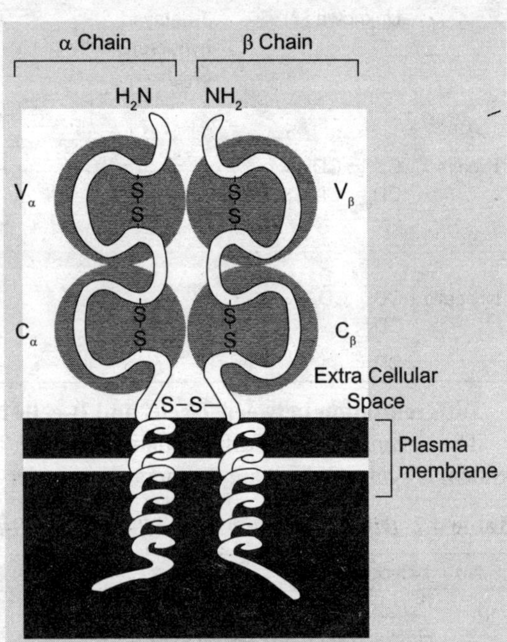

Fig. 4.6 *The T-cell Receptor Heterodimer*

CD_3-Complex: It has been amply evidenced that invariably **all T-cells** do have CD_3 molecules in their membranes that go a long way in the stabilization of the *T-cell antigen receptor*. Besides, a T-cell receptor is observed to be always intimately associated usually with a set of **transmembrane proteins** that are more or less stable and static in nature. In reality these rather rigid, stable, and static types of transmembrane proteins are termed as **CD_3-complex.** Importantly, the CD_3 complex predominantly aids not only in the process of '*signal transduction*' but also in the '*transmittance of information*' with respect to the ensuing extracellular binding* characteristic features to the prevailing intracellular signals thereby giving rise to the **activation of T-cells.** As a result of the signal transduction the generated *tyrosine kinases* affords the much desired phosphorylation of a variety of **cellular proteins** *e.g., CD_3 complex* and *phospholipase C-r* (PLC-γ). In short, the released phosphorylated proteins trigger off the most vital activation of the **inositol phospholipid signaling pathway.**

T-cell Co-Receptors (CD_4 and CD_8): It is worthwhile to mention here that the CD_4 and CD_8 molecules indulge in active participation in the T-cell activation, and are known to recognize **MHC gene products**. It has been duly observed that CD_4 molecules solely recognize MHC class II molecules, whereas CD_8 recognize MHC class I molecules exclusively; and simultaneously monitor and guide the T-cell receptor to interact with the antigen appropriately. In fact, the T-cells with their inherent T-cell receptors and CD-complex invariably facilitate the ensuing interaction taking place between the T-cells and the target cells with marked and pronounced peptide MHC complex on their surface. However, such an interaction is neither sufficiently strong nor quite stable; therefore, the

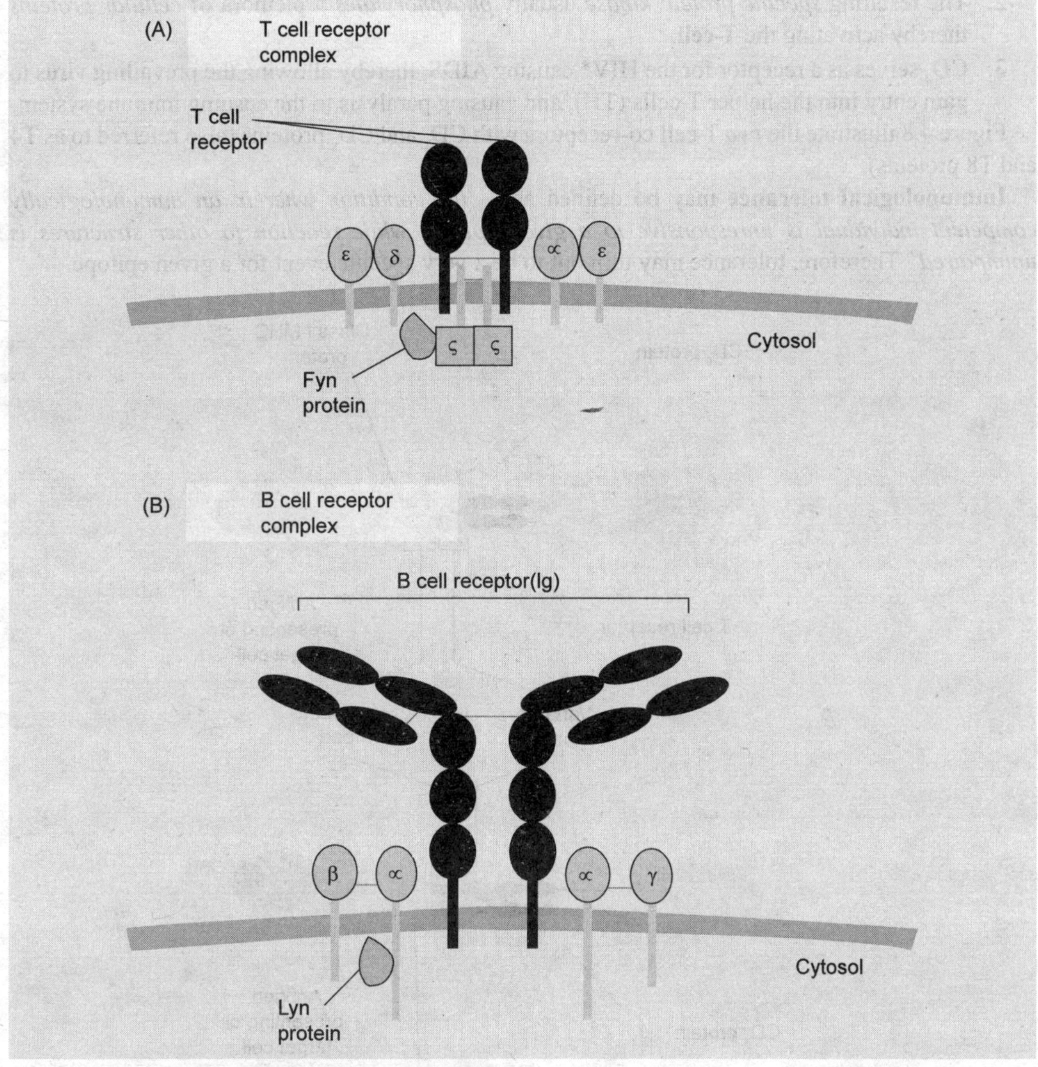

Fig. 4.7 *Comparison of Antigen Receptors on: (A) T-cells; and (B) B-cells*

presence of other *'accessory receptors'* known as **co-receptors** are absolutely necessary to stabilize adequately the interaction *via* **cell-cell cohesion**. Besides, these newer breed of *co-receptors* are found not only in activating the T-cells by producing their own intracellular signals but also required urgently the development of T-cell properly. Importantly, they get bound to the corresponding *non-variable component of the specific MHC* and are thereby rendered **invariant entities.** The *two* CD-receptors are, namely:

a. CD_4 strategically located on **helper T-cells** and **binding class II MHC,** and

b. CD_8 specifically positioned on **cytotoxic T-cells** and **binding class I MHC.**

Salient Features of T-cell Co-Receptors: Following are some of the salient features of the T-cell co-receptors, such as:

1. The two co-receptors are found to be **single transmemebrane proteins.** Besides, their cytoplasmic tail is intimately linked with the members of the Src family of tyrosine specific **protein kinases** known as the **Lck Protein**.

2. The resulting *specific protein kinase* usually *phosphorylates* a plethora of *cellular proteins* thereby activating the **T-cell.**
3. CD_4 serves as a receptor for the HIV* causing AIDS, thereby allowing the prevailing virus to gain entry into the helper T-cells (TH), and causing paralysis to the ensuing immune system.

Figure 4.8 illustrate the *two* T-cell co-receptors with CD_4 and CD_8 proteins (also referred to as T4 and T8 proteins):

Immunological tolerance may be defined as – *'the condition wherein an immunologically competent individual is unresponsive to a given epitope while reaction to other structures is unimpaired'.* Therefore, tolerance may turn out to be a very specific event for a given epitope.

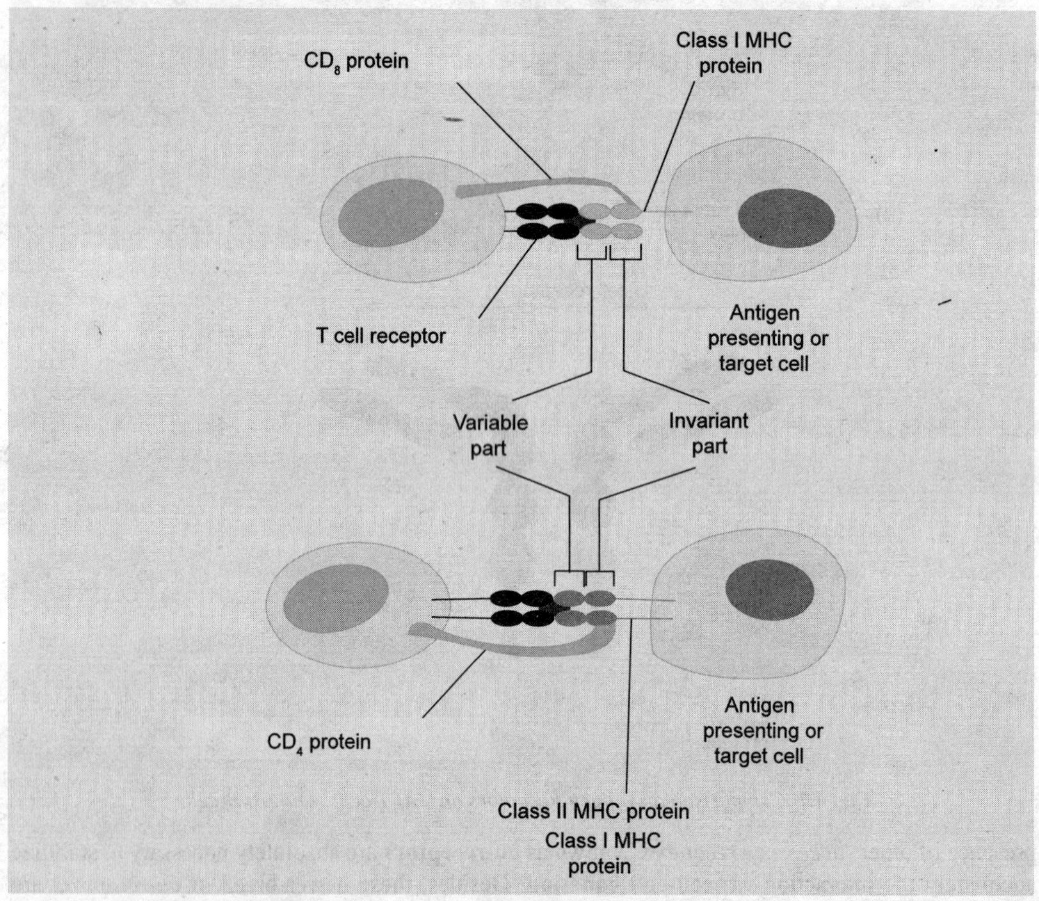

Fig. 4.8 *T-cell Co-receptors with CD_4 and CD_8 proteins*

Autoimmunity: Based on the intriguing observation that the prevailing immune system critically and significantly distinguishes the *'foreign molecules'* from the *'self molecules'*, and subsequently react only against such **foreign molecules.** Thus *two* different probabilities may arise, namely:

a. That an animal may receive genes which encode receptors specifically for *foreign antigens* and not for *self antigens,* and

b. That the immune system of an animal is particularly capable of responding to both foreign and self antigens inherently. However, during the course of the development it learns how to responds to **foreign antigens only;** thereby ascertaining the fact that the ensuing differential response to foreign antigens is nothing but an outcome of an **acquired characteristic property.**

Interestingly, the past two decades have witnessed a remarkable progress in an intensive research in this direction which pinpointed with enough evidence that the second alternative [*i.e.*, (*b*)] holds good and the prevailing **immune system** ultimately succeeds in acquiring the attribute of responding to only the **foreign antigenis.** However, the aforesaid findings were adequately substantiated with the following two observations, namely:

a. Tissues from one particular individual on being transplanted into the living body of another, are always regarded to be as '*foreign*' and hence **destroyed rapidly**, and

b. Genetically different (*i.e., dizygotic*) twins, when cells of one mouse are introduced strategically in the body of another healthy mouse (*i.e., at neonatal stage,* prior to the maturation of the '*immune system*') ; consequently, a little positive response to these foreign cells was ever noticeable for a relatively longer span.

It is pertinent to state at this point in time that a reasonable degree of **'immunological tolerance'** may be accomplished artificially.

Examples:

1. When a '*trimester human embryo*' is exposed adequately to a foreign epitope, it may be rendered tolerant to it, because it usually recognizes it as self. And the exact mechanism by which it is achieved is not understood vividly. It may probably be explained by virtue of the fact that the epitomes which are present strategically at that specific moment when the immune system attains a certain degree of maturity are conspicuously regarded as **self-epitomes,** irrespective of its origin.
2. In *postnatal* subjects the requisite tolerance may also be induced on being administered with massive doses of a immunogen. In this specific instance the *immunocytes* responsible for attributing resistance to the prevailing foreign entities become substantially overwhelmed.

In either of the above two cited instances the follow up exposure to the immunogens is very much needed in case the tolerance has to be maintained adequately and effectively.

Scientists across the globe are making an earnest concerted effort in exploring every possible, viable and feasible means and ways to decepher the exact mechanisms of tolerance so that the accumulated wisdom and knowledge can have application to the development of newer human medicines for a better world of tomorrow.

Amazingly, either IV or IM administration of relatively lower doses of a **highly purified immunogen** has certain undisputable practical applicability. In actual practice, however, the careful initiation of the development of *low-dose-tolerance* has been employed with a thumbing glorious success to afford a prolonged '*graft-survival*' in laboratory animals. Likewise, in the same vein the principle of low-dose tolerance is also-employed to effectively desensitize humans against a host of **immunogens** solely responsible for a wide spectrum of **allergy syndromes**.

As grossly indicated by the ever expanding state of skill, knowledge and excellence in technological advancements in medical sciences (*e.g.*, robotic open-heart surgeries including transplants) evidently suggests that if the real mechanism of tolerance can be unfolded, a very bright ray of hope with respect to *organ transplants* may turn out to be 100% successful without the aid of *immunosuppressive therapy.* Perhaps, the '*organ recipients of tomorrow*' might live perennial normal lives and defend themselves fully and efficaciously against the most common infections that eventually claim the lives of plethora of recepients or ultimately lead to the rejection of the new organ.

Autoimmune Diseases: It has been adequately observed that the prevailing degree of **tolerance of self-antigens** sometimes undergo cessation whereby the T-cells or B-cells or both start interaction with their own antigens effectively. This particular phenomenon *in vivo* largely is responsible for producing disease conditions which is described as **autoimmune diseases.**

A few such predominant **autoimmune diseases** *vis-a-vis* their respective **supramolecular complexes** involved are duly enumerated in Table 3 as under:

Table 4.3 *Organ Specific Autoimmune Diseases Involving Supramolecular Complexes*

S.No	Auto Immune Diseases	Supramolecular Complex
1.	Myasthenia gravis	ACh1 receptor: All subunits
2.	Multiple sclerosis (MS)	Myelin: MBP protecolipid protein; myelin oligodendroglial protein; αβ-crystalline.
3.	Thyroiditis	Thyroid stimulating hormone receptor; thyroglobulin; thyroperoxidase;
4.	Insulin-dependent diabetes mellitus (IDDM)	Islet antigens: GAD; heat-shock protein 65
5.	Primary biliary cirrhosis	Mitochondrial branched-chain keto acid dehydro-genase complexes.
6.	Uveitis2	Photoreceptor-interphotoreceptor retinoid-binding protein; S-antigen of rout outer segment

1. Acetycholine; 2. A nonspecific term for any intraocular inflammatory disorder. **Equilibrium: Autoimmunity Vs Tolerance:**

A striking balance between the limits of tolerance and immunity is virtually attainable and actually maintained in an immune system which is quite evident in the following Fig. 4.9.

Explanation: To accomplish equilibrium between tolerance and immunity the involvement of *positive* and *negative selections* is an absolute necessity; the former takes care of survival, activation and expansion of one class of T-cells; while the latter involves the inhibition and elimination of another class of T-cells. Importantly, any slightest apparent shift in the aforesaid balance on either side ultimately gives rise to prevalent resistance or noticeable susceptibility to an autoimmune disease as stated in Table 3.

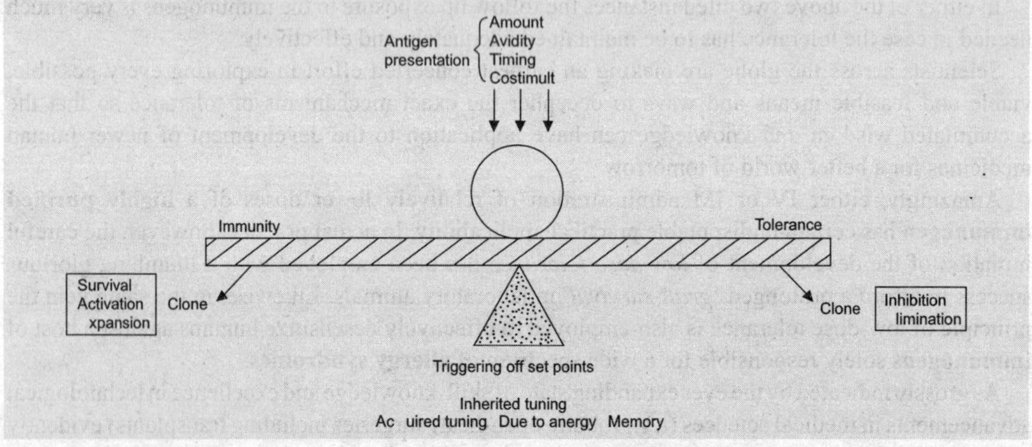

Fig. 4.9 *An Equilibrium between Autoimmunity Vs Tolerance*

4.4.2.1.5 Class II MHC (Major Histocompatiability Complex) Proteins

The articulated and geometrical progression development specifically in the field of **major histocompatiability complex** (MHC) came into being from the extensive and intensive studies carried out solely upon *transplantable tumours* that are capable of growing in nearly 100% of either *homologous* or *allogenic recipients*. In fact, this particular observation was anchored as a solid and strong evidence not only towards the *host-tumour compatibility* but also for the high levels of resistance attainable by different types of immunization characteristics more or less strengthened the belief that tumour cells invariably are associated with both extremely specific and apparently strong foreign antigens. Surprisingly, the aforesaid observation was not found to be correct and genuine based on the in-depth study of *highly inbred strains of mouse.* It was, however, further revealed that such '*tumours*' which either are produced or propagated *via highly inbred strains* do not necessarily afford active support to the various prevailing immunization procedures.

The advent of the knowledge of '*immunogenic laws of tissue transplantation*' that virtually led to the identification of the Mendelian segregation of the dominant genes. The resulting genes were duly designated as '**histocompatibility factor**' or **H-genes** and found to govern the transplantability of both normal tissues and neoplastic ones in experimental laboratory animals. In reality, the transplantable tumours attempt to grow freely across the genetic barriers by avoiding the host response directly and not due to any shortage/availability of the specific histocompatibility antigens. Elaborated experiments being conducted on the *initiation of pre-immunization against their H-antigens* amply gives evidence of the **rejectibility of such tumour lines absolutely.** Such a quick and a premature inference drawn was found to be not so authentic and true, and hence rejected. Further substantial evidences generated showed that the actual population of T-cells (specifically TC) really direct their activity against the **antigens** of the tissue cell surface usually, termed as the **major histocompatibility** complex (MHC complex) region of the genome.**

Classification of MHC-Complex. Studies have revealed that there exist *two* kinds of MHC complexes (molecules), namely: (*a*) **Class I MHC Complexes** (molecules); and (*b*) **Class II MHC Complexes** (molecules). Interestingly, either of the above two complexes categorically represent

transmembrane heterodimers the extracellular-NH_2 terminal regions which get bound to the peptide fragment of the prevailing antigen for logical presentation to the corresponding available T cells. The salient and characteristic features of the aforesaid *two* kinds of MHC complexes are briefly summarized in Table 4 as under:

Table 4.4 *Characteristic Salient Features of Class I and Class II MHC Molecules*

S.No.	Class I MHC	S.No.	Class II MHC
1.	– Seen on all nucleated cells – Involved in bondage of peptide fragment from **virus** (*i.e.,* intracellular antigens) – Present cells to cytotoxic T cells (T_C)	1.	– Seen on highly specialized cells *viz.,* B cells and thymus cells. – Involved in binding endocytosed or extracellular peptide segments. – Present cells to helper T cells (T_H).
2.	Comprises essentially of: 2. (*a*) *single polymorphic transmembrane polypeptide chain* termed as 'α' (made up of 3 domains viz., α_1: α_2: α_3). (*b*) β_2-microglobulin i.e., an extracellular invariant protein.	2.	Comprises of two **transmembrane** polymorphic polypeptides α and β each made up of two extracellular domain pairs α_1 and α_2; and β_1 and β_2.
3.	β_2-Microglobulin; **not** coded in MHC 3. – Neither glycosylated nor covalently linked with 3 domains of α (α_1, α_2, α_3)	3.	– Either chains viz., α, β, are usually encoded in MHC – Either chains are duly glycosylated and this found is non-covalently linked status.
4.	– Immunoglobulin (Ig) resembles 4α_3 and β_2.	4.	– Immunoglobulin (Ig) resembles α_2 and β_2.
5.	– α_1 and β_2 the two outermost domains 5. are polymorphic in nature and help in binding – Bonded peptide has a chain of 8-10 amino acids	5.	– α_1 and β_2 the two outermost domains represent polymorphic features and form the groove for binding. – Bound peptide has a chain of 15-24 Amino acids.
6.	– **Genetic Loci:** In humans: HLA– A; B and C ; In Mice: H-2K, 2D ; and 2L ;	6.	– **Genetic Loci:** In humans: HLA–DP; -DQ, -DR; In mice: H-2A, -2E clusters.

Figure 4.10 illustrates the H-2 (mouse) and human leucocyte antigens (HLA) gene complexes, showing clearly the most preferred location of gene loci encoding the various transmembrane units

of class I and II MHC proteins. For more details on these genetic loci please refer to serial number '6' in Table: 3.

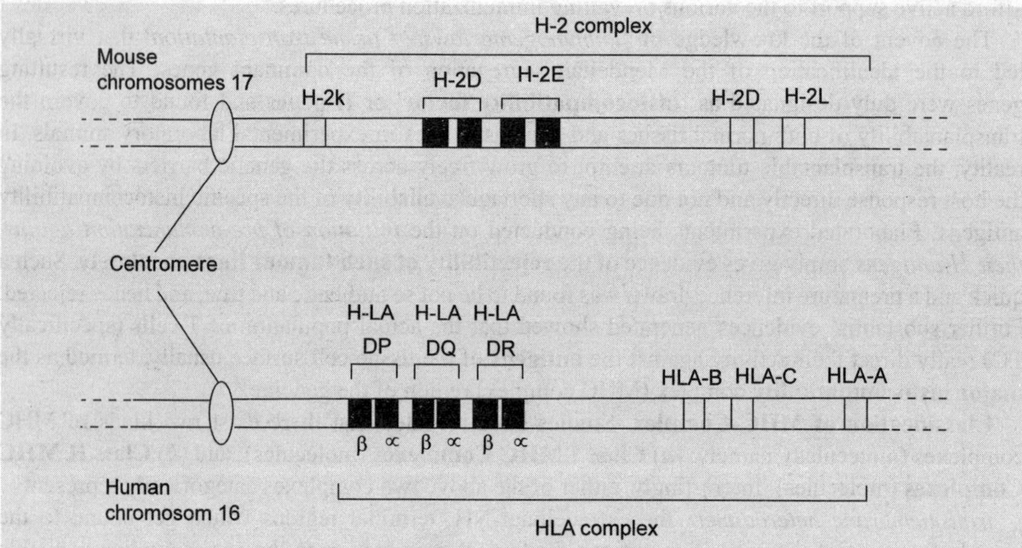

Fig. 4.10 *Showing H-2 (Mouse) and HLA (Humans) Gene Complexes, and the Exact Location of Gene Loci Encoding the Transmembrane Units of Class I and II MHC Proteins*

Explanations of Class I MHC and Class II MHC. A brief explanation of each class of MHC I and MHC II shall be undertaken in the section that follows:

Class I MHC. The various important cardinal aspects are:

a. Its gene invariably *encodes a single polypeptide* known as 'α' as that essentially has the following *three* distinct domains, such as:

i. **Intracellular domain** – comprises of *carboxy terminal*

ii. **Transmembrane** – consists of α-*helix*, and

iii. **Extracellular globular domains** – three in all *viz.*, α_1, α_2, and α_3.

b. An **individual polypeptide** is duly linked (non-covalently) with a specific β_2**-microglobulin** that happens to be extracellular in nature. However, it is duly coded by a **'gene'** which is strategically positioned outside the most predominant MHC gene conglomerate as shown vividly in Fig. 4.11(*a*) and 4.11(*b*).

c. Importantly, two individual domains of class I MHC, *e.g., first* β_2 and α_3 are found to be homologous to an immunoglobulin (Ig) domain; and *secondly,* α_1 and α_2 usually gives rise to the formation of a pocket (or groove) that critically affords the bondage of peptide segments (consisting of 8-10 amino acids length) of the ensuing antigen entitiy.

Class II MHC. This specific molecule also happens to be a **heterodimer** with α and β polypeptides. Importantly, each of these polypeptides to possess a particular immunoglobulin (Ig) like domain (α_2 and β_2) that are observed to be in the vicinity of the membrane ; and the amino-terminal domains (α_1, β_2) positioned far away from the membrane, whereby allocating an appropriate site exclusively for the binding of antigen-peptide segment as depicted in Fig. 1.8. However, the strategic presence of Ig-like domains explicitely offers a plausible explanation for the existence of a common evolutionary genesis (origin) of MHC molecules, T-cell receptors, and antibodies. Recently, even the **3Dstructures** of class I and II MHC molecules have also been proposed.

Thus, it was demonstrated beyond any reasonable doubt that the pocket (groove) of class I MHC caused by α_1 and α_2 domains of a polypeptide [as shown in Fig. $8_{(a)}$ and $8_{(b)}$], do comfortably accommodate **8-10 amino acids,** whereas the pocket (groove) of the class II MHC molecule, obtained from $\alpha 1$ and $\beta 1$, can comfortably accommodate **15-24 amino acids.** In short, the variety observed in both class I and II MHC molecules is capable of getting bound to a wide spectrum of peptides and present them to either T_C or T_H cells accordingly.

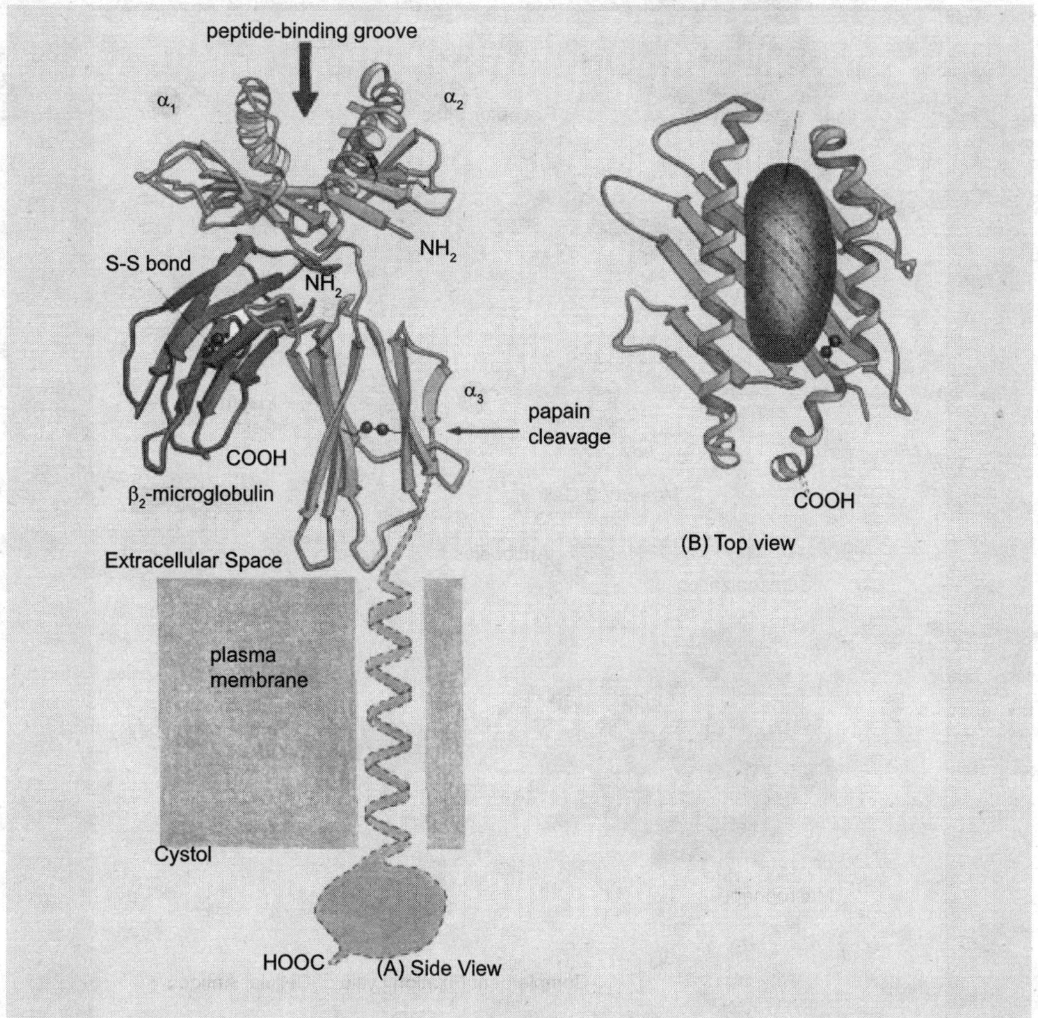

Fig. 4.11 (a) & (b) *Structures of a Human Class I MHC Protein as Determined by X-Ray Diffraction Analysis*

Figure 4.12 represents a comprehensive summary of the **'humoral immunity'** which is essentially mediated by *antibodies* in the body fluids, such as: plasma or lymph. These antibodies are duly synthesized and secreted by B cells, which protect the body against infection or reinfection by common pathogenic organisms (*e.g.,* streptococci and staphylococci). B cells are specifically stimulated by direct contact with a foreign antigen and differentiated into *plasma cells* (which produce antibodies against the antigen) and *memory cells* (which enable the body to quickly produce these antibodies if the same antigen appears at a later time). B cell differentiation is also stimulated by interleukin–2 (IL-2), secreted by T_4 *cells*, and by foreign antigens processed by macrophages. [*Synonym: B-cell mediated immunity*].

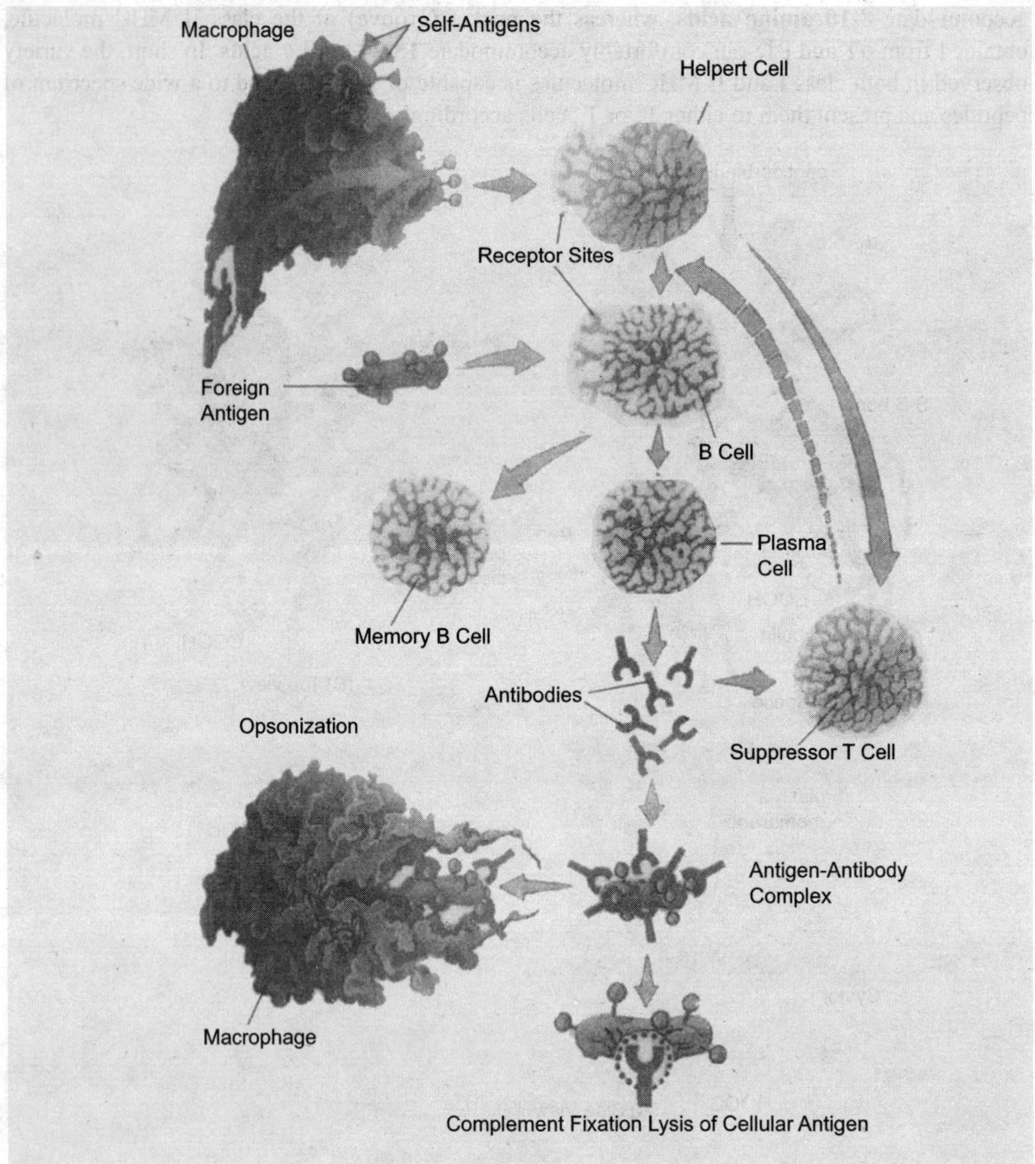

Fig. 4.12 *Comprehensive Summary of Humoral Immunity*

4.4.2.2 Cell-Mediated Immunity (CMI)

The **cell-mediated immunity** (CMI) essentially involves the particular system that is directly responsible and associated with not only the critical '*rejection of certain organ transplants*' (*e.g.*, heart, kidney, liver, eyes etc.,) but also the *'defense mechanisms'* against intracellular microorganisms, endogenous neoplastic (tumour) growths, and host cells infected with various viruses. Importantly, this specific classification of the relatively huge immune system, *e.g.*, humoral immunity, depends heavily and exclusively upon the ensuing **immunogen (antigen) stimulation** for it's much desired activation.

Another school of thought explains CMI as inadequacy and insufficiency of antibody mediated immune response that may eradicate effectively infections caused by a host of pathogenic microorganisms, parasites, and viruses as well that would ultimately develop within the host cells, eventually offered a tremendous impetus to scientists across the globe in the specialized field of '**immunology**' to evolve a *corrective response mechanism* that could go a long way in the management and control of such most dreadful and serious infections. Therefore, justifiably the prevailing mechanism is invariably termed as the '**cell-mediated response**' that not only effectively controls fatal infections emanated by viruses, microorganism and protozoa that multiply within the host cells significantly, but also affords paramount attraction of non-specific immune cells by **lymphokines** solely secreted by lymphocytes. In a nut shell, the effectiveness of the cell-mediated immune response must be **adequately normal** because it predominantly is responsible for providing general and overall protection to these critical situations, namely: transplantation immunity, hypersensitivity reactions, auto-immunity and neoplastic immunity as well.

Genesis of CMI

T-effector cells which is solely responsible for CMI, in fact, originate from the *precursor cells* (stem cells**) generated in bone marrow, very much akin to the instance of the antibody-forming cells in humoral immunity (see section 4.2.1). Interestingly, in CMI, the effector cells should precisely complete the differentiation process taking place in the thymus before undergoing circulation more or less freely in the vascular net work or regional lymph nodes or collecting in the spleen eventually.

Differentiated cells thus produced are essentially of different types that are exclusively dependant upon the type and nature of the prevailing cell-mediated response; besides, the extraordinary T-cell receptor (T_CR) structures invariably observed on their surface, that is genuinely acquired *via* **random genetic recognition** is the ensuing course of differentiation at two distinct sites, namely: (*a*) in bone marrow; and (*b*) maturation in thymus.

In actual practice, however, one may divide **CMI responses** into *two* distinct major categories based on the realistic requirement of *different effector cell populations*, namely:

A. Based on the Requirement of T_C cells being converted to Cytotoxic T Lymphocytes (CTLS) having Direct Toxic Effect on Target

The CMI essentially engaging CTLS is found to be profusely effective as a reasonably solid defense against a plethora of neoplastic (cancerous) growths, virus infections, and also tissue transplants.

On a serious note one may observe that the prevailing **'immune system'** fails to realize that CTLS are virtually meant to protect the body, and must not destroy it in the long run.

Salient Feature: The various silent features are namely:

1. CTL-response may be sub-divided into two distinct phases *eg., (a) sensitization phase ;* and *(b) effector phase.*
2. *Sensitization phase:* Usually commences when a **macrophage** or other **antigen-presenting cell** (APC) specifically detects cells sloughed off from the growing tumour (neoplasm) transplanted tissue, or previously killed by the infective virus. It is quite normal for any dead, damaged, partially damaged or even changed cells to become disconnected from the parent tissue, and travels ultimately to either liver or spleen for final destruction.
3. APC will afford phagocytization of the '**target cell**' as it would duly take cognizance of the *viral, tumour* or *foreign epitopes* available on the surface of the cell in its normal passage *via* the *vascular* or the **lymphatic systems.**

B. Based on the Requirement of Modified TH Cells Adopted for a Delayed Type Hypersensitivity (DTH) Reaction:

Salient Features: The various salient features involved in the necessary requirement of modified TH cells adapted for a DTH-reaction are as follows:

1. APC would save *immunodominant peptides* containing the epitopes of the target cell, as could be seen in HI (humoral immunity), and subsequently present them to the most suitable

T_H cells *via* the prevailing class II MHC. However, the activated T_C cell secretes IL-2, that eventually gives rise to **enhanced activation** and **duplication of T_H cells.**

2. Consequently, the higher activated T_H cells now secrete a larger number of **cytokines** which act in a concerted manner exerting localizing, chemotactic and stimulatory, effects on a variety of entities, such as: neutrophils, macrophages, and earlier unstimulated cytotoxic T cells (usually termed as T_C, effector T cells, or CD_8 cells).
3. T_C cells are selectively and strategically positioned to an area of the *viral infection, growing neoplasm,* or *foreign organ* (*e.g.,* kidney, heart, eyes), and those with T_CR_S found to be quite specific for the epitopes of the target will ultimately get bound with the **target cell** which distinctly shows the foreign tumour or virus epitopes along with its **Class I MHC surface structures.**
4. As a result the IL-2 receptor get duly activated that were previously recruited and attached to T_C cells. Besides, IL-2 generated by T_H cells critically and prominently **activates, proliferates,** and also **differentiates** T_C cells, thereby converting them to CTL cells. And perhaps this initiates overwhelmingly the **EFFECTOR PHASE** of the prevailing *immune response* appreciably.

4.4.2.2.1 Immunosuppression

Immunosuppression may be defined as – *'a phenomenon wherein an organism's ability to form antibodies in response to an antigenic stimulus is substantially reduced or suppressed'*.

As on date a good number of *'immunosuppression drugs'* are being used in order to enhance and prolong the '*life-expectancy*' of a **transplanted organ** *e.g.,* heart, kidney, eyes etc. It has been duly observed that when small doses of immunosuppressive drugs are employed, the recipient's immune system usually overcomes the drug, and **rejection** is indicated vividly by the gradual loss and efficiency of '*organ function*' based on the following common symptoms and actions irrespective of the organ, namely:

a. Fibrous thickening of the innermost small arteries of the transplant,

b. Consequent administration of relatively larger doses of immunosuppressive drugs as an extreme alternative measure, and

c. For each individual patient an altogether different and suitable *'immunosuppressive therapy programme'* is usually slated for.

However, another perception of '*immunosuppression*' legitimately promulgates the ensuing '*immune response*' as a coordinated mechanism essentially involving the due recognition of antigen exclusively by the **immunocompetent cells**, termed as *anti-T lymphocyte serum* (**ATS**); besides, occasionally the *macrophages* that are found to function as an **antigen-presenting cells** (APC).

Immunosuppressions are of *two types:* (*a*) non-specific; and (*b*) specific, which will be treated separately in the section that follows:

(A) **Non-Specific Immunosuppression.** It invariably takes places particularly in the natural instances related to immuno-deficiency disorders, uremia* etc., or may even be inducted by gradual depletion of lymphoid tissue, or by the administration of **immunosuppressive drugs.** It has been observed adequately that the undue exposure to radiation gives rise to significant depletion of lymphocytes, and thus may cause impairment of the antigens present on the macrophages thereby producing **immunosuppression.** Interestingly, non-specific immunosuppression can also be induced by **antilymphocyte globulin (ALG)** that specifically affects the T-cells by causing inhibition of their normal functionalities or by depleting T-cell dependent areas in the strategically located lymphoid tissue.

(B) **Specific Immunosuppression.** Broadly speaking the *specific immunosuppression* is usually induced either by *antigen* (immunogen) or **antibody**. Based on adequate experimental evidences it is quite feasible and plausible to induce **specific immunosuppression** measures that may be enumerated briefly as under:

1. In actual practice involving tissue transplantation the frequent usage of certain drug combinations are employed, for instance: **Azathiopurine** [Immuran[(R)]] and **corticosteroid**

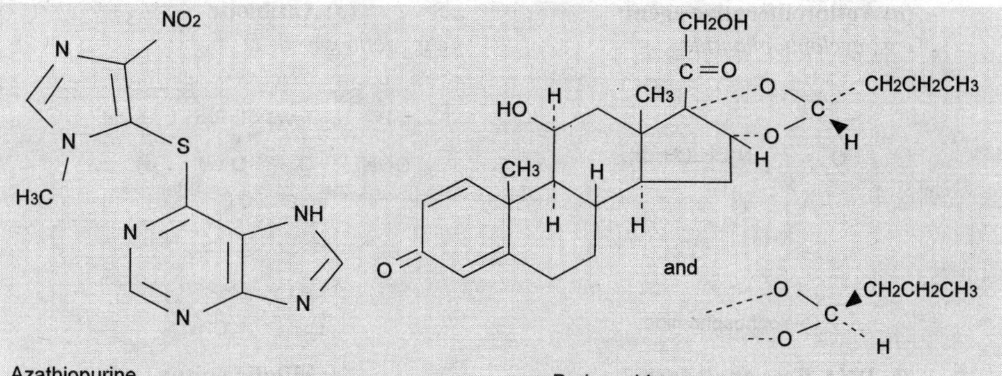

Azathiopurine

Budesonide

[Budesonide (Rhinocort([R]))]; so as to inhibit cell-mediated immunity (CMI). It has also been found that the drug **'cyclosporine'** is extensively employed in **immunosuppressive therapy.**

2. In certain particular instances the response of a host to a specific antigen is substantially eliminated to accomplish **'tolerance'**. In other words, it is a particular instance of **immunosuppression** wherein an *antigen (immunogen)* itself behaves as an **immunosuppressive agent.**

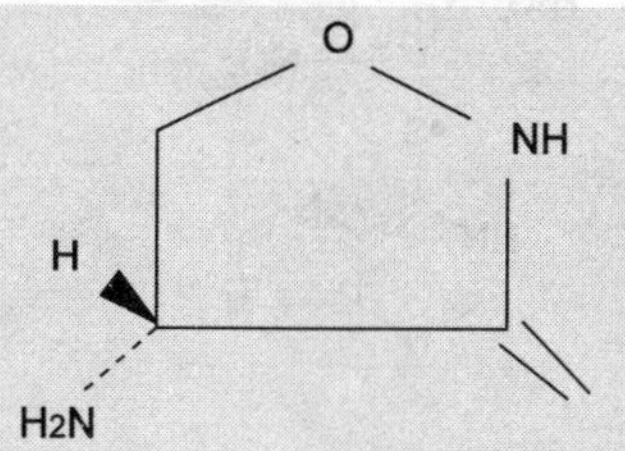

[Synonym: Cycloserine] [Seromycin (R) (Lilly)].

3. The body when exposed to ionising type of radiations it gives rise to the **suppression of lymphocyte proliferation** in the *haemopoetic system.* The overall net effect is **non-specific** in nature and causes impairment of haemopoiesis; and, therefore, periodical inoculation of the synergetic bone marrow cells in the animal has got to be carried out by all means.
4. In order to impair the prevailing **'immune response'** of the host *i.e.,* CMI, predominantly a specific class of **endogenous corticosteroids** are employed extensively and profusely, such as: hydrocortisone, testosterone, corticosterone, prednisone and prednisolone as shown below:

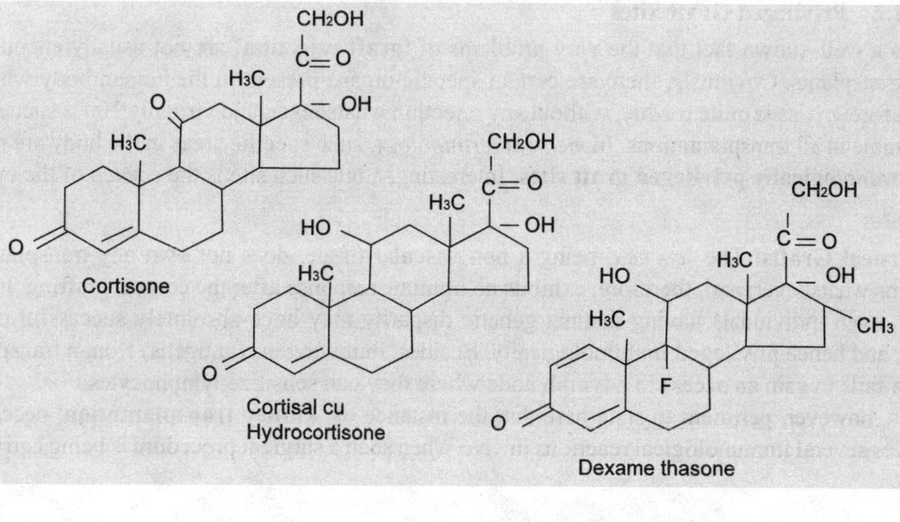

Cortisone

Cortisal cu
Hydrocortisone

Dexame thasone

5. A few other several '*drug substances*' derived from natural sources or of synthetic origin also find their enormous usage as *immunosuppressive agents*, such as:

   (*a*) **Antiproliferative agent:**
   e.g., cyclophophamide

   (*c*) **Antibiotic**
   e.g., actinomycin-D

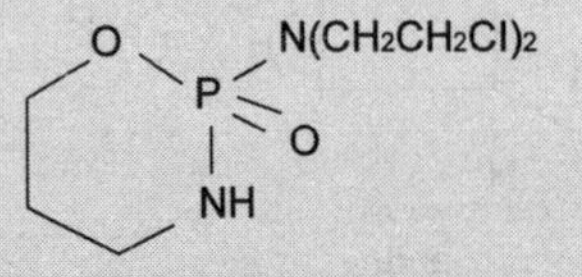

Cyclophosphamide

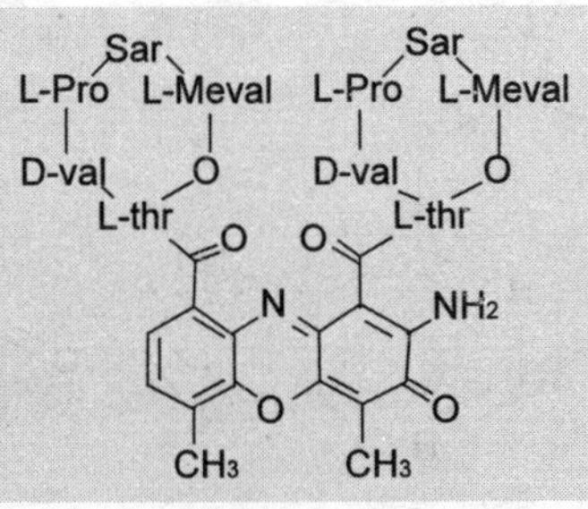

   (*b*) **DNA-Base analogues:**
   e.g., 6-merceaptopurine and its derivatives

   (*d*) **Mitotic poison**
   e.g., mitomycin C

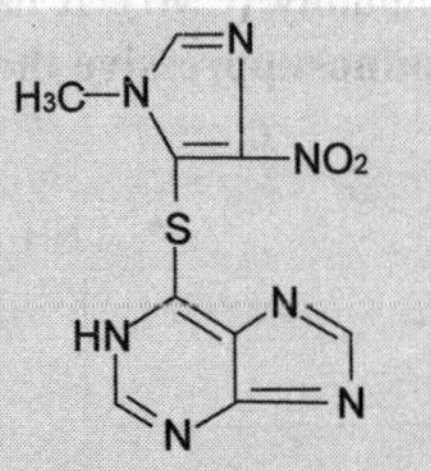

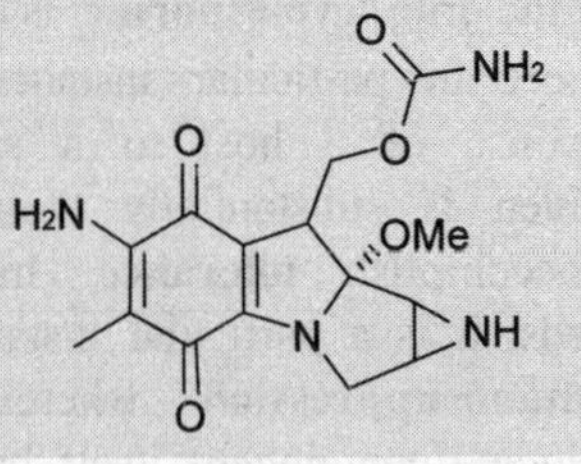

6. **Antilymphocyte Serum** (ATS) is also commonly used to combat specific immunosuppression. It happens to be a T cell inhibitor confined to the recirculating peripheral lymphocytes; however, the lymphocytes that are present within the lymphoid organs remain virtually unaffected.
7. Nevertheless, in the process of tissue/organ transplantation the underlying procedure of inhibiting CMI by the help of **homologous humoral antibody** is invariably termed as '*enhancement*'. In reality, the only way to enhance the survival period of transplants is to infuse a particular antibody to weaken phenomenon of CMI, whereas the formation of the humoral antibodies is protected duly.

4.4.2.2.2 Privileged Graft Sites

It is a well-known fact that the very problems of **'graft rejection'** are not usually encountered in all transplants. Obviously, there are certain specific organs present in the human body which do accept foreign tissue quite readily, without any rejection whatsoever, and virtually 100% success rate achievable in all transplantations. In *medical terminology*, such specific areas in the body are termed as **immunologically privileged graft sites.** Interestingly, one such site is the *cornea* of the eye.

Examples

Corneal Grafts: The '*cornea*' being a non vascular tissue, does not own any transplantation antigens whatsoever; and, therefore, exhibits no immune response after the corneal grafting. In other words, even individuals having distinct genetic disparity may have absolutely successful corneal grafts, and hence privileged immunologically. Besides, immunogens (antigens) from a transplanted cornea fails to gain an access to a lymph node where they can sensitize lymphocytes.

It is, however, pertinent to state here that the instance of **'kidney transplantation'** necessarily involves several immunological reactions in vivo when such a surgical procedure is being carried out from one individual belonging to the same species to another. In fact, it has been amply demonstrated that the tissues of virtually all mammals, except those who are **isogeneic** (or **syngeneic**) *viz.,* **identical twins,** are entirely different; and, therefore, the antigens of the donor stimulate an antibody response in the recipient (host) almost exactly in the same manner an **'antibody response'** in the humans gets elicited by appropriate injection of a **'foreign antigen'**. The aforesaid statement of facts and realities may be further expatiated based on the **'sequence of reactions'** in the typical example of kidney transplantation as detailed below:

Kidney Transplantation

In **kidney transplantation,** the various sequences of reactions involved may be outlined as shown in Fig. 4.13. Below:

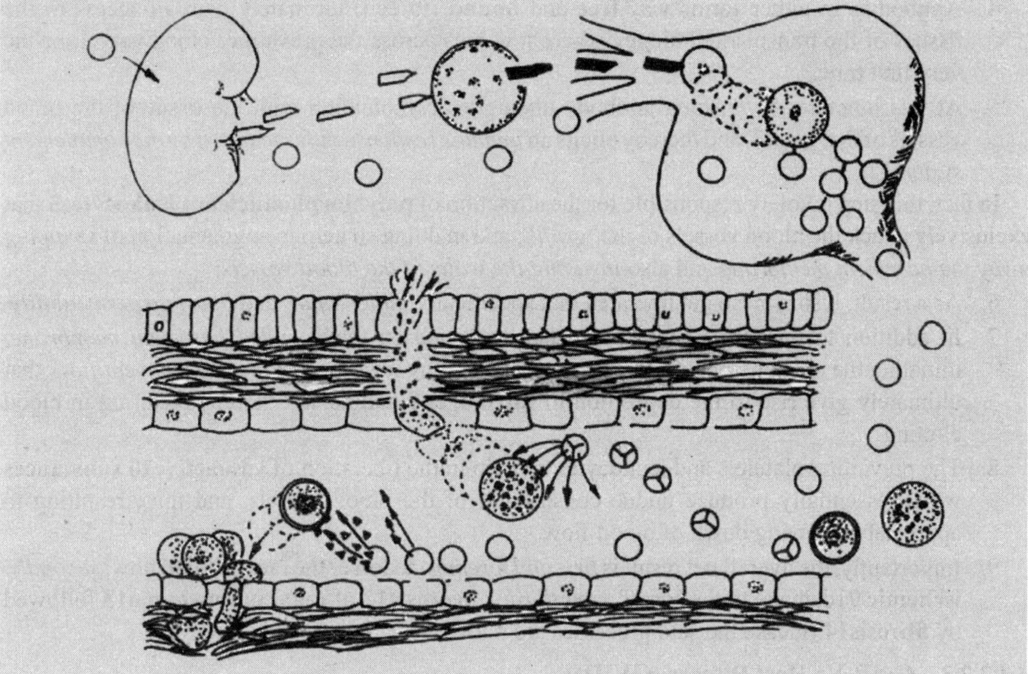

Fig. 4.13 *Various Sequence of Reactions Involved in a Kidney Transplant*

A = Sensitization of circulating lymphocyte;
B = Lymphocyte gains entry into the kidney;
C = Antigens (immunogens) emanating from the donor kidney;
D = Antigens (immunogens) being processed in the microphage;
E = Availability of processed antigen;
F = Formation of lymphocyte;
G = Emanation of lymphoblast;
H = Production of sensitized-antibody containing lymphocytes;
I = Emergence of free antibody globulin;
J = Formation of polymorphonuclear leucocyte;
K = Conversion to macrophage;
L = Representation of a complement sequence, and
M = Evolution of migration inhibiting factor (MIF).

The various procedural steps involved in '**kidney transplantation**' are enumerated below in a sequential manner:

1. Donor kidney emanates *antigen* which is duly processed by a macrophage into a biological entity that is capable of stimulation of the recipient's lymphatic system *viz.,* spleen and lymphatic nodes.
2. The lymphatic system subsequently gives rise to small lymphocytes that ultimately develop into *lymphoblasts*1 that eventually divide into a host of smaller lymphocytes which in turn get sensitized against the prevailing tissues of the graft.
3. These emanating lymphocytes give rise to antibody that may either be available in the '*free state*' in the circulating plasma or subsequently get attached to the overwhelmingly sensitized lymphocytes2.
4. Antibodies in either forms *viz.,* **free** and **bound** (to cell) ultimately gain an access to the tissues of the transplanted kidney where it comes across the prevailing blood vessel for the very first time.
5. At this juncture the ensuing antibody undergoes combination with the tissue of the blood vessels of the '*graft*3, and thereby elicits an *immune response duly mediated by the complement system.*

In fact, this step is solely responsible for the attraction of **polymorphonuclear4 leukocytes5** that exclusively attack the blood vessels of the '*graft*' ; and in doing so help in augmentation of *stripping away the basement membrane* and also *invading the walls of the blood vessels.*

6. As a result, lysozymes6 get liberated that specifically *inflict injury* and *boost up permeability.*
7. In addition to this, the platelets are also deposited on the *denuded basement membrane,* initiating the phenomenon of aggregation followed by liberation of *thermogenic entities*7 that ultimately give rise to the deposition of **fibrinogen8** and *fibrin*9 thereby resulting in blood clotting.
8. The prevailing platelets and leukocytes do help in the liberation of **vasoactive10 substances** which essentially produce undue constriction of the blood vessels, and thus, resulting in appreciable slowing down of blood-flow.
9. Importantly, the overall net result is *first and foremost* to lower the rate of blood flow; *secondly,* **ischemic** 91damage to the '*graft*'; and *thirdly,* **necrosis12** of **renal parenchyma13** followed by **fibrosis14** (incase the said processes are allowed to continue indefinitely).

4.4.2.2.3 Graft-Vs-Host Disease (GVHD)

Keeping in view the prevalent common situation whereby the recipient happens to reject the '**donor graft**', the reverse may also take place when the said donor graft essentially comprises of immunocompetent cells. In immunological environment this specific phenomenon is invariably known as **graft-Vs-host disease (or reaction).** The net result is normally displayed and characterized by the *'graft'* **immunologically rejecting** the '*host*'.

Examples: The above very commonly occurring phenomenon may be explicitly explained with the help of the following typical example:

1. A patient being administered with **fresh bone marrow** from a *non-identical donor,* evidently in such a situation the patients existing **immune cells** shall attack the '*grafted cells*', whereas the grafted bone marrow cells will attack normal body tissues very much present within the patients body. Hence, in this specific instance it is absolutely necessary to first completely destroy the entire immune cells of the patient by subjecting him to **whole-body X-Ray irradiation treatment** just prior to his receiving the *bone-marrow graft* so as to protect the **'graft'** from any external attack. Besides, it is equally important and vital that the patient's tissues may also have to be adequately protected from attack by the prevailing **immune cells** in the bone marrow graft. If by any chance this

protection to the patient's tissues is not accomplished duly, there could be a serious lethal condition developed ultimately usually termed as **graft-Vs-host disease (GVHD).** In order to avoid, manage and control this condition from the very grass-root that pre-operative corrective measures should be swung into action to suppress the **immune responsiveness of the grafted cells** by the help of **appropriate 'drugs'**. However it is quite necessary and important that the dosage regimen of the drug must be reduced slowly and gradually over a certain length of time till the **'graft'** is rendered **fully tolerant** and totally acceptable in its new environment.

Ultimate prevention of GVHD essentially needs an extremely sensitive and careful balancing of the immunosuppressive drugs therapy for relatively longer span wherein the patient is required to be confined in an isolated sterile environment.

It has been observed that the immunosuppressive drugs do possess two serious drawbacks, namely: (*a*) rendering the patient quite vulnerable to infection; and (*b*) exerting enormous unpleasant side-effects. However, the discovery of a new drug **cyclosporine** A has considerably eased the situation which is found to be both more effective and having relatively fewer side-effects.

2. Leukemia and GVHD: **Leukemia** has been pronounced as one of the most dreadful diseases; and the extension of longevity *vis-à-vis* a positive hope of complete cure particularly in adults may be accomplished successfully by replacing the patient's *abnormal bone marrow* with healthier cells. It has been duly observed that only a small fraction of the patient's bone marrow actually made up of **malignant** (*i.e.,* **cancerous**) cells. Therefore, logically and ideally such a grave condition may be tackled by adopting the *three* vital steps in a sequential manner, namely: (*a*) removal of the bone marrow; (*b*) destruction of the leukemia cells; and (*c*) replenishing the healthy cells to the original subject. In fact, such a streamlined meticulous stepwise operation shall not only minimize drastically the higher chances of survival and the utmost danger of GVHD, but also to negate the requirement for inducing *immunosuppression.*

Though substantial break through have already been accomplished and reported, such as: cleaning up of bone marrow by employing *monoclonal antibodies* to **neoplasm** (tumour) **determinants** which are strategically attached to toxins, *radioisotopes* or *magnetic beads,* that could be detached and removed subsequently along with the *cancerous cells* to which they get intimately bound by means of the electromagnets. In nut shell, one has to travel a long zig-zag path to hit bull's eye *i.e.,* to lay its hands on to an absolutely fool-proof, doubly sure and efficient means of **'immunotherapy'**.

Figure 4.14 designates the summarized form of the **'cell-mediated immunity'** whereby the regulatory and the cytotoxic activities of T cells during the specific immune response. This process requires approximately 36 hours reaching its full effect. Unlike B cells, T cells cannot recognize foreign antigens on their own. A foreign antigen is normally recognized by a macrophage that engulfs it and displays part of the antigen on its surface next to a histocompatibility or *"self"* antigen (*i.e.,* macrophage processing). The very presence of these two markers together with the secretion of a cytokine, interleukin-1 (IL-1) by macrophages and other antigen-presenting cells (APCs) activities specifically CD_{4+}/CD_{8-} T cells [helper T cells (TH)], that modulate the activities of other cells involved in the ensuing **immune response** significantly.

4.4.2.3 Innate (or Natural Immunity)

Natural immunity of an animal is also invariably termed as *innate immunity* or *native immunity* or *inherited immunity.*

Natural immunity may be defined as – *'an inherited (in built) resistance to infection(s) and is concerned with species, races or individuals'.*

In fact, as to date the exact mechanism of its defense has not yet been fully established and understood explicitly, inspite of its *natural presence* in an individual and not acquired through any prior exposure to the infectious agent. In other words, the **natural immunity** solely related to a general or non-specific type of resistance that ultimately affords prevention of infection caused by different kinds of *pathogenic microorganisms* (or **pathogens**). Interestingly, the degree and extent of the prevailing **'natural immunity'** largely differs in *various organisms,* which may be expatiated further with the help of the following typical examples;

Examples: **Mumps** may be infected in humans, whereas the kennels like *dogs* and *cats* are practically immune to this disease.

NOTE: The extent of *'natural immunity'* may alter between various species, races, strains, and sexes ; and, may be controlled by nutrition, hormones and a large number of other factors.

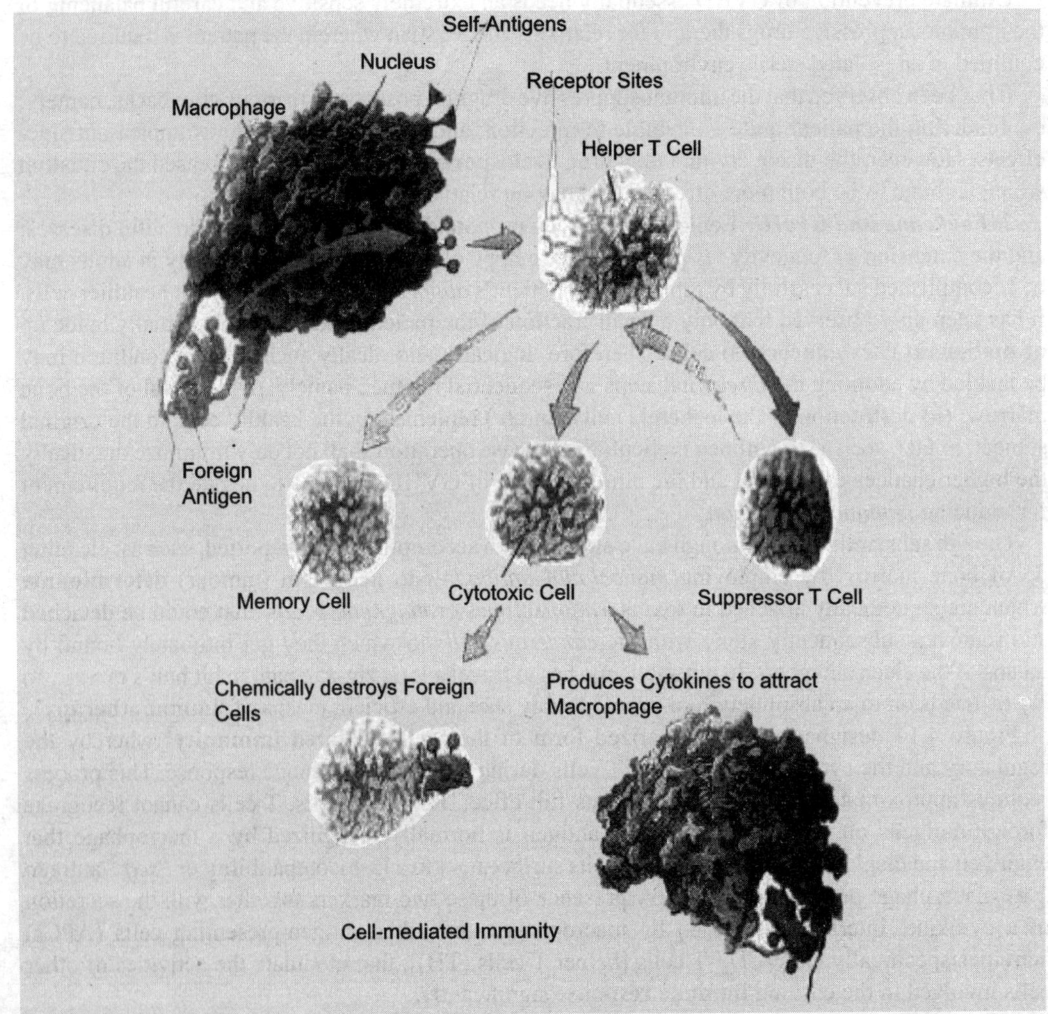

Fig. 4.14 *Summary of Cell-Mediated Immunity*

4.4.2.4 Acquired Immunity

Acquired immunity is a type of immunity which develops in an individual subject in response to an **immunogen** (antigen). It may, however, be acquired naturally by intentional or accidental exposure to an infectious disease or artificially acquired by *receiving active immunizing agents,* such as: **vaccines.**

It has been observed that *'acquired immunity'* usually gets developed during the *life-span* of an individual and hence critically refers to the immunity that a particular individual predominantly exhibits against a specific pathogen. Interestingly, it is quite often related to the very existence of either **antibodies** or **interferon's** (ITFs) present in the circulating blood *in vivo*.

The **acquired immunity** may be justifiably classified into two distinct categories solely based on the **antibodies**, for instance:

(*a*) Actively acquired immunity, and

(*b*) Passively acquired immunity.

These *two* special types of acquired immunities shall now be dealt with individually in the section that follows:

4.4.2.4.1 Actively Acquired Immunity

The **actively acquired immunity** could be either due to, '*natural*' or '*artificial*' derived sources.

a. Actively acquired natural immunity (AANI): It is precisely caused due to any disease-producing infection (*i.e.*, pathogenic organism based) from which a human being recovers ultimately.

It is observed that during the course of infection, the *quantum of antibody production* for the causative specific pathogenic entity gets stimulated in vivo to such an extent so that when there is a subsequent infection either by the same or *antigenically compromised* or *antigenically related pathogen,* the **resultant antibodies** thus generated do assist overwhelmingly in boosting up the body's defense mechanism profile appreciably.

b. Actively acquired artificial immunity: It is regarded universally as the most widely accepted and common mode of accomplishing immunization of *'vaccination'*. In actual practice, the antigens (immunogens) are administered into the body in a meticulously controlled amount as to stimulate the production of immunoglobulin (Ig). With the advent of geometrical progression of research in the field of immunology based on ultra-modern preparation and screening/evaluation methodologies, both attenuated and killed strains of microorganisms and viruses are being employed both intensively and extensively for affording immunization against a plethora of dreadful diseases in man, for instance: *small pox, typhoid, measles, poliomyelitis,* yellow fever and the like.

Vaccines are being developed and prepared by the aid of a large variant of methods and technologies involving the well known **'recombinant DNA technology'** (treated elsewhere in this text book comprehensively).

4.4.2.4.2 Passively Acquired Immunity

As a striking coincidence the **passively acquired immunity** can also be acquired *either by natural* or *artificial* manner.

(*a*) *Passively acquired immunity for 'natural' means.* It essentially involves the actual progressive transfer of antibodies from **mother** to her yet unborn baby in the womb via the placenta in the course of the '*latter stage of pregnancy*'.

(*b*) *Passively acquired immunity by 'artificial means'*. It specifically concerns to the original production of *'antibodies'* in some altogether different entity (*humans* or *lower mammals*); and subsequently followed by the calculated dosage regimens of these '*antibodies*' in affected patients *via* sterile injection. Some renowned organizations *viz.,* **Hoffkine Institute,** Mumbai; **Central Vaccine Institute**, Kasauli ; and several other **Drug Manufacturing Units**, are actively engaged in the commercial production of **'antibodies'** in *horses* and *cows* by active immunization for subsequent usage for **passively acquired immunity in humans.**

4.4.2.5 Non Specific Immunity

The vertebrates, particularly the mammals, are not only privileged but also fortunate enough in possessing a primitive immune system that essentially confers in them **non-specific immunity.** It is, however, pertinent to state here that the *cells* as well as the macromolecules of the prevailing system may render a clear cut basic distinction between either **self or non-self determinants.** Furthermore, these self and non-self determinants fail to distinguish specifically one **antigen** (immunogen) from another ; and, therefore, are perhaps in a better and more vulnerable position to attack '*foreign material*' in a non-specific manner. Interestingly, the cells that are particularly engaged in causing **non-specific immunity** are nothing but white blood corpuscles (cells) [WBCs), but do specialize in the process of **phagocytosis**, as illustrated in Fig. 4.15. below:

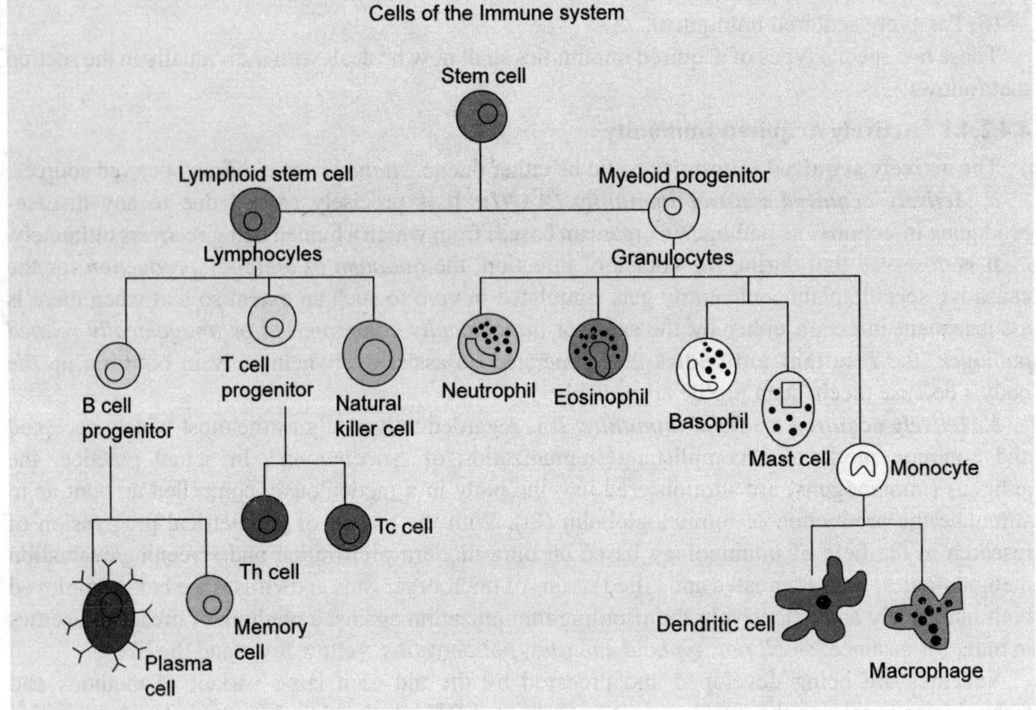

Fig. 4.15 *Model Exhibiting an Overview of Non-Specific Mechanisms that Essentially Contribute to an Immune Response System.*

Nevertheless, the *non-specific immunity* may also be categorized into *two* predominant divisions, namely: (*a*) **humoral immunity** (HI. (discussed under section 4.2.1); and (*b*) **cell-mediated immunity** (CMI) (discussed under section 4.2.2) as illustrated in Fig. 4.16.

4.5 Antigen Antibodies Reactions and their Applications

Euphorically, even thousands of years ago man commenced to explore, exploit and utilize biotechnological processes, phenomena and principles in both development and production of wonderful foods and exotic beverages, such as: beer, apple cider (*brewing*) ; bakery products like breads, biscuits, cookies, short-cakes, cakes (*baking*) ; and red wine, dry wine, white wine (*wine-making*). With advent of its deep roots in the tradition, legendary, and supported by an enormous progress and advances of the modern '*molecular biology*', biotechnology has legitimately undergone a sea change and secured a world-wide recognition in the past few decades. Amalgamated with copious skill, knowledge, and wisdom a few innovative areas like: genetic engineering, novel immunotechniques, biosensors, and protein engineering in the most recent era appear at the leading edge of biotechnology in either research or practical applications.

However, in the recent years it is not only felt strongly but also realized understandably that in a world with ever expanding populations *vis-à-vis* limited resources, a calculated reasonably acceptable expenditure on the prevention of a '**disease**' is certainly more productive logically than a sizable enhanced expenditure on its cure. In other words, it always sounds sensible and sane to '*acquire immunity*' against a specific disease rather than waiting for the disease to appear and cure it subsequently. Evidently, there are quite a few glaring examples widely publicized world-wide in the recent times as the stringent **'Statutory Requirements'** and **'Warnings'** with regard to the following several important.

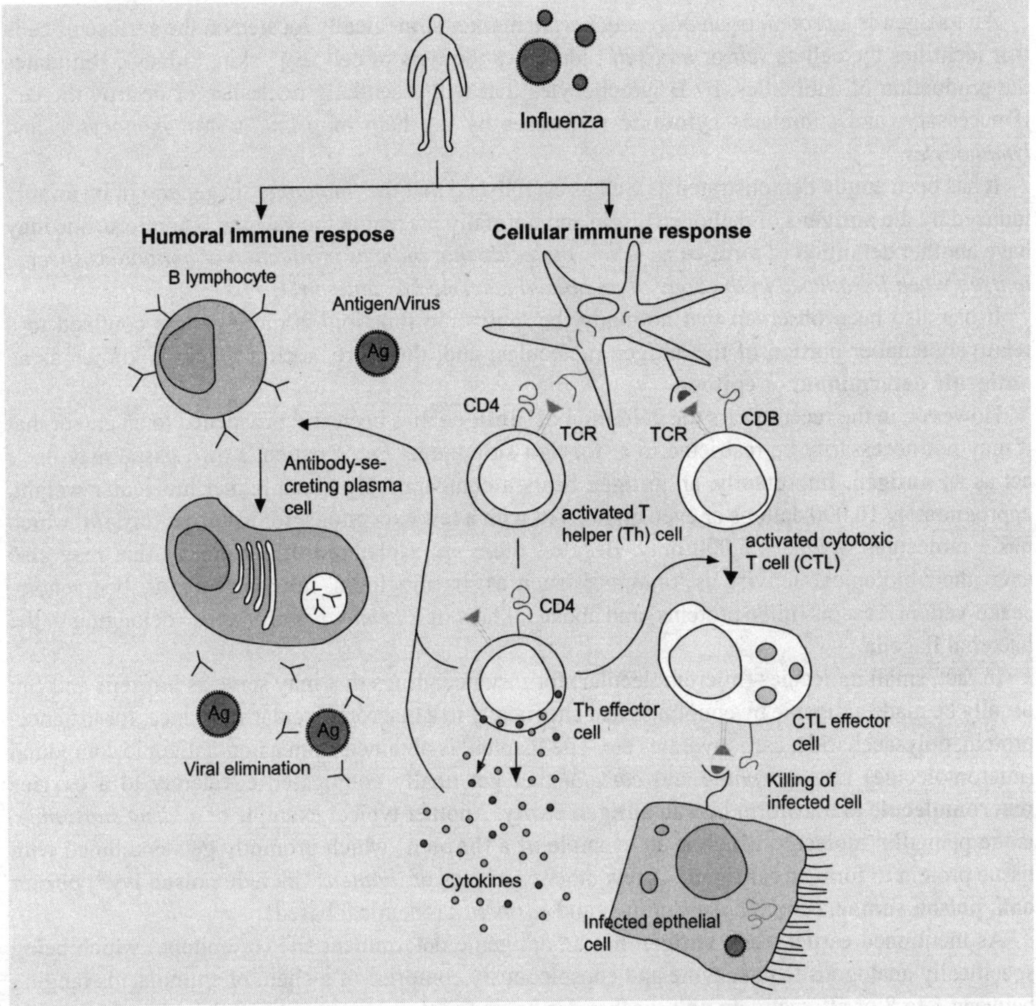

Fig. 4.16 *Subdivisions of Non-Specific Immune Response*

In the light of the above cited dire necessities to improve upon the **'quality of life and longevity'**, an immense galloping, progress has been duly accomplished in the highly specialized field of **'immunobiology'** together with a much deeper and better understanding of **'immunogenetics'** that have virtually opened the blood gates of comparatively altogether newer avenues in a host of meticulous industrial technological, advancements in the production of life-saving **'antibiotics'**, **'vaccines'** and **pharmaceuticals** having an enormous clinical application.

Kohler and Milstein** in 1975, instituted for the first time the wonderful and spectacular discovery of the **'hybridoma' technology** which ultimately turned out to be the fundamental basis of the ever-increasing potential of monoclonal antibodies (Mabs) to revolutionize the methodologies in **'biosciences'**.

4.5.1 Antigen Antibodies Reactions

In order to have an explicite concept of the **antigen-antibodies reactions,** one may understand vividly what are *'antigens'* and *'antibodies'*; and their specific roles *in vivo.*

4.5.5.1 Antigens

An **antigen** is a *protein* or an *oligosaccharide* marker strategically located on the surface of cells that identifies the cell as *self* or *non-self*; identifies the type of cell, *e.g.,* skin, kidney ; stimulates the production of antibodies, by B lymphocytes that will essentially neutralize or destroy the cell if necessary; and stimulates **cytotoxic responses** by the help of *granulocytes, monocytes,* and *lymphocytes.*

It has been amply demonstrated as well as established that the *'immunity'* in general in invariably induced by the **antigens** of pathogen origin and normally present in the vaccine. Therefore, one may have another definition of **antigen** as – *'any molecule that induces production of antibodies specific to itself when introduced in the body of an animal is termed as antigen'.*

It has also been observed that normally the 'antigenic function' is more or less confined to a relatively smaller portion of the antigen molecules; and, therefore, such a region is known as an **antigenic determinant** or **epitope.**

However, in the recent years the definition of **'antigen'** has been still broadened to an extent that it may not necessarily be restricted to a **'foreign substance'** *i.e.,* a patient's own tissue may itself act as an **antigen.** Importantly, an **antigen** bears a comparatively much higher molecular weight, approximately 10,000 daltons or even higher, but with a few exceptions, for instance: '*insulin*' which has a molecular weight ~ 6,000 only. Besides, there are a plethora of substances that may also exert their biological activity as '*antigens*', such as: haemoglobin, microbial toxins, bee-venom, snake-venom, caseins (milk-proteins) and above all host of *'chemical constituents'* belonging to the bacterial flagella.

In fact, small molecules (micromolecular) for instance; drugs that may serve as **haptens** and can usually be made antigenic by coupling them chemically to a macromolecular substance, for instance: protein, polysaccharide, carbohydrates etc. The 'hapten' is obtained from a non-antigenic compound (micromolecule) *viz., morphine* and *cartelol* that get finally conjugated covalently to a **carrier macromolecule** to transform into an **antigen entity**. Another typical example of a *'drug substance'* is the penicillin molecule which is an example of a **'hapten'** which promptly gets combined with tissue protein to form an **'antigen'**. A few other examples of *'haptens'* include **poison ivy*, poison oak, poison sumac,** certain *chemical dyes* and *cosmetics* (chemical based).

As mentioned earlier, each **antigen** has an antigenic determinant site (or epitope) which being specifically analogous to coenzyme and conspicuously comprise of a chain of amino acids ranging between 6 to 8 or alternatively polysaccharides having molecular weight 750 dalton as depicted in Fig. 4.17, which illustrates the molecular configuration of an **'antigen'.**

It is pertinent to state at this point in time that a *specific substance* can only be recognized as an *'antigen'* in case it should undergo the phenomenon of **'degradation'** by the **host's macrophage** as completely as possible.

Classification. In a broader perspective the **'antigens'** are duly classified depending upon their **origin** and **action** as given under:

i. Autoantigens,
ii. Allogenic antigen,
iii. Alpha-fetoprotein antigen, and
iv. Carrinoembryonic antigen.

These variants of **'antigens'** shall now be discussed briefly below:

a. Autoantigens: These represent an individual's own proteins together with *other biochemical's* which evidently elicit adequate **'immune responses'** only in the event or circumstances when the prevailing self-tolerance mechanism either collapses or breaks down completely or partially.

b. Allogenic Antigen: An *antigen* that occurs in some individual's of the some species. A glaring typical example is the human blood group antigens.

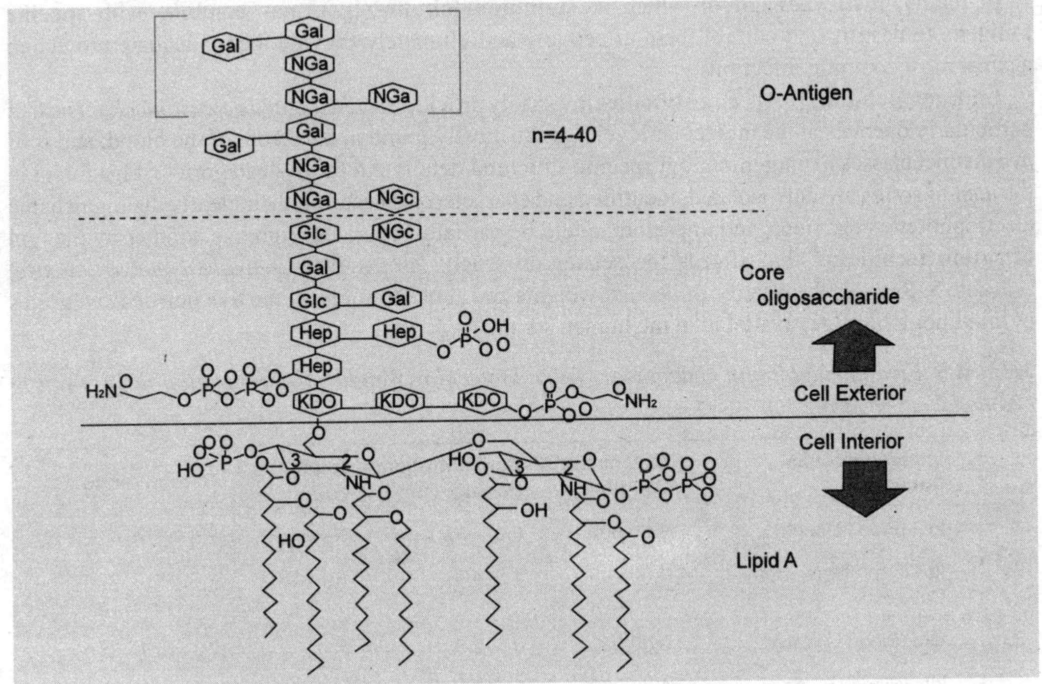

Fig. 4.17 *An Antigen Showing its Molecular Configuration*

c. Alpha-fetoprotein Antigen [AFP-Antigen]: It is an *antigen* present in the *human fetus*, and also in certain pathological conditions in the adult. The material serum level can be evaluated at 16-18 weeks of pregnancy to detect *fetal abnormalities*. Elevated levels indicate the possibility that neural tube defects are present in the fetus. Decreased levels may indicate an enhanced risk of having a baby with **Down syndrome.** In case, an abnormal level of AFP is found, further tests, such as: **ultrasound** or **amniocentesis** will need to be done. Elevated serum levels are found in adults with certain hepatic carcinomas or chemical injuries. Test results may also be abnormal in patients having *diabetes, multiple pregnancies,* or *obesity.*

d. Carcinoembryonic Antigen [CEA]: One of a class of antigens normally present in the fetus. Originally isolated from colon neoplasm's (tumours), they were thought erroneously to be specific for those tumours. In a situation when the previously elevated CEA level gets back to normal after surgery, removal of the **colonic tumour** is thought to be complete and successful.

4.5.1.2 Antibodies [Synonym: Immunoglobulin (Igs)]

In the recent past the entire field of **'biotechnology'** received a thumping broadening and redefining of concepts and ideas that actually helped in exploring the intricacies of various reactions taking place *in vivo*. It has been well established that the conglomeration of major macromolecules particularly associated with the immune response mechanisms are indeed a unique family of protein molecules commonly termed as **'antibodies'.** But in the biochemical conditions accepted these prevailing molecules are invariably known as **'immunoglobulin'** that in fact go a long way to explain vividly their structural relationship with the globular proteins. Therefore, in *'pharmaceutical biotechnology'* both these terminologies are used generously and hence interchangeable.

Antibody may be regarded as any of the complex glycoprotein's generated by B cells in response to the presence of an **antigen.** A single antibody molecule comprises of four polypeptide chains, two of which are light and two heavy, but all of them are duly joined by **disulphide bonds.**

In reality, *antibodies,* all of which are **immunoglobulin** (Igs), may combine with **specific antigens** to destroy and control them effectively and ultimately provide them adequate protection against most common infections.

Immunoglobulins [Igs] *i.e.,* **antibodies** invariably provide a *sophisticated defense mechanism* that particularly operates at the molecular level. Igs-are mostly found in the serum of the blood; and is of *five* distinct classes having minor but specific structural details. All the *five* categories of Igs found in the *human serum* are duly isolated, identified and characterized based on their clearly distinguishable electrophoretic behaviour; and, therefore, could be partially separated from one another by the **'gel filtration technique'** that affords the separation strictly as per their *individual molecular size.*

Table 5. Records the relative molecular weights and concentrations of the **five** purified categories of immunoglobin (Igs) available in the human serum:

Table 4.5 *Five Immuglobulin Categories: Their Molecular Weights, Concentration of Ig, Total Ig (%) and Carbohydrate %).*

S.No	Immunoglobulin Category	Molecular Weight	Concentration Per mg. cm^{-3}	Total Ig (%)	Carbohydrate (%)
1.	IgG (Blood Lymph)	1,50,000	8.0 – 16.0	80	2.9
2.	IgA (Secretions, Body Cavities.	1,60,000	1.5–4.0	13	7.5
3.	IgM (Blood Lymph)	9,00,000	0.6–2.0	6	7.7–10.7
4	IgD (Blood Lymph)	1,80,000	0.03	1	12
5	IgE (Blood Lymph)	1,80,000	0.0003	0.002	10.7

In other words, a **single antigenic determinant entity** is capable of provoking the ultimate synthesis of the above *five* altogether different classes of immunoglobulin molecules; and this categorical display of heterogeneity is prevalent of the **antibody** response to **antigen.** This perhaps is the fundamental basis by which an **antigenic determinant** could be overwhelmingly **attacked** by various categories of an **antibody molecule,** thereby giving rise to the very existence of a reasonably powerful defense mechanism within a living system (*i.e.,* humans and animals).

Salient Features of the Antibody – Synthesizing Cell

These are as stated below:

1. Each antibody-synthesizing cell may cause the production of only antibodies that will eventually combine with one specific determinant on the antigen.
2. Importantly, the antibody-synthesizing cells do possess the unique ability to switch the *category of antibody* (*e.g.,* Ig_G, Ig_A, Ig_M, Ig_D and Ig_E) without altering the specific site of combination for the respective antigen.
3. Interestingly, this particular portion of the *'antibody'* belonging to a given specific Ig-class is observed to be altogether separate from the portion essentially containing the site of combination for the antigenic determinant.

Fig. 4.18 illustrates schematically the sketch of an **'antigen'** displaying evidently several vital characteristic features *viz.,* number of antigenic determinants ; Igs of different categories binding to the same determinant ; portions of the antibody molecule having separate zones that determines the type of Ig ; and the part which precisely determines the **best fit** between an **antibody** and a corresponding **antigen determinant**.

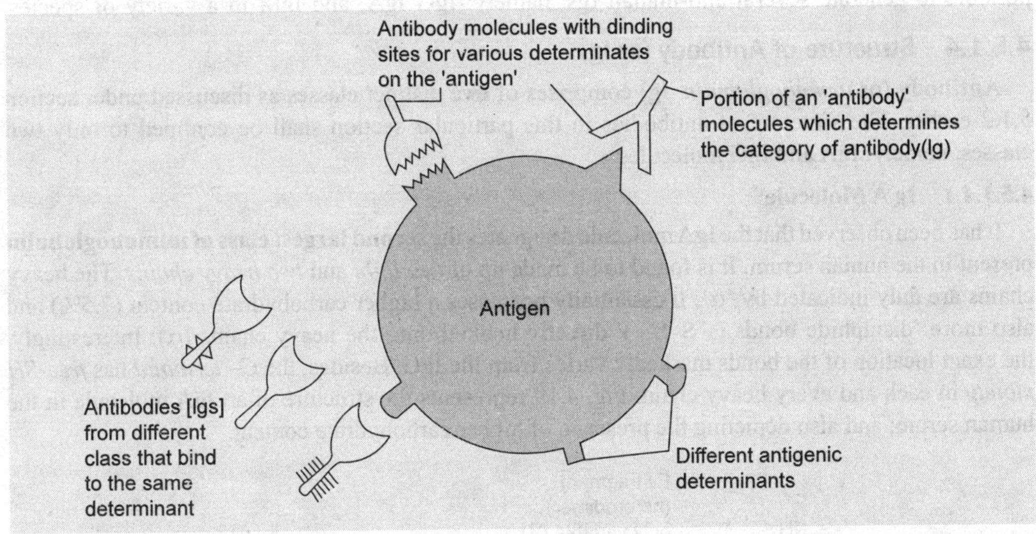

Fig. 4.18 *A Schematic Sketch of a Antigen Exhibiting a Plethora of Antigen Determinants.*

Conclusions. It has been duly observed that approximately 108 different antibody molecules (*i.e.,* Igs) may be synthesized in the human body. In other words, almost the same quantum of the *'antigenic determinants'* may be eventually recognized by the system. From these actual sequences of events taking place *in vivo* one may safely conclude that it is invariably possible that antibodies of the same category having combining sites of the same antigenic determinant will display varying degrees of affinity for that particular determinant.

4.5.1.3 Immunoglobulins as Antigens

After having a detailed discussion on the *two* important terminologies *viz.,* **antibodies** (or immunoglobulin, Igs) and **antigens,** one may raise a very important and crucial question at this junction, whether the *former entities* can actually behave as the *latter entities*. So far it is quite vividly expressed that the **Igs** are invariably and abundantly located in the **human serum.** It has so far been adequately demonstrated and proved that the five variants of Igs found in humans are also available in all the mammalian species ; however, it is quite pertinent to state here that though there exists certain fundamental close similarities amongst the said categories of Igs there also exists some mild but apparent differences in their prevailing structures. Interestingly, the **immunologists** exploited these subtle differences that ultimately resulted in the evolution of **anti-antibodies** or **antiglobulins** which find their enormous use for diagnostic purposes.

It is well established that the *'immune system'* in humans happens to be very sensitive to foreign substances; and, therefore, Ig derived from one mammalian species and subsequently injected into an altogether different mammalian species shall predominantly prove to be **immunogenic** *i.e.,* capable of inducing an immune response, in character.

Example

The IgG molecular entities derived from a *'rabbit'* and then injected into *'sheep'* shall behave as a foreign substance due to the fact that *minor differences* which essentially prevail in the heavy chain fragment crystallisable (F_c) regions. Although there are *significant differences* amongst the *Igs belonging to the same class* but derived from altogether different species that are strategically located in the heavy-chain F_c tail portions of the molecule. Eventually, the recipient species generates Igs which predominantly combines with this region. And the resulting products *i.e.,* **antibodies-against-antibodies** are usually termed as **'antiglobulins'.** In reality, it is indeed quite feasible as well as possible to generate several anti-human Igs, namely: IgG IgA, and IgM in a variety of species.

4.5.1.4 Structure of Antibody (or Ig)

Antibody (or *immunoglobulin,* Ig) comprises of **five** distinct classes as discussed under section 5.1.2 earlier. The structure of antibodies in this particular section shall be confined to only two classes, namely: IgA and IgG molecules.

4.5.1.4.1 Ig A Molecule

It has been observed that the IgA molecule designates the **second largest class of immunoglobulin** present in the human serum. It is found to be made up of *two light* and *two heavy chains*. The heavy chains are duly indicated by 'α'. It essentially possesses a higher carbohydrate content (7.5%) and also more 'disulphide bonds (– S–S–)' directly hooked onto the heavy chains (α). Interestingly, the exact location of the bonds markedly varies from the IgG. Besides, the *C– terminal* has *free-SH moiety* in each and every heavy chain. Fig. 4.19 represents the structure of an IgA molecule in the human serum; and also depicting the presence of higher carbohydrate content.

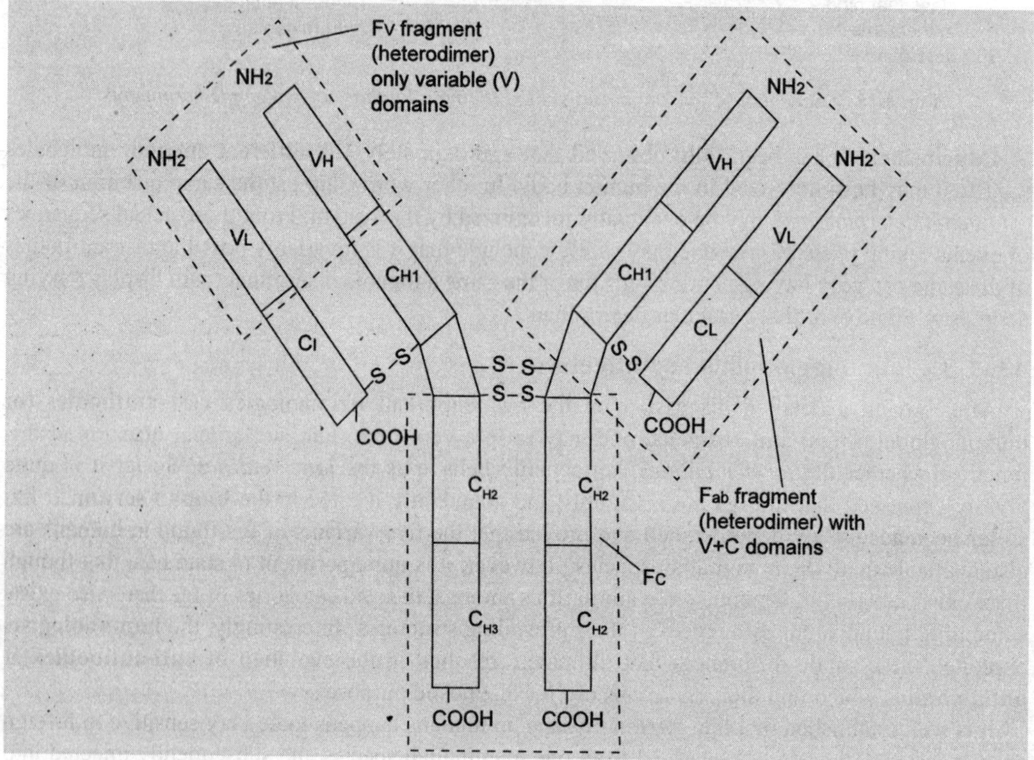

Fig. 4.19 *Structure of IgA Molecule Present in Human Serum.*

4.5.1.4.2 IgG Molecule

In order to have better in-depth knowledge and vivid concept of the ensuing relationship between the basic structure of IgG and its biological activities, an intensive exploration investigative was carried out on patients specifically suffering from a disease termed as **mycloma.**

This situation is regarded as a neoplastic condition of the cells whereby they are capable of synthesizing an enormous quantum of both heavy and light chains that are generated almost monoclonally. However, the patients generally secrete excessive quantities of Igs having light chains in the urine. Because they invariably show up as identical entities, the variable segment of the fragments undergo *polymerization,* that ultimately give rise to the formation of **amyloid fibrils,** with specific characteristic features, and found in **urine**.

V_L-Type amyloid fibrils. Found in patients excreting **Bence Jones Proteins** which is only possible by the application of **antizidiotypic sera** appropriately.

It has been duly observed that the paired light (L) and heavy chains (H) do exhibit an appreciable variation *i.e., variable region* **'A'** in amino acid sequence at the N-terminals ; and maintaining a farily reasonable constancy in the rest of the portion. Interestingly, the *constant region* **'B'** do posses a plethora of *'homologous segments'* that are found to be very much identical **which an IgG molecule** and also **between different IgG molecules.**

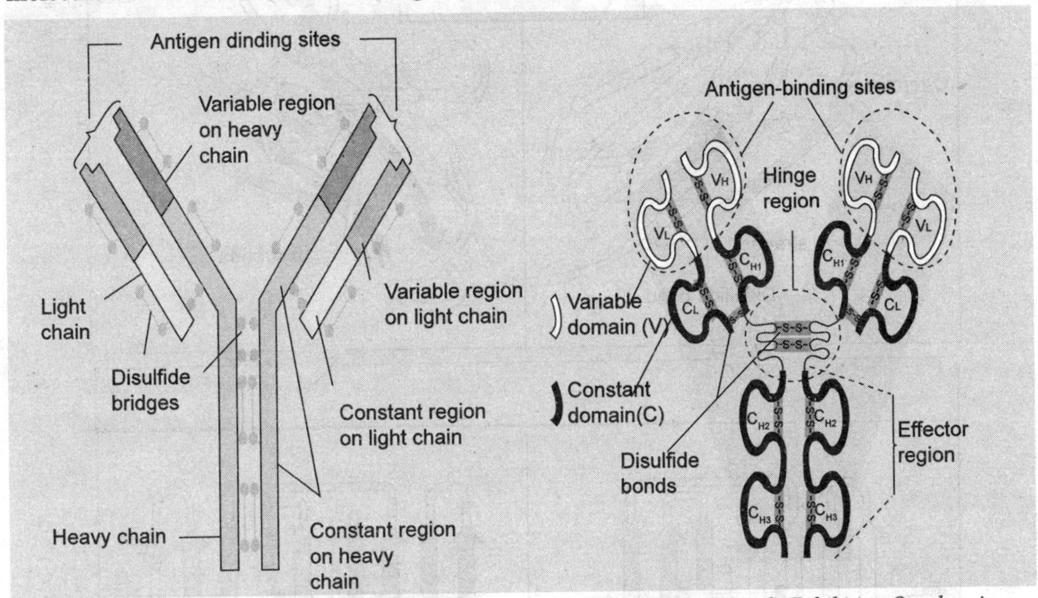

Fig. 4.20 *Schematic Structure of an IgG Antibody*

Fig. 4.21 *An IgG Molecule Exhibiting Overlapping Domains Comprised of β-Pleated Sheets.*

Figure 4.20 illustrates the schematic structure of an IgG antibody wherein the *antigen-binding sites, disulphide bonds, light chain, heavy chain, complement binding sites* and an *antibody* have been ear-marked explicitly.

Figure 4.21: designates an IgG molecule exhibiting the overlapping domains comprised of essentially the β-*pleated sheets*. Importantly, the *heavy chains* consists of primarily four vital segments *viz.,* $V_{H,}$ C_H1, C_H2 and C_H3 ; whereas, the light chain cosists of only segment, namely: V_L. The three predominant zones are: (*a*) antibody combining site; (*b*) fragment antibody binding site (Fab); and (*c*) fragment crystallisable site (F_C). The coupling of C_H1 and C_H2 designated as the hinge region. The two hinges are strategically joined with each other by a disulphide bond.

Figure 4.22 reveals explicitly the spectacular analysis of Bence-Jones light chains (L) by the help of X-ray crystallographic studies whereby it was virtually established that the IgG molecule essentially possessed three dimensional (3D) configurations. Furthermore, it predominantly comprised of two distinct segments usually known as: (*a*) *variable domain,* designated by V_L; and (*b*) *constant domain,* designated by C_L. Interestingly, either these domains (or regions) have **β-pleated sheets** that were meticulously joined together by the help of short and irregularly folded chains. In fact, these two above mentioned regions are commonly termed as **'structural domains'.**

It is, however, pertinent to state here that the *variable domain* (V_L) is essentially comprised of light chain (L); and the *constant domain* (C_L) is distinctly connected by the help of β-pleated sheets, thereby eliciting a marked and pronounced similarity in the folding patterns of these *two domains* specifically.

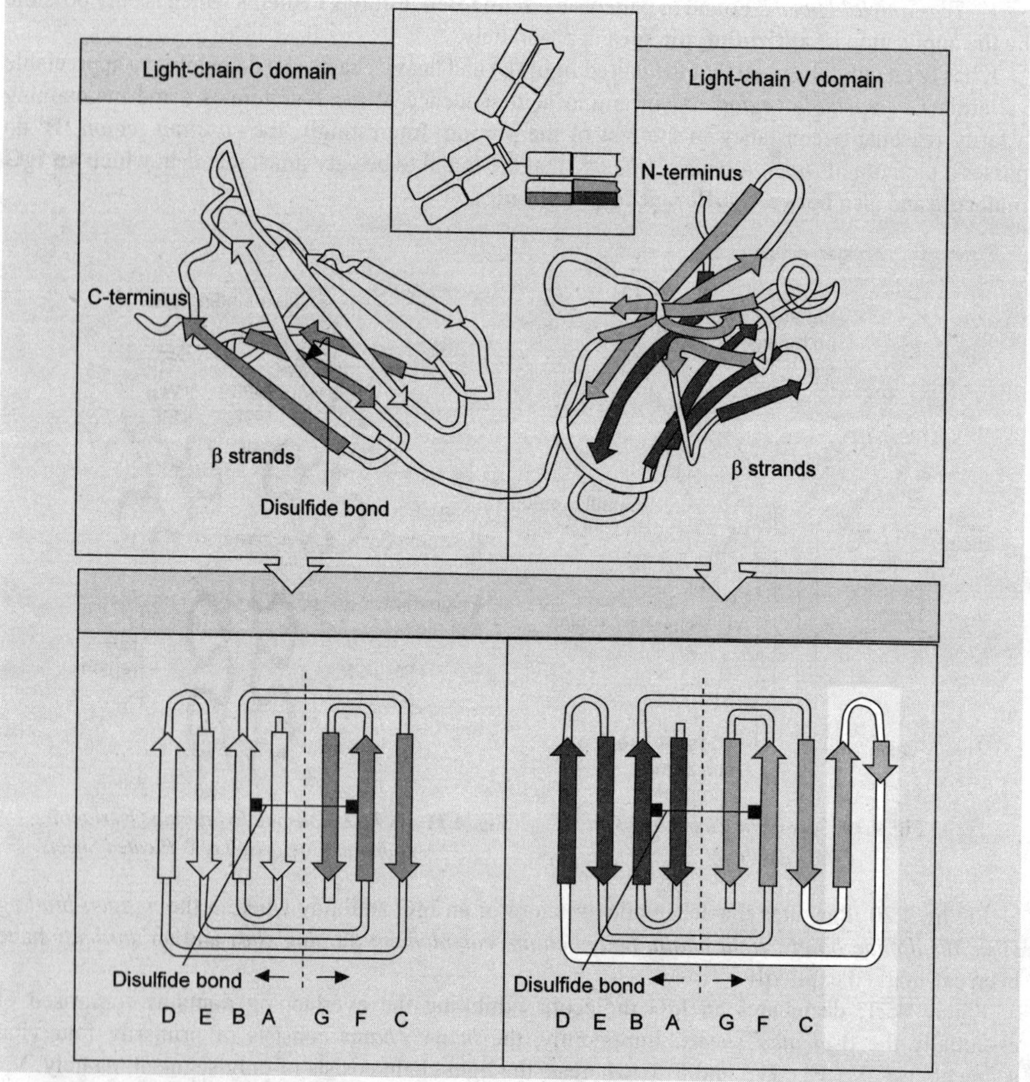

Fig. 4.22 *3D-Conformation Variable and Constant Domains of a Single Light Chain (L) of IgG Molecule*

Though there exists several points of differences in the basic structure of these two domains, yet in the prevailing 3D-structure there are several points of similarities that the predominantly due to:

(*a*) Glaring stabilizing influence of **single intra-chain disulphide bond** (see Fig. 19) in each domain; and (*b*) partially by virtue of the presence of a huge quantum of 'hydrophobic' amino acid residues strategically located within the interior of the folds.

It has been amply observed that a good number of *'glycyine residues'* are located wherever the chain is involved in the process of *'folding back on itself'*. Therefore, it has been duly advocated that the ensuing degree of **flexibility** prevailed upon by the presence of rather small side chain (*e.g.*, H-atom) in glycine [H_2N-CH_2-COOH] is an absolute necessity to enable and execute the phenomenon of the folding pattern.

4.5.1.4.3 Glycosylation of Antibody (IgG)

Generally, an '*antibody*' gets **glycosylated**, invariably carrying carbohydrate residues specifically located in the CH_2 region. It has been established that the carbohydrate portion of the Ig is essentially an oligosaccharide loaded with several '*monosaccharide units*'. It may include rather **complex N-acetyl lacto amine rich segments** as depicted in Fig. 1.23 given below:

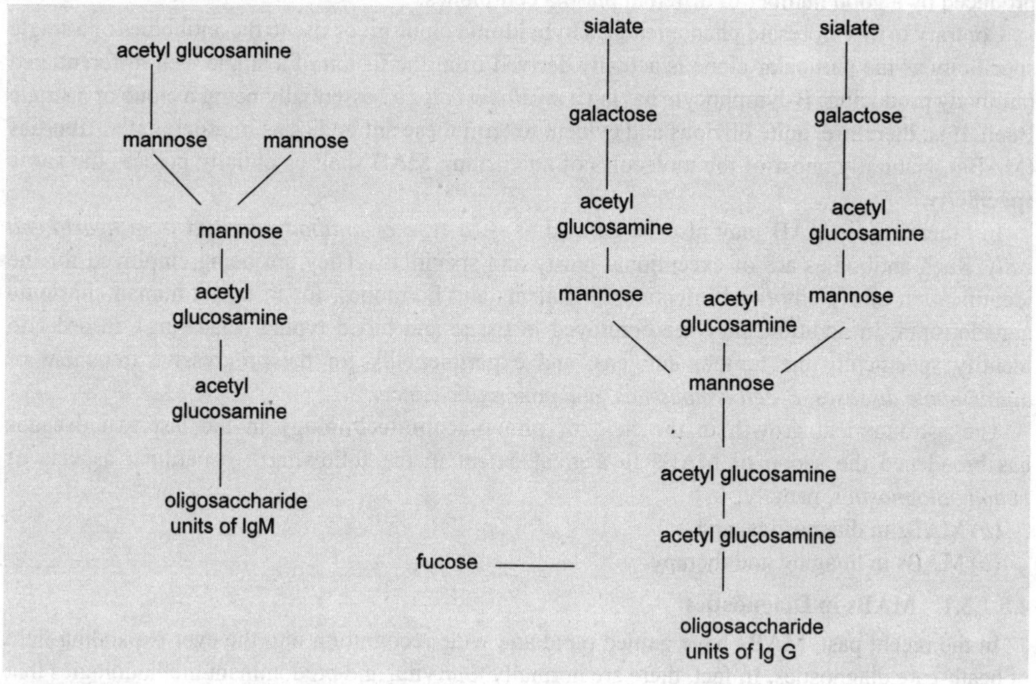

Fig. 4.23 *Structure of Carbohydrate Moieties (Oligosaccharide Segments) Observed in the Antibody IgG.*

However, it has been found that in IgG, the presence of the '*carbohydrate segment*' extends upto 2.5% of the entire molecule ; and, besides, it is practically equally divided between the prevailing **two γ- heavy chains (H),** that are strategically linked *via* two specific *amino acids*, namely: **threonine** and **aspartic acid** residues present in the **polypeptide chains.** It has been adequately proved that there exists no *'glycosylation'* in the fragment antibody binding (F_{ab}); and this perhaps puts across a logical explanation that glycosylation exerts practically little effect on the **antigen binding property of antibody.**

However, it affords an influence upon the effector function duly controlled particularly by the fragment crystallisable (F_C) component.

4.5.1.5 Monoclonal Antibodies (MABs)

In a broader perspective, an antigen (or immunogen) molecule predominantly possesses antigenic determinants of more than one specificity. In other words, different determinants shall undergo viable interaction with altogether different antibodies. In reality, each separate antigenic determinant of the antigen will have a tendency to get bound to a fully mature B-cell whose surface immunoglobin (SIg) specifically matches the characteristic features presented by the concerned determinant. Consequently, a single antigen thus produced may essentially activate the B-cells having more than one SIg specificity. The resulting activated B-lymphocytes (cells) of each SIg specificity shall precisely *divide* and *differentiate* to produce **clones** of the respective plasma cells thereby generating antibodies having more or less the same specificity. Interestingly, it has been observed that a '*single antigen*' would usually induct more than once distinct clones of the prevailing plasma cells; and, therefore, it will give rise to the production of **'antibodies'** bearing variant specificities. Most logically, the serum of an animal adequately immunized by a single antigen shall definitely comprise *antibodies* with *various specificities,* but **reacting particularly to the same antigen.** These specific varieties of antibodies are invariably termed as **polyclonal antibodies** because they are eventually produced by a good number of different plasma cell-clones.

Contrary to this aforesaid phenomenon, a **hybridoma** clone gives rise to the antibodies of a single specificity as the particular clone is actually derived from the fusion of a single well differentiated (antibody producing) B-lymphocyte having a *mycloma cell i.e.,* essentially being a clone of a single Bcell. It is; therefore, quite obvious and evident to term these antibodies as **monoclonal antibodies** (MABs). Naturally, most of the molecules of an ensuing MAB shall essentially possess the **same specificity.**

In other words, MAB may also be defined as – '*a type of antibody derived from hybridoma cells*. Such antibodies are of exceptional purity and specificity. They are being employed for the identification of a plethora of infectious organisms and hormones, for instance: human chorionic gonadotropin. In addition, they are employed in tissue and blood typing (matching), in order to identify specifically the tumour antigens, and experimentally for the progressive treatment of *autoimmune diseases, B-cell lymphomas, and pancreatic cancer.*

The astronomical growth in the field of **pharmacobiotechnology** in the last two decades has broadened the scope of MABs to a great extent in the following *two* cardinal aspects of *immunodiagnostics,* namely:

(*a*) MABs in diagnostics, and

(*b*) MABs in imaging and therapy.

4.5.1.5.1 MABs in Diagnostics

In the recent past, MABs have gained rapid and wide recognition into the ever expanding field of heath-care diagnostics. In fact, there are normally *four* vital and predominant methodologies that find their enormous applications in '*diagnostics*', for example:

4.5.1.5.1.1 Immunoassays

Most immunoassays are carried out by the application of radioactive antibodies [*i.e.,* radio immunoassays (RIAs)] whereby the sample exhibiting radioactivity shall be retained onto the sample.

However, the underlined and prescribed stringency and authencity of RIA tests largely restrict it to centralized specialist diagnostic facilities exclusively.

4.5.1.5.1.2 Enzyme Immunoassays (EAI)

In this specific instance a particular colour-producing enzyme is coupled to the antibody. Thus, the outcome of the results may be read either directly by a naked eye or spectrophotometrically.

4.5.1.5.1.3 Enzyme Cascade Technique

Here, a number of enzyme reactions are taking place are coupled strategically to produce an appreciable amplification of the original binding signal that is either read by a naked eye or spectrophotometrically, and

4.5.1.5.1.4 Fluorescence Immunoassays (FIA) and Luminescence Immunoassays (LIA)

Precisely, these are more or less inter-related techniques wherein the **'lable'** either gives rise to fluorescence or light respectively.

Examples:

1. **Pregnancy Dipstick Test.** It is solely based on MABs ; the pregnancy dipstick test determines the pregnancy either at home or in a clinical laboratory.
2. **Ovulation Dipstick Test.** Another type of dipstick test based on MABs that essentially ascertains the positive or negative ovulation on a subject, and
3. **AIDS test.** MABs based AIDS test kit is abundantly available to identify its presence in donated blood samples.

Notes. *Therefore, each and every blood sample must be tested for AIDS test before the actual blood-transfusion is carried out onto a healthy patient.*

4.5.1.5.2 MABs in Imaging and Therapy

It is, however, quite pertinent to state here that the most acute and major observed hinderances ever encountered in the management and subsequent treatment of cancer virtually lies in the fact that the *malignant cells* have a very close resemblance to the *normal cells*. Therefore, it is quite evident and possible that such '*therapeutic agents*' which are solely intended to cause complete destruction of the cancerous cells would also destroy invariably the '*normal cells*' as well perhaps by virtue of their close resemblance. However, it has already been well established that the surfaces of the malignant cells do differ in certain respects from those of the normal cells. But we have seen earlier that MABs exclusively recognize specific *antigens* on cells, they ar being fully *exploited to image* cancerous tumours particularly in an intense on-going clinical research undertaking, and also in therapy against a variety of malignancies, namely: colon and breast cancer; lymphomas; and melanomas.

A few typical examples have been adequately detailed below, namely;

1. **Gastrointestinal Cancer.** MABs is used alone to combat gastrointestinal cancer. The underlying principle being that when the antibodies opt to bind to the turnover, they invariably exhibit a tendency to attract the cells of the immune system to act against the prevailing cancerous tissue.
2. **Lung, Breast, Prostate, and Pancreas Cancer.** It is, however, pertinent to mention here that enough research activities have triggered off in the recent past towards the development of monoclonal conjugates of *two* important class of drugs, such as:

i. Anthracycline Drugs. Such as antibodies having quinones and related structures *e.g.*, Adriamycin(R) (Adrio); Bufex(R) (Bristol).

ii. Desacetyl Vinblastine. When desacetylvinblastine *i.e.*, a chemical entity obtained either from the plant source or produced by plant cell culture, is conjugated to a monoclonal which consequently acts specifically on lung, prostrate, breast and pancreas malignant cells.

4.5.1.5.3 Production of Monoclonal Antibodies (MABs):

It is well established at present that – *'monoclonal antibodies are invariably produced from hybridoma clones ; whereas each hybridoma clone is meticulously derived by the actual fusion of a mycloma cell together with an antibody producing lymphocyte, and ultimately the hybridoma clone producing the desired antibody is adequately isolated and subsequently identified.'*

In actual practice the *'hybridoma cells'* are **mass cultured** for the overall production of MABs with the help of one of the following two methods, namely:

(*a*) Culture in Peritoneal Cavity *i.e., in vivo* peritoneal cavity of mice, and

(*b*) Mass *in vitro* culture *i.e., in vitro* large scale culture vessels.

The above *two* methodologies shall now be discussed individually in the section that follows:

4.5.1.5.3.1 Culture in Peritoneal Cavity

In this developed, tested and tried methodology the '*hybridoma cells*' are strategically transplanted into the peritoneal cavity of a suitable and highly purified strain of mice, and subsequently the *ascitic fluid* derived from the animals is duly harvested and the MABs are purified meticulously.

Importantly, this particular technique positively yields between 50-100 times higher quantum of the **'desired antibody'** in comparison to the usual traditional in vitro culture of the hybridomas.

It is however pertinent to state here that there are *three* important characteristic features of this technique, namely:

(*a*) Generally, the ensuing *'antibody preparations'* happen to be a **lower purity** than those obtained from the corresponding cell cultures, particularly if, **serum-free media are employed,**

(*b*) Methodology involved is predominantly a **labour-intensive** one, and

(*c*) Unconditionally and absolutely **pathogen-free animals of particular genotypes** are essentially required.

4.5.1.5.3.2 Mass in vitro Culture

One may accomplish the commercial/large-scale culture of the *'hybridoma cells'* by adopting any one of the *three* methodologies, namely: (*a*) *Bioreactors with frequent stirring device* ; (*b*) *Aircraft fermentors;* and (*c*) *Specific vessels based on immobilized cells.* In actual practice, the culture systems making use of specifically **immobilized cells** are responsible for the progressive cultivation of cells at very high densities that markedly increases the production of **'antibody'** *in vivo.*

Examples:

There are *two* typical examples to expatiate the above process i.e., mass in vitro culture, namely:

(*a*) **Hollow fibre cartridges** (*i.e.,* a culture system) – found to yield 40 g MABs *per month*; and

(*b*) **Special ceramic cartridges** (i.e., an optical system) – found to yield 50 g MABs *per day*.

Future Scope. An extensive and intensive research towards the futuristic developments and progress in the area of immobilized culture systems may ultimately give rise to an increased production of MABs in a significant manner and therapy markedly and pronouncedly minimize the cost of their mass production from the cell cultures.

Production. The various steps that are intimately involved in the *production of monoclonal antibodies* (MABs) are represented sequentially in Fig. 4.24 as below:

The various steps that are involved sequentially in the production of MABs and polyclonal antiserum (Fig. 4.24) are as follows:

1. A very specific *'antigen'* (immunogen) comprising of **four epitopes** was injected into mice where B cells have already commenced generating **antibodies** against that antigen.
2. The same mice (pure strain of albino mice), received another **'booster dose'** of the same antigen so as to accomplish a much desired **'secondary response'.**
3. The **'spleen'** of the treated mice was duly removed after a gap of 3-4 days that essentially comprised of B cells active enough in the process of synthesizing **'specific antibodies'.**
4. The isolated spleen was adequately macerated and the resulting *spleen cells* thus obtained in the form of a suspension consisting of B cells giving rise to **four distinct cell lines** *i.e.,* one cell line representing a specific *antigenic determinant (epitope).*
5. The resulting spleen cells were meticulously mixed with the *mycloma cells* of the mice derived from the bone marrow and incubated in a culture medium containing polyethylene glycol (PEG).
6. Quite a few of the *'spleen cells'* were adequately **fused with neoplasm** (*tumour*) **cells** to result into the formation of **hybrid mycloma cells.**
7. The spleen cells thus obtained are **hypoxanthine phosphoribosyl transferase** (HPRT) – positive and fuse with myeloma cells to give rise to hybridomas [see (6) above] ; besides, utilize *hypoxanthine* categorically to generate *purines* and *pyrimidines.*
8. The **hybrid myeloma cells** (*hybridomas*) do survive and continue to multiply indefinitely thereby producing a good number of **'specific antibodies'** against the **'specific antigens'**.
9. Each hybridoma cell is isolated meticulously and duly cultured individually to allow them to multiply in a clone of *daughter cells.*

10. It has been observed that such **'hybridomas'** are absolutely uniform and permanent characteristically; and, therefore, when *cloned through several generations,* invariably give rise to **only one type of antibody** having specific feature of the parent B cell, hence termed as **monoclonal antibodies** (MABs).

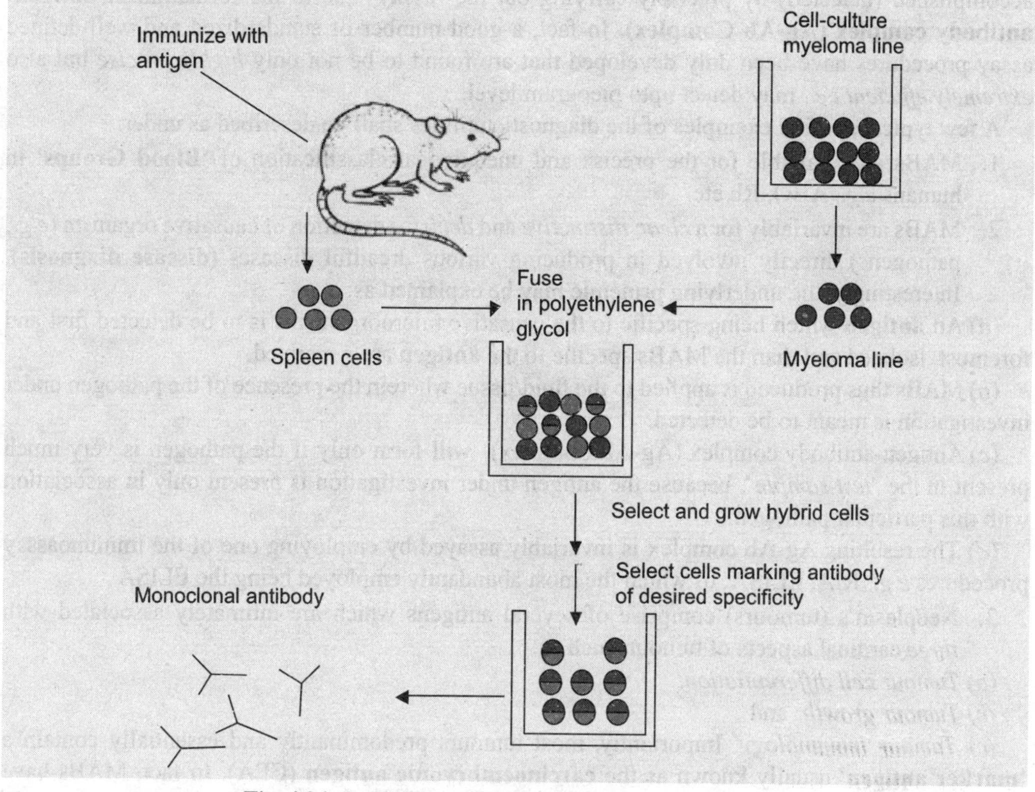

Fig. 4.24 *Production of MABs and Polyclonal Antiserum.*

4.5.1.5.4 Application of Monoclonal Antibodies (MABs)

The most spectacular major advantage of the monoclonal antibodies (MABs) is that most of the antibody molecules present in a *single preparation* strategically undergo reaction with a **single antigenic determinant** or a **single epitope.**

Consequently, the outcome of results achieved by the aid of MABs are not only significant but also explicite and devoid of any ambiguity because there prevails absolutely little confusion which may eventually come into existence by virtue of the presence of antibodies essentially displaying other specificities in the instance of *conventionally employed antisera.* However, in the light of above diversified multiple and wide spectrum applications of MABs, these may be classified judiciously into the following *four* categories, namely:

(*a*) Diagnostic Utilities,
(*b*) Biological Reagents in Diversified Disciplines,
(*c*) Therapeutic Usages,
(*d*) Immunopurification, and
(*e*) Miscellaneous Applications.

These categories of applications of MABs shall now be dealt with separately in the section that follows:

4.5.1.5.4.1 Diagnostic Utilities

Diagnostic utilities are mainly focused when MABs are employed to detect and identify the very presence of either a particular antigen (immunogen) or of antibodies specific to an antigen in a sample or samples. It is, however, pertinent to mention here that the presence of antigen is invariably accomplished (detected) by precisely carrying out the **'assay'** due to the formation of **antigen-antibody complex (Ag-Ab Complex).** In fact, a good number of standardized and well-defined assay procedures have been duly developed that are found to be not only *highly precise* but also *extremely efficient i.e.,* may detect upto picogram level

A few typical specific examples of the diagnostic utilities shall be described as under:

1. MABs are available for the precise and unequivoeal classification of **'Blood Groups'** in humans *e.g.,* ABO, Rh etc.
2. MABs are invariably for a *clear, distinctive* and *decisive* detection of causative organism (*e.g.,* pathogens) directly involved in producing various dreadful diseases (**disease diagnosis**). Interestingly, the underlying principle may be explained as:

(*a*) An **antigen** which being specific to the causative microorganisms is to be detected first and foremost, isolated and than the MABs specific to the **antigen** are generated.

(*b*) MABs thus produced is applied to the fluid/tissue wherein the presence of the pathogen under investigation is meant to be detected.

(*c*) Antigen-antibody complex (Ag-Ab Complex) will form only if the pathogen is very much present in the *'test sample'*, because the antigen under investigation is present only in association with this particular pathogen.

(*d*) The resulting Ag-Ab complex is invariably assayed by employing one of the immunoassay procedures *e.g.,* RIA, ELISA; of which the most abundantly employed being the ELISA

3. Neoplasm's (tumours) comprise of several antigens which are intimately associated with *three* cardinal aspects of tumour, such as:

(*a*) *Tumour cell differentiation;*

(*b*) *Tumour growth;* and

(*c*) *Tumour immunology*. Importantly, most tumours predominantly and essentially contain a **'marker antigen'** usually known as the **carcinoembryonic antigen** (CEA). In fact, MABs have been specifically produced for CEA together with certain other tumour-linked antigens.

In actual practice, the application of such tailor-made MABs in *histochemical assays* allows the clear-cut identification of such vital information, for instance:

(*a*) The nature of tumour cell type,

(*b*) The malignant and benign king of neoplasm's, and

(*c*) The early instances of *melastasis*.

Note. (1) Radioimmunoassay may detect even small tumours to the extent of 0.5 cm in size that are otherwise not detectable conveniently.

(2) Immunological assays are capable of detection of cancerous cells at a very early stage which is of immense help and advantage in 'cancer chemotherapy'.

4. MABs may be effectively and accurately used for the detection of *'particular chromosomes'* of a given species.

It may be accomplished by adopting the following steps:

(a) Raising MABs against particular proteins that are duly encoded by the genes present in different chromosomes of a specific *viz.,* for the *amylase inhibitors* encoded by the **genes in chromosomes 1 and 6 of wheat.** The actual quantum of Ag-Ab formation in the tissues, such as: seed, extracts, from various individuals may be employed to ascertain in case an individual is found to be:

Nullismic : *i.e.,* **no** Ag-Ab complex formed:

Monosomic : *i.e.,* **low** quantum of Ag-Ab complex formed;

Normal Disomic : *i.e., intermediate* amount of Ag-Ab complex formed;
Trisomic : *i.e., high* quantum of Ag-Ab complex formed.
Specific for the **'concerned chromosome'.**

4.5.1.5.4.2 Biological Reagents in Diversified Disciplines

The most pivotal, major and extremely important major applications of MABs in the capacity of **'biological reagents'** in a number of diversified disciplines are provided in Table 6 as under.

Table 4.6 *Applications of MABs as Important Biochemical Reagents in Diversified Disciplines*

S.No	Discipline	Applications
1.	Bacteriology	Identification of microorganism, and their respective pathogenicity (ie., disease producing organisms)
2.	Cytology	Cell separation by employing flourescent antibodies, carcinoma cells etc.,
3.	Diagnostics	Diagnosis of viral hepatitis, typhoid, filariasis, amoebiasis, breast cancer, HIV-infections, pregnancy tests, haemolytic diseases, genetic disorders, Japanese encephalitis, autoimmune and immunodeficiency disease.
4.	Forensic science (Criminology)	Characterization of Blood stains.
5.	Immunology	Immunoassays, characterization antibody, molecules, antigenic determinants, neoplasm antigens, analysis and identification of T-cell subsets, cytotoxic drug conjugated with MABs against tumour antigens to act as **'magic bullets'**.
6.	Medicine	Identification of blood group, tissue typing, *human leucocyte antigen typing* (HLA-typing), blood clotting factors.
7.	Pathology	Test for allergens in vivo.
8.	Pharmacology	Estimation of drug substances e.g., barbiturates, antibiotics, antineoplastic agents etc.
9.	Virology	Detection and identification of viruses, expression of viral antigens in infected cell-membranes etc.

4.5.1.5.4.3 Therapeutic Usages

The therapeutic usages essentially and prominently make use of MABs to combat *two* vital aspects: *first*, the management and treatment of a disease condition; and *secondly,* to afford a reasonable protection from a disease profile. A few typical examples eliciting certain exemplary developments in this specialized field are enumerated as under:

a. Immunotoxins with 'Ricin'. Antibodies specific to neoplasm cells (i.e., a cell-type) may be linked with a particular toxin polypeptide thereby giving rise to a conjugate molecule normally termed as **immunotoxin.** It has been amply demonstrated that the antibody segment of the prevailing immunotoxin shall be strategically bound to the **'target cells'**; and, therefore, the attached toxin will categorically kill the ensuing cells. Interestingly, the immunotoxins with **'ricinin'** have been prepared successfully and evaluated subsequently by accessing their ability to kill the *'neoplasm cells'* with commendable success. The resulting toxin is observed to be very much effective against both *dividing* and *non-dividing* cells because it helps in the inhibition of protein synthesis to a considerable extent. Importantly, the conjugate derived from **antibody-Ricin A** has been shown to reduce protein synthesis particularly in mouse B-cell neoplasm's. Besides, the antibody employed in forming the conjugate was found to be absolutely specific to the *'antigen molecules'* present on the surface of the prevailing target neoplasm cells as shown in Fig. 4.22.

Note. The *'immunotoxin with Ricin'* failed to exhibit any binding affinity to either other neoplasm cells or the normal cells.

b. Radioactivity to Target Tumour Cell. Based on the identical principle it has been adequately exploited to deliver radioactivity particularly to the target tumour cells. Interestingly, in this specific instance, radioactivity caused by virtue of ^{131}I (iodine), ^{90}Y (yitrium), ^{67}Cu (copper), ^{212}Pb etc., is strategically incorporated (or inducted) right into the neoplasm specific antibody (*i.e.,* **toxin is not used**). Consequently, the prevailing **radioactive antibody entity** exclusively gets bound to the tumour cells that in turn *express the particular antigen.* Thus, the radiation ultimately emitted by the isotopes helps to kill the neoplasm cells and also their neighboring cells.

Broadly speaking, this particular approach is commonly known as **'radio imaging'** to solely detect *neoplasm cells* for which the *antibodies* are more or less extremely specific.

Examples:

A few typical examples of the radio-labeled antibodies that have been used extensively as therapeutic purposes are:

For Hepatoma: Human T-cell leukemia/lymphoma virus-1 (HTLV-1); and Adult T-cell leukemia (ATL).

c. The proper activation of T-cells (lymphocytes) by virtue of their adequate *proliferation, maturation* and *antibody secretion* achieved due to their **interleukin-4 [IL-4] dependence profile.** Perhaps the aforesaid observation would certainly go a long way to put forward a solid explanation that both *tissue* and *bone marrow* explant rejections are significantly mediated by T-cells. Therefore, quite evidently an overwhelming strategy to lower the probability of rejection of '*grafts*' from other individuals (*i.e.,* **allograft**) in particular shall be aimed at to eradicate the T-cells from either bone marrow or circulatory system (*viz.,* blood stream) by employing **T-cell specific MABs.** In general, T-cells do display many *antigens* (immunogens), but it has been observed that CD3, CD4, CD8 etc., have been the most preferred targets for the development of MABs.

Methodology. The various steps involved in the bone-marrow transplantation are enumerated briefly as under:

1. Bone marrow cells of the recipient are adequately inactivated by appropriate radiation.
2. Donor bone marrow cells are meticulously subjected to the T-cell specific antibodies to cause destruction of the T-cells present in them; and, subsequently, the residual treated cells are transplanted into the recipient.

d. Passive Immunity against Diseases. MABs may be employed to cause an efficacious and preventive '*passive immunity against diseases*'. It has been squarely proved that the **'active immunity'** duly inducted in an immunized individual by itself generates the antibodies against the concerned pathogenic microorganisms (*pathogens*); whereas, interestingly in the specific instance of **'passive immunity'** antibodies that are actually produced elsewhere are adequately introduced into the body of an individual to make the **required and desired provision of immunity** against the *concerned pathogens.*

e. MABS are found to be extremely beneficial in affording the purification of antigens that are particularly specific to the '*concerned pathogens*'. In short, these '*highly purified antigens*' are invariably employed as **vaccines** *e.g.,* polio vaccine, cholera vaccine, small pox vaccine etc.,

4.5.1.5.4.4 Immunopurification

The highly specific and critical interaction of an *'antibody'* to an '*antigen*' is largely employed for the purification of antigens that are essentially present in small quantum in the form of a mixture along with several kinds of other molecules; and this phenomenon is termed as **'immunopurification'**.

The various kinds of immunopurification usually encountered are discussed as under briefly:

1. The specific structure of a *MAB molecule* should be largely compatible to the antigen that needs to be purified; and the latter is invariably fixed to an *insoluble matrix,* such as: *dextran* [Macrodex$^{(R)}$] or *agarose beads, strategically joined together by a cross-linking* agent like *cyanogens bromide* in such a fashion that its **inherent antigen-binding** ability is least affected. The aforesaid beads are suitably packed into a column *via* which the solution consisting of the '*antigen*' is made to elute under standard specified conditions. The *antibody molecules* present in the system do interact

appropriately with the *antigen molecules* thereby giving rise to the formation of Ag-Ab complex that is obviously held up in the column whereas the residual molecules (smaller in size) get eluated rather freely without any inconvenience whatsoever. Now, appropriate washing processes are adopted so as to collect the **'purified antigen'** retained as Ag-Ab complex in the column. This prevailing technique is commonly known as **'affinity chromatography'.**

Note. *Exactly the reverse of the above phenomenon is skillfully used for the purification of MABs i.e., in this specific instance the '**purified antigen**' is duly fixed onto the beads adequately packed in a column via which the antibodies are passed. Consequently, the MABs from the ensuing Ag-Ab complex are meticulously recovered in its purest form.*

2. MABs have been frequently utilized in the isolation of mRNA* via encoding the particular protein entity to which the MABs are eventually specific.

Methodology:

The different steps involved are as follows:

(*a*) Almost one dozen of *ribosomes* are intimately associated with the *'active protein synthesis' in vivo* being supported by one mRNA molecule. Consequently, one ribosome is closely linked to a molecule of the corresponding *polypeptide* undergoing synthesis; and this very resulting new structure is usually termed as polysome.

(*b*) The ensuing *'preparation of polysomes'* on being treated with antibodies, undergo instant interaction with the *highly specific nascent polypeptides* closely linked with the ribosome's thereby affording ultimate precipitation of the prevailing **'polysomes'.** This phenomenon evidently suggests that a specific MAB shall only precipitate such *'polysomes'* that are critically engaged in the synthesis of **polypeptide** for which the MAB is articulately specific.

(*c*)Subsequently, the **'precipitated polysomes'** are normally recovered by standard procedures, and the mRNA is isolated carefully.

(*d*) The resulting mRNA is found to be extremely pure in nature; and, therefore, predominantly aids in the process of encoding the protein for which the specific MAB was initially engaged in the precipitation of the *'polysome'*.

3. MABs are invariably utilized for several vital operations, such as: identification, isolation of cells exhibiting a particular 'antigen' on their surface.

Methodology: The various steps involved are as stated below:

a. MAB which is specific to the *'concerned antigen'* being articulately conjugated with a fluorescent molecule.

b. The MAB very much specific to the concerned antigen is conjugated with a *'fluorescent molecule'*; and thereafter, added to the corresponding *cell suspension* to facilitate Ag- Ab complex production.

c. The resulting *'antibody conjugate'* shall ultimately get bound to those cells only which prominently display the 'concerned antigen on their surface; and, therefore, such cells will exhibit fluorescence under suitable conditions.

d. In actual practice, these specific cells are easily identified and subsequently separated from the others by virtue of their *'fluorescence characteristics'*. Hence, for this precise measurement one may make use of highly sophisticated **'fluorescence activated cell sorters'** (FACS) to afford a rather prompt and rapid sorting out of such characteristic cells.

4.5.1.5.4.5 Miscellaneous Applications

There are quite a few miscellaneous applications of MABs which would be discussed in the section that follows:

1. Drug Delivery and Targeting. The most vital and exemplory application of MABs in therapeutic domain is to precisely direct and guide a drug adequately conjugated with MABs against the neoplasm (tumour) antigens strategically positioned on the target cells. In other words, a **'toxic**

drug entity' is very selectively and precisely delivered to the target cell (*i.e.*, neoplasm cells) without causing any affect on the normal cells. Hence, in the latest therapeutic (pharmacologic) terminology such highly specific **drug-conjugated MAB** invariably act as **'Magic Bullets'.**

Advantages: The various advantages of **'Magic Bullets'** are as follows:

(*a*) The desired *'toxic-drug'* entity is solely prevented from circulation in the body, whereas a **'small dosage'** may be administered most precisely to the *'desired target'* in a rather effective manner; and

(*b*) The aforesaid technique is found to be an extremely useful one for the meticulous administration of *anti-neoplastic agent's viz.,* **methotrexate, busulfan, phosphoramide mustard, lomustine** and the like, without resulting into any serious side-effects whatsoever.

Notes: *The most challenging and difficult aspect of the entire exercise is the problem of raising MABs which shall get bound to* **'neoplasm cells'** *rather than the* **'normal cells'**.

2. Identification of Lymphocyte Subpopulations. A major break through and spectacular advancement in the application of MABs has been critically focused towards the identification for the sub-populations of lymphocytes by the help of **Fluorescence-Activated Cell Sorter** (FACS).

Methodology: The various steps involved are as follows:

(*a*) The fluorescent dye-labeled MABs absolutely specific for cell-surface antigenic determinants are made to interact with the ensuing lymphocytes.

(*b*) The resulting cells are subsequently passed through a *thin stream of culture medium via* an electric field.

(*c*) Consequently, the fluorescent cells pick-up charges accordingly; and, therefore, may be isolated from the non-flurescent ones conveniently.

Importance: The aforesaid technique is abundantly utilized not only to differentiate but also to segregate the fluorescent cells so as to pin-point effectively the prevalent and relative abundance of various kinds of **immune cells.** Therefore, the above delicate phenomenon may be exploited as a viable, dependable and trustworthy **'diagnostic tool'** for various **autoimmune diseases** and **immune deficiency disease conditions.**

3. Autoimmune and Immunodeficiency Diseases. It has been proved and well established beyond any reasonable doubt that in both *autoimmune* as well as *immune-deficiency diseases* the prevalent helper and suppressor T cell subset ratio gets disturbed appreciably. Therefore, the overwhelming T cell deficiencies may be monitored precisely and accurately by the aid of MABs-directed against the specific *T cell immunogens* (antigens).

4. Detection of Surface Molecules. MABs have been skillfully and purposefully employed to probe the **surface of immunocompetent cells.** Besides, MABs have also been used in *mapping* the actual prevailing *distribution of the membrane determinants, e.g., major histocompatibility complex* (MHC) *antigens* and a plethora of macromolecules. It is, however, a well known fact that the ensuing *T cell subsets* essentially comprise of various surface markers that are *predominantly antigenic in nature.*

In the therapeutic armamentarium the particular role and unique ability to *deplete a specific T cell subset* in a patient by the induction of MABs that have the capability and vulnerability to get bound selectively to one specific determinant of the aforesaid subset.

Example: The above critical situation may be further expatiated by specifically discarding the cytotoxic T cells in patients that might have been provided with a kidney transplantation from a donor, whereby the chances of *kidney rejection* (or *graft rejection*) in the **recipient** (*i.e.*, **new host**) **is minimized substantially.**

5. Veterinary and Plant Diagnostics. It has been duly recommended that the MABs could be employed extensively towards the diagnosis of Foot and Mouth disease in animals. They are also beneficial in the measurements of reproductive hormone levels in the animals. Interestingly, the utilization of MABs in *plant viral diseases* is not so quite predominantly recognized as in humans or animals.

In nut shell, the above applications are representatives of the numerous applications of MABs the technological advancement of which is advancing in an astronomical speed as well as momentum.

4.6 Hypersensitivity Reactions

Hypersensitivity may be defined as – '*an abnormal sensitivity to a stimulus of any kind*'. Invariably, a situation may crop up when an *antigen* specifically interacts with a *sensitized* host thereby giving rise to tissue **damage;** and this is usually termed as **hypersensitivity reactions.**

In other words, one may lodge an explanation that immune reactions are particularly responsible for not only managing but also tackling adequately the invasion by a host of so called *'foreign antigens'* necessarily comprising of various types of viruses, microorganisms, chemicals, drug substances, allergens etc., and ultimately render reasonable protection to the human body as a whole. Therefore, a majority of prevailing *immune responses* are overwhelmingly useful for the human body; however, there are quite a few *immunological reactions* that significantly afford an almost **adverse reaction** ultimately resulting into undersirable, painful, and harmful effects. In true sense, these untowards hypersensitivity reactions are mostly characterized by a *highly specific antigen-antibody reaction (Ag-Ab reaction)*, and these are of *three* cardinal categories as **detailed below:**

i. When no visible reaction takes place even after the very first exposure to an '*agent*'. Evidently, the symptoms commence soon after *i.e.,* normally within a short span of a few days only after drug therapy begins,

ii. when the desired effects of an immunologic reaction utterly fail to resemble the pharmacological actions of the '*drug substance*' ; besides, such responses normally occur at dose levels much below the therapeutic limits (*i.e.,* the effective dose level), and

iii. When the prevailing immunologic reactions usually afford a restricted quantum of allergy related syndromes embracing only a small patient population.

There are ample evidences whereby certain therapeutic agents *i.e., 'drugs'*, quite often responsible for acute or severe adverse reactions (or allergic reactions), such as: penicillins, sulpha drugs, corticotrophin, erythromycin; besides several blood products. However, apparently most of these hypersensitive conditions *i.e.,* allergic reactions, may be observed on account of the '*inflammation*' occurring at the *very site of the Ag-Ab reaction.*

4.6.1 Types of Hypersensitivity Reaction

In actual practice, one may come across a variety of '*adverse reactions*' that may be conveniently categorized into the following *five* types, solely based on the prevailing underlying *immunologic mechanism,* namely:

(*a*) Type-I: Anaphylactic hypersensitivity,
(*b*) Type-II: Antibody-dependent cytotoxic hypersensitivity,
(*c*) Type-III: Complex mediated hypersensitivity,
(*d*) Type-IV: Cell-mediated or delayed type hypersensitivity, and
(*e*) Type-V: Stimulatory hypersensitivity.

The five aforementioned types of hypersensitivity reactions ('*a*' through '*e*') shall now be dealt with individually in the section that follows:

4.6.1.1 Type-I: Anaphylactive Hypersensitivity

Anaphylactic hypersensitivity exclusively based upon the reaction of '*antigen*' with a particular IgE antibody intimately bond *via* its *crystallisable fragment* (Fc) to the corresponding *mast cell* there by leading to the ultimate release from the granules of the mediators '*histamine*', **slow**

reacting substance of **anphylaxis** (SRSA) **platelet activating factor,** and above all an **eosinophil chemotactic Factor.** It has been observed that the ensuing eosinophils evidently neutralize the prevailing mast cell mediators.

Examples: **Extrinsic asthma** and **hay fever** are the two most glaring examples which represent the most common *atopic allergic disorders.* The most critical and offending antigen being identified by the specific '*intradermal prick tests*' thereby providing instant **wheal and erythema reactions** or by *provocation testing.*

Preventive Measures: Most common symptomatic therapy essentially involves the usage of *mediator antagonists* or such agents the intracellular cAMP (*i.e.,* cyclic adenosine monophosphate), and thereby help in stabilizing the mast cell granules.

(2) Regular dose related therapy of '**antigen injection**' may also desensitize by causing either blockade of IgG or IgA antibodies or by switching off IgE production almost completely.

Interestingly, the anaphylactic hypersensitivity reactions are found to be extremely rapid and hence causes excessive inflammations which could be either localized or generalized ones ; and they have a series of critical stages as enumerated below in sections ('*i*' to '*v*')

i. Triggering off '*antibody generation*' *i.e.,* the initial sensitization takes place first and foremost on being exposed to a particular '*drug substance*'.
ii. IgE is produced liberally and profusely in the course of the *inductive phase.* Consequently, the antibodies under rapid circulation *in vivo* and get fixed onto the surface of the mast cells throughout the body,
iii. The '*allergen*' *i.e.,* the **antigenic drug** subsequently gets bound intimately to the prevailing IgE antibodies on the mast cells,
iv. The phenomenon of '**degranulation**' of mast cells commences with the corresponding release of a huge excess of **mediators,** for instance; *SRS-A* and *histamine,* and
v. A predominant peripheral vasodilation followed by a substantial enhancement of vascular permeability by virtue of the release of '*histamine*' ultimately gives rise to **apparent vascular congestion and edema.** Besides, the bronchiolar smooth muscles also get constricted significantly.

Broadly speaking, the **anaphylactic hypersensitivity reactions** quite often give rise to a host of serious allergic manifestations in humans, such as: (*a*) *asthma* (lower respiratory tract allergy);

(*b*) *Rhinitis* (upper respiratory tract allergy); and (*c*) *skin allergy* or *dermatological allergy* (causing eczema etc.).

Example: **Immunopathologic conditions of asthama:** The various sequential stages involved in the immunopathologic conditions of asthma are as stated under:

i. An inflammatory response which specifically initiates airway obstruction,
ii. As a consequence releases mediators from the mast cells which particularly render bronchial smooth muscle to become spasmodic,
iii. This event gives rise to '*bronchioconstriction*' *i.e.,* narrowing the passage bronchial airways, and
iv. Bronchioconstruction in turn gives rise to blood-vessel engorgement followed by infiltration of the corresponding inflammatory cells (*i.e.,* **neutrophils**).

Mechanism: The '*airborne antigen*' (*viz.,* pollen) first enters the airway and soon after gets bound to a receptor strategically located on a mast cell. Activation of the mast cell commences thereby influencing a distinct enhancement in cAMP, an influx of Ca^{2+} ions, spontaneous release of performed mediators (*e.g.,* **histamine**), and ultimately the synthesis of no performed mediators [*e.g.,* **prostaglandin** D_2 (PGD_2)]. However, the *performed mediators* essentially comprise of various vital and important components, such as: histamine, heparin, eosinophil chemotactic factor of anaphylaxis (ECFA), neutrophil hemotactic factor (NCF), and above all certain other enzymes. Likewise, the *nonperformed mediators* invariably consist of certain highly critical constituents, for instance: prostaglandin D_2 (PGD_2), platelet activating factor (PAF), and importantly the so called **leukotrienes C_4 and B_4** which are presently recognized to be the essential components of the slow-reacting substance of anaphylaxis (SRS-A). In utshell, these *two* different types of *'mediators' viz.,* performed and nonperformed ones do serve as the ajor cause of the overwhelming **bronchoconstriction, airway-edema,** and **excessive mucous production.** The various interesting aspects of the immunopathologic events and sequences of asthama are illustrated in Fig. 4.25 as under:

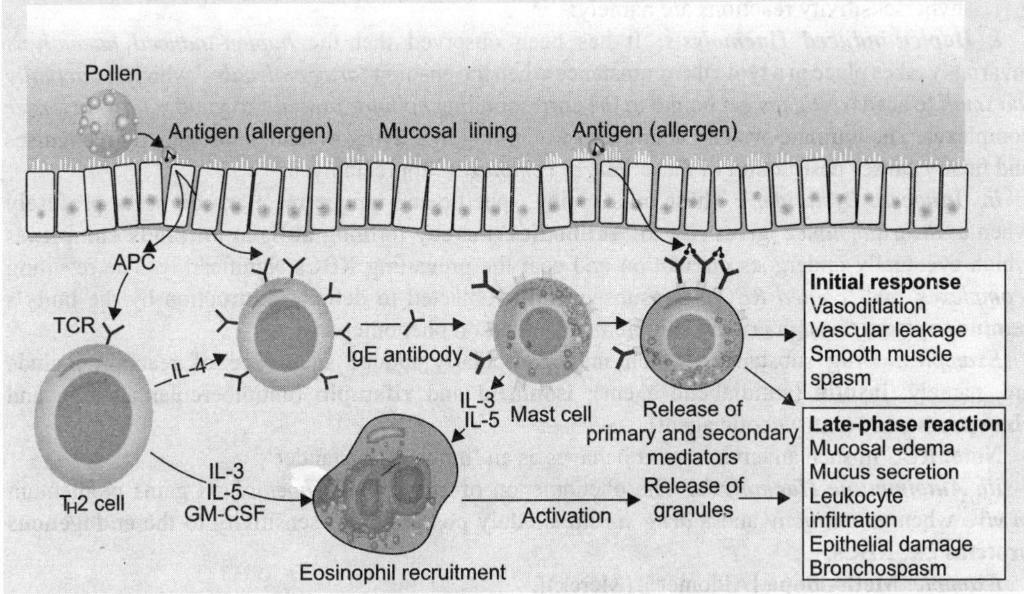

Fig. 4.25 *Immunopathological Sequence of Events in Asthma.*

[IgE = Immunoglobulin E; 5′ AMP = Adenosine-5-monophosphate; cAMP= Cyclic adenosine onophophate; ATP = Adenosine Triphosphate; cGMP = Cyclic guanine monophosphate; PGD_2= Prostaglandin D_2.]

4.6.1.2 Type-II: Antibody-Dependent Cytotoxic Hypersensitivity

Antibody-dependent cytotoxic hypersensitivity essentially involves the ultimate death of cells bearing *antibody* that are intimately attached to a *surface antigen*. These ensuing cells may be engulfed by the prevailing phagocytic cells to which they get adhered *via* their actual coating of either IgG or C_{3b} or eventually lyzed by the operation of the full complement system. However, these ensuing cells critically bearing IgG may face fatal consequences due to either the *mycloid cells* (*i.e.,* polymorphos and macrophages) or by virtue of the non-adherent lymphoid K cells through an extracellular mechanism (*i.e.,* antibody dependent cell-mediated cytotoxicity).

Examples: The various examples are as stated below:

i. *Transfusion reactions i.e.,* when blood groups are not matched properly,
ii. *Haemolytic disease* concerning the newly born babies *via Rhesus incompatibility,*
iii. *Graft destruction or rejection i.e.,* antibody-mediated '*graft*'** destruction or rejection.
iv. *Autoimmune reactions* usually directed against the formed elements of the blood, and the kidney glomerular basement membranes, and
v. *Hypersensitivity* as a consequence from the coating of *erythrocytes* or platelets by a specific **'drug molecule'.**

In other words, the main characteristic features of the antibody-dependent cytotoxic hypersensitivity reaction may be expatiated as under:

a. Reactions invariably take place in a situation where IgM or IgG antibodies (see section 5.1.2) undergo interaction with antigen on the cell surface thereby giving rise to either cell destruction from phagocytosis or cell lysis,

b. Progressive activation of the prevailing complement system ultimately leading to either the *destruction of RBCs* or the *specific target cells*, and

c. Recognition of three predominant categories of Type-II antibody-dependent cytotoxic hypersensitivity reactions are namely:

i. Hapten-induced Haemolysis: It has been observed that the *hapten-induced haemolysis* invariably takes place in a typical circumstance when the ensuing '*drug molecules*' which are *actually too small* to act as *antigens* get bound to the corresponding *cellular proteins* to yield *relatively larger* complexes. The immune system, acting as a watch-dog in a living system, subsequently recognises and finally causes destruction of these *'larger complexes'* appreciably.

ii. 'Innocent Bystander': These outstanding, specific and unique reactions do occur profusely when a *'drug substance'* gives rise to **'antibodies'** thereby forming **antigen antibody complexes** which eventually undergoes circulation and coat the prevailing RBCs significantly. The resulting '*complexes*' and '*coated RBCs*' are subsequently subjected to definite destruction by the **body's immune system** through critical complement activation phenomenon.

Examples: Drug substances which may particularly induce such tyoe of reaction include are, namely: **insulin** (antidiabetic agent); **isoniazid** and **rifampin** (antitubercular agents); and **chlorpromazine** (antisychotic agent).

Note: RBC in such an environment behaves as an 'innocent bystander'.

iii. Autoimmune Haemolysis: The phenomenon of *autoimmune haemolysis* gains momentum *in vivo* when an *antibody* and a *drug substance* duly possess cross-sensitivity to the **endogenous proteins** *i.e.*, RBCs.

Example: **Methyldopa** [Aldomet(R) (Merck)].

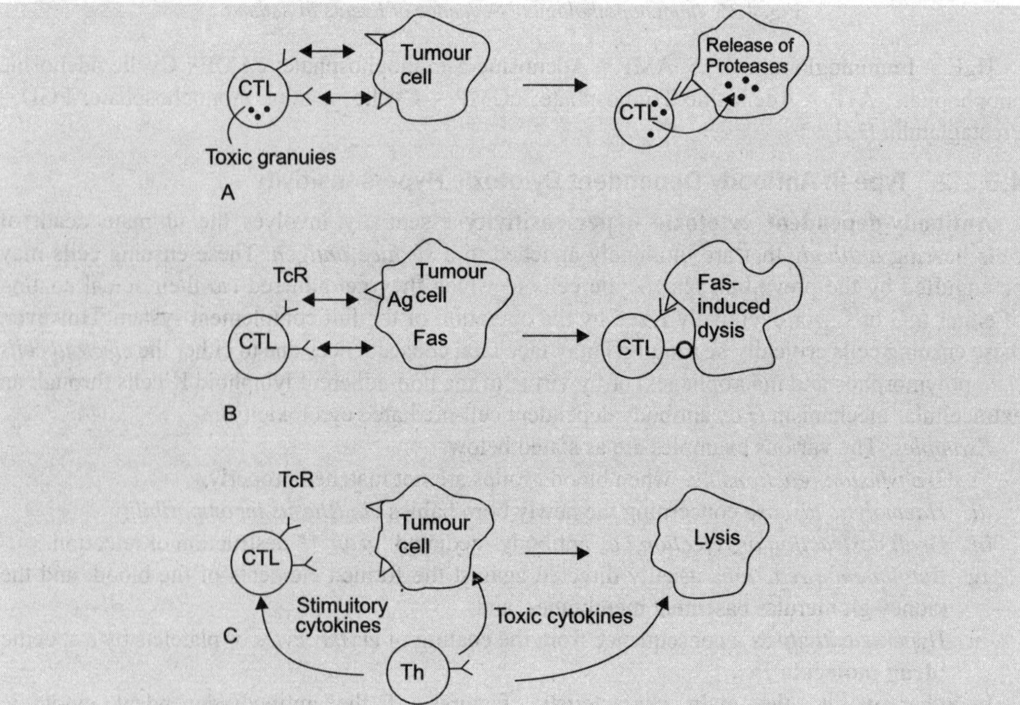

Fig. 4.26 *Type II-Antibody-Dependent Cytotoxic Hypersensitivity. [(a), (b) and (c)].*

Methyl dopa is capable of inducing the autoimmune haemolysis process in the body. Fig. 23 illustrates the typical '*Type II-antibody-dependent cytotoxic hypersensitivity*' that takes place in three different stages, such as:

a. Acute phagocytic activity: i.e., when the normal tissue cell more or less functions as an antigen (or allergen) that essentially gets bound to the prevailing fragment antibody binding (Fab) region strategically located on the antibody. Thus, the fragment crystallisable (Fc) segment remains virtually in the Free State to bind the compliment, phagocytes or the K cells accordingly.

b. Complement activation and phagocytosis: i.e., the phenomenon when the 'normal cells' are first and foremost adequately coated with the corresponding antibodies so that they may be killed (lysed) either by the prevailing complement cells or the K cells, and get phagocytosed eventually, and

c. Development of antibody-dependent cytotoxicity: i.e., another typical mechanism whereby only the K cells are specifically involved via IgG and Fc receptor towards the ultimate and precise development of antibody-dependent cytotoxicity.

4.6.1.3 Type-III: Complex Mediated Hypersensitivity

The *complex mediated hypersensitivity* reaction is an outcome of the prevalent and pivotal **antigen- antibody complexes** *via* **two cardinal phenomena** taking place *in vivo,* such as: (*a*) most articulated activation of complement as well as attraction of *polymorphonuclear leucocytes* that help in the release of '*tissue damaging enzymes*' upon instant contact with the prevailing complexes; and (*b*) most predominant *aggregation of platelets* that would afford microthrombi and vasoactive amine release.

At this junction *two* clearly perceptible situations may arise:

1. Relative antibody excess:

In this specific instance the *antigen* is adequately precipitated very close to the site of entry into the human body; and the ultimate reaction in the skin is invariably exhibited by the *polymorph infiltration, oedema,* and **erythema maximal** within a range of 3-8 hours (also known as *Arthus reaction*).

Examples: There are *two* critical and specific examples:

i. *Farmer's Lung Disease i.e.,* a form of hypersensitivity alveoli is caused by exposure to moldy hay that has fermented. The two causative microorganisms are *Actinomyces micropolyspora faeni* and *Thermoactinomyces vulgarisms.*

ii. *Pigeon Facier's Disease i.e.,* a type of sensitivity whereby the inhaled antigens from the bird usually provoke high antibody levels in humans.

2. Relative antigen excess:

In this particular case the resulting **complexes** duly formed are found to be soluble, also circulate and are ultimately deposited at some most preferred strategical sites, such as: kidney glomerulus's, skin, joints and *choroid plexus*.

Detection: The detection of '*complexes*' may be accomplished by carrying out the following steps sequentially:

i. Immunofluorescent staining of tissue biopsies,

ii. Analysis of serum for the *cryoprecipitates*, *raised antiglobulins* and *immunoconglutinin,*

iii. Abnormal peaks on ultracentrifugation,

iv. High molecular weight IgG or C_3,

v. Reaction with rheumatoid factors or C1q,

vi. Alternations in C_3 and C_{3c},

vii. Inhibition of K-cell activity, and

viii. Competition for Fc receptor binding upon the prevailing macrophages and lymphoid cell lines.

Examples: The various examples belonging to this category are:

i. Serum sickness immediately after injection of large quantum of foreign protein *in vivo*,

ii. Glomerulonephritis associated with systemic lupus or contract infections with *streptococci*, malaria (due to *Plasmodium* sps.) and other parasites.

iii. Neurological disturbances in systemic lupus and subacute sclerosing *panencephalitis*,

iv. polyarteritis nodosa associated with *hepatitis B virus*,

v. crythema nodosum in leprosy and syphilis,

vi. Hemorrhagic shock in *Dengue viral* infection, and

viii. An element of the *synovial lesion* in rheumatoid arthritis.

In other words, the complex mediated hypersensitivity reactions invariably and essentially involves three components, namely: *antigens, antibodies,* and *complement.* These reactions strategically take place within the body's capillaries between two vital entities *viz.,* **soluble antigen** and **circulating antibodies** thereby generating due formation of *antigen-antibody complexes* adequately indicated by apparent inflammatory responses.

Salient Features: Following are the salient features of these reactions:

a. Antigen-antibody complexes mostly circulate and eventually become fixed in comparatively smaller blood vessels (*viz.*, kidneys) or other target tissues as well,

b. Resulting intravascular complexes specifically help in the activation of the prevailing *complement system* which ultimately gives rise to a *predominant inflammatory reaction* that causes tissue destruction.

c. An immune complex manifestation causes '**serum sickness**' wherein the ensuing deposition of the said complex in the vascular system gives rise to *vasculitis*. A few apparent abnormalities may crop up in the various organs of the body *e.g.,* development of specific lesions inside the glomerular wall thereby causing permanent impairment of glomerular tissue. Besides, it may also give rise to two ciritcal situation *e.g., proteinuria* and *hematuria* whereby an enhanced noticeable permeability of the '*glomerular basement membrane*' take place in the long run.

d. Two prominent processes occur invariably in human body, namely; (*i. complement activation*; and (*ii. antibody precipitation,* which ultimately produce an **acute localized vasculitis.** This is usually termed as **Arthus reaction**, whereby both necrosis and cellular inflammation are accomplished at the very site of antigen injection in an already sensitized patient.

e. Very much akin to specific '*drug reactions*' it produces **systemic lupus erythematosus.**

Figure 4.27 illustrates the outcome of the complex mediated hypersensitivity reactions producing distinct inflammations that may initially behave almost as normal; however, at a later stage, when *antigen* is found to be in excess, it has been observed adequately that the evolution of **Ag-Ab-complement complexes** commense the process of circulation and finally get deposited specifically in various tissues in the human body. Importantly, the target organs are invariably found to be kidneys, joints, and skin that get damaged not only physiologically but also irreversibly. *Complement* loaded with various components particularly attracts the '*phagocytes*' which subsequently undergoes degranulation of the mast cells in that specific region. Therefore, the final cause of **local inflammation** is solely based upon two vital processes *viz. first*, engulfing of the complexes by the prevailing phagocytes; and *secondly*, releasing of the chemicals from the congregation of the mast cells.

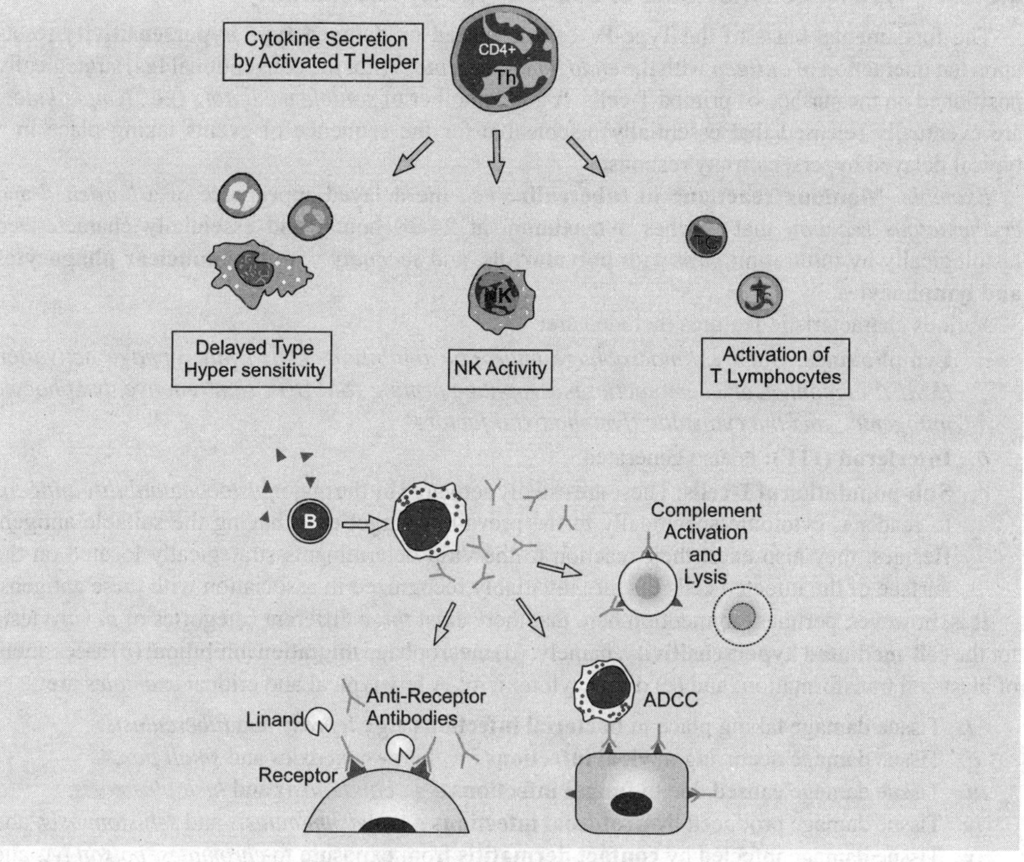

Fig. 4.27 *Type III Complex Mediated Hypersensitivity*

A few typical examples of Arthus Reactions (or Arthus Phenomenon) are provided in Table 7 given below:

Table 4.7 *Type III-Complex Mediated Hypersensitivity and Their Causation.*

S.No	Nomenclature of Disease	Causation
1.	Cheese Washer's disease	– *Pencillin casei* spores
2.	Crohn's disease	– Intestinal tissue injuries
3.	Elephantiasis	– *Wauchereria bancrofit* in lymphatic vessels.
4.	Farmer's Lung	– Infection produced by *Actinomycetes* spores
5.	Furrier's Lung	– Fox fur proteins
6.	Glomerulonephritis	– Deposition of immune complexes and infections caused by *Pneumococcal* and *Streptococcal* species.
7.	Lymphocytic leukemia	– Injuries in tissue by virtue of deposition of immune complexes in blood vessels.
8.	Pigeon Fancier's disease	– Dried excreta of pigeons.
9.	Serum sickness	– Foreign blood serum.
10.	Systemic Lupus Erythematosus (SLE)	– Complexes deposited in kidney, skin and CNS.

4.6.1.4 Type-IV: Cell-mediated or delayed Type Hypersensitivity

The fundamental basis of the Type-IV **cell-mediated or delayed type hypersensitivity** resets upon the interaction of *antigen* with the *endogenous receptors* (not the conventional Igs) strategically positioned on the surface of primed T-cells. A good number of *soluble mediators* (*i.e., lymphokines*) are eventually released that essentially responsible for the sequence of events taking place in a typical delayed hypersensitivity response.

Example: **Mantoux reaction* to tuberculin:** *i.e.,* the delayed appearance of a *hardened* and *erythematous reaction* that reaches a maximum at 24-28 hours; and essentially characterized histologically by infiltration, *first* with **polymorphs**, and *secondly* with **mononuclear phagocytes and lymphocytes.**

Various characteristic features included are:

a. **Lymphokines:** Such as: *macrophage migration inhibition; (MIF) macrophage activation (MAF); mononuclear chemotactic; macrophage arming (SMAF) ; skin reactive, lymphocyte mitogenic ; and the cytostatic (lymphotoxin) factors.*

b. **Interferon (ITF):** is also generated.

c. **Sub-population of T-cells:** These are usually activated by the major *histocompatibility antigens* to render it cytotoxic specifically to the prevailing target cells having the suitable antigen. Besides, they also exert their reaction to the viral determinants strategically located on the surface of the infected cells that are invariably recognized in association with these antigens.

It is, however, pertinent to mention here that there exist *three* different categories of *in vitro* tests for the **cell-mediated hypersensitivity,** namely: (*a*) macrophage migration inhibition; (*b*) assessment of blast cell transformation; and (*c*) direct cytotoxicity. A few typical and critical *examples* are:

i. Tissue damage taking place in **bacterial infections** *e.g., leprosy* and *tuberculosis,*

ii. Tissue damage occurring in **viral infections** *i.e.,* herpes, *measles* and *small pox,*

iii. Tissue damage caused due to **fungal infections** *e.g., candidiasis* and *histoplasmosis,*

iv. Tissue damage produced by **protozoal infections** *e.g., leishmamiasis* and *sehistomiasis,* and

v. Tissue damage infected by **contact dermatitis** from exposure to *chromates, poison ivy,* and *insect bites.*

In other words, the Type IV-cell-mediated or delayed type hypersensitivity reactions mostly take place specifically '*on the skin*', brought about by microorganisms and chemicals. In actual practice, the TDH cells (*i.e.,* delayed hypersensitivity T-cells) are found to be closely associated with not only in '*graft rejections*' but also function primarily by secreting many types of '*lymphokines*'.

Examples: The most befitting instance of such reactions is that of '**contact dermatitis**' which gets developed exclusively, when the skin being exposed to certain '*chemical substances,* namely: *para*-amino benzoic acid (PABA) ethylene diamine, methyl and ethyl parabens (preservatives), neomycin (antibiotic), and hair dyes (aniline-dyes). In fact, the said chemicals give rise to apparent **itching** and **inflammation** of skin when they happen to come in contact with it. Perhaps such reactions are mainly due to the interaction between the **skin proteins** and the **chemical substances** thereby triggering T cells.

4.6.1.5 Type V: Stimulatory Hypersensitivity

The Type V-stimulatory hypersensitivity reactions quite often take place whereby the antibody undergoes specific reaction with a key surface component e.g., hormone receptor and subsequently 'switches on' the cell.

Example: An interesting and extremely typical example being the thyroid hyperactivity in Grave's disease by virtue of a thyroid-stimulating autoantibody.

As a summarization the comparison of various types of hypersensitivity reactions may be explicitly grouped individually as given in Table 4.8 below:

Table 4.8 *Comparative Characteristic Features of Various Types of Hypersensitivity Reactions*

S. No	Characteristic Features	Type-I Anaphylactic	Type-II Cytotoxic	Type-III Complex Mediated	Type-IV Cell- Mediated	Type-V Stimulatory
1.	**Antibody mediating reaction**	Homocytotropic Ab - mast-cell binding	Humoral Ab ± CF (*i.e.,* complement fixation.	Humoral AB ± CF	Receptor on T-cell	Humoral AB Non-CF
2.	**Antigen**	Usually exgenous (*e.g.,* grass pollen.	Cell-surface	Extracellular	Extracellular or cell-surface	Cell-surface
3.	**Response to intradermal antigen: Max. reaction**	30 minutes	–	3-8 hours	24-28 hours	–
	Appearance	Wheal and flare	–	Erythema and oedema	Erythema and induration	–
	Histology	Degranulated mast cells; oedema; eosinophils;	–	Acute inflammatory reaction; - predominant polymorphs.	Perivascular inflammation: polymorphs migrate out leaving predominantly mononuclear cells.	–
4.	**Transfer sensitivity to normal subject**	–	Serum antibody	–	Lymphoid cells Transfer factor	Serum antibody
	Examples	Atopicallergy *e.g.,* hay fever.	Haemolytic disease of newborn (Rh.	Complex glomerulo nephritis Farmer's - lung	Mantoux reaction TB ; Skin - homograft rejection	Thyrotoxicosis

4.7 Vaccines: Preparation, Standardization and Storage

4.7.1 Definitions

The term **'vaccine'** was originally derived from the Latin word **"vacca"** meaning *cow*.

Vaccine may be defined as – *'pharmaceutical suspension or solution of an immunogenic substance or compound(s) that is intended to induce active immunity'*.

Importantly, in the older days it was quite common to limit the term to such specialized products that essentially comprised of whole microorganisms but as on date the *'terminology'* may be broadly applied to *'all active immunization agents'* and the process of active immunization is invariably termed as – **'vaccination'**.

BP defines *vaccines* as – *'preparations containing antigenic substances that have been shown to be capable of inducing a specific and active immunity in man'*.

In general, vaccines and sera are the pharmacological active preparations usually employed in **'immunology'** and both may be for the prevention of infectious disease.

Vaccines may also be regarded as therapeutic agents that are particularly derived directly or indirectly from the *'pathogenic microorganisms'*, or are effective because of an immunological reaction as none of the significant groups of chemotherapeutic agents including *antibodies* are effective against many viral types of infections.

Another school of thought defines **vaccine** as – *'any preparation that is normally used to confer active immunity, and active immunization involves the use of antigenic preparations which, when administered, stimulate the body to produce antibodies specific to the antigen administered.'*

According to Wagner *et at*. (1991) the **vaccines** are antigenic material invariably obtained from *microorganisms* and *viruses* and also specific T-cells, as discussed earlier, which may be viewed as specific agents that are solely responsible for regulating the **immune system**. Besides, there are plethoras of purely synthetic as well, as physiological factors that may essentially cause and afford substantial modifications in the prevailing *immune response.* It has been duly established that quite a few '*natural products*' and their corresponding *synthetic structural analogues* could be 'hormonal' in nature, for instance: *cytokines*, and **steroid hormones;** which in reality go a long way not only in influencing the development of immunologically reactive cells but also in carrying the reactions intimately associated with them. Importantly, there are other *'natural'* and *'synthetic'* products that may characteristically cause induction with regard to overwhelming transformations and adequate activation of specific cells (lymphocytes) closed involved in clonal expansion. However, in totality the ensuing *'immune response'* appears to be largely to 'protective nature'. Perhaps this could register a very solid support for the 'immune response' with respect to the immense **survival effect** ; and therefore, is exclusively responsible for the ability of the host to adapt to the surrounding rather '*hostile environment*'.

4.7.2 Historical

The modern prophylactic treatment against small poinx is more or less the same as that used by Edward Jenner, a Gloucestershire medical practitioner, who in 1798 critically observed that milkmaids who incidentally acquired and developed '*cowpox*' became ultimately immune to '*small pox*'. There exists now an ample evidence and support to the view that *vaccinia* or *cowpox virus* is nothing but **variola** or **small pox virus** that has been adequately modified, and, therefore, rendered less virulent.

Later on, Jenner laid the foundation of **vaccinology** *i.e.,* the science of treating millions of potential victims from a plethora of dreadful and defastating diseases, using a technique invariably termed as '**vaccination**'. Subsequently, Jenner successfully demonstrated and proved that an infection duly caused with the cowpox virus duly protests an individual against a subsequent infection contracted with small pox virus. Louis Pasteur made another spectacular and revolutionary advancement by developing the technique of '**attenuation**'. The bacteria and virus utterly responsible for diseases and inoculating individuals with these weakened disease-producing agents. Most current '*vaccines*' available for mass inoculation essentially are found to be either '*live*' but either attenuated forms of the parasite or totally killed (*i.e.,* inactivated) infectious microorganisms. Nevertheless, invariably these '*vaccines*' are highly successful but they have an inherent limitation with regard to their *efficiency* and *safety* profile. However, the attenuated vaccines certainly carry a risk by virtue of the fact that the '*weakened pathogen*' may at any time revert to a harmful entity *in vivo.*

4.7.3 Classification of Vaccines

The '**vaccines**' may be classified on the basis of the '*type of preparation*' actually employed for their production, namely:

(*a*) Toxoids derived from bacterial toxins,

(*b*) Suspensions of inactivated (killed) bacteria or viruses, and

(*c*) Suspensions of non-activated (live but attenuated) bacteria or viruses.

Keeping in view the tremendous and geometrical advancemement in the field of technology, integrated research and utmost skill in the past 3 to 4 decades the safety, longevity, and quality of life in humans, almost *two dozens* of various potential, efficacious, and safer vaccines have been designed, developed and delivered for mass protection as well as specific applications, such as:

i. Synthetic peptide vaccines

ii. Multivaccine system

iii. Bacterial vaccines

iv. DTP-vaccine

v. Typhoid-paratyphoid A and B vaccine
vi. Other bacteria vaccine
vii. Typhoid and tetanus vaccine
viii. Anthrax vaccine
ix. Q-Fever vaccine
x. Leprosy vaccines
xi. Whooping cough vaccine
xii. Diphtheria vaccines
xiii. Varicella-Zoster Vaccines
xiv. Viral and Rickettsial vaccines
xv. Smallpox vaccine
xvi. Vaccines for special protection
xvii. Rabies vaccine
xviii. Influenza vaccine
xix. Inactivated Influenza vaccine
xx. Polio Vaccine
xxi. Cancer vaccine
xxii. Birth control vaccine for women
xxiii. AIDS-vaccine
xxiv. Pneumococcal vaccine
xxv. Measles Vaccine, live
xxvi. Meningococcal Polysaccharide Vaccine
xxvii. Future Development scope of vaccines:
- *a.* Vaccine against Alzheimer's disease
- *b.* Vaccine for Meningitis C
- *c.* Super vaccine
- *d.* Immunomodulators
- *e.* Vaccination with Gas-Lighter
- *f.* Vaccine against cervical-cancer
- *g.* Vaccination without needles

The above broad and specific classifications of **'vaccines'** shall now be treated individually along with their method(s) of preparation in the sections that follows:

4.7.3.1 Synthetic Peptide Vaccines

In fact, the production of **inactivated** (killed) **vaccines** essentially involves the culture of huge amount of *live* and pathogenic (disease producing) forms of the '*parasites*' that ultimately pose the danger of infections. This specific observation has virtually paved the way for a whole new generation of vaccines entirely based on the much improved understanding of the molecular structure of *'harmful microorganisms'*. One such approach is to identify the specific regions of the pathogens that are though not so harmful, yet would elicit a definite protective immune response of the body. Interestingly, the short chains of amino acids (*peptides*) representing these regions are generally a part of a large protein on the surface of the parasite. Nevertheless, these peptides may be prepared either by *chemical synthesis* or *biological synthesis*.

It is, however, worthwhile to state here that the **chemically synthesized peptides** are usually obtained in the purest form having almost little contamination; and are termed as **synthetic peptide vaccines.** Unfortunately, they are produced only in small quantities. Large scale (commercial) synthesis of these **'peptide vaccine'** may be accomplished by using the latest technique of **'genetic engineering'.**

Preparation: Various steps involved are as follows

1. An appropriate '*carrier*' is selected that could be either a **plasmid** *e.g.* a tiny circular double stranded molecule of DNA, or a **virus** *e.g.*, a bacteriophage.
2. Gene which essentially encodes that peptide of interest is subsequently inserted into this '*carrier molecule*' strategically.
3. Resultant recombinant molecule thus obtained is subsequently made to enter its host cell that happens to be bacterium, for instance: *E. coli.* Once inside the host, the exact number of copies (replicas) of this recombinant carries enhances as the bacterium undergoes multiplication.
4. For commercial production of the desired peptide, the bacterial host comprising the recombinant plasmid/virus is allowed to grow in *'grow fermentors'* strictly under controlled conditions of temperature, pH, aeration etc., whereby the *'peptide of interest'* is subsequently accomplished by breaking the walls of the host and further detachment of the ensuing peptide from the carrier molecule. This is invariably known as a **subunit vaccine.**

Note: *Though this particular technique gives rise to the desired peptide in appreciable quantum, but it is not absolutely free from* **contaminants** *i.e., the end-product cannot be obtained in its purest form.*

4.7.3.2 Multivaccine System

It represents another latest generation of vaccines and being designated as the **multivaccine system** solely based on r *DNA technology*. In this specific instance, the '*immunogenic peptides*' of more than one pathogen are normally incorporated together into the same carrier. Interestingly, the 'carrier' is not the conventional *plasmid* or virus but instead another 'strain' of another pathogen whose disease causing abilities have been destroyed significantly. In actual practice, however, *two* crippled bacterial strains, namely: (*a*) BCG-the attenuated strain of tuberculosis organism employed as TB vaccine; and (*b*) weakened strains of the pathogen *Salmonella,* that essentially causes *typhoid*, are extensively employed at the experimental stage only. However, these two aforesaid strains may be readily manipulated to carry genes coding for different antigens of more than one pathogen. The weakened form of the *smallpox virus, viccinia* invariably offers similar prospects.

A few highlights of the *'Multivaccine System'* may be enumerated as under:

- Based on the above techniques vaccines are being developed for use against *hepatitis* (a virus disease) that affects millions of people in the tropical countries, against the malarial bug, *Plasmodium*, targeted exclusively to interfere with the different kinds of the parasite.
- *A human-birth control vaccine* (HCG) is being developed at the National Institute of Immunology (NIT), New Delhi, to prevent pregnancy without causing any physiological disturbances. This particular vaccine is not only *safe* but is also *reversible*. It consists of a *small fragment or submits of HCG protein hormone* which essentially plays a vital role in the implantation of the embryo in the womb and also helps in the maintenance of the on-going pregnancy. It has been observed that an antibody titer of more than 50 mg.L^{-1} [nanogram (ng), one millionth of a gramme] raised against the peptide, derived from HCG, eventually ensued contraception. Strategies to synthesize this peptide in a commercial scale by employing r DNA technology are being worked out progressively.

4.7.3.3 Bacterial Vaccines

Bacterial vaccines are usually made either from the whole microorganisms or from the exotoxins, which have been shown responsible for the clinical symptoms of the disease. However they may be categorized under *two* heads, namely:

a. Live attenuated vaccines e.g., Bacillus Calmette Guérin (BCG) vaccine; Typhoid vaccine; and

b. *Inactivated vaccines e.g.,* Anthrax vaccine ; Cholera vaccine; Hemophilus Influenza Type B vaccine; Lyme Disease vaccine; Meningococcal Polysaccharide vaccine; Plague vaccine ; Pneumococcal vaccine ; and the like.

Some of these *'vaccine'* shall be dealt with appropriately under section 7.3. In this chapter.

4.7.3.4 DTP-Vaccine

The *diphtheria and tetanus toxoids and pertussis* vaccine (DTP) are invariably adsorbed in the vast majority of the products in which they occur and this is so noted on the label. The main purpose is to immunize against the three fatal diseases with minimum number of injections, doses similar to diphtheria and pertussis vaccines *(a triple vaccine)*. The adsorbed diphtheria toxiod is also available alone or in combination with absorbed tetanus for use in special circumstances. Importantly, these preparations of *diphtheria toxoid* should not be employed in adults. A dilute (low dose) preparation is also available for adults who need to be immunized or to have their immunity boosted against diphtheria. It may specifically to be given to such personnel's who are entrusted as health workers and laboratory workers, especially those serving in the '*infectious disease units*' ; besides, clinical professionals traveling abroad to discharge their duties in 'hospital' where diphtheria is quite common and prevalent essentially require this immunization. It has also been observed that *certain types of skin infections with diphtheria bacilli* (**non-faucial**) invariably occur in some warm countries.

4.7.3.5 Typhoid-Paratyphoid A and B Vaccine [TAB-Vaccine]

Typhoid fever (enteric fever) is an acute generalized infection caused by *Salmonella typhi*; whereas, *paratyphoid* fever is caused by *Salmonella paratyphi A* and *Salmonella paratyphi B.*

Preparation

1. The vaccine is prepared by the general process and contains the following in each millilitre: Typhoid bacilli (*Salmonella typhi*): 1000 million Paratyphi A bacilli (*S. paratyphi A*) and Paratyphi B bacilli (*S. paratyphi B*): 500 or 750 million.
2. The smooth strains of the *three* organisms known to produce the full complement of O somatic antigens should be used. This specific strain of S. *typhi* must contain the *virus associated antigens* (Vi-antigen).
3. It has been duly established that when the organisms were killed with 75% ethanol and the resulting vaccine preserved with 22.5% ethanol, the potency of the **alcohol treated vaccine** was found to be almost double to that of the **heat-treated vaccine,** there by minimizing the possibility of both local and *constitutional* reaction with the relatively smaller dose. Besides, alcohol treated vaccines did possess definitely and predominantly **longer life** under the optimal storage conditions [*viz.*, storage between 2-4°C without allowing the vaccine to freeze].

Variants of TAB-Vaccine: There are *two* prevailing variants of TAB-vaccine, namely:

a. *Typhoid-paratyphoid A, B and C vaccine (TABC-Vaccine):* It is identical in all respects to the *TAB-vaccine,* but containing an additional 500-750 million *S. paratyphi* C organisms per millilitre, and
b. *Typhoid-paratyphoid A, B and Tetanus Vaccine (TABT):* It is a *'mixed vaccine'* essentially containing per millilitre the following *three* components:
   i. *Salmonella typhi*: 500 or 1000 million;
   ii. *S. paratyphi* A and B: 250 or 500 million;
   iii. Tetanus vaccine: 0.9 ml;

Usually present in a single solution. The TABT-vaccine is normally prepared from the smooth strains having the full complement of O and H somatic antigens, and also in the case of *S. typhi* the Vi antingen.

Notes:

1. In this vaccine the bacterial cells potentiate the activity of the toxoid.
2. Both TAB and TABC vaccines are called the polyvalent vaccines and used as prophylaxis in 'enteric infections'.
3. TAB vaccine sometimes mixed with 'cholera vaccine' when it is termed as 'TAB and cholera vaccine'.

4.7.3.6 Other Bacteria Vaccines

The '*other bacteria vaccines*' invariably include those made from the species of *Staphylococcus* or *Streptococcus* or other such microorganisms that are believed to be intimately associated with the respiratory infections either singly or in combination. Mixed vaccines containing *Staphylococcus; Streptococcus*; *Diplococcus; Klebsiella pneumoniae; N. catarrhalis;* and *H. infuenzae* have been employed profusely and extensively in the past not only for the prevention but also for the treatment of *secondary respiratory infections*.

4.7.3.7 Typhoid and Tetanus Vaccine

It is a mixture of suspension of killed *Salmonella typhi* and *tetanus formol* (*i.e.,* formaldehyde solution) *toxoid;* and contains in 1 ml either 1000 or 2000 million typhoid bacilli *viz., S. typhi.*

Preparation: The various steps that are involved in the preparation of *typhoid and tetanus vaccine* are as follows:

1. The suspension of *'bacteria'* is prepared from one or more strains of *S. typhi* that are smooth and have the full complement of O, H, and Vi-antigens.
2. The bacteria rekilled by treatment with HCHO (formaldehyde solution) or phenol or by heating the above suspension.
3. The **typhoid bacilli** are identified by *agglutination* by means of **specific typhoid antiserum.**
4. The **toxoid portion** is identified by *centrifuging the bacteria* and *adding tetanus antiserum* to the supernatant when flocculation takes place
5. For specific toxicity the vaccine is injected either *sub-cutaneougly* (SC) or intraperitoneally (IP) into guinea pigs. None of the animals shown symptoms of or dies from tetanus within 21 days.
6. **Potency** may be determined by injecting the vaccine into guinea pigs and examining the sera of the guinea pigs for *tetanus antitoxin* after a stated period.

4.7.3.8 Anthrax Vaccine

Anthrax is an acute and highly infectious disease caused by *Bacillus anthracis,* usually attacking cattle, sheep, horses, and goats. Humans invariably contract it from contact with animal hair, hides or waste. Workers who handle raw wools and hides, and manufacture brushes are commonly affected. Immunization with a cell-free vaccine is recommended for persons handling potentially contaminated industrial raw materials.

Anthrax may also be contracted in humans who are directly involved in carpet, tanning and wool industries; and may take the form of *cutaneous* or *pulmonary anthrax.*

Anthrax can be treated with antibiotics, such as: *penicillin, tetracycline* and *erythromycin,* but those with **high-risk segment** a vaccine consisting of killed organisms are prepared for overall protection and immunization.

Preventions:

1. Killed bacterial preparation is usually employed for the protection of those who may be exposed to the risk of '*anthrax*' at work.
2. Stringent, better and improved industrial legislations with regard to handling procedures have more or less reduced these risks to an appreciable extent ; however, personnel's involved at

the particular stage of predisinfection of certain essential processes *e.g.,* production of '*bone meal*' from imported bones need additional and vital protection of immunization.

4.7.3.9 Q-Fever Vaccine

A **Q fever vaccine*** consisting of a purified killed suspension of *Coxiella burnetti.* It is a recognized occupational hazard of abattoir workers, farm workers; besides, cardiothoracic surgical teams who invariably operate on patients with cardiac complications of Q fever endocenditis. In such a situation Q fever vaccine is used.

Preparation: It is usually prepared from **Phase I Hanzerling** strain of *C. burnetti* grown meticulously in the yolk sacs of embryonated eggs. A single 0.5 ml subcutaneous dose of the Q fever vaccine is normally administered for the active immunization in individuals at high risk of Q fever. These may also include veterinarians as well as various laboratory workers that are actively engaged in handling potentially infected tissue.

4.7.3.10 Leprosy Vaccines

These are vaccines meant for chronic mildly contagious infectious disease, leprosy, caused by pathogenic organisms *Micobacterium leprae* as well as other mycobacteria. Several drug substances are duly recommended for its management, control, and treatment, such as: *Sulphones* (*e.g.,* dapsone); and thio-semicarbazones or ethyl mercaptan derivatives. Besides, BCG-vaccine (see section 7.3.3) has also given adequate encouraging results.

Development of Leprosy Vaccines: Several attempts have been made to develop a vaccine against leprosy that are solely based upon the assumption that induction of a cell-mediated immune response to *M. leprae* will ultimately lead to protection against the bacillus. A certain extent of success has been accomplished with BCG vaccine, and with a vaccine prepared from killed *M. leprae* grown in armadillos. In fact, a possible combination of these two vaccines was apprehended to be more promising; and, therefore, and *extensive field studies were* duly conducted to compare the effect of: (*a*) BCG- killed *M. leprae* vaccine; and (*b*) BCG vaccine alone. It has been observed **unfortunately**, based on the preliminary results in *Venezuela*, that there was no substantial proof or evidence to show that the combined vaccine afforded a marked and pronounced protection than did BCG alone (although the study population were not immunologically naive and hence such results may not be applicable to different zones of the globe. Interestingly, vaccines from more easily cultivated non-pathogenic species of mycobacteria, *viz., Mycobacterium* w., are under active investigation in India where the incidence of leprosy is still prevalent.

Importantly, the '**leprosy vaccines**' are broadly used in *two* manners, namely:

(*a*) *As immunoprophylaxis: i.e.,* to prevent infection with *M. leprae.* and

(*b*) *As immunotherapeutic: i.e.,* to prevent disease in infected individuals.

Nevertheless, one may observe beneficial responses from the immunotherapeutic application of *Mycobacterium* w vaccine in combination with standard multidrug therapy. The WHO has suggested that the *immunotheraphy use of vaccines* may ultimately prove to be more clinically relevant than the immunoprophylactic use, and eventually high compliance with immunotherapy seems to be attainable.

4.7.3.11 Whooping cough Vaccine (Syn: Pertussis Vaccine)

Whooping cough (or **Pertussis**) is an acute, infectious disease characterized by a catarrhal stage, followed by a peculiar paroxysmal cough ending in a whooping inspiration. It may be prevented by immunization of infants beginning at 3 months of age. The disease is caused by a small, non-motile Gram-negative bacillus, *Bordetella pertussis.* The incubation period is 7-10 days. Treatment is symptomatic and supportive. Antibiotic are administered to prevent the secondary bacterial pneumonia particularly in infants and children.

Importantly, it is the whole cell preparation of killed *Bordetella pertussis* organisms; and it is the **third component of DTP-triple vaccine.** In fact an early protection against whooping cough has long been recognized by virtue of the fact that the said disease being the most dangerous one specifically to very young children.

It is, however, pertinent to mention here that the '*protective antibody against pertussis*' is not invariably demonstrable in the **adult sera**. As such little protection is passed on from a mother to her unborn baby. Hence, the time for DTP vaccination has been duly brought forward to 3 months with 2 additional doses during the first year of life.

However, the recognized **common adverse reaction to DTP vaccine** includes episodes of *crying, screaming* and fever. Nevertheless, the overall protection afforded by the **whole cell pertussis** is quite significant. Studies on the use of **cellular pertussis vaccine** are being made. They essentially comprise of '*various fractions of pertussis culture*' in semi-purified preparations and are definitely presumed to be **more protective** and **less reactogenic** in comparison to the conventional whole cell preparations being employed for general purposes.

Preparation: The various steps involved are as follows

1. A sterile suspension of *B. pertussis* in the specific culture condition known as '*phase-I*', prepared from the cultures of organisms dried soon after isolation from a patient.
2. It is usually prepared by the general process ; and each ml contains at least 20,000 million organisms.
3. The organism(s) isolated from patient by the well-known '*cup-plate method*', and subsequently harvested when they are in a *smooth* and *virulent form* usually termed as *Phase-I*. It has been duly observed that in *Phase-I* the organisms present are rather smooth but when they are grown on unfavorable media then a S → R variation takes place quite frequently with the *loss of important antigens*. The fully developed rough form corresponds with Phase- IV
4. The organisms are invariably grown in **Bordet-Gengou Blood Agar Medium,** and subsequently incubating from 24-74 hours.
5. After suspending in NaCl injection the resulting suspension is centrifuged and the bacterial mass transferred to NaCl injection containing **0.01 to 0.02% thimerosal** *i.e.,* a bactericide known not to alter the prevalent antigenic properties.
6. The concentrated preparation is stored in the refrigerator for approximately 3 months so as to lower its toxicity; and subsequently diluted with sufficient NaCl injection to opacity greater than twice that of the standard preparation in a final concentration of 0.01% of thimerosal. Thus, the organisms are killed by thimerosal. Importantly, it is not a heat-treated vaccine. Labeling, requirements are as per the '**general stipulated guidelines**'.

4.7.3.12 Diphtheria Vaccine: [Syn: Adsorbed Diphtheria Vaccine (ADV. BP 1993]

It is a preparation of diphtheria formol toxoid absorbed on a mineral carrier.

Absorbed Diphtheria Vaccine (ADV) may be defined as – '*a preparation from the diphtheria formal toxoid containing 1500 lines floculatainis [Lf] per mg of protein nitrogen and a mineral carrier, which is hydrated aluminium hydroxide or aluminium phosphate or calcium phosphate, in a saline solution or another suitable solution isotonic with blood*'.

Preparations: The various steps involved are as follows:

1. The formal toxoid is prepared from the toxin produced by the growth of *Corgynebacterium diphtheriae* and contains not less than 1500 Lf per mg of protein nitrogen.
2. Hydrated $Al(OH)_3$, $AlPO_4$, or $Ca_3(PO_4)_2$ may be employed as mineral carrier, and the resulting ultimate mixture is isotonic with blood.
3. The antigenic characteristic properties are found to be adversely affected by certain antimicrobial preservatives, specifically those of the '*phenolic type*' and, therefore, these must not be added to the vaccine.

4. ADV-BP-1993 contains not less than 30 units per dose; and it must be stored at 2-8°C, not be allowed to freeze, and be protected from light.

Note. Under these stringent storage conditions 'ADV-BP-1993' may be expected to retain its potency for not less than 5 years from the date on which the potency test was begun (or conducted).

Variants of Diphtheria Vaccines: Following are the *three* variants of diphtheria vaccines duly included in *official compendia viz.,* BP-1993; USP-XXIII, and USP-XXIII as detailed under:

a. **Adsorbed Diphtheria Vaccine (ADV) for Adults and Adolescents (BP-1993) [Dip/Vac/Ads (Adults)]**. It contains not less than 2 units per dose (*i.e.,* 2.0 Lf per dose).

b. **Diphtheria Toxoid (DT) (USP XXIII).** It is a sterile solution of the formaldehyde-treated products of growth of *Corynebacterium diphtheriae*. It contains a non-phenolic preservative. It should be stored at 2°C and 8°C and not be allowed to freeze.

c. **Diphtheria Toxoid Adsorbed (DTA) (USP XXIII).** It is a sterile preparation of plain diphtheria toxoid which has been either precipitated or adsorbed phosphate as adjuvants. It must be stored between 2–8°C and not be allowed to freeze.

Special Note on Diphtheria Toxin. It has been amply proved and established that the **'diphtheria toxin'** is **'fairly unstable'**. Furthermore, when it is adequately stored in the refrigerator for duration of six months at a stretch, the toxins undergo maturation and a major portion of it gets converted to the corresponding toxoid. However, an addition of 0.4% formaldehyde solution (or formalin), followed by incubation at 37°C for a period of 30 days may help in the conversion of the entire *toxin* into the corresponding *toxoid.* The resulting product thus obtained is termed as the **'formal toxoid'** which is predominantly and precisely *free from any toxicity* but remarkably *retains the same degree of antigenicity.* Thus, the filtrate essentially containing toxin may be purified at this stage and subsequently toxoided either by HCHO (formalin) or toxoided before any purification is commenced. The actual process of purification involves the careful precipitation by ammonium sulphate $[(NH_4)_2SO_4]$ with a view to accomplish a **'highly immunizing antigen'** that is prominently devoid of any untoward reactions whatsoever. The **'purified toxoid'** obtained in this meticulous manner is now employed in the preparation.

Properties of Diphtheria Toxin and Toxoid. The various properties of the ensuing *diphtheria toxin* and *toxoid* are as enumerated below in Table 9.

Table 4.9 *Properties of Diphtheria Toxin and Toxoid*

S.No	Properties	Diphtheria Toxin	Diphtheria Toxoid
1.	Toxicity	Highly toxic.	No specific toxicity.
2.	Reactions	Causes an inflammed around the site of injection.	Area Causes local reactions specifically in elderly subjects.
3.	Stability	Not quite stable.	Quite stable at room temperature (2 ± 2°C) for at least 2 years.
4.	Antibody formation	Stimulate the formation of antibodies upon injection.	Stimulate the formation of antibodies upon injection.
5.	Combination with antitoxin	Positive	Positive.

Toxoid-Antitoxin Floccules [TAF]. The toxoid-antitoxin floccules (TAF) were duly obtained as a precipitate when the two components were mixed in appropriate neutralizing quantities. The floccular precipitate was separated, washed and suspended in NaCl injection. These floccules were almost free from *broth constituents and non-specific proteins;* and, therefore, were used as an efficient prophylactic having substantially reduced local effects. In actual practice, however, the most preferred, effective and best prophylactic were found to be toxin wherein the *diphtheria formal toxoid* were duly adsorbed on a '*mineral carriers*'.

Alum-Precipitated Toxoid (APT). APT is duly prepared by adding 1% of **potash alum** to formol toxoid. Importantly, the slight alkalinity caused due to the toxoid preparation ultimately eased the precipitation of a basic aluminum salt onto which the toxoid is **adsorbed selectively.** The precipitate is washed to get rid of the non-antigenic constituents of the toxoid and is subsequently resuspended NaCl injection. Thimerosal is added as a bacteriostatic. The aluminium-toxoid complex is only very sparingly soluble at the sight of the injection. Therefore, the toxoid ATP gets adsorbed very poorly and gradually thereby prolonging the immunity stimulus. In fact, the desired immunity is accomplished much earlier (approximately within a span of two months) specifically with this preparation in comparison to other preparations of the prophylactic. In general, the production of the immunity is very effective with APT; but with '*adults*' there is a possibility of '*local reaction*' at the site of injection.

Purified-Toxoid-Aluminium-Phosphate [PTAP]. PTAP is mostly prepared by the addition of *formal-toxoid* to a *suspension of hydrated aluminium phosphate in saline.* However, it was claimed to be '*antigenically*' as potent as APT having both good storage conditionality and good properties but producing appreciably less reaction profiles relative to APT is rather sensitive subjects. Thimerosal (0.1% w/v) was duly used as a bacteriostatic.

4.7.3.13 Varicella-Zoster Vaccines [Syn: Varicella Vaccine, Live BP 1993]

Varicella-Zoster vaccine is a suspension of the OKA *attenuated strain* of *Hypesvirus varicella* grown in the cultures of the human diploid cells. The culture medium may contain appropriate antibiotic at the smallest effective concentration. It is prepared immediately before use by reconstitution from the '*dried vaccine*'; and it may contain a stabilizer. The vaccine contains not less than 2000 plaque forming units per dose. Importantly, the dried vaccine must be stored between 2-8°C and not allowed to freeze. It should also be protected from light.

Varicella vaccine, live BP 1993, may be used for active immunization against varicella *(chickenpox)* in persons considered to be at high risk of either contracting the infection or to be highly susceptible to any complications that it may cause subsequently *e.g.,* patients having *leukemia or those receiving immunosuppressant therapy.*

The usual dose of a live attenuated vaccine (Oka strain) is 2000 plaque-forming units administered by the subcutaneous (SC) injection.

It may be useful as an adjunct to varicella-zoster immunoglobulin (Ig).

4.7.3.14 Viral and Rickettsial Vaccines

The **viral and rickettsial vaccines** are suspensions of *viruses* or *rickettsiae* grown in animals, in embryonated eggs, in appropriate cell cultures or in suitable tissues that contains essentially live or inactivated virus or rickettsiae or there immunogenic components. They are invariably presented as freeze dried preparations. Living viral vaccines are normally prepared from strains of the *'specific virus'* that are of the attenuated virulence. Nevertheless, the viral vaccine may usually vary in opacity according to the type of preparation. They may even be colored in case they happen to contain a pH indicator, for instance: *phenol red.*

The typical example(s) of: *Rickettsial vaccine* is **typhus vaccine;** and *viral vaccines* are **measles vaccine** and **mumps vaccine.**

These vaccines shall now be dealt with adequately in the section that follows:

Typhus Vaccine [Typhus Vaccine BP 1993]:

Typhus vaccine is a sterile suspension of killed epidemic typhus rickettsiae (*Rickettsia prowazekii*) prepared in the yolk sacs of embryonated eggs, rodent lungs, or the peritoneal cavity of gerbils. It must be stored between 2-8°C, not be allowed to freeze, and be protected from light. Under these specific conditions it may be expected to retain its potency for at least 1 year.

Special Remarks. These are as follows:

a. **Killed vaccines** give very *limited protection* but may modify the disease.

b. A vaccine used in the USSR contains **live rickettsaie** (E strains) as well as **soluble antigen** but is awaiting trial under the field conditions.

c. A **live attenuated vaccine** made from the E strain has been adequately tested under the field conditions; and a much lower rate of late reactions than previously described has been reported.

Preparation: The **typhus vaccine** may be prepared by either of the two methods described as under:

Method I. The virulent rickettsiae are carefully injected into the yolk-sacs of embryonated eggs that have been duly incubated for seven days. After heavy yolk-sac injective has been established (normally within a span of 9-13 days), the yolk-sacs are meticulously collected under perfect aseptic conditions as soon as practicable. Dead or moribund eggs are harvested. The yolk-sacs are subjected to appropriate treatment to liberate the maximum number or rickettsiae and the material is suspended in a saline or other suitable solution isotonic with blood to which formaldehyde solution has been added so that the concentration of formaldehyde ranges between 0.2 to 0.5%. The suspension so obtained contains from 10-15% (w/w) of yolk-sac tissue. It may be further purified by treatment subsequently with ether or trichlorofluoroethane; and the aqueous middle-layer of the resultant mixture is collected.

Method II. The '*typhus vaccine*' may also be prepared from the lungs of small rodents in which *rickettsial pneumonias* have been adequately inducted by the inhalation of **massive doses of virulent rickettsiae,** or from the peritoneal cavities of gerbils that have received previously *intraperitoneal (IP) injections of rickettsiae.*

Measles Vaccine, Live: Measles Vaccine, Live is a specific preparation containing a suitable modified strain of live measles virus grown in cultures of chick embryo cells or in other appropriate approved cell cultures.

It is prepared immediately before use by reconstitution from the dried vaccine with the liquid stated clearly on the label itself. However, the vaccine is free from any added antimicrobial preservative.

Preparation. The various steps involved are as follows

1. The virus is grown with the necessary aseptic precautions in the primary cultures of chick embryo cells or other suitable cells.
2. The chick embryos are derived from a healthy flock free from avian leucosis and the cell cultures are shown not to contain extraneous microorganisms.
3. Animal serum may be employed in the medium for the initiation of cell growth; however, the medium for maintaining the cell cultures in the course of virus multiplication contains absolutely no protein at all.
4. Nevertheless, the cell culture medium may contain an appropriate *pH indicator e.g.,* **phenol red,** and also suitable *antibodies* at the smallest possible effective concentrations.
5. The temperature of incubation is accurately controlled during the growth of the virus.
6. The virus suspensions are usually harvested at a time suitable to the strain of virus used and are tested for identity, sterility and freedom from extraneous viruses.
7. Virus harvests which strictly comply with these tests are subsequently pooled and clarified to remove cells. At this stage a suitable stabilizer is added to the clarified vaccine, which is **freeze-dried** to a moisture content shown to be favorable to the ultimate stability of the vaccine.

Mumps Vaccine, Live: Mumps Vaccine, Live is a preparation containing a suitable live modified strain of mumps virus (*Paramyxovirus parotitidis*) grown in chick-embryo cells or other suitable cells. It is invariably prepared immediately before use by reconstitution from the dried vaccine with the solvent stated on the label. The vaccine does not contain any added antimicrobial preservative.

Preparation. The different steps involved are as follows:

1. The virus is grown using the necessary aseptic precautions in the primary cultures of chick embryo cells or other precautions appropriate cells shown not contain extraneous microorganisms.
2. When employing chick-embryo cells, the embryos are derived from a healthy flock usually free from specified pathogens. Animal serum may be used in the medium for initial cell growth but the medium employed for maintaining the cell cultures in the course of virus multiplication must not contain any protein.
3. The concentration of serum carried over into the final vaccine does not exceed one part per million. However, the cell-culture medium may contain a pH indicator *e.g.,* phenol red, and suitable antibodies preferably at the smallest effective concentrations.
4. The viral suspensions are harvested at a time suitable to the strain of virus being employed and tested for identity, sterility, and total freedom from extraneous agents.
5. The virus harvests that comply with these tests are normally pooled and clarified to remove cells.
6. An appropriate stabilizer is added to the clarified vaccine that is **freeze-dried** subsequently to a content shown to be favourable to the final stability of the vaccine.

4.7.3.15 Smallpox Vaccine

Smallpox is an acute highly infectious disease by the *variola virus*. It has been established beyond any reasonable doubt that **'passive immunization'** with adequate doses of *γ-globulin* prepared from plasma of recently vaccinated donors may be expected to protect unvaccinated household contacts of smallpox or persons last vaccinated previously.

Earlier *smallpox vaccine* was known as *vaccine lymph* on account of the original method of preparation. However, the vaccine may be prepared from one of the following modes, namely:

(*a*) From *lesions** produced on the skin of suitable *living mammals,*

(*b*) In the membranes of *chick embryo,* and

(*c*) In cells of suitable tissue by inoculation of *vaccinia virus.*

Method-I (From Free-Living Animals): In this particular instance healthy calves or sheep may be employed for the production of the vaccines. Because **sheep-vaccine** is an active as *calf-vaccine* and since sheep are more easily kept clean and tidy they may also be used abundantly. Besides, the method of preparation is virtually the same in either of the two methods (cases). The various steps followed are as given below:

1. The animal is '*quarantined*' for a fortnight and after a thorough health examination to exclude any possible communicable disease(s), the animals, *flank* and *abdomen* are adequately scrubbed and disinfected, shaved, rescrubbed and redisinfected. Most preferred zone selected is the area from the shoulder to the hip-joint and from the centre-line of the back to the underline of the belly. Subsequently, the shaved and cleaned area is then scarified (*i.e.,* scrubbed lightly with a comb-like device without causing bleeding).

2. The '*seed virus*' of the known potency is now rubbed thoroughly into the scratches with a sterile spatula. The treated sheep is then retired to a special place for an incubation period ranging between 4 to 5 days whereupon vesicles containing the virus developed all along the lines of the **'scarification zone'.** Throughout the span of incubation all necessary precautions must be taken to maintain and keep the inoculated areas aseptically clean.

3. The animal is sacrified, *exsanguinated* (*i.e.,* to blood to the point at which life can no longer be sustained) and washed. The contents of the vesicles *i.e.,* the lymph, are removed by *curretage* (*i.e.,* by scrapping with a special '*valkmanna's* spoon that has a very sharp edge to the bowl). The pulp thus obtained is transferred from the spoon to a '*sterilized jar*', which is then maintained at

–10°C until ready for grinding in a '*tissue grinder*'. In fact, each batch of pulp is usually ground individually (**homogenized**) in a specially designed grinding machine. It is absolutely necessary to carry out a postmortem examination judiciously made on the sacrificed animal's carcass to ensure the absence of infectious diseases.

4. As it is not practically feasible to entirely prevent the possible contamination with extraneous microorganisms, the lymph should be treated adequately to kill pathogens completely and also to reduce the number of residual bacteria to very low ebb. Previously it was normally carried out by grinding with an equal volume of glycerin and storing for a long time at –10°C. Importantly, a relatively more convenient, efficient and feasible method adopted nowadays is as stated under:– 'The *lymph is extracted with a protein solvent like trichlorofluoroethane. Presence of protein lowers the efficiency of the bactericidal agent. Phenol is added to produce a concentration of 0.4% and the material is incubated at 22°C for duration of 48 hours or until the bacterial count is is low enough*'.

The '**viruses**' especially are unharmed by this particular treatment because they are much more resistant than bacteria to phenol. *Glycerol* and *peptone* are eventually incorporated to afford concentrations of 40% and 1% respectively. In fact, glycerin assists the bactericidal action of phenol during the subsequent storage at –10°C. Besides, glycerin renders the product a viscosity very much similar to the earlier preparations that were treated previously with glycerin alone; – a viscous preparation being always easier to use for vaccination.

5. **Peptone** specifically helps to preserve the viability of the viruses, particularly if the product is meant to be '**freeze dried**'. Sometimes, incorporation of either **Brilliant Green** or another appropriate colouring substance is added to mark the area of application of the vaccine. Tests are usually carried out to ascertain the presence of the number of living extraneous microorganisms not exceeding more than 500 ml since the product from the free living animals could not attain the requisite target because of its virtually unavoidable contamination with the living organisms.

Method-II (From Chick-Embryo): This **smallpox vaccine** may also be prepared from virus grown on the *chorioallantois membrane** of fertile hens eggs and this methodology is being adopted in certain parts of USA. In actual practice, well-defined '*tissue-culture methods*' making use of **calf-embryo skin** or **chick-embryo cells** have also been developed and products appear *antigenically equivalent* to vaccines from other sources. However, the major advantages of these methods are that a sterile preparation can be obtained; and the resulting products should comply with the '*official tests for sterility*'.

Note: Freeze-dried Smallpox Vaccine. *The* ***'liquid preparation'*** *retains its potency for 12 months at –10°C, but definitely possesses much lower stability at higher temperature, specifically if it is not adequately protected from light.* ***Example:*** *The exact storage life at 10–20°C and 2–10°C stands at 1 and 2 weeks respectively. Importantly, the freeze-dried product is much more stable and keeps definitely below 10°C, for a year at 22°C, and for a month at 37°C. Therefore, it is particularly advantageous in tropics and in situations where it is absolutely necessary to maintain 'emergency stocks'. And after reconstitution, it is found to retain its potency for a week if stored below 10°C. The freeze-dried product is available in multiple dose containers together with appropriate volumes of reconstituting fluid. There are ample information's available with respect to purity, potency, storage, labeling and containers.*

Method-III (From Vaccinia Virus). In this particular instance the lymph is carefully incubated at 22°C for 48 hours during which period the bacterial count of contaminants gets reduced significantly. The resulting product is then tested bacteriologically as required essentially by the **Therapeutic Substances Act and Regulations.** Two portions of *glycerin* are now added and the product tested for conformity to the laid down *official standards.*

The lymph is invariably dispensed either in *capillary tubes* for single dosage with the aid of a vacuum device or *in ampoules* for multi-dosage forms. The thermally sealed containers are then stored at a temperature ranging between –10 to –15°C until used actually.

Interestingly, one fully-grown healthy sheep may yield approximately *500 ml of liquid smallpox vaccine* which is equivalent to *350,000 doses*. It is, however, pertinent to state here that the vaccine thus obtained normally comprises of a high concentration of **vaccinia virus particles that** may be regarded broadly to be almost **equivalent to an attenuated smallpox strain,** and obviously in a limited sense it is still, therefore, infectious and pathogenic in character.

Note. *In actual practice, the* ***'freeze-dried material'*** *is dispensed in the form of multiple dose ampoules along with an appropriate volume of reconstituting fluid. The 'Label' carries complete information with regard to purity, potency, storage conditions, expiry date etc.*

Advantages of Smallpox Vaccine Prepared from Chick-Embryo:

The cardinal advantages of smallpox vaccine prepared from chick-embryo *vis-à-vis* from lesions produced on the skin of live animals, such as: *calves* or *sheep's* are as enumerated under:

1. The **'chick-embryo'** is virtually *free from latent viruses*, whereas live animals (*e.g.*, mammals) may serve as hosts for a plethora of pathogenic viruses. Therefore, evidently a virus culture is prominently less prone to be contaminated by a majority of '*unwanted viruses*' when grown on '*chick-embryo*'. Besides, it is definitely much convenient and easier to maintain and sustain the product free from the contaminating microorganisms.

Note:

a. Since several years it was believed that 'chick-embryo' was not a natural carrier of viruses; however, now it is more or less well established that avion leucosis may be present.

b. The virus causes tumours in birds and although there is no substantial/concrete evidence of transmission to humans; besides, the eggs from avion leucosis free flocks are being employed for measles vaccine.

2. The viruses grown on the *chorioallantois membrane* of the chick-embryo produces lesions that differ widely in size and structure from one virus to another one. Consequently, contamination by such an '*unwanted virus*' is detected fairly easily.

3. *Multiplication of a viral culture* in an animal tissue is sometimes rather difficult to accomplish on account of immunity of the prevailing tissue; and perhaps this could affect the yield significantly. Importantly, the chick-embryo is unable to develop such antibodies against a virus at the age of its usage. The viruses either grown in yolk-sac or *embryo-sac* are usually separated by the **'grinding process' (homogenization)** ; as a result, certain traces of egg protein creep into the vaccine and thus may give rise to **'untoward reactions'** in the recipient very much akin to those produced by the injection of *'serum proteins'*. Therefore, when either of these two regions (*viz.*, yolk-sac and embryo-sac) is employed, the egg must not be more than 10-11 days old; and if the harvesting is performed even before its due time its proteins are not sufficiently developed to produce **hypersensitivity reactions.**

4. *Undesired anaphylactic reactions* in humans just following administrations of a second dose of a viral vaccine grown on *chick-embryo* are virtually unknown as on date.

5. *Viral vaccines grown on the skin of living mammals* (*e.g.*, calves, sheep's) may be heavily contaminated with bacteria. However, with the advent of suitable aseptic technique the viral vaccines produced in the *chick-embryo* are absolutely **free from bacterial contamination.** It has been duly observed that the *allantoic and amniotic cavities* strategically located in the chick-embryo are capable of destroying **light bacterial contamination** due to their inherent anti-bacterial nature, but they fail to cope up with **heavy bacterial infection.** The yolk-sac provides a highly nutrient medium for bacteria. As such the material infected right into the yolk-sac should be free from bacterial contaminants. Therefore, it is quite necessary to maintain stringent aseptic technique throughout the operational procedures so as to prevent bacterial contamination squarely.

6. Interestingly, there are certain viruses which cannot be grown on *chick-embryo e.g., poliomyelitis virus.* In such cases, other methods should be employed for their cultivation.

7. *Virulence of a plethora of viruses* is reduced appreciably by repeated passage through the *chick-embryo* from egg to egg. When a **living vaccine is required,** steps must be adopted accordingly to maintain the *virulence of the virus.* The virus may become adapted to embryo tissue and become less virulent for its natural host. To ensure an adequate supply of virus having satisfactory virulence, the *vaccinia strains* is grown in quantity in one batch of eggs and then freeze-dried or stored at a low temperature so that the same virus can be employed for many batches of vaccine. The eggs for vaccine production must be examined in front of a bright light so as to confirm that the embryos are still very much alive. The spontaneous movement or well-defined blood vessels invariably indicate the presence of a **living-embryo**.

8. *Chick-embryo* is found to be more satisfactory in the growth of certain specific viruses, such as: **attenuated measles virus,** and **cowpox virus.**

4.7.3.16 Vaccines for Special Protection (For People at Special Risk)

There are several vaccines that find their immense usage in causing immunization to humans who are exposed to special risk(s), such as: Hepatitis B ; Rabies ; Yellow Fever ; Anthrax ; Plague ; Japanese B encephalitis ; Bird's Flu ; Hongkong Flu ; Q-Fever, Typhoid ; Smallpox etc., which shall be discussed appropriately in this section.

4.7.3.17 Rabies Vaccines (Rabies Vaccine BP-1993)

Rabies Vaccine is a suspension of an appropriate strain of *fixed rabies virus* grown in *human diploid cells* (HDCV) and inactivated by β-propionilactone. HDVC may also be used for active immunization of those considered at risk (pre-exposure vaccine). In actual recommended practice two doses are administered at an interval of one month, and then followed by a **'booster dose'** one year later. Nevertheless, it is also used for the post-exposure treatment in combination with **human rabies immunoglobulin (HRIG)**. It has been duly observed that *neuroparalytic* and *hypersensitivity* reactions are intimately associated with the vaccines that are derived exclusively from either animal nerve tissues or duck-embryos; in reality, such vaccines are still used in the developing world. Most developed countries use such vaccines prepared in cell cultures, frequently HDCV. Interestingly, the usual hypersensitivity reactions are significantly less frequent with these (HDCV) preparations.

Rabies being an acute infection of mammals caused by rabies virus. However, the clinical rabies (*viz.,* **hydrophobia**) is proved to be fatal in man. Infection normally has a 'long incubation period' after introduction of virus through the bite of a *rabid-animal e.g.,* dog, jackal etc. If a high degree of immunity can be stimulated while the virus is slowly traversing centrally *via* the peripheral nerves its ultimate penetration and subsequent establishment in the brain may be prevented adequately.

Modern immunotherapy procedures invariably combine both **passive** and **active immunization** in order to accomplish a rather effective *high concentration* as well as *a high level of antibody as rapidly as possible in vivo.*

a. Passive Immunization

Pre-exposure immunization is also recommended for such subjects who frequently handle or administer modified live rabies virus vaccines intended for animals because of the unavoidable possibility of exposure via either needle pricks or sprays, animal handlers, laboratory workers, and even veterinarians.

b. Active Immunization

Post-exposure immunization may be inducted due to the rabies vaccination whereby antibody production commences within a span of 7-10 days and the duration of protective effect lasts for 2 years or even beyond that. It is indicated for post exposure immunization against rabies infection.

Preparation. It may be prepared from different methods as stated below:

Method-I (Seed-Lot System): The various steps involved are:

1. The virus used in the final vaccine represents not more than five cultures from the seed lot employed for the actual production of the vaccine on which were carried out the laboratory and clinical tests that ascertained the strain to be suitable.

2. Animal serum may be used in the medium for the initial cell growth; however, the medium employed for maintaing the cell cultures during virus multiplication contains no protein.
3. The concentration of serum carried over into the vaccine does not exceed one part per million.
4. The cell culture medium may contain a suitable pH, indicator, such as phenol red, and '*appropriate antibiotics*' usually present at the **smallest effective concentrations.**
5. The virus suspension is invariably harvested on one or more occasions during incubation. In actual practice, multiple harvests from a single cell lot may be pooled and regarded as a *single virus suspension.*
6. The resulting suspension is meticulously and carefully tested for *identity*, *bacterial sterility* and above all complete freedom from *extraneous viruses.* In case, suspension legitimately complies with these *three extremely vital tests*, it is inactivated subsequently; and hence, may be finally purified and concentrated.
7. It is absolutely necessary to carry out the '*amplification test*' for the **residual infectious rabies virus** in cell cultures derived from the same species as those employed in the production of the vaccine to confirm effective inactivation of the rabies virus. The quantum of virus used in the above test is equivalent to not less than 25 human-doses of the vaccine.
8. *Test for Live Virus:* Samples of the cell-culture fluids are inoculated into mice. No live virus is detected.
9. The resulting thoroughly tests **'Rabies Vaccine'** are distributed aseptically into sterile containers and freeze-dried. The containers (*e.g.,* ampoules) are sealed hermetically. The inherent residual moisture content is sufficiently low to ensure the stability of the vaccine.
10. **Potency Test:** The maintenance of potency is duly verified in an **'accelerated degradation test'** wherein the '*vaccine*' is stored at 37°C for 4 weeks at a stretch.

Method-II (From Chick and Duck Embryos): Rabies vaccine should be prepared from such tissues that are devoid of essential the *encephalitogenic* material specifically. Therefore, for this particular reason the **rabies virus strains** have been duly adopted to grow either in '*chick*' or in '*duck*' embryos. Furthermore, the viruses grown in duck-embryo are usually inactivated by β-propionilactone which process is found to be effective reasonably.

Method-III (From Brains of suckling mice, rats, rabbits and sheep): The Rabies vaccines prepared from the brains of sucking mice, rats, rabbits and sheep must conform to the requisite potencies by standard usual tests satisfactorily. The 'Pharmacopoeal Method' advocates the rabbits and sheep may be infected *intracerebrally* with the '**fixed rabies virus**'. Once they distinctly exhibit typical symptoms after a span of 24 hours and become paralyzed completely, they are killed and their brains are duly harvested and homogenized in NaCl injection. The resulting viruses are inactivated adequately. Phenol is the 'chemical of choice' and hence often preferred; however, treatment with other chemical substances, such as: formaldehyde solution (formalin), β-propionilactone or UV-light has also been equally successful. The **'preparation'** is diluted to contain an appropriate amount of the brain material.

Salient Features of Rabies Vaccines Production

Following are some of the salient features with regard to the production of *Rabies Vaccines*:

1. Human subjects, immunized with rabies vaccine prepared from brains, invariably developed higher concentrations of the **'neutralizing antibody'** in comparison to the '*controls*' immunized with the conventional nerve-tissue vaccines.
2. Rabies vaccine containing nerve-tissue may give rise to serious allergic response in the brain leading to nerve cell deterioration and ultimately rendering complete paralysis.
3. The reactions described in (1) and (2) above are found to be rare when the vaccines are prepared either in **'fertile hen'** or **'duck-eggs'**. The latter are normally preferred because the yields are definitely better.

4. β-Propionilactone is mostly used as a normal inactivated agent.
5. In actual practice, the usage of **live-avianized vaccine having attenuated virulence** are seldomly done because of the difficulties encountered in producing batches of *uniform and adequate potency.*
6. Active immunization against **'rabies'** remains absolutely and mainly unsatisfactory unless and until extremely potent and highly safe inactivated vaccines are available abundantly.
7. Proper application of **'human diploid-cells'** and other types of cell cultures of substrates for the growth of very high concentrations of '*rabies virus*' is showing adequate cognizance and great promise.
8. A plethora of **'human diploid-cell rabies vaccines'** are mostly produced from **Wilstar's Pitman-Moore** or **CL-77 strain** of *rabies virus* grown in **MRC-5 human diploid cell culture.** The resulting 'vaccine virus' is duly concentrated and then inactivated by β-propionilactone.
9. **Rabies vaccine** adsorbed is prepared from the **CVS Kissling / MDPH strain of rabies** virus grown in a **diploid cell line** actually derived from **fetal rhesus monkey lung cells.**
10. The vaccine virus is duly inactivated and later on concentrated by adsorption to aluminium phsophate [AlPO4].
11. USP officially recognizes the following two variants of rabies vaccine, namely:
    a. cell-culture vaccines for **intradermal usage** (*e.g.,* into the intracutaneous); and
    b. cell-culture vaccines for **intramuscular injection** (*e.g.,* into the **deltoid viz., triangular muscle**).
12. As a precautionary measure the **'Rabies Vaccines'** must be administered immediately following reconstitution or the reconstituted vaccine must be discarded.

4.7.3.18 Influenza Vaccine: [Syn: Flu Fever Vaccine]

Influenza is an acute, contagious respiratory infection characterized by the sudden onset of fever, chills, headache, myalagia, and sometimes prostration. Coryza, cough and sore throat are common. The incubation period ranges between 1 to 3 days. It is usually a self-limited disease that invariably lasts from 2 to 7 days. The preferential and differential diagnosis includes **typhoid fever, cerebrospinal meningitis,** and, rarely **pulmonary tuberculosis.**

In actual practice, both killed and live attempted vaccines are used but assessment of their value is complicated by the appearance of antigenic variants to different virus strains. Interestingly, within a span of 24 years *i.e.,* between 1933 and 1957, antigenic variations of the influenza strain were legitimately recognized when both epidemics and *pandemics* surfaced predominantly in a few countries across the globe. Consequently, classifical strains like A1 [*A Primer*], A2 [*Asian Virus*] strains were isolate and identified duly.

Historical Background. In the year 1940, the causative virus for influenza in New York was observed to be a **Type B virus** and the antigenic variants for these strains were also recognized soon after.

Later on two cases of Type B virus infection have been duly isolated and recognized. Subsequently, another Type C strain was also isolated. These critical observations and findings, in fact afforded the preparation of a *'satisfactory prophylactic for influenza'* that is rendered complicated by the capacity of the virus for the prevailing range of variation. It is quite well-known and established that most influenza outbreaks are duly produced by one or two different types of viruses.

Type A Virus: Mainly responsible for spreading rapidly major epidemics that are sometimes worldwide. It specifically shows considerable lack of stability in antigenic characteristics.

Type B Virus: Particularly gives rise to small localized outbreaks; and, therefore, occasionally gives rise to a wide-spread epidemic outbreaks.

It is, however, pertinent to mention here that there exists almost **little cross-immunity** amongst any of the *five* recognized classes or types of viruses *viz.,* Type A, A1, A2, B and C. Perhaps, it is, feasible as well practicable to afford **'protection against influenza'** by providing a **'polyvalent vaccine'** that will certainly give blanket coverage. Besides, one may acquire sufficient relevant and valuable information(s) with regard to the antigenic composition of such a strain that might cause the next outbreak, in time to prepare a specific vaccine for it. However, the formal preparation may prove to be beneficial only if the prevailing antigenic components of the virus are confined to a certain limit. Interestingly, in USA preparations of this kind containing one or more strains of each of A, A1 and A2 and B have been employed for many years.

Attenuated Nasal Spray Vaccine. The development of a novel attenuated vaccine meant to be administered via nasal spray has claimed to be more effective because it specifically cause stimulation in the production of antibodies at a place where different flu viruses gain entry quite easily.

Advantages: The various advantages of this nasal vaccine are:

i. It may be easily administered to children who show aversion to injection which is the usual method recommended for the **'killed vaccine'**.

ii. Best suited for children who contract flu at least 2-10 folds more than elderly people; besides, they invariably get the infection at least 2-3 times before they attain the age of 5 years.

iii. The flue contracting children are not so dangerous (whereas the elderly people may sometimes prove to be quite dangerous).

iv. Vaccines need to be administered twice a year to children so as to prevent and arrest the spread of the said disease *i.e.,* flu.

Preparation. In a broader perspective the production of an effective **'Influenza Vaccine'** prophylactic essential requires the inclusion of strains of both Types A and B normally isolated particularly *'during the most recent epidemic'* unless a new variant appears.

The various steps involved are as follows:

1. The **'influenza vaccine'** is prepared in the embryonated hens eggs.
2. The virus is inoculated in the *allantoic cavity* for 2-3 days, and subsequently the eggs are adequately chilled between 2-8°C in a refrigerator for a day. This kills the embryo and thus prevents any possible hemorrhage creeping into the allantoic fluid in the course of harvesting.
3. The outer-shell is carefully removed from over the air sac, and the underlying membranes are cut away meticulously whereby the allantoic fluid is finally drawn off into a flask.
4. Pools of the fluid from relatively smaller batches of eggs are tested individually for their sterility.
5. All the sterile batches are pooled and the virus is purified by centrifugation, initially at a *low speed* to separate a flocculent precipitate of proteins followed by a *very high* speed to throw out the **viruses** due to the centrifugal forces. These viruses are removed subsequently to an appropriate vehicle; and the suspension is subjected to concentration preferably under sterile and reduced pressure.
6. The resulting concentrated suspension is treated with requisite amount of 0.01% formaldehyde between 0–4°C for 2 to 3 days so as to inactivate the *virus* that is ultimately suspended in a neutral buffered saline solution containing *thimerosal* or other appropriate bactericide.
7. **Poly-valent vaccines** are usually prepared by mixing together *purified* and *inactivated suspensions* of each strain. The components of prior to dilution and standardized by **haemagglutination titrations** both virus types are blending into a vaccine.
8. The *'Official Vaccine'* is an aqueous suspension; whereas, the *'commercial products'* essentially contain a material carrier or oil adjuvant that are observed to afford predominantly **higher antibody responses.**
9. It has been further demonstrated and established that by rendering the emulsification of the *'aqueous suspension'* with mineral oil employing a *W/O emulsifier* may help a lot in the

potentiation of the antigenic effect of the vaccine. The mineral oil perhaps stimulates the creation of a granuloma (*i.e.,* a small harmless growth of cells) at the very site of injection. This specific phenomenon not only protects the *virus* but also *delays its destruction* appreciably. The overall *'not result'* appears as an improved level and also the prevailing duration of immunity.

Living Attenuated Influenza Virus. In Russia, it has been a practice to spray the living attenuated influenza virus right into the nose. The vaccine is an egg or cell culture preparation of a strain passaged in *eggs* or *cell cultures* and adequately selected because of its ability to **multiply in the nose** and appear subsequently in the **nasal secretions.**

Salient Features: The various salient features are as follows:

i. Unlike the *killed vaccine* this *specific live prophylactic vaccine* is said to be effective even when employed during an **influenza epidemic.**

ii. Clinical reactions are *bare minimal in adults* but may be *quite acute and severe in children.*

iii. Isolated haemagglutinin of the virus is immunogenic and does not produce any *febrile* and *toxic reactions soon* after vaccination with the whole live attenuated influenza virus.

iv. Active immunity to influenza undergoes development rather rapidly between 10-14 days.

v. One injection is administered only, as there is little improvement noticeable in the **'antibody response'** from a second one. The actual attainable protection however is prominently short-lived and lasts for almost six months duration only.

4.7.3.19 Inactivated Influenza Vaccine

The *official compendia include two* variants of inactivated influenza vaccine, namely:

(*a*) Inactivated Influenza Vaccine (Split Virion), and

(*b*) Inactivated Influenza Vaccine (Surface Antigen)

First of all the simple Inactivated Influenza Vaccine shall be discussed as under:

Inactivated Influenza Vaccine is a sterile aqueous suspension of *a suitable strain or strains of influenza virus,* Types A and B either individually or mixed*, duly inactivated so that they are noninfective but predominantly retain their antigenic characteristic features. Importantly, the vaccine strains employed must possess those **haemagglutinin** and **neuraminidase antigens** likely to render protection against the prevalent influenza viruses. The vaccine contains an approved quantity of haemagglutinin.

Preparation: The different steps involved are as stated below:

1. The virus of each strain is grown adequately in the allantoic cavity of 10-13 day-old embryonated chicken eggs derived from a healthy flock. The allantoic fluid is harvested after incubation for 2-3 days at a temperature appropriate for the optimal growth of the strain of virus employed.
2. The resulting viral suspensions of each type are pooled individually and inactivated duly by a process shown to *inactivate* not only the *influenza virus without destroying its immunogenicity,* but also any *contaminating virus.*
3. The virus thus obtained is purified by centrifugation or other suitable means and finally suspended in a buffered solution that may contain a suitable antimicrobial preservative.
4. The vaccine may also be issued as an adsorbed vaccine. The adsorbed vaccine is prepared as described above with the addition of an appropriate adjuvant.

The following *three* tests, as given in BP-1993, need to be carried out before adsorption, namely:

i. Identification Test 'A',

ii. Ovalbumin Test (for Viral inactivation), and

iii. Haemagglutinin content.

4.7.3.19.1 Inactivated Influenza Vaccine (Split-Virion)

The **Inactivated Influenza Vaccine (Split Virion)** is a sterile aqueous suspension of a suitable strain or strains of influenza virus, Types A and B either individually or mixed, *wherein the integrity of the virus particles has been disrupted.* The vaccine strains employed should possess essentially those haemagglutinin and neuramindase antigens that are likely to provide adequate protection against the currently prevalent influenza viruses. The vaccine contains an approved quantity of haemaglutinin.

Preparation. The various steps that one essentially involved are as stated under:

1. The virus of each strain is grown in the allantoic cavity of 10-13 day old embryonated chicken eggs derived from a healthy flock. The allantoic fluid of live eggs is harvested after due incubation for 2-3 days at a temperature found to be suitable for optimal growth of the strain of virus used.
2. The viral suspensions of each type are pooled individually and inactivated subsequently by a process shown to inactivate not only influenza virus, without destroying its immunogenicity, but also any contaminating virus.
3. The resulting virus is purified by centrifugation or other appropriate means and the **virus particles are disrupted by suitable surface-active agents.**
4. The *disrupted particles* are adequately suspended in a buffered solution that may contain an appropriate antimicrobial preservative.
5. The vaccine may also be employed as an '*adsorbed vaccine*'. The '*adsorbed vaccine*' is prepared as described above with the addition of a suitable adjuvant.
6. The following *three* tests, as given in BP-1993, require to be performed before adsorption, namely:
   i. Identification Test-A,
   ii. Ovalbumin Test (for Viral inactivation), and
   iii. Haemagglutinin content.

4.7.3.19.2 Inactivated Influenza Vaccine (Surface Antigen)

The **Inactive Influenza Vaccine (Surface Antigen)** is a sterile aqueous suspension of the immunologically active haemagglutinin and neuroaminidase surface antigens of a suitable strain or strains of influenza virus. The virus strain or strains used, which may be Types A or B either individually or mixed, should essentially possess antigens likely to provide protection against influenza viruses currently prevalent or likely to be prevalent and should have been inactivated that they are non-infective but retain their immunogenic properties.

Preparation. The vaccine may be prepared by the following method:

1. The virus of each strain is grown in the allantoic cavity of 10-13 day-old embryonated eggs derived from a healthy flock. The allantoic fluid of live eggs is harvested after incubation for 2-3 days at temperatures suitable for optimal growth of the particular strain.
2. The viral suspensions of each strain are pooled individually and treated by a process shown to inactivate not only the influenza virus while maintaining its antigenicity but also any contaminating virus.
3. The resulting virus is purified by centrifugation or other suitable means, the virus particles are disrupted by treatment with **suitable agents** and the surface antigens are duly separated from other virus components by approved procedures and suspended in a buffered solution containing a suitable preservative.
4. The vaccine contains an approved quantity of haemagglutinin antigen which is measured by an approved technique, such as: **immunodiffusion** using antiserum to purified haemagglutinin and comparing the vaccine with a **homotypic antigen reference preparation.**

5. The *'vaccine'* may also be issued as an *'adsorbed vaccine'*, which is prepared as described above with the addition of a suitable adjuvant or mineral carrier. Nevertheless, the test for antigen content may be performed before the addition of the adjuvant or mineral carrier.

4.7.3.20 Polio Vaccine

Polio (*or acute anterior poliomyelitis*) – is an acute infections inflammation of the anterior horns of the gray matter of the spinal cord. In this acute systemic infections disease, paralysis may or may not occur. In the majority of patients, the disease is mild, being limited to respiratory and gastrointestinal symptoms, such constituting the minor illness or the abortive type, which lasts only a few days. In the major illness, muscle paralysis or weakness takes place with loss of superficial and deep reflexes. In such instances characteristic lesions are found in the gray matter of the spinal cord, medulla, motor area of the cerebral cortex and the cerebellum.

It has been observed that probably 90% of infections caused no symptoms and only 1% lead to actual paralysis.

Explanation. The causation of the disease is due to the fact that the virus first invades the cell of the oropharyngeal and the intestinal mucosal; and in most individual remains here until it gets eliminated by cell replacement completely. In a rather small percentage of infections, however it finds its way *via* the lymphatic route and the blood cell to the CNS where it produces the ensuing **'degenerative changes'** which ultimately is responsible for causing paralysis.

The *first* successful prophylactic was due to the inactivated vaccine which is administered parenterally and thereby stimulates the production of antibodies in the blood. As the virus pass through the blood stream on its way from the alimentary canal to the CNS; it gets neutralized subsequently thereby providing the protection. However, it fails to prevent establishment of the infective virus in the mucosa. Interestingly, the individual actively immunized with this type of vaccine might act as a **'carrier for virulent virus'** and hence infect others.

The *second* successful type of vaccine contains *'attenuated organisms'* which on being administered to an individual orally (*e.g.*, on a *sugar lump*) invariably invade by the normal route ; and in the mucosa of the alimentary canal to check and prevent the establishment of the infective virus by stimulating the production of antibodies locally and possibly through the interposal production. In this case also the antibodies develop in the blood stream.

In short, both these types of vaccines are duly represented in the **Indian Pharmacopoeia** (IP); however, in actual practice the **'Live Oral Vaccine'** is largely preferred.

Variants of Polio Vaccine: There are in all *five* recognized variants of the **'polio vaccine'**, namely:

(*a*) Oral Polio Vaccine (OPV),

(*b*) Salk Type Polio Vaccine,

(*c*) Sabin Type Polio Vaccine,

(*d*) Inactivated Poliomylitis Vaccine [or Inactivated Polio Vaccine BP-1993], and

(*e*) Poliomyelitis Vaccine Live (Oral) [or Polio Vaccine Live (Oral) BP-1993].

These different variants of **'Polio Vaccine'** shall now be treated individually in the section that follows:

4.7.3.20.1 Oral Polio Vaccine (OPV)

It was initially developed by Sabin, after the American Researcher, and is a mixture of *'live attenuated strains'* of the *three polio viruses viz.*, Type 1, 2, and 3.

- An oral dose of the mixture is given to the children at 3 months age; 4 ½ to 5 months; and finally at 8 ½ -11 months of age. These doses are usually administered at the same time as and when the initial course of injections of triple DTP vaccination is given to a child.
- A booster dose is administered orally at 4 to 5 and again at 15-18 years of age.
- The viruses invariably grow in the *'lymphoid tissue'* associated with the gut epithelium and thus generate local and humoral immunity.

- As fecal excretion of the vaccine strains may actually persist for some weeks, the nearest family members of the children given OPV must be advised with respect to the '*hygienic handling and proper disposal of napkins / diapers etc.,*' any non-immune immediate family members should preferably be immunized simultaneously.
- *Vaccine associated poliomyelitis* takes place very rarely (less than one in a million); however, the benefits of the vaccine outweighs this enormously.
- OPV must not be administered to **hypogammaglobulinaemic** children specifically.
- Absorption of *antigen* or *preformed antibodies via* the alimentary canal has not been of much interest in the therapeutic armamentarium until recently because of the major reason that the 'prevailing digestive process' invariably gives rise to severe wastage.

4.7.3.20.2 Salk Type Polio Vaccine

The **Salk Type Polio Vaccine** (or **Salk filled vaccine**) is a formaldehyde inactivated mixture of the *three* **types of polio virus** and it is also found to be very effective. It was subsequently replaced more or less by the *'Sabin type polio vaccine'* (see section 7.3.20.3) in a good number of countries based on the following predominant plus points, namely:

- If refrigeration is assured adequately, OPV may be more conveniently delivered to communities; and that too at a reasonably, economically viable and cheaper cost.
- Local gut immunity associated with OPV coupled with the possibility of the vaccines' spread and separation of wild virus in the community is an additional advantage.

The **Salk type polio vaccine** is, in fact, an inactivated vaccine baptized after the American 'virologist' who first developed it.

Preparation. The various stages involved in its preparation are as follows:

1. The *three* types of polio vaccines (*e.g.,* Type 1, 2 and 3) are grown individually in either suspended or fixed cell cultures of monkey kidney tissue; and for these *Rhesus monkeys* are employed generally.
2. Rhesus monkeys are usually quarantined on arrival and checked meticulously for TB and other '**communicable diseases**' both before and after death.
3. The '*monkey kidney cell*' must not have been propagated in series and are invariably obtained from a continuous line of cell. This exclusion, however, is entirely based on the possible fear that because it has been easier to '**produce continuous lines of malignant cell'** in comparison to the '**normal cell'** ; all this vividly depict the ability to maintain a line of the latter which is indicative of a transformation towards malignancy in the cells.
4. For both types of vaccines, the inclusion of *serum* is strictly forbidden in the culture media employed for maintaining cell growth in the course of *'virus propagation'*; however, it may be included in media used to initiate the process of growth of tissue cells. It is so done in order to prevent the *'serum reactions'* when such preparations are subsequently administered. In fact, it is virtually more important in the inactivated vaccine which is usually given parenterally; and for this purpose there is a prescribed limit of 1 ppm of serum in the final product.
5. Healthy Rhesus monkeys are duly anaesthetized and their kidneys are removed and decapsulated. The 'cordical tissue' is coarsely disintegrated and suspended in No: 199 substrated.
6. The chopped tissue is then treated with several lots of dilute, warm trypsin solution each at 0.5% concentration at pH 7.6 for a span of 20 minutes. This treatment, in fact, partially hydrolyses the tissue frame-work; and further helps in separating the cells into a rather free suspension without affecting their **viability** and **efficacy.**
7. The cells are subsequently centrifuged, washed and resuspended in a complex medium to a density of 3 × 105 mL^{-1}. The medium could be either an admixture of *No: 199 substrate plus calf-serum* or an admixture of *lactoalbumin hydrolysate plus serum.*

8. The resulting suspension is then inoculated into relatively larger vessels and incubated for a duration of 5 days to allow the cells to become adequately established as a '*monolayer*' on the **glass surface.**
9. When optimal growth has taken place, the liquor is poured off and the cells are washed with BSS-medium. After adding fresh medium, a small inoculation with one specific strain on the **'virulent stock'** virus is made.
10. Separate batches for each of the *three types* are made and all are incubated for approximately three days or until such a time the full effect of the virus degeneration has actually taken place. By this time the medium invariably contains a high concentration of the *'free virus particles'*.
11. Debris is centrifuged off and the supernatant layer is cooled adequately. In case, these are not required immediately, the deep frozen strains may still be kept separately which can now be batches to larger volume(s) as and when required.
12. Once this harvesting step is over, the resulting virus suspension is tested meticulously to confirm that only the **correct strain of polio virus** is present ; and also that the virus liter is above certain specified bare minimum level and in addition free from *viral, bacterial* and *fungal contaminants as* far as possible.
13. Consequently, the suspension is made to pass through the filters having increasing fineness so as to remove any remmants of tissue cells and ultimately *'bacteria'*. The former could some of the virus from the inactivating agent.
14. The liquors containing the virus particles are separately treated with dilute (0.01% v/v) formaldehyde under accurately controlled conditions of pH and temperature and making use of a magnetic stirrer. However, the removal of tissue cells and finally bacteria is duly accomplished within a span of 6 days, but in actual practice at least twice this duration is allowed (*i.e.,* 12 days) to ascertain almost 100% absence of any **'active virus'**.
15. In usual practice, the suspension may be *refiltered* at the half-way stage *i.e.,* after nearly 7 days. The rate at which the phenomenon of inactivation takes its normal course is followed meticulously for several days at a stretch on regular intervals; and subsequently almost between the 9th and 12th days larger samples are tested precisely for the total and absolute absence the infecting virus.
16. The formalized and sterile viral solution is now subjected to dialysis and checked thoroughly. The *'univalent vaccines'* of the three strains are now blended adequately to give rise to the desired **'trivalent product'.** At this critical stage large number samples are rechecked once again for freedom from the infective virus ; and finally the added formaldehyde solution is carefully neutralized with the addition of sodium metabisulphite.
17. A requisite quantum of **'thimerosal'** is added to serve as a bactericide. An aliquot of soluble disodium edetate is also included with a specific purpose to **sequester heavy metals** (as **'chelates'**) that would catalyze the decomposition of thiomersal to such products which are **'toxic'** to the virus.
18. The entire sequential procedure right from the very beginning to the final stage usually takes about 120 days. Importantly, the *'toxoid'* is prepared for IM-injection by subjected it to due emulsification with the aid of mineral oil essentially containing **3% highly purified Manito monoleate** in almost equal proportions together with 0.01% thimerosal as preservative.

4.7.3.20.3 Sabin Type Polio Vaccine

Interestingly, the vigorous activity in this direction has revived once again with the advent of enormous development and broad-scale usage of **oral polio vaccine** (OPV) that essentially comprises *of living attenuated strains of the virus.* However, the principle of its action is that these virus particles have the ability to proliferate in the gut and consequently release their modified toxins that are in turn getting absorbed directly into the blood stream; and thus induce the formation of specific antibodies.

Preparation the various steps involved are as follows

1. The overall manufacturing procedure is essentially as that of the **'Salk Vaccine'** (see section 7.3.20.2) except in one aspect that once the attenuated strains prepared by rapid passages through tissue cultures of monkey kidney cells are employed exclusively.
2. The virus in the *'final vaccine'* must not represent more than three sub-cultures from a strain that laboratory and clinical test have shown to be satisfactory. This, however, drastically reduces the chance of using a vaccine which has been rendered either **more virulent** or **lost antigenicity.**
3. Here exists practically no *'activation stage'* in this specific vaccine.
4. Besides, testing for freedom on the extraneous *bacteria, molds,* and *viruses,* special tests are absolutely predominantly necessary because the virus in the vaccine is living so as to confirm as well as ascertain the absence of virulent polio virus.

4.7.3.20.4 Inactivated Poliomyelitis Vaccine [or Inactivated Polio Vaccine BP-1993]

The **Inactivated Poliomyelitis Vaccine** is an aqueous suspension of appropriate strains of poliomyelitis virus, types 1, 2, and 3, grown in suitable cell cultures and inactivated by a suitable method. It is invariably obtained as a **'clean liquid'**.

Preparation. The various steps followed sequentially are as described under:

1. It is solely based on a **'seed-lot system'.** The virus used in the final vaccine represents not more than ten subcultures from the seed lots used for the production of the vaccine on which were carried out the laboratory and clinical tests that showed the strains to be suitable.
2. Animal serum may be employed in the medium for the initial cell growth but the medium for maintaining cell culture during virus multiplication contains no protein. The concentration of serum carried over into the vaccine does not exceed one part per million.
3. The million may contain a suitable pH indicator, such as: *phenol red*, and suitable *antibodies at the* smallest effective concentrations.
4. Each virus suspension is tested for identity, for bacterial sterility and, after neutralization with *'specific antiserum'*, for affording freedom from extraneous viruses.
5. The virus suspension is passed through a suitable filter and may then be concentrated and purified.
6. The suspension should contain at least 7.0 log10 CCID 50 mL^{-1} for each type of virus.
7. Within a suitable period of time of the last filtration, preferably within 24 hours, appropriate chemical substances that inactivate the *'virus filtrate'* without destroying its antigenicity are added. During the process of inactivation a suitable filtration is carried out. If necessary, the inactivating substance is later neutralized.
8. Each of the monovalent suspensions is shown by appropriate tests in cell cultures to be free from infective poliomyelitis virus and other human and simian (*i.e.,* monkey like) viruses.
9. The *'trivalent vaccine'* is prepared by mixing suspensions of each type.
10. Before the addition of any antimicrobial preservative, the *'trivalent suspension'* is shown to be free from infective poliomyelitis virus and other human and simian viruses.

4.7.3.20.5 Poliomyelitis Vaccine, Live (Oral) [or Polio Vaccine Live (Oral) BP-1993]

Poliomyelitis Vaccine, Live (Oral) is an aqueous suspension of suitable live, attenuated strains of poliomyletis virus, types 1, 2 or 3, grown in suitable, approved cell cultures. It may contain any one of the three virus types or mixture of two or three of them. It is a clear a *'clear liquid'*. The vaccine should be shown to be stable.

Preparation. The various steps involved are as enumerated under:

1. It is based on a seed-lot system. The '*final vaccine*' represents not more than three subcultures from the vaccine on which were made the laboratory and clinical tests that showed the strains to be suitable as approved by the appropriate authority.
2. The virus of each type is grown in cultures that have been shown not to contain extraneous microorganisms.
3. Animal serum may be used in the medium for initial cell growth but the medium for maintaining the cell cultures during virus multiplication contains absolutely no protein.
4. The cell culture medium may contain a suitable pH indicator *e.g.*, phenol red, and also appropriate antibodies at the smallest effective concentrations.
5. The virus suspension is harvested and is adequately tested for *identity, bacterial sterility* and freedom from *extraneous viruses.*
6. Virus harvests that pass these tests are pooled and filtered through a **bacteria-retentive filter.**
7. The filtered virus harvest is tested in cell cultures for identity, for growth capacity at different temperatures and for virus concentration.
8. A test for neurovirulence is carried out by intraspinal injection into *Macaca irus* (cynomolgus monkey) or equally susceptible animals. The vaccine and a *reference homotypic vaccine* are examined simultaneously in monkeys from the same quarantine batch.

4.7.3.21 Cancer Vaccine

Extensive work was carried out to develop a vaccine against the most dreadful disease **'cancer'.** The advent of tremendous progress accomplished *via* **newer genetic engineering techniques** over the past couple of decades have made it possible to produce the **'cancer vaccine'** on a large scale rather cheaply. The Cancer Research Compaign in Great Britain who developed the said vaccine over whelmingly hopes that it would certainly provide legitimate and adequate protection against the following three forms of the cancer related diseases, namely:

(*a*) **Glandular Fever.** It is usually caused by **Epstein Base Virus**, which is found to be an important component in triggering the cancer of the *terrat*,

(*b*) **Naso-Pharyngeal Cancer.** It has claimed to be mostly fatal in Asia and South China, and

(*c*) **Cancer of Jaw.** It is invariably confined to children specifically *viz.*, **Burkett's lymphoma;** and it kills thousands of children in Central Africa each year.

However, it was believed that the 'cancer vaccine' do possess the substantial potential to afford protection to millions of people throughout the world form largely fatal EBV related cancers. EBV is assumed to be closely associated with the Hodgkin's disease thereby causing death of thousands of children in Africa and China.

4.7.3.22. Birth Control Vaccine for Women

Scientists at the National Institute of Immunity (NII), New Delhi (INDIA) developed a **'birth control vaccines for women'** based on the concept of terminating the pregnancy by inactivating the hormone, **human chorionic gonadotropin** (HCG), produced by a woman at the time of conception. This vaccine is termed as the **Hill Vaccine,** and strategically makes use of the purified β-subunit of HCG as the **'antigen'**. However, there exists one extremely vital potential risk attributed to this '*vaccine*' by well-known researchers in the West was that the **'antibodies'** raised by β-HCG cross reacted predominantly with the **lutenising hormone** which critically controls the menstrual as well as the *ovulation* cycles significantly.

It is, however pertinent to mention here that the Indian scientists at NII still maintain that the aforesaid claim by the Western Scientists was not adequately substantiated by experimental evidences; besides, the original investigators at NII legitimately maintained that the '*impairment of ovulation*' has not been observed in any of the immunized women in trials conducted either in India or elsewhere.

World Health Organization (WHO) scientists opined that the vaccine actually intended for healthy women must be not only **absolutely safe** but also **100% free cross-reactivity.** Therefore, they almost abandoned working with whole β-HCG hormones several years ago.

The **WHO developed vaccine** is nothing but a *'synthetic peptide'* representing a small fragment (36 amino acid C-terminal sequence) of β-HCG hormone which is specific to HCG and hence does not react with the lutenising hormone (LH). This particular vaccine (WHO) was claimed and pronounced to be safe; however, the former vaccine (WHO) was claimed and pronounced to be safe; however, the scientists at NII (India) made a starting revelation that the former vaccine (*i.e.,* WHO-vaccine) helps in the induction of **reactions against the pancreatic tissue** which is believe to be still more dangerous and harmful in comparison to the *LH cross reactivity*. The WHO scientists hope to overcome this problem sooner. Furthermore, the Indian scientists (NII) proclaimed that the WHO developed vaccine is a very poor **'antigen'**, because it produces 20-30 folds lesser anti-HCG antibodies than the NII-developed vaccine; and maintained that the latter one is safer and effective. The trials are going on to evaluate the efficacies of the said two vaccines in due course of time.

4.7.3.23 AIDS-Vaccine

Preamble: Sometimes in 1980s, it was proclaimed that the cause of acquired-immuno deficiency syndrome (AIDS) has been discovered and that an AIDS-vaccine was almost round the corner. Unfortunately, as on date there has been no remarkable break through. It has been duly observed that under certain **'idealistic experimental parameters'** employed even some of the best results have practically demonstrated only 50% protection in animal experiments using specifically whole killed human immunodeficiency virus (HIV). One prevailing recognized glaring *concept* is that HIV is a **'retrovirus'**; however, it predominantly integrates into the host DNA and thereby gets carried around forever and hence could be activated by a whole number of vital factors. In other words, one may suggest that a vaccine can stimulate on the **high memory B cell litres.** Importantly, the constantly circulating B cells invariably act as the **'immune system watchdogs'**, perpetually looking for the **'pathogens'** vigorously they might have encountered before. The mechanism solely rests on the fact that once a HIV-particle gets recognized, the B cell immediately triggers off the **'signal'** to kill HIV-particle. Interestingly, this particular phenomenon gives rise to antibodies-producing response which essentially produces a good number of *HIV-particle specific antibodies i.e.,* a process which normally takes approximately seven days before they are rendered effective completely. In fact, a **'vaccine'** that blocks HIV would in turn stimulate this *humoral response* so as to recognize the infecting strain before it could cause or spread out infection.

There are member of HIV strains that have been duly identified world-wide, but researchers used specifically the **'III-strain'** because it was relatively easier to grow without looking into the fact whether the III-strain was actually the most preferred representative of the HIV commonly found in the infected population. It has been duly reported that there are in all **'five recognized families of HIV'** world wide. Besides, the virus is diverse in US; and the HIV strain dominates 66-70% of those individuals actually screened and tested but no individual strain accounts for more than 50% of the remainders. Perhaps, the prevailing existence of the **'high-viral mutation rate'** has been legitimately blamed and hence responsible for the utter failure to produce a **'traditional vaccine'.** At this point in time, it was even suggested that possibly a **'vaccine cocktail'** might be conceived and duly formulated which could be capable of binding together the *principle neutralizing determinants.* In fact, this postulated strategy predominantly necessitates **'updated booster shots'** at regular intervals to update the antibodies *titer values* high enough to protect as well as vaccinate against every recognized newer HIV mutations.

Paradoxically, on one hand the Western nations of the world categorically live with the illusion that HIV has been to a certain extent contained specifically well within the population of the homosexuals and IV drug users (*viz.*, morphine and narcotic drugs addicted individuals), whereas on the other the heterosexuals spread of AIDS in Asia and Africa overwhelmingly constitutes an epidemic that not only threatens but also affects every fabric of the society. By the end of the year 2000 AD, it was logically believed, projected, and estimated that approximately 40 million men, women and children will be affected with AIDS across the globe.

WHO opines vehemently that the looming pandemic due to AIDS critically threatens the socioeconomic development and also the survival of the whole communities in the world. A few vital aspects are as follows:

- Unusual homosexual practices
- Usage of dirty (unsterilized) needles amongst drug users
- Careless attitude of a large segment of men and women sleeping together at night without having the least worry about coutracting a **'lethal virus'**.
- Prevalently in Asia and Africa the deadly virus spreads widely with surprisingly fearsome ease wither from men to women or from women to men.
- Interestingly the issue of HIV spread through a highly unlikely means *via* physician to patient or *vice versa, e.g.,* the case where a female patient was exposed to HIV at the hands of her '*dentist*' in the course of an *'ordinary dental procedure'*.

Recently, a conglomerate of fifteen US and European pharmaceutical companies have agreed to share information and also to prompt the supplies of drugs so as to expedite and augment the eventful search for the combination of drug therapy that may be employed jointly in a concerted manner to fight other similar gresuome ailments.

In fact, several pharmaceutical companies including the manufacturers of the *three* **antiviral drugs** that have been duly licensed to control HIV in the US, such as:

i. **Zidovudine** (AZT): Manufactured By-Burroughs Welcome (**UK**);
ii. **Didansonine** (DDL): Manufactured By-*Bristol Meyer Squibb* (**US**); and
iii. **Zalcitabine** (DDC): Manufactured by *Hoffmann-La Roche* **(Switzerland)**.

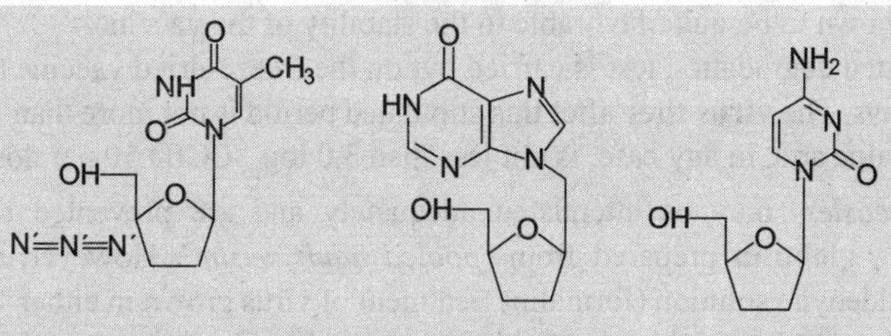

Zidovudine Didansonine Zalcitabine

4.7.3.24 Pneumococcal Vaccine

Pneumococcal Vaccine is a – *'a polyvalent vaccine containing polysaccharide capsular antigens representing 23 pneumococcal types.'* This vaccine is usually available for such patients that are particularly deemed to be at a special risk of pneumococcal infection, such as: *spleenectomized patients.*

- A '*single dose*' is found to afford adequate protection against the range of types represented in the '**pneumococcal vaccine**' for upto a duration of five years.
- The vaccine must **not** be administered to children below the age of two years.

4.7.3.25 Measles Vaccine, Live (BP-1993)

Measles-represents a highly communicable disease characterized by fever, general malaise, sneezing, nasal congestion, brassy cough, conjunctivitis, spots on the buccal mucosa (Koplik's spots), and a maculopapular eruption over the entire body caused by the **rubella virus.** Interestingly, the occurrence of measles before the age of 6 months is relatively uncommon, by virtue of the fact that the infant gets passively acquired maternal antibodies from the immune mother.

Measles Vaccine, Live is a preparation containing a suitable modified strain of live measles virus grown in cultures of the *chick embryo cells* or in other suitable approved cell cultures. It is normally prepared immediately before use by reconstitution from the dried vaccine with the liquid mentioned on the label. The vaccine does not contain any added antimicrobial preservation.

Preparation. The various steps involved in the preparation of the **Measles Vaccine, Live** are as enumerated under:

1. It is based on an approved seed-lot system from virus known to be free from neurovirulence. The final vaccine represents not more than ten subcultures from the vaccine on which were made the laboratory and clinical tests that showed the strain to be suitable.
2. **Dried Vaccine.** It may be prepared by the following method:

a. The virus is grown with the necessary aseptic precautions in primary cultures of chick embryo cells or other appropriate cells.

b. The *'chick embryos'* are derived from a healthy flock free from *avian leucosis* and the cell cultures are shown not to contain extraneous microorganisms.

c. Animal serum may be used in the medium for initial cell growth but the medium for maintaining the cell cultures during the virus multiplication contains no protein.

d. The cell culture medium may contain a suitable pH indicator *e.g.,* **phenol red**, and also suitable antibodies at the smallest effective concentrations.

e. The temperature of incubation is accurately controlled during the growth of the virus.

f. The viral suspensions are harvested at a time appropriate to the strain of virus used and are subsequently tested for identity, sterility and freedom from extraneous viruses.

g. Virus harvests that comply with these tests are first pooled and then clarified duly to remove cell.

h. An appropriate '*stabilizer*' is added to the clarified vaccine, which freeze dried to moisture content is shown to be quite favorable to the stability of the vaccine.

i. An accelerated degradation test is carried out on the freeze-dried vaccine by heating at 37°C for seven days. The **virus titer** after this stipulated period is not more than 1 log10 lower than the initial value and, in any case, is not less than 3.0 $\log_{10}$ CCID 50 per dose.

In general, *'measles'* may be attenuated adequately and are prevented completely by the administration of γ-**globulin** prepared from '*pooled adult serum*'. However, a **'killed vaccine'** prepared by formaldehyde solution (formalin) treatment of virus grown in either *'monkey kidney'* or *'dog kidney'* cell cultures invariably showed low degree of antibodies responses, but was certainly able to protect against the rash and febrile reactions caused by the administration of a **live attenuated vaccine.** Besides, it has been observed that the concentration of the killed vaccine and specifically addition of a mineral carrier immensely improved upon the prevailing *antibody response;* however, the overall duration of the immunity was of rather short duration.

Later on, efforts were geared towards the preparation of '*live vaccine*' with **attenuated strains of reduced pathogenicity** that essentially prolonged: (*a*) lower incidents of reaction; and (*b*) good antibody responses for many years.

Variants of Measles Vaccine. There are two known variants of the **'measles vaccine'**, namely: (*a*) Measles, mumps and rubella (MMR) vaccine, and (*b*) German measles (Rubella) vaccine. These *two* variants of measles vaccine shall now be treated individually as under:

4.7.3.25.1 Measles, Mumps and Rubella (MMR) Vaccine

The **measles, mumps and rubella vaccine** mainly aims to iradicate the diseases in a combined vaccine and invariably administered to children with an age ranging between 12-18 months.

It is also given to children between the ages 4-5 years. In other words, the **MMR-vaccine** virtually replaces the traditional **measles vaccine** to a considerable extent. It is, in fact, a mixed preparation comprising of suitable live attenuated strains of *measles virus, mumps virus* (*Paramyxo virus, Parotitidis*) and the *rubella virus*. These viruses are grown in chick-embryo cells or in suitable approved cell cultures as found suitable. The vaccine is normally prepared immediately before use by reconstitution from the dried vaccine with liquid mentioned on the label itself. The vaccine does not contain any added antimicrobial preservative (*e.g.,* thiomerosal). Each of the individual viral components is produced employing an **approved seed-lot system** for the individual component vaccine. After the viral cultures are grown adequately and clarified to recover cells, the clarified preparations of the individual viral components are mixed; a suitable stabilizer is incorporated and ultimately freeze-dried.

At the conclusion of the accelerated degradation test, the mixed vaccine must not contain less than 3.0 for the measles component; 3.7 for the mumps component; and 3.0 $\log_{10}$ CCID 50 per dose of the rubella component.

Notes: (1) Tests for identification, virus titer storage, and labeling conditions are almost similar to those described under *'measles vaccine'*.

(2) The label should essentially mention that it must not be administered to pregnant mothers.

4.7.3.25.2 Germanl Measles (Rubella) Vaccine

The **German measles (Rubella)** – is an exanthematous contagious disease specifically caused by the German measles virus. It has been duly observed that during the first three months of pregnancy, maternal rubella may result in **miscarriage, still-birth** and congenital deformities, for instance: **mental retardation, deaf mutism, cardiac abnormalities** and **cataract.** In such a situation, γ-globulin is not so effective in the treatment of infected cases but it will certainly prevent infection in contacts if administered promptly in appropriate doses. Importantly, the administration of γ-globulin is absolutely unnecessary after the first 3 months of pregnancy as **'rubella virus'** seldomly cause infection of the fetus in the later months.

Nowadays, the **German measles vaccines** are available prepared from any of the three strains as given below:

(*a*) **Attenuated PHV77 Strains** – obtained by repeated passage in *African green monkey kidney cell cultures,* was further attenuated in either duck embryo fibroblast cells or dog kidney cells,

(*b*) *Cendehill Strains* – isolated in monkey-kidney tissue and attenuated in rabbit kidney cells, and

(*c*) **RA 27/3 Strains** – isolated and attenuated in human diploid embryonic lung fibroblast cell cultures.

It is worthwhile to state here that all the three aforesaid vaccines give rise to an appreciable antibody response with little reaction in children and the inducted protection even lasts for several years at a stretch.

4.7.3.26 Meningococcal Polysaccharide Vaccine [BP-1993]

The **Meningococcal Polysaccharide Vaccine** consists of one or more purified polysaccharides obtained drom appropriate strains of *Neisseria meingitidis* group A, group C, group Y and group W135 that have been adequately proved to be capable of producing polysaccharides that are absolutely safe and also capable of inducing the production of satisfactory levels of specific antibody in humans. The vaccine is prepared immediately before use by reconstitution from the **stabilized dried vaccine** with an appropriate prescribed sterile liquid. It may either contain a single type of polysaccharide or any mixture of the types.

N. meningitidis group A polysaccharide – consists of partly O-acetylated repeating units of **Nacetylmannosamine,** linked with 1 → 6 **phosphodiester bonds.**

N. meningitidis group C polysaccharide – consists of partly O-acetylated repeating units of **sialic acid,** linked with 2 → 9 **glycosidic bonds.**

N. meningitidis group Y polysaccharide – consists of partly O-acetylated alternating units of **sialic acid,** a **D-galactose,** linked with 2 → 6 and 1 → 4 glycosidic bonds.

The polysaccharide component or components stated on the label together with Ca^{2+} ions and residual moisture invariably account for not less than 90% of the weight of the preparations.

Preparation. The various steps adopted are as stated under:

1. The preparation of the vaccine is based on a seed-lot system. Each seed-lot is subjected to microbiological examination by culture in an appropriate media and microscopic examination of Gram-stained smears.
2. The polysaccharide shown to be free from contaminating bacteria is precipitated by the addition of cetrimonium bromide and then purified.
3. Each polysaccharide is dissolved under aseptic conditions in a sterile solution containing lactose or another suitable stabilizing medium for freeze drying.
4. The solution is blended, if appropriate, with solution of the polysaccharides of any or all of the other groups and passed through a bacteria-retentive filter.
5. Finally, the filtrate is freeze dried to a moisture content shown to be favorable to the stability of the vaccine.

4.7.3.27 Future Development Scope of Vaccines

The constant relentless endeavor directed towards the future development scope of vaccines is gaining momentum across the globe with a view to improve upon the quality of life of such patients who are suffering from Alzheimer's disease, meningitis C, and the like.

A few cardinal aspects for the futuristic development of newer vaccines shall be discussed in the section that follows:

4.7.3.27.1 Vaccine against Alzheimer's disease

The American researchers suggest that a **vaccine against Alzheimer's disease** may be possible and accomplished. They have adequately demonstrated in their intensive studies on mice, which were genetically modified to come down with an Alzheimer's like condition, compete with altered **β-amyloid**– a protein that specifically causes the build up of sticky insoluble deposits usually termed as **'plaque'**, found in the brains of Alzheimer's patients.

The researchers based on the above clue used **β-amyloid** itself to *stimulate the immune response* thereby preventing the plaque formation in 6-weeks old mice; besides, reduced plaque formation in relatively older mice.

4.7.3.27.2 Vaccine for Meningitis C

There in all *three* types of **meningitis** that are prevalent, identified, and recognized so far that invariably give rise to inflammation to the specific lining of the brain and in certain cases proved to be even fatal, such as:

(a) Hemophilus Influenza Type B (HIB):

These are the most common cause of bacterial infection particularly confined to the *under fives-only* was eliminated both radically and virtually by the introduction of **HIB-vaccine** in 1992.

(b) Pneumococcal Meningitis Vaccine:

It is found to be less common and affect particularly the very *young, elderly,* and *immuno-compromised* subjects that almost kill 150-200 persons a year.

(c) Meningcoccal Meningitis (or Meningitis C Vaccine):

It essentially includes *septicemia/ blood poisoning* and is found to be equally prevalent and predominant; and, therefore, is considered to be the most common virus. Initially, 2/3rd of the cases recorded belonged to '*group B*' and *1/3rd to 'group C'*; however, this ratio has changed quite recently. As one date the '*group C*' is actually responsible for approximately 40% of all cases in UK thereby causing death of youngsters between the age limits ranging between 15 and 17. It has been observed duly that the two major recognized risk-factors are: *(a) passive smoking;* and *(b) damp and cold environment*.

Meningitis C Vaccine – an altogether new and most efficacious vaccine has been produced against the most virulent strain of the disease **meningitis C** that is presently employed to immunize the babies, school children and students (age group 16-18) going to the Universities. In UK alone, 150 deaths occurred in the year 1998 in both schools and universities. The rate of illness is catching up speedily and rapidly in the recent past having touched the peak-level specifically in '*semi-closed communities*' during winter. The new vaccine *i.e.,* Meningitis C Vaccine provides adequate protection against the group C meningitis virus but certainly not against the group B infection for which a vaccine is still being sought. Interestingly, in babies the vaccine does trigger an immunological memory that must attribute to the desired long-lasting protection profusely. More than 4500 children and young persons in UK were tested with the **'new vaccine'**.

Combating Meningitis. The scientists in UK worked out the so-called **'genetic blue-print of the bacterium'** actually responsible for the most dangerous form of meningitis. By meticulously sequencing together the prevailing two million units of its DNA, they actually prepared the legitimate well-defined ground for developing the new vaccines to prevent the illness and also in preventing the '*causative bacterium*' from harming the people. Britain plans to launch an altogether '*new vaccine*' against **group C meningitis** that is expected to cut dramatically the enormous death-toll caused by this harmful disease. The existing vaccine only afford protection for upto two years, and fail to show any response in infants under two years of age. Importantly, the '*new vaccine*' is expected to overcome these problems and initially be targeted at young children and teenagers. However, 10% of the meningitis cases in Britain are of the slightly less deadly *group B vaccine* against these organisms are under investigation, but are unlikely to be available for yet several years.

4.7.3.27.3 Super Vaccine

Various scientists across the globe vehemently believe and opine that the well-known **cowpox virus vaccinia,** the '*vaccine*' of which caused protection to millions from smallpox could also be enlisted in the fight against the host of diseases usually encountered, namely: *cancer. AIDS* and *hepatitis*. It has been critically observed that the said '*vaccine*' possesses an excellent safety record and the genome that of the virus has an ample and adequate room to accommodate rather large genes as such. It was, therefore, most logically thought that the virus could be genetically engineered to prime the prevailing '*immune system*' against other virus and even the cancer cells to a considerable extent. Unfortunately, the greatest problem normally encountered is that immunization with vaccinia against the smallpox renders the prevailing immune system categorically ignore the **'newer genetically engineered viruses'**. However, the scientists observed, at the National Institute of Health (NIH): Washington DC, that experimental mice injected with vaccinia primed immune responses in their *lymph tissue specifically,* but not in the mucous membrane sites *viz.,* nose or rectum. It has been duly observed that when on HIV vaccine containing engineered vaccinia was delivered to mice *via* rectum, they usually developed immunity throughout their immune systems. Interestingly, the injection of the engineered vaccine right into the blood-stream of animals failed to provoke an immune-response. From this study one may legitimately infer that if **engineered vaccinia-vaccines** for HIV are particularly delivered through a mucous membrane, the earlier smallpox vaccinations would pose a rather serious problem.

4.7.3.27.4 Immunomodulators

The National Institute of Immunology, New Delhi, (India) developed a **'leprosy immuno modulator'**, known as **LEPROVAC.** This specific immunomodulator when used either alone or with *Multi Drug Therapy* (MDT) ultimately led to *four* vital biological phenomena, namely:

- Histopathological upgrading,
- Rapid clearance of thermal granuloma,
- Flattening of lesions, and
- Regression of lesions.

It has been observed that this type of treatment invariably stimulates cell-mediated immunity, accelerates bacteriological clearance, and above all minimises drastically the chances of reaction relapse noticeably. MDT is found to be absolutely inadequate for such diseases.

4.7.3.27.5 Vaccination with Gas Lighter

It is a well established fact that normally a large-scale vaccination not only involves an enormous strain but also an appreciable expenditure. Noted scientists at the National Institute of Immunology (NII), New Delhi, (India) meticulously developed an easy and rather cheap (inexpensive) method of vaccination by means of a small Piezo-electric (PE) gas lighter. In a actual practice, large number of farm animals was vaccinated quite easily with these improvised techniques that practically needed no syringe at all. In fact, the *membrane-electroporosis technique* is proved to be rather costly in comparison to a direct DNA, amino acid molecules or protein into cells on the skin; however, the process is easy with the help of a small PE-generator. In the kitchen-lighter (PE-generator) each time a friction is developed within a few seconds a voltage of 18 kW of is generated. Eventually, adequate experiments were conducted to create electropolation into cells with the help of the ensuing voltage pulse thus generated. Medical experts overwhelmingly hailed the above results which ultimately paved the way to an altogether newer approach in the prevailing **'vaccination techniques'.**

4.7.3.27.6 Vaccine against Cervical Cancer

The **vaccine against** cervical cancer may be soon on the anvil. It is regarded to be a most important, vital, and abundantly found cancer in women particularly next to breast cancer. In the context of nearly three lakh deaths taking place the world over due to the cervical cancer alone and this represents almost 80% of the total death. Furthermore, about five lakh new cases are being recorded the world over every year. Importantly, the cervical type amongst the total incidence of cancers usually ranged from 3- 5% in North America and Western Europe; between 20-25% in Latin America, South West Asia, and Sub-Saharan Africa.

Causation of Cervical Cancer: The **cervical cancer** is an exclusively sexually transmitted disease (STD) caused by a virus known as **Human Papilloma Virus (HPV).** Infection invariably commences in the early years of usually sexual activity, but it takes almost upto 20 years for it to undergo complete development into a **fully grown malignant tumor.** Interestingly, most of the vaccines that are under aggressive stages of development are solely based upon the genetically engineered virus *viz.,* particles composed of the outer structural protein of the virus.

4.7.3.27.7 Vaccination without Needles

In general, the **vaccine** that are entirely based on the *fragments of DNA* are found to be **more stable, cheaper** and **relatively less risky** in comparison to the host of **conventional vaccines** made solely from *disease-causing organisms.* It may further be observed that the most of the so-called **'conventional vaccine'** essentially involved the usage of needless **(except the oral polio**

vaccine). Dedicated and world recognized scientists at the **Palo Alto Health Cow System, Palo Alto, (California)**, advocated that certain DNA-vaccines may be effective 100% even when applied directly to the normal-skin conditions.

However, fruitful attempts to deliver immunizing agents *via* skin-surface predominated involves such simple procedures as: shaving with a sterile razor, threading, or clinically treating the skin-surface. In actual practice, all these processes leave pathways for infection and hence they are not entirely satisfactory. The scientists tried *two* distinct types of DNA-sequences, namely:

(*a*) Encoded for bacterial sequence, and

(*b*) Portion of the surface of the hepatitis B virus.

The solutions of these two different types of DNA sequences were carefully administered to '*experimental mice*' either by dripping them cautiously onto the animal skin or through injection. Importantly, both groups of mice tested with the bacterial protein reacted equally strongly. In the case of hepatitis D DNA, the mice tested with '*skin affection*' reacted comparatively less strongly than those tested with injection of a conventional vaccine comprising of the same DNA, but still at a level likely to have a therapeutic effect.

It was further demonstrated that the effect of '*immunization*' was related to the presence of '*hair*' on the skin which was explained duly that **DNA-fragments** gained entry into the skin via the oil producing cells in *hair follicles.* This observation articulately supports the fact DNA-vaccine may be delivered *via* '**unprepared skin**' which is evidently important and vital for those who are afraid of needles. Besides, it also eliminates completely the possible cause infection and the risks associated intimately within the more **invasive techniques.** One would certainly appreciate that providing clean sterile needles poses usually the most challenging and expensive task of a mass vaccination programme.

Questions

1. Cellular humoral immunity. (JNTUA-May 2009)
2. Antigen-antibody reaction. (JNTUA-May 2009)
3. Immunization and immunological tolerance. (JNTUA-May 2009)
4. Immunological tolerance. (JNTUA-Nov 2010)
5. Standardization and storage of polio vaccine as per I.P (JNTUA-Nov 2010)
6. Write note on monoclonal antibody production and explain with suitable example. (JNTUA-Nov 2010)
7. Passive Immunization. (JNTUA-Nov 2010)
8. Describe in detail antigen-antibody reactions. (JNTUA-May 2009)
9. Explain their application with suitable example. (JNTUA-May 2009)
10. What are vaccines? Explain. (JNTUA-May 2009)
11. Describe the production of vaccines along with a neat flow diagram. (JNTUA-May 2009)
12. Immune system. (JNTUA-May 2009)
13. RBC. (JNTUA-May 2009)
14. Human fibrinogen. (JNTUA-May 2009)
15. Explain cellular immunity and add a note on interferons. (JNTUA-Nov 2010)
16. Explain antigen-antibody reactions. (JNTUA-Nov 2010)
17. What is passive immunization? Explain. (JNTUA-Dec 2009)
18. Describe the preparation of vaccine with a suitable example. (JNTUA-Dec 2009)
19. Whole human blood. (JNTUA-Dec 2009)
20. Hyper sensitivity. (JNTUA-Dec 2009)
21. Discuss transformation and transduction. (RGUHS–Mar 2009)

22. Turbidometeric method of assay of antibiotics. (RGUHS–Apr 2008)
23. Methods of standardization of vaccines. (RGUHS–Apr 2008)
24. Enumerate various antigen-antibody reactions. Discuss in detail the agglutination tests? (RGUHS–Oct 2007)
25. Classify types of immunity. (RGUHS–Oct 2007)
26. Taxolids. (RGUHS–Oct 2007)
27. Outline the production and purification of monoclonal antibodies. (MGRU Apr- 2004)
28. Briefly discuss about antigen antibody interaction. (MGRU Apr-2004)
29. Production and purification of hepatitis-B vaccine. (MGRU Apr-2004)
30. Different type of hypersensitivity. (MGRU Apr-2004)
31. Define antigen and antibody. (MGRU Apr-2004)
32. How an antibiotic can be assayed by one level and two levels. (MGRU 2003)
33. What is MIC? What is the significance of it. (MGRU 2003)
34. How monoclonal antibodies are produced. (MGRU 2003)
35. Classify immunity with example. (MGRU 2003)
36. What are the methods that are usually adopted to produce viral vaccines. (MGRU 2003)
37. Write a note on MMR group of vaccine. (MGRU 2003)
38. Quality control test for vaccines. (MGRU 2003)
39. Write the production of BCG vaccine. (MGRU 2003)
40. Differences between exotoxin and endotoxin. (MGRU 2003)
41. Differences between toxin and taxoid. (MGRU 2003)
42. Differences between active immunity and passive immunity. (MGRU 2003)
43. Differences between an antiseptic and disinfectant. (MGRU 2003)
44. Cholera vaccine. (MGRU 2004)
45. Monoclonal antibodies. (MGRU 2004)
46. Differentiate between active immunity and passive immunity. (MGRU 2004)
47. Define Haptens with suitable example. (MGRU 2004)
48. Define immunity and distinguish active with passive immunity. (MGRU 2003)
49. Explain the production and evaluation of BCG vaccine. (MGRU 2003)
50. Differentiate between toxins and toxiods with examples. (MGRU 2003)
51. Give a brief account of containerization vaccines. (MGRU 2003)
52. Write the applications of monoclonal antibodies. (MGRU 2003)
53. Write a short note with application of immunoglobulin. (MGRU 2003)
54. Write stability studies described for official vaccines. (MGRU 2003)
55. Write in detail about autoimmune disorders. (MGRU 2003)
56. Describe in detail about production of any one bacterial killed vaccine. (MGRU 2002)
57. Define immunity and clarify. (MGRU 2002)
58. Conversion method of toxin to toxoid. (MGRU 2002)
59. Brief introduction about Diptheria toxoids. (MGRU 2002)
60. Explain about the standards of penicillin injection. (MGRU 2002)
61. Role of adjuvants in vaccines and write the example. (MGRU 2002)
62. Define acquired immunity. (MGRU 2002)
63. Define monoclonal antibodies. (MGRU 2002)
64. Explain immunity and production of BCG vaccine. (MGRU 2002)

65. Oral polio vaccine. (MGRU 2002)
66. Diptheria toxoids. (MGRU 2002)
67. Monoclonal antibodies. (MGRU 2002)
68. Whole human blood. (MGRU 2002)
69. Define immunity and differentiate between active immunity and passive immunity. (MGRU 2001)
70. What are the applications of monoclonal antibodies. (MGRU 2004)
71. Discuss in detail the production of Rabies vaccine. (MGRU 2004)
72. Discuss in detail the production of Tetanus toxoid. (MGRU 2004)
73. Outline the preparation of Diphtheria antitoxin. (MGRU 2004)
74. Outline the storage conditions for vaccines. (MGRU 2004)
75. Haptens. (MGRU 2004)
76. Give an example for attenuated and killed bacterial vaccine. (MGRU 2004)

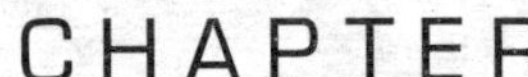

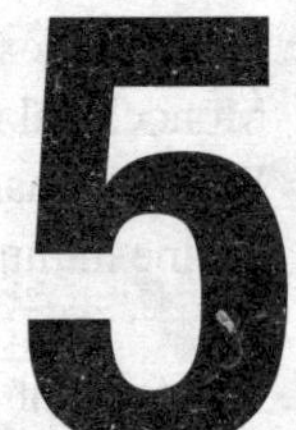

Enzyme Immobilization

5.1 Introduction

Microbial enzymes are most extensively employed in the food and beverage industries across the globe to meet the ever increasing demand for nutritionally superb and high-value products. Importantly, the predominant utilization of the enzymes in an industrial environment has been drastically restrained and limited by virtue of the fact that a large number of enzymes are not only relatively unstable but also involve exorbitantly high-cost of isolation, purification, and recovery of '*active enzymes*' from the reaction mixtures after the due completion of the ensuing catalytic on-going process. In actual practice, the soluble enzymes engaged in '**batch operations**' is found to be not-so-economical due to the fact that the *active enzyme* is virtually lost (not recovered) after each viable reaction.

Therefore, in order to combat and overcome such a non-productive, economically not feasible, and deleterious effect the **enzymes have been ultimately immobilized;** and the process is termed as **enzyme immobilization.** Hence, it may be defined as — '*confining the enzyme molecules to a distinct phase from the one wherein the substrates and the products are present*'.

5.1.1 Salient Features

Some of the vital and important salient features of **enzyme immobilization** are enumerated as under:

1. Enzymes are more or less physically confined in the course of a definite continuous catalytic process. They may be suitably recovered from the reaction mixture and used over and over again thereby gainfully improving the economic viability of the entire process.
2. It may be accomplished by fixing the enzyme molecules to or within certain appropriate substance.
3. It should be absolutely critical that both the *substrates* and the *products* migrate quite freely in and out of the phase to which the specific enzyme molecules are actually confined.

4. Certain enzymes which are as such readily inactivated by heat (*i.e.,* **thermolabile**), may be rendered heat-stable by attachment to inert polymeric supports.
5. Utilization of whole beads are invariably employed for a wide spectrum of catalytic functions thereby ascertaining the fact that *immobilized enzymes* do have an edge over their soluble counterparts overwhelmingly.
6. *Immobilized enzymes* may be recycled, rapidly controlled, operated continuously, product(s) easily separable, and above all the enzymatic properties (*i.e.,* stability, activity) altered favorably.
7. *Immobilized enzymes* seem to be fairly compatible with **multienzyme procedures** that essentially make use of *enzyme-based cofactors*.

5.1.2 Carrier Matrices

The substances that are solely employed for the immobilization of enzymes are known as **carrier matrices** *e.g., inorganic materials* (salts), and *inert polymers.* An ideal **carrier matrix** has the following characteristic features, namely:

a. Cost effectiveness,
b. Inertness,
c. Reasonable physical strength,
d. Adequate stability,
e. Regenerability after the gainful lifespan of the immobilized enzyme,
f. Enhancement in specificity of enzyme,
g. Reduction in product inhibition,
h. A possible shift in optimum pH for enzyme activity to the desired value for the process, and
i. Appreciable reduction in non-specific adsorption and microbial contamination.

It is, however, pertinent to state here that a large segment of carrier matrices do possess inherently only a few of the aforesaid characteristic features ('*a*' through '*i*'). In the light of the above statement of facts one should always remember that the **carrier matrix** for the immobilization of an enzyme need to selected with utmost care and wisdom bearing in mind the *characteristic features* as well as *the prevailing limitations* of various matrices.

5.2 Methods of Immobilization

The immobilization methods are of *four* distinct types depending solely upon the **physical relationship** of the catalyst being used to the **carrier matrix,** such as: (*a*) adsorption; (*b*) covalent bonding; (*c*) entrapment; and (*d*) membrane confinement.

Importantly, the *carrier matrix* selected for the process must enhance the operational stability of the immobilized enzyme purification. The carriers should be either porous or nonporous matrices belonging to the **organic** (natural or synthetic) or **inorganic** domain. The *four* various types of methods of immobilization as stated above (*i.e.,* '*a*' through'd') shall now be described individually as under:

5.2.1 Adsorption Method

Adsorption of an enzyme may be accomplished by allowing the contact of the *enzyme* and the *polymer support* either by percolating* the enzyme *via* a packed bed, tube, membrane formed from a support material or in a stirred bioreactor. In other words, in the particular instance of *adsorption,* the enzyme molecules evidently get adhered to the surface of a *carrier matrix* on account of the spectacular combination of **hydrophobic effects** and the **critical formation** of *several salt-linkages* per enzyme molecule as shown in Fig. 5.1.

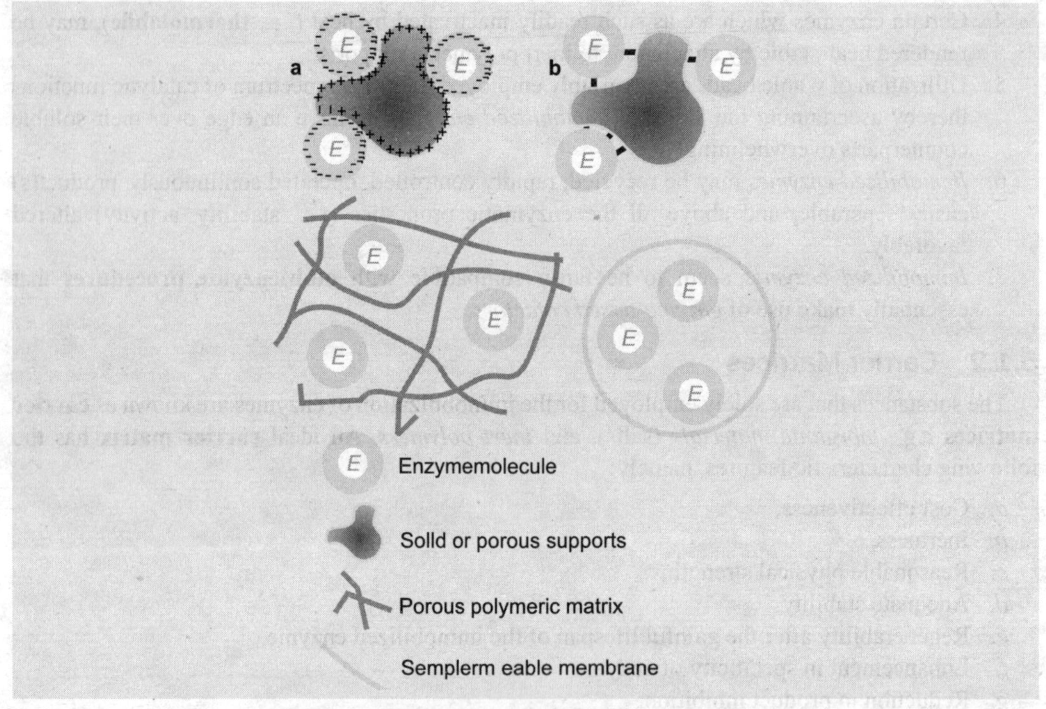

Fig. 5.1 *Enzyme Immobilization by Adsorption Method*

In usual practice, a variety of specific and non-specific forces come into play in the **adsorption method** *viz.,* hydrophobic, electrostatic interactions or affinity bondage to certain specific ligands duly attached to the carrier matrix. However, a predominant influence being exerted upon the quantity of enzyme adsorbed exclusively depends upon the enzyme concentration per unit surface of the carrier matrix. Consequently, the overall activity gets enhanced with an increasing enzyme concentration — approaching a targeted saturation value — having a noticeable decline in the specific activity.

It has been duly observed that the process of binding of the prevailing carrier matrix to the available enzyme molecules is invariably quite strong but it may be weakened during actual usage by several vital factors, namely: pH, ionic strength, and addition of substrate. Therefore, it is always advisable to pick up the carrier matrix with great care, wisdom, and judicious manner from such substances as: porous carbon clays, hydrous metal oxides, polymeric aromatic resins, glasses, and ion-exchange matrices.

Methodology: The actual methodology involved in the adsorption of enzymes to the matrices is quite simple, easy, and employed largely. The appropriate enzyme is adequately mixed with a right adsorbent usually under *appropriate pH parameters* as well as the *desired ionic strength.* After incubation for a stipulated duration, the carrier matrix is washed thoroughly to get rid of the entire *unabsorbed enzyme molecules,* whereby the **'immobilized enzyme'** is ready for actual usage. Interestingly, this specific method invariably gives rise to a high loading (nearly 1 g enzyme per g matrix) of the enzyme.

Note: Ion-exchange carrier matrices are relatively costlier; however, they may be regenerated easily and rapidly (*i.e.,* at the end of the active life of the absorbed enzyme) by a rather absolutely simple operation *viz.,* carefully washing off the absorbed enzyme by means of a concentrated salt solution.

The various enzymes that may be immobilized by adsorption on respective carrier matrix are summarized as under:

S.No	Enzymes	Carrier Matrix
1.	α-Amylase	Calcium phosphate
2.	Amyloglucosidase	Agarose-Gel; DEAE-Sephadex
3.	Catalase	Charcoal (activated)
4.	Glucose oxidase	Cellophane (followed cross linking with glutaraldehyde, inorganic adsorbents)
5.	Invertase	Charcoal (activated); DEAE- Sephadex
6.	Subtilisn	Cellulose.

5.2.2 Covalent Bonding

In this particular instance the **'enzyme molecules'** in questions are duly attached to the carrier matrix by the formation of **covalent bonds.** Consequently, the actual strength of bondage happens to be quite strong; and hence, there is absolutely no loss of enzyme during usage. The formation of covalent bond usually takes place particularly with the side chains of amino acids present in the enzyme; however, their actual strength of reactivity being exclusively linked to the status of 'charge' present in them as given below:

$$—S^- > —SH > —O^- > —NH_2 > —COO^- > —OH >> —NH_3^+$$

Thus, the various functional moieties mostly present in enzyme which actively take part in the formation of the numerous viable chemical bonds are: sulphide, sulphhydril, oxide, amino, carboxyl, hydroxyl, ammonium, imino, amide, methylthiol, guanidyl, imidazole, and phenol ring.

The **covalent bonding** of an enzyme may be accomplished either by activating the polymer with a *reactive moiety* (*i.e.,* copolymerization with ethylene, anhydride of maleic acid) or by effectively employing the bifunctional reagent to serve as a bridge between the two entities: enzyme and polymer, whereby 3D-network may be obtained by cross-linking with low molecular weight bifunctional agent(s). In doing so, the enzyme invariably may get *inactivated* because the reactions normally engage a functional moiety strategically located at the 'active site' of the enzyme. Thus, the overall net effect being the substantial loss of **enzymatic activity**. Importantly, such an overwhelmingly loss in the enzymatic activity may be overcome by judiciously carrying out the '**enzyme immobilization**' either in the presence of a *competitive* inhibitor or an *enzyme substrate*.

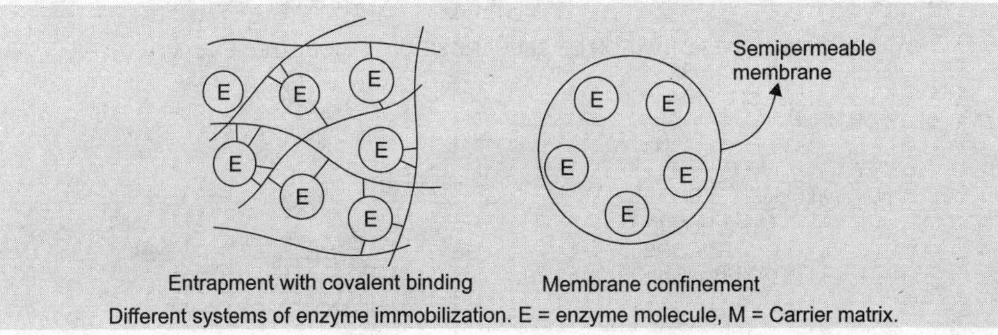

Different systems of enzyme immobilization. E = enzyme molecule, M = Carrier matrix.

Fig. 5.2 *Covalent Bonding and Cross Linking of Enzyme Immobilization*

Figure 5.2 illustrates the covalent bonding and cross linking explicitely.

The activated polymers that are solely employed are: **hydrogels** duly incorporated with a host of typical chemical entities, such as: *azide group; diazo group; carbodiimide group.* The various enzymes immobilized by **covalent bonding** using typical *carrier matrix* and *binding reaction* are summarized below:

S.No	Enzymes	Carrier Matrix Used	Binding Reaction Involved
1.	α-Amylase	DEAE-Cellulose	Direct coupling
2.	Amyloglucosidase	–do–	Cyanuric chloride
3.	Cellulase	Polyurethane	Isocyanate
4.	Glucose Isomerase	–do–	–do–
5.	Glucose Oxidase	Porous Glass	Isothiocyanate
6.	Pectinase	Polyurethane	Isocyanate
7.	Pronase	CM-Sephadex	Carbodiimide Activation

Advantages of Covalent Bonding: The various important advantages of the covalent bonding in enzyme immobilization are as enumerated below:

1. Adsorption of enzymes to the carrier matrices is quite easy and convenient, and hence used extensively.
2. Covalent bonding attachment is not reversed by pH, ionic strength or substrate.
3. Relatively broader spectrum of bonding reactions, and of matrices with functional moieties capable of either having covalent bondage or prone to be activated to yield such groups renders this method into a highly acceptable one.
4. **Support with Functional groups:** Various typical examples using support with functional groups are:

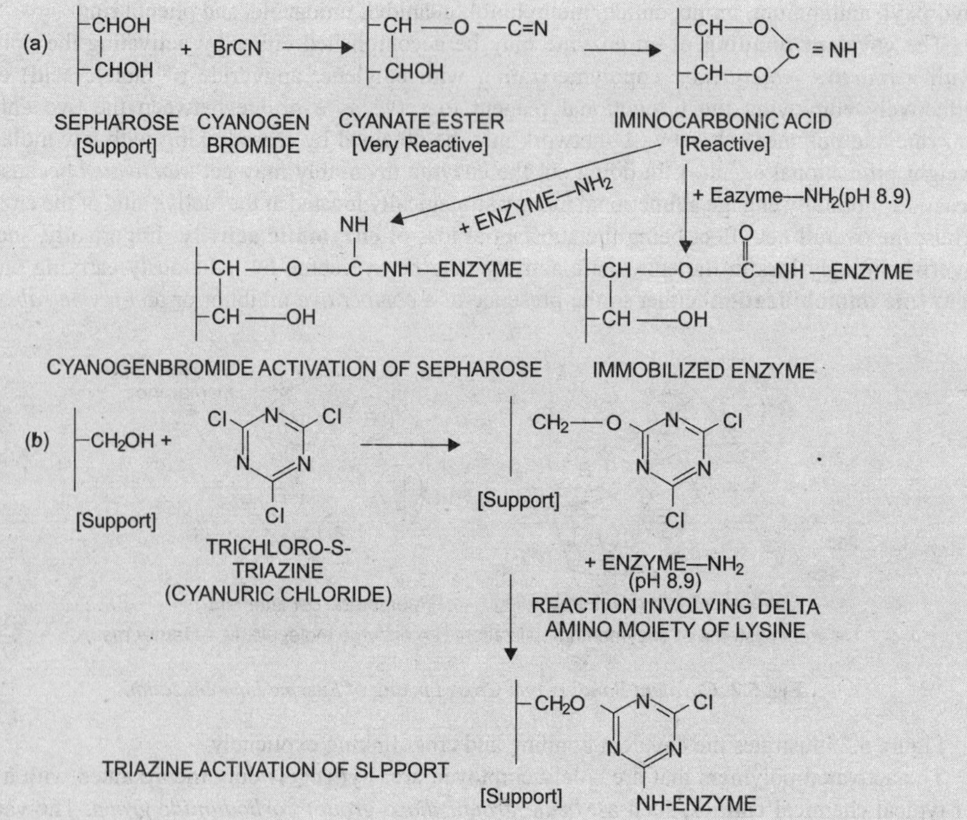

Fig. 5.3 *Immobilization of Enzymes; Using Supports with – OH Moieties that are activated by Covalent Bonding with: (a) Cyanogen Bromide; and (b) Triazine*

a. **With – OH Group:** Supports of this type may be activated specifically for the **covalent bonding** by subjecting it to treatment with either *cyanogen bromide* or triazine as illustrated in Fig. 5.3(a) and (b). The reaction with the enzyme protein in each instance involves the –NH_2 moiety of **lysine.**

b. **With – COOH Groups:** Carboxymethyl cellulose (CMC) may be activated either *via* acyl-isourea formation or azide derivative formation as given in Fig. 5.4(*a*) and (*b*) below. The reaction essentially involves the participation of amino (– NH_2) moiety present in lysine; besides, a host of other amino acids *viz.,* cysteine, serine, tyrosine — are also made use of in the covalent bonding phenomenon.

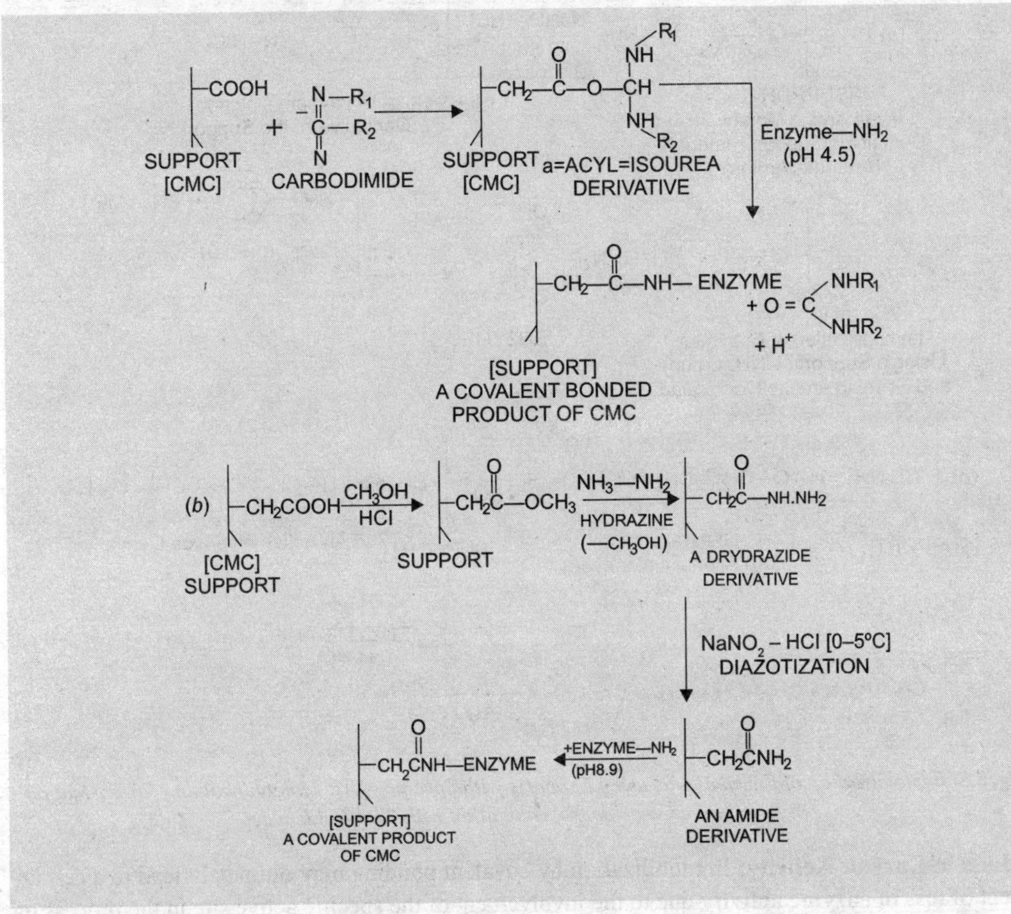

SUPPORT [CMC]–COOH + R_1–N=C=N–R_2 (CARBODIMIDE) → SUPPORT [CMC]–CH_2–CO–O–CH(NHR_1)(NHR_2) (a=ACYL=ISOUREA DERIVATIVE)

Enzyme—NH_2 (pH 4.5)

→ [SUPPORT]–CH_2–CO–NH– ENZYME + O = C(NHR_1)(NHR_2) + H^+

[SUPPORT] A COVALENT BONDED PRODUCT OF CMC

(*b*) [CMC] SUPPORT–CH_2COOH —(CH_3OH, HCl)→ SUPPORT–CH_2CO–OCH_3 —(NH_3—NH_2 HYDRAZINE, (—CH_3OH))→ –CH_2CO–NH.NH_2 A DRYDRAZIDE DERIVATIVE

$NaNO_2$ – HCl [0–5°C] DIAZOTIZATION

→ –CH_2CONH_2 AN AMIDE DERIVATIVE —(+ENZYME—NH_2 (pH8.9))→ –CH_2CONH—ENZYME [SUPPORT] A COVALENT PRODUCT OF CMC

Fig. 5.4 *Immobilization of Enzymes using CMC Supports Having —COOH with — NH_2 Group or with Hydrazine (NH_2–NH_2) Group via Covalent Bondage Involving: (a) Acyl Urea; and (b) Azide Derivative*

c. **With – NH2 Group:** The amino functional moiety containing support material may be converted easily to the corresponding **diazonium chloride** salt by suitably treating with a mixture of sodium nitrite ($NaNO_2$) and diluted hydrochloric acid (HCl) between 0–5°C (*diazotization*). The enzyme protein gets hooked up with the resulting diazotized derivative thereby establishing an appropriate azo-linkage involving the corresponding the **tyrosine residue of enzyme protein** as illustrated in Fig. 5.5(*a*). In certain specific instances one may make use of **glutaraldehyde** (*i.e.,* an aliphatic aldehyde) to strategically activate the support material essentially having the $-NH_2$ functional group. Thus, the reaction predominantly involved as **Schiff's base** formation between two entities, namely: (*i*) *amino moiety* of the support material; and (*ii*) *amino moiety* of one of the amino acids present in the protein, as depicted in Fig. 5.5(b).

Interestingly, it has been observed that the exact number of bonds existing between the **support material** and the corresponding **enzyme molecule** in the course of the very covalent bondage is distinctly variable, such as: **papain molecule** has 17 covalent bonds; and **subtilopeptidase** immobilized duly on semialdehyde starch analogue possesses 8 covalent bonds.

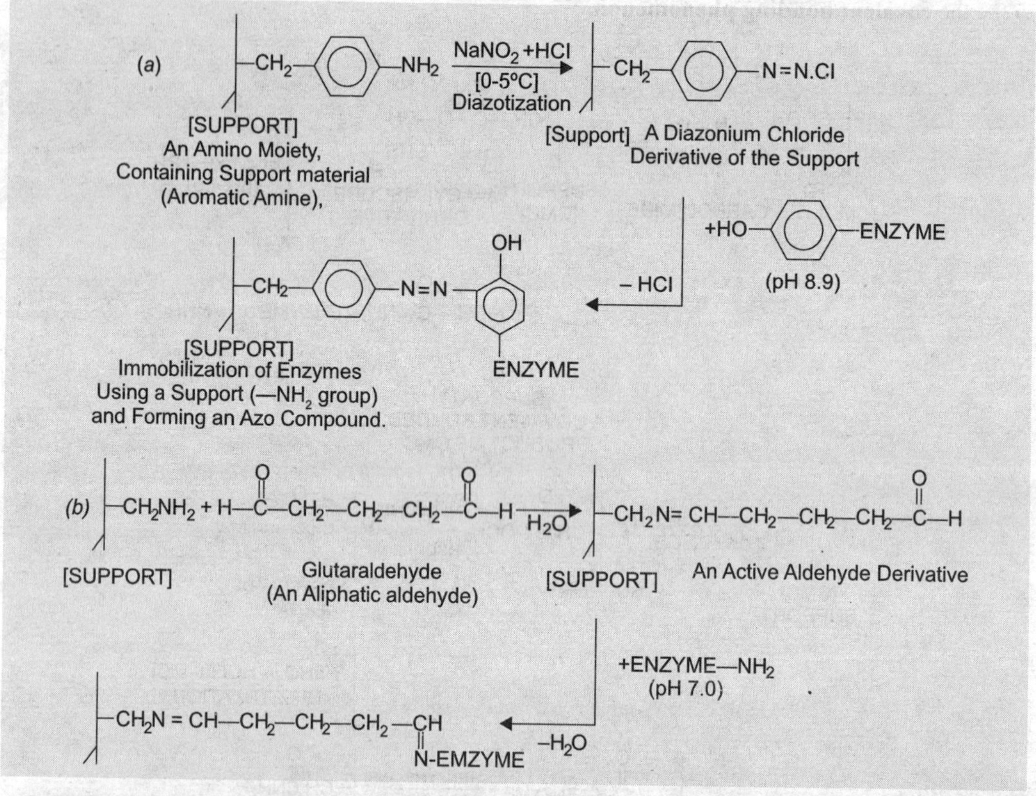

(*a*) $-CH_2-C_6H_4-NH_2$ $\xrightarrow[\text{[0-5°C] Diazotization}]{NaNO_2 + HCl}$ $-CH_2-C_6H_4-N{=}N.Cl$

[SUPPORT] An Amino Moiety, Containing Support material (Aromatic Amine),

[Support] A Diazonium Chloride Derivative of the Support

+HO—C₆H₄—ENZYME (pH 8.9), – HCl

$-CH_2-C_6H_4-N{=}N-C_6H_3(OH)-ENZYME$

[SUPPORT] Immobilization of Enzymes Using a Support (—NH_2 group) and Forming an Azo Compound.

(*b*) $-CH_2NH_2 + H-C(=O)-CH_2-CH_2-CH_2-C(=O)-H \xrightarrow{H_2O} -CH_2N{=}CH-CH_2-CH_2-CH_2-C(=O)-H$

[SUPPORT] Glutaraldehyde (An Aliphatic aldehyde) [SUPPORT] An Active Aldehyde Derivative

+ENZYME—NH_2 (pH 7.0), $-H_2O$

$-CH_2N = CH-CH_2-CH_2-CH_2-CH{=}$N-EMZYME

Fig. 5.5 *Immobilization of Enzymes was using Supports with Specific* $-NH_2$ *Moiety Involving (a) Formation of Diazonium Chloride; (b) Activation with Glutaraldehyde*

Loss in Enzyme Activity: Immobilization by covalent bonding may ultimately lead to a certain extent of **loss in enzyme activity** due to the involvement of the specific active site in the process of immobilization. Another school of thought suggests that immobilization of the enzyme in a particular orientation affords either a distortion of the active site or renders it more or loss unavailable. However, the ensuing *loss in enzyme activity* may be minimized to a considerable extent by adopting the following methods, such as:

a. Immobilization of the enzyme in the presence of its substrate at a saturated concentration only, and

b. Incorporation of a '*competitive inhibitor*' (*i.e.*, it gets bound to the active site).

The above possible effects of **enzyme mobilization** exclusively by the help of **covalent binding** upon the enzyme activity may be illustrated explicitely in Fig. 5.6.

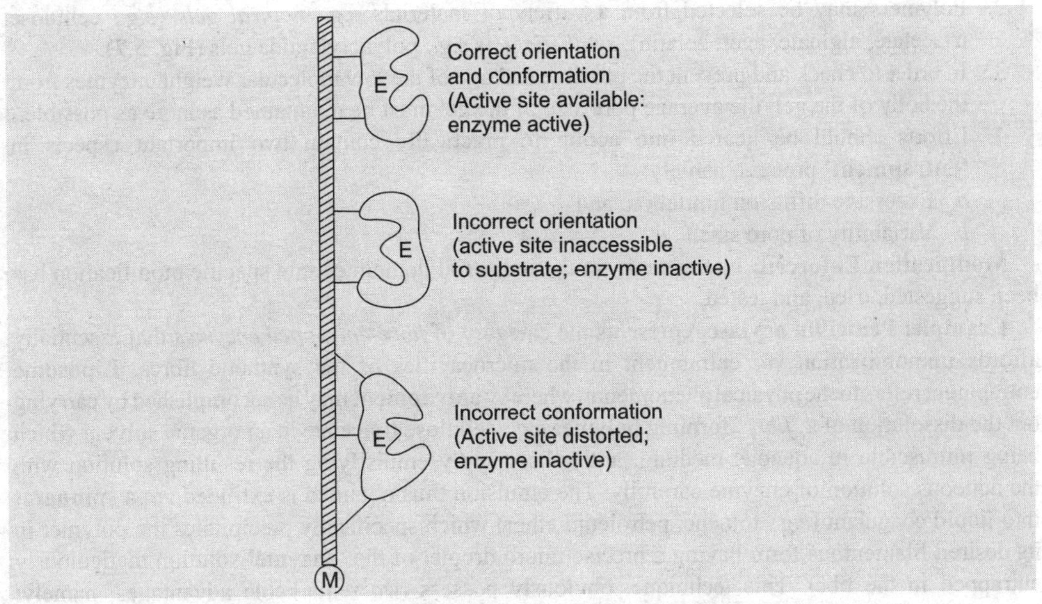

Fig. 5.6 *Enzyme Immobilization: Probable Effects by Covalent Bonding upon the Enzyme Activity*

5.2.3 Entrapment

Entrapment refers to the phenomenon whereby the *enzyme molecules* are either held or entrapped within the appropriate *fibers* or *gels*. Nevertheless, this entrapment may or may not necessarily be accomplished *via* covalent bonding existing between the enzyme entities (molecules) and the carrier matrix. Obviously the phenomenon pertaining to a non-covalent entrapment would be regarded as putting the '**enzyme molecule**' virtually in a **molecular cage** very much akin to a caged-bird or a caged-animal. In a situation when the covalent bonding is also needed, evidently the *enzyme molecules* essentially required to be treated with synthetic reagents *e.g.*, acryloyl chloride, cellulose acetate etc.

Examples:

1. **Lysine residues** may be prepared by employing *acryloyl chloride* resulting into the formation of the corresponding **acryloyl amides.** The acryloyl amides are *first* copolymerized, and *secondly* cross-linked with either acrylamide and bisacrylamide to give rise to the formation of the desired '**gel**' which comprises of the '**entrapped enzyme**' that may be further exploited in the form of a *thin film* on a solid support or as *small beads.*
2. **Cellulose acetate fibres** also find their application for the entrapment of enzymes. Enzyme and cellulose acetate is blended together to obtain an '**emulsion**' preferably in an organic solvent, methylene chloride. The resulting emulsion is subjected to the process of '**extrusion**' to obtain fibres into a solution of an aqueous precipitant. **Calcium alginate** is the material of choice used for the entrapment of *microbial, plant cells,* and *animal cells*.

Mechanism: Entrapment is exclusively based upon the coupling enzymes specific to the lattice of a polymer matrix or enclosing them in semi permeable membranes to check and prevent the release of proteins but permitting the adequate diffusion of substrates and products. Besides. **Entrapment** does not allow the binding of the enzyme itself either to the *gel matrix* or the *membrane.* Therefore, practically negligible inactivation of the ensuing '**biological activity**' of the enzyme takes place in comparison to the *coupling method.*

Methodology: The various steps involved in '**entrapment**' are as stated below:

1. The enzyme(s) may be dissolved in a solution of the polymer's precursors.

2. Polymers may be selected from a variety of materials *e.g., natural gels* (*e.g.,* cellulose triacetate, alginate, agar, gelatin); *synthetic gels e.g.,* polyacrylamide gels (Fig. 5.7).
3. In order to check and prevent the possible leakage of the low molecular weight enzymes from the body of the gel, the average pore size of the gel must be maintained as large as possible.
4. Efforts should be geared into action to practically contain two important aspects in **'entrapment'** process, namely:
   a. Excessive diffusion limitation, and
   b. Variability of pore size.

Modification Enforced: Interestingly, in the industrial domain certain specific modification has been suggested, tried, and tested.

Example: Penicillin acylase represents the category of *fibre-entrapped enzymes* that essentially affords immobilization *via* entrapment in the microcavities of the synthetic fibres. **Liposome** entrapment refers to the physical phenomenon whereby **entrapment** may be accomplished by carrying out the dissolution of a *'fibre'* forming polymer *e.g.,* cellulose triacetate in an organic solvent which being immiscible in aqueous medium, and subsequently emulsifying the resulting solution with the aqueous solution of enzyme carefully. The emulsion thus obtained is extruded *via* a **spinneret** into liquid coagulant (*e.g.,* toluene, petroleum ether) which specifically precipitates the polymer in its desired filamentous form having a precise micro droplet of the **'enzyme'** solution meticulously entrapped in the fiber. This technique, obviously possess *two* remarkable advantages, namely:

a. Minimises the diffusion limitation, and
b. Relative surface to volume ratio is appreciably high.

Figure 5.8 depicts the manner 'liposome entrapment' actually takes place.

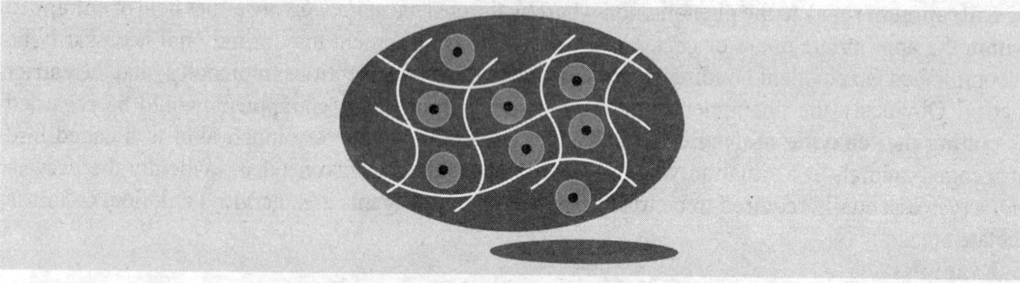

Fig. 5.7 *Enzyme immobilization via Polymer Entrapment*

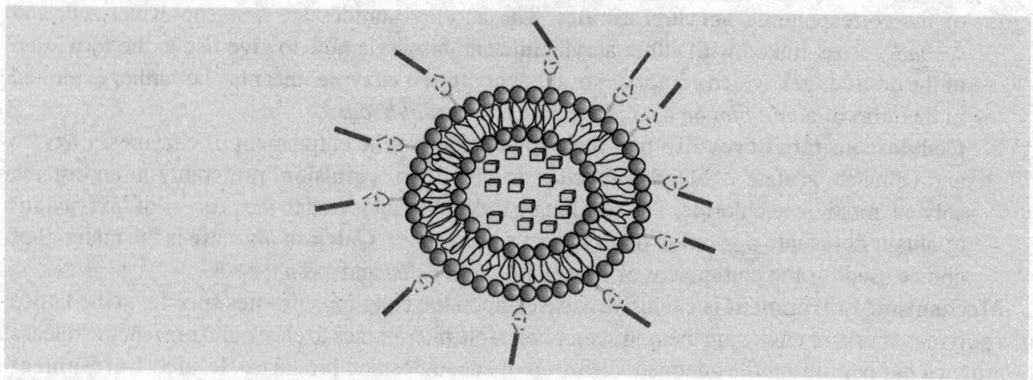

Fig. 5.8 *Enzyme Immobilization via Liposome Entrapment*

Another way to elaborate explicitely the manner whereby the *'enzyme'* may be entrapped inside a cross-linked gel matrix by allowing the formation of the gel very much in an aqueous medium having one or more than one enzymes. Thus, the **polymerization of the gel** is invariably performed in the presence of enzyme(s) which ultimately gets entrapped physically very much within the matrix; and, therefore, fail to escape *via* permeation at all, as shown in Fig. 5.9 below:

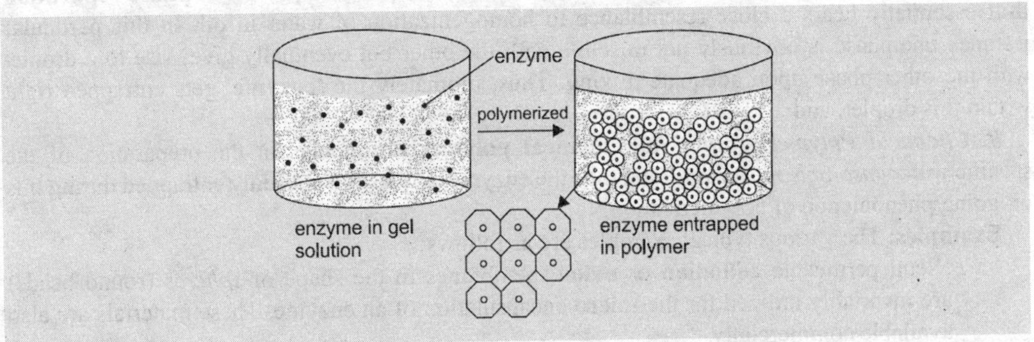

Fig. 5.9 *Entrapped Enzyme Inside a Polymerized Gel*

It has been observed that the **substrate molecules,** which are smaller in size, have a tendency to diffuse in, may be acted upon by the enzyme, and ultimately may diffuse out of the matrix. The most important and vital matrices for entrapping enzymes are **polyacrylamide, silicone rubber gel,** and **purified starch gel.** Nevertheless, the observed immobilization of enzymes afforded by such an *entrapment method* is invariably linked with *three* distinct kinds of difficulties, namely:

a. Continuous leakage of the entrapped enzyme by virtue of its abnormal wide pore-size distribution in the gel,

b. Significantly *lowered substrate accessibility* to the respective enzyme, and

c. Certain extent in the *'loss of enzyme activity'* on account of the **free radicals** generated frequently in the course of the polymerization process of the ensuing gel.

5.2.4 Encapsulation [Micro encapsulation; Membrane Confinement]

Encapsulation or **micro encapsulation** or **membrane confinement** is another versatile and effective approach in the field of *enzyme immobilization* specifically by entrapping technique. In this method the *enzyme molecules,* invariably taken up in an aqueous medium, may be strategically confined very much within a semi permeable membrane that ideally permits an almost absolute *'free movement'* of the enzymes in either direction to the products and substrates but fails to allow their migration and escape, eventually as depicted in Fig. 5.10(*a*) and (*b*). In other words, the enzyme immobilization prevailing in **encapsulation** method predominantly occurs well within the **microcapsules** meticulously prepared from organic polymers in order that the ensuing enzymes are prevented from the *'great escape'*; and, of course, the comparatively low molecular weight products and substrates do have a tendency to either **enter** or **leave** the *'capsule'* by diffusion *via* the membrane sooner or later.

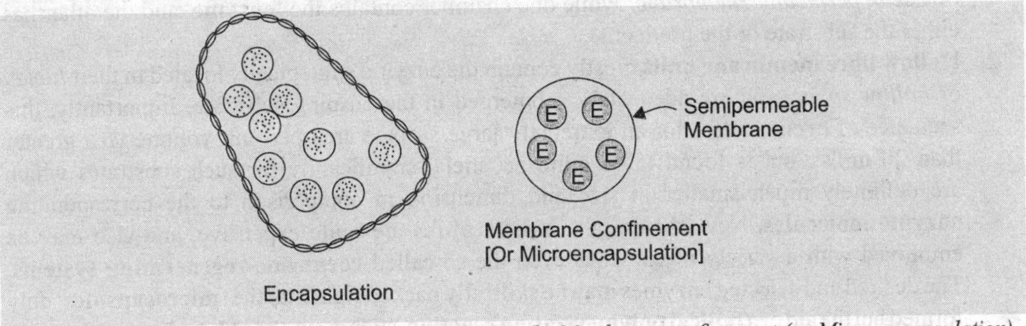

Fig. 5.10 *Enzyme Immobilization: (a) Encapsulation; (b) Membrane confinement (or Micro encapsulation)*

In actual practice, there are *two* well-known general methods for preparing the membranous capsules for **enzyme entrapping**, namely:

a. Phase Separation: Membranes are usually made by adopting the process of **phase-separation that** essentially bears a close resemblance to homogenization of water in oil. In this particular instance one phase is obviously not miscible with the other but eventually gives rise to a droplet with the other phase upon adequate mixing. Thus, ultimately the '**enzyme**' gets entrapped right within this droplet, and

b. Chemical Polymerization: The **chemical polymerization** aids in the preparation of the specific *water-insoluble membrane,* and thus the enzyme in question gets duly entrapped during this on-going phenomenon of polymerization.

Examples: The various typical examples are as follows:

i. Semi permeable **collodion** or **nylon** membranes in the shape of *spheres* (round beads) are invariably utilized for the **micro** encapsulation of an enzyme. These materials are also available commercially.

ii. Fibres of **cellulose triacetate** may also be employed for the entrapment of enzymes within this synthetic material. However, these fibres may be either woven into a suitable fabric or packed into the columns carefully.

Choice of Method: The choice of method exclusively depends upon the degree of immobilization corresponding to the specific enzyme involved, and its subsequent application. In fact, a rather broad spectrum of variation has been duly cited in the literature with respect to the actual level of retention of the ensuing enzyme activity (%) upon the immobilization to various commercially available support materials as summarized under:

Enzyme	Support	Method of Enzyme Immobilization	Retention of Enzyme Activity (%)
Aminocyclase	AE-Cellulose	Cross-linked with Glutaraldehyde	0.6
	CN Br-Activated Sephadex	Covalent Bonding	1.0
	CM-Sephadex C-50*	Ionic Bonding	0
	DEAE-Cellulose	–do–	55
	DEAE-Sephadex A-59	–do–	56
	Nylon	Encapsulation	36
	Polyacrylamide	Entrapment	53

A plethora of *viable, feasible,* and *tangible* strategies have been judiciously used for carrying out the phenomenon of **encapsulation** *(membrane confinement)* that may be enumerated briefly as under:

1. **Bioreactor** or **'reaction vessel'** may be partitioned into two separate compartments by means of a *semi permeable membrane;* while one chamber contains the '**enzyme**' and the other has either the substrate or the product.
2. **Hollow fibre membrane units** mostly contain the enzyme strategically located in their *lumen* or *hollow space,* and are adequately submerged in the ensuing substrate. Importantly, this sequence of events caters for an extremely large surface area per unit volume *viz.,* greater than 20 m^2L^{-1}, but is found to be quite beneficial significantly for such substrates which are definitely much smaller in size and dimension in comparison to the corresponding **enzyme molecules.** Nevertheless, the **hollow fibres** are quite expensive, and also may be employed with a variety of enzymes even the so-called **coenzyme-regenerating systems.**
3. The desired and selected enzymes may be skillfully packed right into the '**microcapsules**' duly formed but the aid of a **typical polymerization reaction,** such as: usage of **1, 6-diaminohexane.**

In conclusion, one may critically observe that each immobilization strategy does possess certain *strengths* and *weaknesses* that may be adequately summarized in Table 5.1. below:

Table 5.1 *Comparisons of Characteristic Features of Immobilization Techniques*

S.No	Characteristic Features	Immobilization Techniques			
		Adsorption	Covalent Bonding	Entrapment	Encapsulation
1.	Matrices (examples)	Clays; Glasses, Ion- exchange matrices	Acrylamide; Cellulose; Sepharse	Acrylamide; Cellulose acetate etc.	Semipermeable membranes via., hollow fibres, liposomes etc.
2.	Preparation	Simple	Difficult	Difficult	Simple
3.	Immobilization mechanism.	Hydrophobic effects; salt links etc.	Covalent bonds;	Trapping in gel or fibre;	Confinement in semi permeable membrane
4.	Binding force	Variable	Strong	Weak	Strong
5.	Enzyme loading	High (Ca. 1g/g matrix)	Low (Ca. 0.2g/g matrix)	—	—
6.	Enzyme leakage during usage	Yes	No	Yes	No
7.	Applicability	Wide	Selective	Wide	Very wide
8.	Problems encountered during operation	High	Low	High	High
9.	Matrix influences on enzyme	Yes	Yes	Yes	No
10.	Diffusional barriers to substrate and product molecules	Absent	Absent	Significantly large	Significantly large
11.	Protection from microbial attack	No	No	Yes	Yes
12.	Cost factor	Low	High	Moderate	High

Advantages of Enzyme Immobilization

It has been amply researched, proved, established, and recognized as well that **'enzyme immobilization'**, discussed under section 5.1.3.1 through 5.1.3.4, do afford a spectacular qualified success and remarkable advantages as stated under:

1. **Enzymes** being quite expensive and also having the unique ability to be used repeatedly only in a situation when these may be recovered completely from the accomplished reaction mixtures. In true sense, **immobilization** distinctly and specifically allows their repeated usage by virtue of the fact that *such enzyme preparation* may be separated conveniently from the reaction system involved.
2. Importantly, the final desired product should be readily from the *enzyme.* It goes a long way in affecting reduction and saving upon the cost of **'downstream processing'** of the ensuing end-product.
3. Non-aqueous systems (*i.e.,* using organic solvents exclusively) are found to be fairly compatible with the **immobilized enzymes** particularly, and this may be regarded to be extremely desirable in certain typical and specific instances.
4. *Immobilized enzymes* may be used predominantly in most **continuous production systems;** and, of course, this not absolutely feasible and possible with the *'free-enzymes'*.

5. *Immobilized enzymes,* a few selected ones, may exhibit **thermo stability** of the highest order, *viz.,* the free-enzyme **glucose isomerase's** usually gets denatured only at 45°C in solution; however, when **immobilized suitably** the enzyme is found to be stable enough upto 1 year at 65°C.
6. Importantly, the ultimate recovery of **'immobilized enzyme'** would drastically minimize the high effluent disposable problems (which is quite acute in several fermentation industries).
7. *Immobilized enzymes* may be employed at a much higher concentration range in comparison to the corresponding *free enzyme.*

Disadvantages of Enzyme Immobilization

Immobilized enzymes do offer several disadvantages which are briefly discussed in the section that follows:

1. *Enzyme immobilization* evidently gives rise to an additional bearing on cost. Hence, this improved technique is got to be used only in such an event when there prevails a sound economic viability, feasibility, safety, and above all a positive edge over the corresponding '*soluble enzymes*'.
2. Immobilization of enzymes invariably affects the **stability** and/or **activity** adversely. In order to circumvent such typical instances one may have to adhere strictly to the laid down developed **immobilization protocols.**
3. Practical utilization of the '*immobilized enzymes*' may not prove to be of any use or advantage when one of the substrates is found to be insoluble.
4. Certain *immobilization protocols* do offer a good number of serious problems with respect to the diffusion of the ensuing substrate to have an access to the corresponding *enzyme.*

Essential Requirements for Commercial Application of Immobilized Enzyme Systems:

The potential and enormous application of the **immobilized enzymes** gained a world-wide recognition in various industries particularly during the period 1970–'80. It is indeed worthwhile to mention here that during the late 1970s the specific **immobilized isomerase** turned out to be a grand and spectacular success in the commercial production of **high-fructose corn syrup (HFC - Syrup).** This product find its immense utilization particularly in the soft-drinks industry (*e.g.,* Coca-Cola; Pepsi, Campa-Cola, etc.).

The outcome of concerted research has made it abundantly possible for the skilful and gainful utility of *immobilized enzymes* and *whole cells,* as on date, for a broad-spectrum of industrially viable processes across the globe, a few typical examples are enlisted in the following Table: 5.2.

Table 5.2 *Typical Applications of Immobilized Enzymes and Whole Cells*

S.No.	Enzyme System Involved	Commercial Process
1.	**Immobilized Enzyme Systems:**	
	α-Amylase	Corn-Syrup production
	L-Amino acid oxidase	D-Amino acid production
	Flavoprotein oxidase	N-oxidation of drugs containing hydrazine Moieties
	Glucoamylase	Glucose production from corn syrup
	Invertase; Inulinases	Conversion of sucrose into glucose and fructose
	Lipases	Hydrolysis of oils
	Pectinase	Treatment of fruit juices
	Proteases	Hydrolysis of whey protein; cheese ripening.
	Ribonuclease	Nucleotide production from RNA
	'Δ Steroid hydrogenase	Production of prednisolone

	Tannase	Hydrolysis of tannins
	Urease	Estimation (assay) of urea
2.	**Whole Cell Systems:**	
	L-Arginine deaminase	Production of citrulline
	Aspartase	Production of L-aspartic acid
	Fumarase	Production of L-malic acid
	Glucose isomerase	Conversion of glucose to fructose
	L-Histidine ammonialyase	Production of urocanic acid
	Penicillin amidase	Production of 6-amino penicillinic acid (6-APA) for semi synthetic pencillns
	Yeast cells	Production of fuel ethanol (from molasses), and silent spirit from 'malt wort' in making alcoholic beverages (e.g., Scotch Whiskies etc.); removal of lactose from milk; primary beer fermentation.

Important Features: It must be grossly recognized and fully appreciated that in the perfect development of an immobilized enzyme system only a fraction of the total cost involved is actually implicated. In doing so, if one is able to maintain a justifiable and favorable **cost: benefit ratio,** one may go ahead not only towards the development, but also the commercial exploitation of the said immobilized enzyme system with full vigor and total confidence to accomplish 100% assured profitability.

5.3 Factors Affecting Enzyme Kinetics

Enzyme kinetics specifically refers to the in-depth study of '*enzymes in action*'. The abnormally high inherent rate of the induced enzyme-catalyzed reactions enormously obviates and facilitates this study. It has been established beyond any reasonable doubt that the physical and chemical nature of the carrier matrices employed, together with the conformational alterations in the enzyme structure after adequate immobilization, ultimately gives rise to the conversion of the ensuing catalyst to heterogeneous nature having significant changes in its characteristic features. The various effects caused duly by the altered reactivity essentially includes: *activity, pH, stability, optimum temperature, kinetic constants,* and *substrate specificity.*

It has been duly observed that the rate of reaction catalyzed by an enzyme particularly enhances '*linearity*' with the corresponding increase in the substrate concentration generally up to a certain point. However, it soon approaches the maximum value, usually termed as V_{max}; and beyond which there is absolutely no further enhancement in the rate of reaction as shown in Fig. 5.11. It is known as **saturation**.

Just contrary to this, is the rate of a *nonenzymatically catalyzed reaction* that enhances linearly very much across the *entire range of attainable substrate concentrations.* Importantly, the prevailing 'immobilization phenomenon' does help in the actual conversion of the catalyst from **homogeneous** (*i.e.,* soluble enzyme) nature to the **heterogeneous** one, whereby the enzyme is intimately associated either with a particular **enveloping matrix** or a **supporting matrix.** Nevertheless, in the course of immobilization phenomenon, the activity of ensuing enzyme is virtually lost by virtue of *two* vital reasons, namely: (*a*) various reactions involved in the process; and (*b*) effective occlusion of active sites in the enzyme support complex.

Examples

1. **Hem-containing proteins: Hemoglobin and catalase:** It has been observed that **hemoglobin** gets bound to O_2; and in doing so several O_2-molecules may bind and release during one

minute, while at any material time only one O_2 molecule becomes intimately associated with one hem centre.

Catalase — an enzyme invariably exerts a cumulative effect. In this particular instance, not more than one O_2 molecule gets bound per hem; and when it remains in the '*bound form*' it has a tendency to react progressively. Consequently, one may distinctly observe a very rapid evolution O_2 (*i.e.,* one million molecules per enzyme molecule per minute).

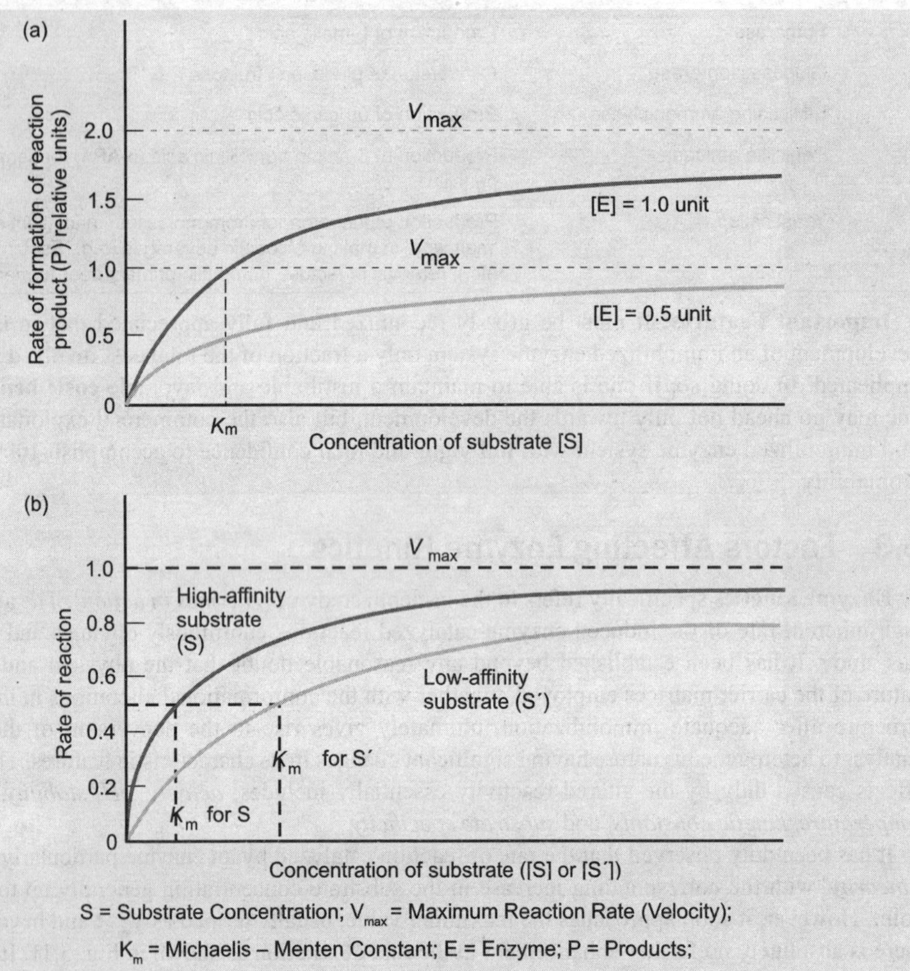

Fig. 5.11 *Effect of Initial Substrate Concentration upon Initial Reaction Velocity of Nonenzymatically [A] and Enzymatically [B] Catalyzed Reactions*

5.3.1 Enzyme Activity

Enzyme refers to an organic catalyst invariably produced by *'living cells'* but capable of acting either outside cells or even *in vitro*. Enzymes are **'proteins'** that change the rate of chemical reactions without needing an external energy source or being changed themselves; an enzymes may catalyze a reaction numerous times. Enzymes are **highly reaction specific** in that they act only on certain substances usually known as substrates. Nevertheless, the enzyme and its substrate or substrates invariably give rise to a temporary configuration, called an **enzyme-substrate complex** that essentially involves *both physical shape and chemical bonding.* The enzyme usually promotes the formation of bonds between separate substrates, or induces the breaking of bonds in a single substrate to form the product or products of reaction. The human body contains thousands of enzymes, each catalyzing one of the many reactions that eventually occur as part of metabolism.

In a broader sense, **enzymes** do carry out a plethora of remarkable and much needed rearrangements as well as chemical modifications both *in vivo* and *in vitro*. A few typical examples are given below to justify its magnanimous utility in the living biological systems, namely:

Rennin

1. Casein [Milk Protein] → Paracasein

Dehydrogenase

2. Ethanol [From Molasses] → Acetaldehyde + O_2 + H_2O

Oxidase

3. Glucose → Hydrogen Peroxide + Gluconic Acid

Catalase

4. Hydrogen Peroxide → Oxygen + Water

Lactase

5. Lactose [Milk Sugar] → Glucose + Fructose

α-Amylase

6. Starch [Barley; Maize] → Glucose + Maltose

β-Amylase

7. Starch [Barley; Maize] → Maltose + Dextrin

Rennin Oxidase

8. Sucrose [Starch] → Glucose → CO_2 + H_2O + O_2 + H_2O

Oxidase

9. Xanthenes → Uric Acid + H_2O

Deaminases

10. Amino Acids [Excess protein hydrolysates] → Removal of $-NH_2$ moieties

Lipase

11. Fatty Acids [Long-chain fatty acids] [Short-chain fatty acids] → Fatty Acids

The enzyme activity exclusively rests on the **'concentration of reactant'**; and, therefore, the rate of enzyme activity gets enhanced progressively with the increase in the concentration. One may observe the enhancement in the reaction-rate to maintain a *genuine linearity* along with increase in the substrate concentration; however, the linearity subsequently levels off at high concentrations, and, ultimately becomes independent of the prevailing concentration (see Fig. 5.11B).

Explanation: The above hypothesis may be explained by putting forward the simple argument explicitely that at high concentrations majority of the ensuing enzyme molecules do have their **'active sites occupied'**. Thus, the overall net rate of enzyme activity solely depends on the rate at which the bound reactants are converted into the respective products. Evidently, any extent of further increases in the '*substrate concentrations*' would exert practically little effect. In fact, the behavioural pattern of enzyme activity in the above context is widely termed as **Michaelis-Menten Mechanism.**

5.3.2 Michaelis-Menten Constant [Km]

Michaelis-Menten hypothesis assumes categorically that an **enzyme-catalyzed reaction** should normally take its course *via* several different stages, for instance:

Stage 1: Binding of enzyme (E) and substrate (S) would result into the formation of **enzyme substrate complex.**

Stage 2: Obvious catalysis takes place by virtue of the actual formation of transient **enzyme substrate (ES) complex.**

Stage 3: In a situation when the *substrate concentration* stands at higher ebb, further incorporation of enzyme would increase the reaction-rate appreciably, till such time the prevailing substrate concentration renders limiting:

Stage 4: Being the last stage the final conversion into product (P) predominantly takes place very much within the ES-complex (see stage-2); and subsequently the desired product gets released, whereas the *original free enzyme* eventually gets regenerated.

Figure 5.11B clearly shows a distinct direct proportionality existing between the reaction rate (V) and substrate concentration (S) till such time the prevailing enzyme concentration becomes limiting. Thus, at certain material time when the substrate concentration (S) affords almost half the maximal enzyme-reaction rate, the specific value is termed as **Michaelis-Menten Constant,** and designated as '$\mathbf{K_m}$'. It is, however, pertinent to state here that the normal observed $\mathbf{K_m}$ values for a large experimental data remain constant, besides found to be absolutely independent with respect to the quantum of enzymes present. Nevertheless, the usual Km-values for a host of enzymes reported so far ranges between 10^{-3} to 10^{-7} molar K_m.

Significance of K_m Values: The various important significance of K_m values are as follows:

1. Indicative of substrate concentration (S),
2. Affinity of enzyme with corresponding substrate,
3. Indicative partially of enzyme-substrate concentration prevailing in the **cellular compartment** *i.e.,* the target where most of the reaction invariably takes place.
4. K_m-values are found to be inversely proportional to the ensuing affinity of the enzyme for its substrate *i.e.,* higher K_m-values give rise to lower stability of the enzyme substrate [ES] - complex apparently.

5.3.2.1 Kinetic Characteristic Features

It is a well known fact, based upon the **'transition state theory'**, that whenever a chemical interaction takes place specifically between two reactant molecules, their free energy level usually should be distinctly elevated much above the threshold level so as to boost them up to an *extremely unstable*, and *high-energy state* termed as the **transition state.** Furthermore, the *'free energy'* essentially required to raise a molecule from its initial *'ground state'* to the attained unstable *'transition state'* invariably known as the **activation energy,** designated as G_0^1 as depicted in Fig. 5.12.

From Fig. 5.12 it is quite evident that the prevailing rate of a chemical reaction solely depends upon the number of available reactant entities (molecules) that do possess enough energy to attain critically the **'transition state'** pertaining particularly to the *'slowest step'* in the entire reaction profile, and is mostly known as the **'rate determining step'**. Importantly, one must take cognizance of the fact that only one-half of all the available molecules ultimately approaching the **transition state** would react to form the desired products; whereas, the remaining half shall be returning safely to the **low-energy ground-state reactant molecules.** Based on a generalized rule, only a rather scanty molecule would gainfully possess enough energy to reach the so called **transition state.**

It is, however, pertinent to mention here that the inherent magnitude of G_0^1 denotes the major factor limiting the rate of a chemical reaction *i.e.,* higher the value of G_0^1 the lower would be the prevailing rate of reaction. Interestingly, the — *'enzymes predominantly minimize the value of* $\Delta\ G_0^1$ *for a specific reaction, thereby overwhelmingly enhancing the ultimate rate of reactions'*, (see Fig. 5.13).

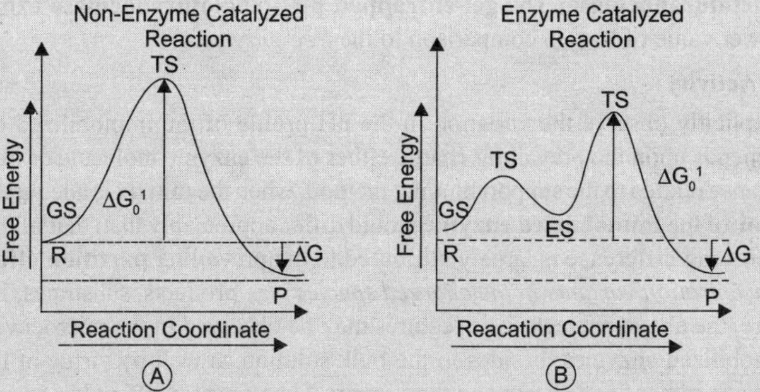

Fig. 5.12 *Reaction Coordinate Diagrams of Non-Enzyme Catalyzed Reaction [A] and a Enzyme Catalyzed Reaction [B]*

Important Points: There are three important points that must be taken into consideration, namely:

1. Energy levels and the stabilities of the products and reactants in a **chemical reaction,** when compared with those in the same reaction but catalyzed by an **enzyme** are more or less identical.
2. Rate of **reverse reaction** is increased by an almost same order of magnitude as that of the **forward reaction.**
3. **Enzymes** when compared to other *innumerable catalysts*, fails to alter the equilibrium ratio of the *reactants* as well as the products.

5.3.2.2 Parameters Governing Enzymatic Reactions

There are several cardinal parameters which categorically govern the enzymatic reactions, such as:

i. Maximum reaction velocity, (V_{max})
ii. pH Activity,
iii. Optimum temperature, (T_{opt})
iv. Stability,
v. Dissociation constants for substrate (K_s) and product (K_p),
vi. Turnover number or Rate constant (K_{cat}),
vii. Michaelis constant, (K_m)
viii. Specifically constant, (K_{cat}/K_m)
ix. Rate enhancement, (K_{cat}/K_{non}), and
x. Catalytic proficiency [$(K_{cat}/K_m)/K_{non}$].

The above parameters shall now be treated individually in the section that follows:

5.3.2.2.1 Maximum Reaction Velocity (V_{max})

The maximum reaction velocity of an *immobilized enzyme* is found to be practically the same as that obtained for the free enzyme. However, the precise effectiveness depends solely upon the ensuing enzyme activity together with diffusion limitation in the course of immobilization.

Examples:

1. **Glucoamylase:** It has been amply proved that the V_{max} value for an **immobilized glucoamylase** in the presence of *maltose as substrate* is 10 fold higher in comparison to the soluble enzyme (*i.e.,* **native enzyme**).

2. **β-D-Fructofuranocidase:** The **gel-entrapped β-D-fructofuranocidase** exhibits almost 10 times lower value of V_{max} in comparison to the *free-enzyme.*

5.3.2.2.2 pH Activity

One may explicitly observe the variation in the pH profile of the immobilized enzymes which prominently depends upon the prevailing charge either of the enzyme molecule or of the support. In the specific instance related to the support binding method, when the **matrix** is adequately charged, the **kinetic behavior** of the **immobilized enzyme** would differ appreciably than that of the free enzyme. However, the ensuing difference is largely attributed to the prevailing **partition effects** which may give rise to *concentration variants in the charged species viz.,* products, substrates, H^+ ion, OH^- ion etc. Furthermore, the above characteristic features may be observed in the microenvironment of the prevailing immobilized enzymes, besides in the bulk solution as well by virtue of the electrostatic interactions bearing rather fixed charges on the support. The **partition effect** has an overall tendency with respect to a corresponding shift in the **pH optima,** essentially exhibiting a definite displacement activity profile of the immobilized enzyme towards alkaline or acidic pH values for the negatively or positively charged matrices respectively.

Salient Features: The various salient features of pH activity profile are as follows:

a. Degree of shift of the pH profile shall entirely depend on the partition coefficient for the respective H^+ ions of the **'polymer matrix'** *e.g.,* for polymer anion the value is > 1; and for polymer cation it is < 1.

b. Broader pH profile may be observed in the event when the enzymes are coupled covalently to the respective support or entrapped in a gel securely. However, enzyme entrapment specifically in **neutral polymers** fails to exhibit any shift at **optimum pH.**

c. H^+ ions exert a marked and pronounced effect upon the enzyme activity; and this depends upon exclusively whether the initial pH is above or lies below the pH optimum.

d. Microenvironment pH would fall in a situation when the accumulation of H^+ ions stands above the pH optimum; and this in turn shall enhance the ensuing rate of enzyme reaction.

e. Substrate diffusion limitation may also induce a recognizable effect in the specific response of an enzyme to change in pH.

5.3.2.2.3 Optimum Temperature (Topt)

It has been duly established that enzymes do possess a **temperature optimum,** designated as Topt; and are found to be fairly active only in a narrow range of temperatures beyond that they are invariably get denatured readily and inactivated ultimately. A large segment of the enzymes are viable between 30 and 80°C.

Arrhenius Equation: Evidently, the *enzyme activity* as a **function of temperature** closely obeys the **Arrhenius Equation:**

$$k = Ae\ H/RT$$

Where, k = Rate of reaction, H = Energy of activation;
T = Absolute temperature; R = Gas constant; A = Arhenius constant;

It has been proved beyond any reasonable doubt that the usual denaturation of enzyme may be adequately protected by virtue of *two* physical phenomena, namely: (*a*) diffusional effects in case of entrapment; and (*b*) binding on porous supports. Obviously, the inherent **optimum temperature** of the prevailing enzymes turns out to be higher than that of the **native enzymes** (soluble enzymes). Diffusional effects that predominantly afford protection to the enzyme against the heat denaturation finally give rise to **deactivation energies** amalgamated with **lower rate of activation.** In reality, these critical **mass transfer effects** enhance with the increase in ensuing temperature. In actual practice, the *immobilized enzymes* accomplished via different means and ways prominently exhibits

lower activation energies, such as: (*i*) entrapment in gel; (*ii*) entrapment in fibre-structure; and (*iii*) support binding upon porous matrix.

5.3.2.2.4 Stability

The actual '*retention of enzyme activity*' for a relatively longer duration under the influence of proper storage conditions is of paramount importance. **Stability,** is governed by several vital factors, namely: (*a*) nature of the surface of '*carrier*' to which it gets bound intimately; (*b*) prevention of conformational inactivation; and (*c*) meticulous protection of *active moieties* on enzymes from the corresponding reactive groups in solutions increases the stability of immobilized enzymes.

Loss of Enzyme Activity: Enzyme activity may be impaired (lost) for several identified reasons, for instance:

1. Under usual operational parameters, the enzyme activity would suffer an appreciable loss on account of *two* distinct counts *viz.,* (*i*) enzyme denaturation; and (*ii*) physical loss from carrier.
2. Loss incurred *via* **matrix** could result either due to **carrier erosion** or from **gel-entrapment matrix** or from **cleavage of existing bonds between enzyme and carrier.**
3. It is an universal truth that *'covalent bonding'* certainly leads to **fairly stable enzyme preparations**; however, in several identified situations *e.g.,* physical absorption, feeble bonding, and ionically bound enzymes—the activity is lost significantly into solutions depending upon temperature, ionic strength, pH, and above all the prevailing physical operating parameters.
4. **Type of 'Bioreactor'** being employed also contributes a major determining factor for stability of enzymes.

Examples: *Abrasion* or *attrition* may tantamount to noticeable loss of activity for the immobilized enzymes strategically positioned on the respective organic support.

5. **Microbial contamination** would give rise to '*loss in activity*' under usual standard experimental parameters. In a specific instance when the immobilized enzymes are critically **diffusion limited,** they will display a rather slower apparent loss of activity in comparison to a situation when almost little **mass-transfer resistance** were present.
6. pH exerts its influence of enzyme stability. The '*partition effects*' may appreciably increase the **pH stability** of an ensuing immobilized enzyme.

Examples: Stability gets increased:

a. Towards 'alkaline range' — with immobilized enzymes on **polyanionic supports,** and
b. Towards 'acidic range' — with immobilized enzymes on **polycationic supports.**

7. **Heat Stability:** The plausible increment in **'heat stability'** may be accomplished either by *entrapment techniques* or *covalent coupling;* whereas, *ionic-linkage technique* or *physical adsorption* methods afford a distinct decline in the heat stability of enzymes.
8. **Storage stability:** The storage stability of enzymes may be enhanced *via* **covalent coupling** invariably at relatively low temperature *i.e.,* 40°C.

5.3.2.2.5 Dissociation Constants of Substrate (K_s) and Product (K_p)

It is a measure of dissociation. The dissociation constant of substrat is designated as Ks, whereas the dissociation constant of the product as K_p. The low values of K_s and K_p invariably give rise to inhibition of enzyme activity.

5.3.2.2.6 Turnover Number or Rate Constant [K_{cat}]

The **turnover number** refers to the specific activity of the enzyme and is usually quantified by K_{cat}. It may be obtained when V_{max} is divided by the enzyme concentration [E]. This designates the number of substrate molecules processed per enzyme molecule per second, and its value is generally 1000 but could be even much greater.

5.3.2.2.7 Michaelis Constant [K_m]

Michaclis constant or Michaelis Menten constant represented as K_m.

5.3.2.2.8 Specificity Constant [K_{cat}/K_m]

The **specificity constant** or **catalytic efficiency** of an enzyme is determined by the maximum specificity constant (K_{cat}/K_m). It precisely indicates the accurate rate of association of enzyme and substrate, besides the specificity for competing substrates.

5.3.2.2.9 Rate Enhancement [K_{cat}/K_{non}]

It has been observed that one may compare the rate constant of a **un catalysed reaction** (K_{non}) with that of the corresponding **catalysed reaction** (K_{cat}), and subsequently calculate the increase in reaction rate which an *enzyme* eventually yields. It is termed as the **rate enhancement** and designated as [K_{cat}/K_{non}].

5.3.2.2.10 Catalytic Proficiency [$(K_{cat}/K_m)/K_{non}$]

The proficiency of the catalytic ability of an enzyme is known as the **catalytic proficiency** and may be represented as [$(K_{cat}/K_m)/K_{non}$].

5.4 Profile of Some Important Enzymes

Quite a few typical human ailments, specifically those intimately associated with hereditary genetic disorders, there could be partial deficiency or even an absolute absence of one or more than one enzymes present in the tissue organs. It has been amply observed that in certain extreme abnormal conditions the unnatural and two much inherent activity of a particular enzyme in vivo could be adequately managed and controlled at times by a **'specific drug substance'** designed to control as well as inhibit its overall *catalytic activity.*

Enzymes are also required for carrying out various synthesis reactions in the living body. Evidently, the articulated synthesis of proteins, nucleic acids, phospholipids for cell membranes, hormones, and glycogen all essentially need at least one if not many enzymes. For instance: **DNA polymerase.** Is extremely needed for carrying out the phenomenon of **DNA replication that** precedes mitosis. Even blood clotting, the formation of angiotensins II to boost up blood pressure, and the transport of CO_2 in the blood also require specific enzymes.

Enzymes may be employed in the replacement therapy whereby either the *'missing enzyme'* or malfunctioning of certain impaired organs are corrected to prolong the life-expectancy of patients. A good number of **hereditary diseases** are caused due to deficiency of certain required enzymes that ultimately gives rise to a host of undesired, abnormal, and useless accumulation of substances in the body which otherwise would have undergone appropriate cleavage, such as; **Gaucher's disease** *i.e.,* a chronic congenital disorder of lipid metabolism caused by a deficiency of the enzyme **β-glucocerebrosidase; Tay-Sachs disease** *i.e.,* an inherited disease caused due to the lack of the enzyme **hexosaminidase** A, which is important in sphinogolipid metabolism; **Fabry's disease** *i.e.,* an inherited metabolic disase in which there is a **galactosidase** deficiency, which leads to accumulation of glycosphinogolipids throughout the body.

Adenosine deaminase deficiency invariably causes **severe combined immunodeficiency (SCID)** which would categorically respond to the desired and much required *enzyme replacement therapy,* wherein the said purified enzyme is first duly stabilized in polyethylene glycol (PEG), and then administered parenterally.

Interestingly, **oxidase-enzyme regenerating systems** or even simple **hydrolase's** may be exploited efficaciously for the enzyme replacement therapy. *Example:* in a typical instance of inherited deficiency of the enzyme **galactokinase,** the required treatments may be instituted by administering through injection the following *two* preparations sequentially:

i. **coencapsulated galactokinase** with ATP/ADP, and
ii. **pyruvatekinase** as an ATP generating system.

Another glaring and befitting example is a drug known widely as **tissue plasminogen activator** (TPA) that predominantly finds its usage to dissolve the *blood clots (i.e., thrombolysis)* which eventually cause occlusion of the arteries in myocardial infarction. TPA usually dissolves blood clots by the conversion of **plasminogen** into **plasmin.** However, TPA with great specificity and precision activities **plasmin** at the ensuing **fibrin clot. Plasmin** being an enzyme which exerts its activity by affording cleavage of the **protein fibrin** that eventually constitutes a major component of blood clot.

A number of vital and important enzymes below shall be discussed in an elaborated manner individually:

i. Hyaluronidase
ii. Penicillinase
iii. Streptokinase
iv. Streptodornase
v. Amylases
vi. Proteases

5.4.1 Hyaluronidase

It is an enzyme found in the *testes* and *semen.* It depolymerizes hyaluronic acid, thereby enhancing the permeability of connective tissues by dissolving the substances that essentially hold body cells together. It acts to disperse the cells of the *corona radiata* about the newly ovulated ovum, thus facilitating entry of the sperm.

The enzyme accelerates specifically the subcutaneous spread of the ensuing particulate matter. *Hyaluronidase* finds its abundant utility as a **dispersion agent** along with the other injected drugs being employed as a therapeutic measure. It is also used as a **potential adjunct** particularly in **subcutaneous urography** for not only augmenting but also markedly improving the *resorption of radiopaque agents*. Besides, it also helps in the enhancement of *'adsorption of drugs'* particularly in *transudates, tissue spaces,* and *oedemas.*

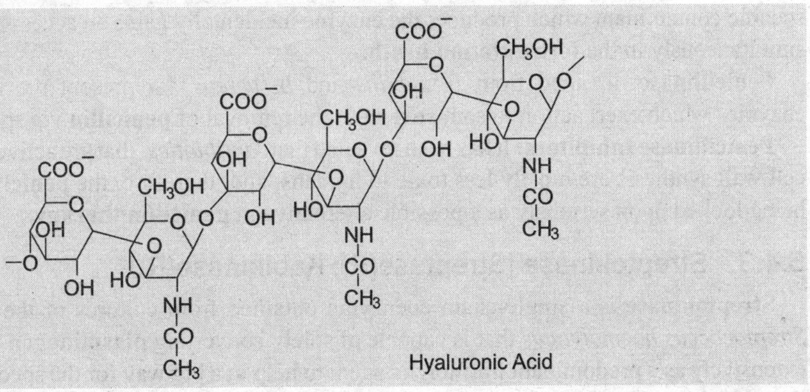

Hyaluronic Acid

Hyaluronidase for Injection [Wydase(R)]: It is obtained as a sterile dry, soluble enzyme product obtained from the mammalian (bovine) testes and capable of hydrolyzing *mucopolysaccharides* of the **hyaluronic acid type.** It usually contains not more than 0.25 µg of tyrosine for each **Hyaluronidase Unit.**

Therapeutic Applications: The various therapeutic applications are as follows:

1. It serves as intercellular cement that essentially binds together the paren-chymal cells. Probably the enzyme, *hyaluronidase* affords the hydrolysis of *hyaluronic acid* by splitting the glucosaminidic bond between C-1 of the glucosamine moiety and C-4 of glucoronic acid.

2. The most prominent clinical usage of *hyaluronidase* is to distinctly facilitate the administration of fluids by the aid of **hypodermoelysis.**

Cautions:

a. It must not be used in infected areas because of the danger of spreading the infection.

b. Its usage with local anesthetics is not recommended.

5.4.2 Penicillinase

Penicillinase is a *bacterial enzyme* that invariably inactivates most but not all *penicillin's.* Importantly, this is regarded as an *extra cellular type enzyme* produced adaptively by members of the coli form group of bacteria, by most *Bacillus* species, and certain strains of *Staphylococcus.* The enzyme exclusively carries out the hydrolysis of **penicillin** to **penicilloic acid** *i.e.,* a dicarboxylic acid as depicted below in Fig. 5.13.

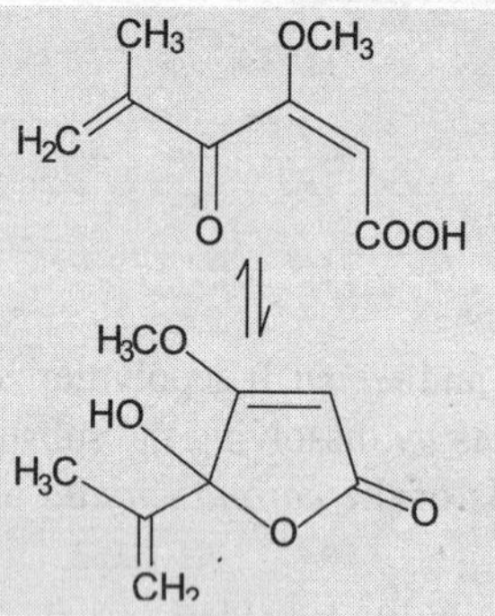

Fig. 5.13 *Hydrolysis of Penicillin to Penicilloic Acid by Penicillinase.*

It has been duly observed that a rather large segment of penicillin-resistant pathogenic strains of *Staphylococcus aureus* invariably comprise of this specific enzyme; and perhaps it overwhelmingly contributes a *major factor* of *penicillin resistance during infection.* Importantly, this enzyme causes an extremely rapid degradation of **penicillin** particularly in **penicillin fermentations** in case a specific contaminant which produces the enzyme incidentally gains an access to and be able to grow simultaneously in the **fermentation broth.**

Penicillinase obtained from *B. subtilis* and *B. cereus*** represent the industrially produced enzymes which exert action to some extent in the removal of **penicillin** *via* specific inactivation.

Penicillinase Inhibitors: It has been revealed that *'antibiotics'* that are active against the microbial cell wall synthesis are mostly less toxic to humans; and, therefore, the **penicillinase inhibitors** are being looked upon seriously as a possible alternative in **penicillin therapy.**

5.4.3 Streptokinase [Streptase(R); Kabikinase(R)]

Streptokinase is a single-chain coenzyme obtained from cultures of the Group C β-strain of *Streptococcus haemolyticus* that is capable of solely converting **plasminogen** to **plasmin.** It is used extensively as a predominant fibrinolytic agent to help in a big way for the specific removal of **fibrin thrombi** from arteries.

The Global utilization of Streptokinase and tPA of Occluded Arteries (GUSTO) trial was designed meticulously to investigate and establish the benefits of a **'front loaded'** dose of **alteplase** (a large initial bolus*** followed by an infusion of the total dose over a span of 90 minutes) when compared with the usual conventional alteplase administration.

Besides, an intensive and extensive study was carried out with respect to the safety and improvement in mortality of combining **alteplase** and **streptokinase** with either agent alone. Interestingly, the outcome of results from these extended investigations appears to exhibit an appreciably favorable mortality rate in patients having been treated with *alteplase* comparison to the *streptokinase* treated subjects.

A mixture of *streptokinase* and *streptodornase*, as produced by a hemolytic *streptococcus* grown in a specific environment of aerated-submerged culture, is used meticulously to clean up the debris from wounds and burns effectively.

Physical Properties: It is a hygroscopic white powder of friable solid. It is freely soluble in an aqueous medium; and quite unstable in concentrations of less than 10,000 IU. mL^{-1}.

Therapeutic Applications: The therapeutic applications of streptokinase are as stated below:

1. It is recommended for the management and control of myocardial infarction (AMI) in *adults* to bring about various therapeutic benefits, such as:
   - Specific lysis of intracoronary thrombi
   - Improvement in ventricular function
   - Remarkable reduction of mortality associated with AMI.
   - Reduction of infarct size and congestive heart failure associated with AMI when administered by the IV route.
2. It is also indicated for the adequate lysis of objectively diagnosed pulmonary emboli, involving obstruction of blood flow to a lobe or multiple segments, with or without unstable haemodynamics.
3. Besides, the **'drug'** is abundantly recommended for the lysis of objectively diagnosed, acute, and extensive thrombi of the **deep veins, emboli,** and **arterial thrombi** respectively.
4. Individuals having quite recent **streptococcal infections** may possess an appreciable quantum of circulating **antisteptokinase antibodies;** and to counteract this situation a *'loading dose'* sufficient to neutralize the prevailing **antibodies** is required urgently.

Streptokinase IP: Streptokinase (SK) — IP refers to a preparation as per the **Indian Pharmacopoeia,** of a specific protein obtained from the culture filtrates of certain strains of *Streptococcus haemolyticus* Group C. It possesses an inherent characteristic property of combining with human plasminogen to form the corresponding tissue-type plasminogen activator (tPA). The resulting product is duly purified to contain 4600 IU of SK activity corresponding to each μg of N before the addition of any **stabilizer** or **carrier.** It invariably comprises of a buffer and may be stabilized conveniently by the suitable incorporation of **human albumin**. It is categorized as a **fibrinolytic enzyme,** freely soluble in water, and may be administered by IV infusion.

Label on the container must clearly state whether or not the preparation is intended for use in the manufacture of injectable preparations.

Limit Tests: IP recommends limit tests for *three* substances namely: **streptodornase, streptolysis,** and the presence of **bacterial endotoxins.**

Biological Assay of Streptokinase: It essentially involves comparing its ability to activate **haemoplasmingen** to form **plasmin** with that of this 'standard preparation' the plasmin generated is obtained by measurement of the time taken to lyse a fibrin clot under the prevailing condition of assay.

Methodology: Three serial dilutions (*each in quadruplicate*) of the standard preparation are duly prepared with the aid of *citro-phosphate buffer* (pH 7.2) containing 3% (w/v) of bovine serum albumin and thrombin, such that the longest clot lysis time is less than 20 minutes. The test dilutions are also made in the same manner. The tubes are placed carefully in a water bath at 37°C, and using an automatic pipette, human euglobulin solution is meticulously introduced into the bottom of the tubes, thus ensuring thorough mixing. The addition is repeated to all the tubes at 5 second intervals. The time in seconds that elapses between the addition of euglobulins and lysis of the clot is measured in each one. Now, using the logarithms of the lysis time the result of assay is calculated by making use of standard statistical methods.

5.4.4 Streptodornase

Streptodornase refers to one of the enzymes produced by certain strains of haemolytic streptococci. It is capable of liquefying fibrinous and purulent exudates. It is also employed sometimes as a **wound debridement** *i.e.,* removal of damaged tissue.

Streptodornase is actually obtained from *Streptococcus haemolyticus* that affords depolymerization of polymerized deoxyribonucleo-proteins. It is used extensively in conjunction with **streptokinase** as desloughing agent to cleanse ulcers and promote the healing process progressively.

5.4.5 Amylases

It refers to a class of enzymes that specifically split or hydrolyze starch. In general, the **amylases** found in the animal kingdom are designated as α-amylases; and the one encountered in plant kingdom are represented as **β-amylases**.

It has been duly observed that a plethora of *bacteria* and *fungi* give rise to **α-amylases,** although the enzymes from these two sources are not identical. The bacterial amylases are relatively heat-resistant with an optimum temperature of ~ 55°C, which is a definite advantage over the corresponding fungal amylases when starch hydrolysis is to be performed at a higher temperature.

Applications of Amylases: The various glaring applications of amylases are as enumerated under:

1. Production of '*sweeteners*' for the food industry *e.g.,* glucose syrup; high mannose sugar; high-fructose syrup etc.
2. **Dextrin's:** The short-chain polymers, **dextrin's,** are produced by the hydrolysis of starch with *amylases,* followed by the disaccharide *maltose,* and ultimately *glucose* (*i.e.,* a monosaccharide).
3. **Maltose Syrup [>80% Maltose]: Maltose** with >80 brix (solids), which is specifically produced primarily in Japan, is of *low viscosity,* weakly hygroscopic, slightly sweet, and not crystallizable; however, possesses two remarkable characteristic features, namely: (*a*) shows good heat stability; and (*b*) fails to undergo browning reactions.
4. **Glucose Isomerase:** It is used invariably to convert **glucose** into **fructose** (*i.e.,* isomer of glucose) because the former is not nearly as sweet as the latter. Therefore, most of the commercial sweeteners based upon **fructose** do possess certain viable economic and manufacturing advantages over the conventional rather more widely used sweetener *sucrose.* The amylases are used commercially for the preparation of **sizing agents,** removal of **starch sizing from woven cloth, starch sizing pastes** for use in paper coatings, **liquefaction of heavy starch pastes** that form during heating steps in the manufacture of corn syrup and chocolate syrup, bread manufacturing, and removal of food spots in the dry-cleaning industry wherein the amylase functions in conjunction with the **protease enzymes.** It is, however, pertinent to mention here that these **'amylases'** may be exploited judiciously as a substitute for *'malt'* for carrying out hydrolysis of starch in the **brewing industry** (*i.e.,* for the commercial production of **'Lager Beer'.**

Based on the copious volume of information's with regard to the utilization of the **'amylases'** in a rather wider spectrum of genuine innovated products one may classify them into *two* well-known categories, namely:

a. α-Amylases, and *b.* β-Amylases.

The aforesaid *two* distinct categories of enzymes shall now be discussed individually in the section that follows:

5.4.5.1 α-Amylases [Diastase]

It is an **amylolytic enzyme** or a mixture of enzymes duly obtained from **fungi,** for instance: *Aspergillus oryzae* or from a nonpathogenic variant of **bacteria,** such as: *Bacillus subtilis;* and having the unique and characteristic highly specific activity of converting starch into *dextrin* and *maltose.* It may even contain certain suitable absolutely harmless diluents *e.g.*, dibasic calcium phosphate [$CaHPO_4$] or lactose.

α-**Amylases,** chemically known as [1,4-α-glucanglucanohydrolases], are basically the extracellular enzymes that specifically **hydrolyze α-1, 4-glycosidic bonds,** In latest literatures these enzymes are known as **endoenzymes,** responsible for affecting the cleavage of the substrate strategically positioned in the interior of the molecule. Interestingly, their action is least inhibited by the presence of α-**1, 6-glycosidic bonds,** although such bonds do not undergo splitting at all.

α-**Amylases** are usually classified based upon a plethora of cardinal characteristic features, such as: saccharogenic effect and/or starch-liquefying activity, temperature range, optimum pH, and stability. One may take cognizance of the fact that the **saccharogenic amylases** specifically give rise to the production of *'free-sugars'*; whereas, the **starch-liquefying amylases** predominantly initiate cleavage of the '*starch polymers*', but not necessarily yield *'free-sugars'*. In fact, there are many organisms which categorically produce several α-**amylases.**

α-**Amylases Producing Bacteria:** A large number of bacteria are particularly responsible for producing α-**amylases**, such as:

Bacillus subtilis; B. cereus; B. amyloliquefaciens; B. coagulans; B. polymyxa; B. stearothermophilus; B. caldolyticus; B. licheniformis; B. acidocaldarius; B. subtills var. amylosaccharaticus; Lactobacillus; Micrococcus; Pseudomonas; Arthrobacter; Eschrechia; Proteus; Thermomonospora; and Serratia.

It has been revealed that there exists *three* very much look-alike (identical) strains producing **saccharogenic** α-**amylases**, namely: *B. natto; B. subtilis Marburg; and B. subtils var. amylosaccharaticus.* However, the particular strain *B. amyloliquefaciens* differs from the other strains by virtue of the fact that it exclusively yields a **liquefying** α-**amylase.** Importantly, it has been well established that the *'substrate-concentration'* source as the determining factors with respect to the degree to which the '*enzymes*' would act in a liquefying or saccharogenic manner.

Besides, there are certain highly specific α-**amylase-producing fungi** categorically belonging to the genera *Aspergillus, Candida, Cephalosporium, Neurospora, Penicillium,* and *Rhizopus*.

Nevertheless, the molecular weights of various α-**amylases** do not necessarily differ widely as stated below:

S.No	Organism	Molecular Weight $\times 10^3$	Comments
1.	*Aspergillus oryzae*	51–52	Narrow difference
2.	*Aspergillus niger*	58–61	–
3.	*Bacillus acidocaldarius*	68	–
4.	*Bacillus amyloliquefaciens*	49	Wide difference
5.	*Bacillus subtilis*	24–100	–
6.	*Thermomonospora curvata*	62	–

Interestingly, all the α-**amylases** do contain a large proportion of **tyrosine** and **tryptophan** in the enzyme protein and most require **calcium as a stabilizer.**

One may observe critically that the most important and vital α-**amylases** are obtained from *Bacillus amyloliquefaciens*, *Bacillus licheniformis,* and *Aspergillus oryzae.* However, in actual practice the application and utilities of *Bacillus amylases* are much more extensive in comparison to the corresponding *Aspergillus amylases*. The extremely important and profusely applicable industrial usages of these *two* aforesaid varieties of α-**amylases** are duly summarized in Table: 5.1 below:

Table 5.1 *Extremely Important Industrial Applications of α-Amylases*

S.No	Name of Industry	Source		Applications
		Bacillus	Aspergillus	
1.	Alcohol [Ethanol]	+	+	Liquefaction of starch before incorporation of 'malt' for saccharification.
2.	Baked Products		+	Increase in the production of fermentable carbohydrates.
3.	Brewing		+	Improved fermentability of grains, and modification of beer characteristics.
		+		Barley preparation, and liquefaction of additives
4.	Feed Products	+		Improvement in utilization of enzymatically treated barley in poultry and cattle up-bringing.
5.	Laundry and detergent	+		Enhancement in 'cleansing power' for soiled clothing's mixed with starch, and additive in 'dishwashing detergents'.
6.	Milling	+	+	Supplementation of α-amylase deficient flour.
7.	Paper	+	+	Liquefaction of starch without sugar production for sizing of paper.
8.	Starch Products	+	+	Liquefaction of starch for production of glucose, fructose, and maltose.
9.	Sugar	+	+	Filterability improvement of cane sugar juice via cleavage of starch in juice.

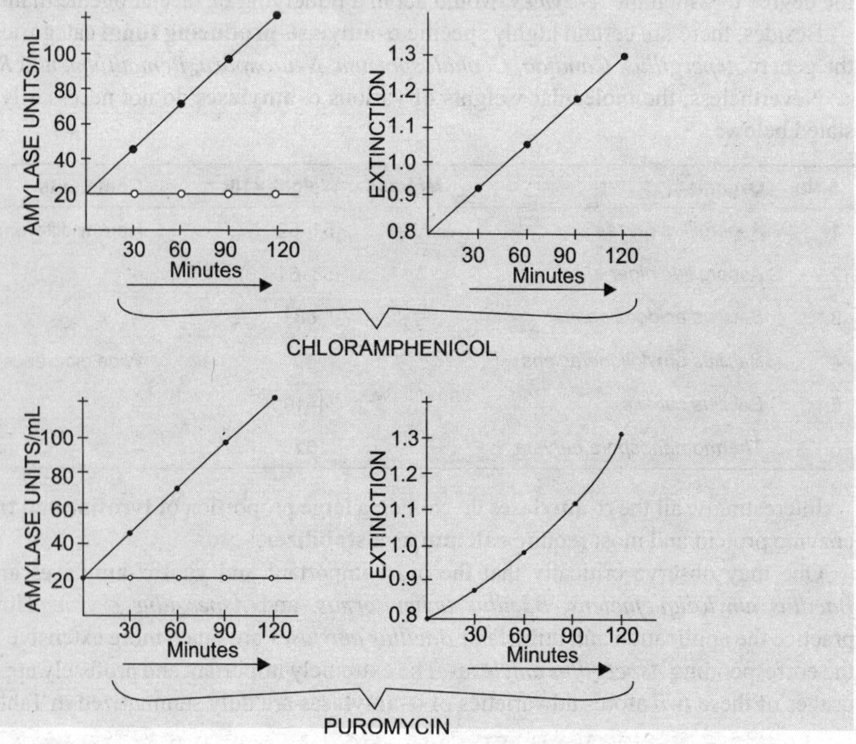

Fig. 5.14 *Effects of Chloramphenicol and Puromycin on the Production of α-Amylase in Bacillus subtilis*

Production of Bacterial α-Amylases: Essentially the production of **bacterial α-amylases** occurs solely due to the function of the normal cell machinery associated intimately with the *protein synthesis*.

Experimental Evidence: The addition of *'specific antibiotic substances'* can be used to prevent and inhibit specifically the protein synthesis in *B. subtilis* in the course of the production of α-**amylases,** thereby the *growth* and production of α-*amylase* cease virtually as shown in Fig. 5.14.

Chloramphenicol

Puroimycin

There are several evidences to ascertain the fact that production of α-**amylases** is meticulously modulated by a host of specific genes that have been only partially characterized till date. Interestingly, the *single-step mutations* invariably enhance productive yields by a factor ranging between 2 to 7, and the mutants have been judiciously selected after *five steps* which give rise to 250 folds higher yields in comparison to the corresponding **wild strain.**

The **industrial production,** α-*amylases* are subjected to either in **fed-batch** or in **batch** fermentation procedures. One may, in fact, observe explicitly that the ensuing 'enzyme-production rate' is exceedingly low particularly during exponential growth in *several actual production strains*; however, just prior to the growth rate gets decreased and spore formation commences, the amylase production enhances progressively as depicted in Fig. 5.15.

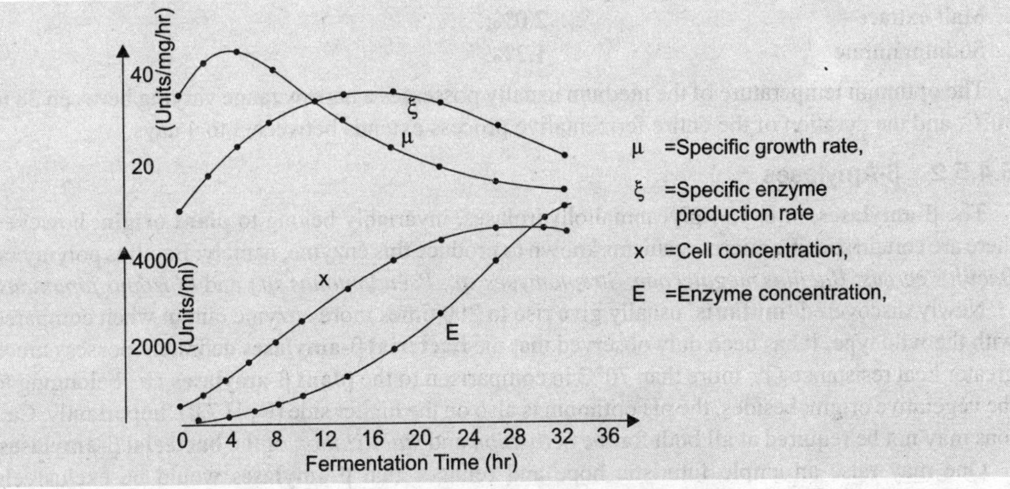

Fig. 5.15 *Production of Amylase in Bacteria Bacillus amylosolvens*

Medium: The composition of the **medium** for the usual production of α-*amylases* in a 100 m^3 fermentor using *Bacillus subtilis* as the organism comprises essentially of the following ingredients:

Ammonium nitrate (NH_4NO_3) : 0.56%;
Calcium chloride ($CaCl_2$. $2H_2O$) : 0.01%;
Peptone : 0.5%;
Potassium acid phosphate (KH_2PO_4) : 0.13%;
Magnesium sulphate ($MgSO_4$. $7H_2O$) : 0.01%;
Sodium citrate : 0.28%;
Starch : 5%;
Yeast extract : 0.2%;
pH : 6.8.

Salient Features: The various salient features are as follows:

1. Maximal specific enzyme formation rate is accomplished with the test strain at a temperature of 45°C after duration of 18 hours.
2. Maximal quantum of enzyme production, up to 3000 units. mL^{-1}, is invariably obtained at an appreciably lower temperature ranging between 27–30°C.
3. Latest newly developed processes make use of highly specific thermophilic strains (*i.e.*, heatloving or heat-stable strains).

Example: *Thermomonospora*, meticulously isolated from *compost*, possesses an optimum temperature of 53°C for the growth and amylase production.

Production of Fungal α-Amylases: It has been established beyond any reasonable doubt that the very production of **fungal amylases** is **constitutive**; however, as in the case of the other enzymes, it may be repressed by regulators.

Medium: The production of fungal α-amylases employing *Aspergillus oryzae* the **'medium'** having the following composition may be used:

Ferrous sulphate : 0.003%;
Potassium chloride : 0.05%;
Potassium basic phosphate [K_2HPO_4] : 0.1%;
Magnesium sulphate [$MgSO_4$] : 0.1%;
Magnesium nitrate [$Mg(NO_3)_2$] : 0.08%;
Magnesium phosphate [$Mg(H_2PO_4)_2$] : 0.05%;
Malt extract : 2.0%;
Sodium nitrate : 1.2%;

The optimum temperature of the medium usually possesses a narrow range varying between 28 to 30°C, and the duration of the entire fermentative process extends between 3 to 4 days.

5.4.5.2 β-Amylases

The β-**amylases**, or α-1, 4-glycanmaltohydrolases, invariably belong to **plant origin**; however, there are certain specific microorganisms known to produce this enzyme, namely: Bacillus polymyxa; *Bacillus cereus; Bacillus megaterium, Streptomyces sp.; Pseudomonas sp.;* and *Rhizopus japanicus.*

Newly discovered **'mutants'** usually give rise to 200 times more enzyme output when compared with the wild type. It has been duly observed that the **bacterial** β-**amylases** definitely possess much greater heat resistance *i.e.,* more than 70°C in comparison to the **plant** β-**amylases** *i.e.,* belonging to the vegetative origin; besides, the pH optimum is also on the higher side (~ pH 7.0). Importantly, Ca^{2+} ions may not be required at all both for the *activation* and *stabilization* of the **bacterial** β-**amylases.**

One may raise an ample futuristic hope and reliance that β-**amylases** would be exclusively exploited for the paramount production of **maltose syrup** to meet the global requirement.

α-**Amylase Preparations:** It is mostly used as a digestive enzyme with a dosage regimen from 200 to 500 mg per dose. The enzyme is found to be sparingly water soluble except when given in conjunction with an insoluble diluent.

Label Claim: The **label claim** of α-amylase (or diastase) preparation should include the following *four* specifications:

a. Nature and source of enzyme *e.g.*, fungal, bacterial,
b. Name of the organism from which enzyme is derived,
c. Amylase activity in terms of Units or Weight in g of starch digested by 1 g of enzyme, and
d. Name of any added diluent.

Assay Method: A specific quantity of the enzyme is triturated with a phosphate buffer of pH 6.0 meant for the **bacterial amylase** or with an acetate buffer of pH 5.0 meant for the **fungal amylase**; and subsequently diluted with the same buffer to give the corresponding **'test solution'**. The sample solution is filtered, if necessary. The filtered solution is carefully distributed into six stoppered test tubes containing the requisite quantum of starch substrate solution duly maintained at 40°C; the *'test solution'* is now added in graded quantities, mixed, and maintained at 40°C. After exactly 60 minutes, iodine solution is Incorporated and mixed thoroughly. The tube containing the lowest volume of test solution, which **does not show a bluish or violet** tinge, is recorded. From this observation the number of grammes of dry *soluble maize* or cornstarch digested by 1 g of the substance being examined is calculated. Ultimately, this gives the number of units of amylase activity pergramme.

5.4.6 Proteases [Proteolytic Enzymes]

Proteases or **proteolytic enzymes** refer to a class of enzymes that exclusively break down or hydrolyze, the peptide bonds [–CO–NH–] which join the array of amino acids in a **protein**. In this manner, the protein is cleaved into its so called **basic building blocks** (*i.e.*, amino acids).

Proteases are usually produced by a host of **bacteria,** for instance: species belonging to *Bacillus; Pseudomonas; Closstridium, Proteus,* and *Serrata;* and by a plethora of **fungi,** such as: *Aspergillus niger; Aspergillus oryzae; Aspergillus flavus;* and *Penicillium roquefortii.* It is, however, partinent to state here that the enzymes intimately associated with the aforesaid microorganisms are, in fact, mixtures of **proteinases** and **peptidases**; and the former usually get excreted right into the fermentation medium during growth phenomenon, whereas the latter are invariably liberated exclusively during autolysis of the cells.

As on date approximately 500 Metric Tonnes (MTs) of these enzymes (*i.e.*, solely based upon the pure protein) are consumed each year.

Commercial Applications of Proteases: The numerous legitimate applications of the **'proteases'** are as given under:

1. Primarily extensively in the **'detergent industry'**.
2. Employed extensively in the **'daily industry'**, *e.g.*, rennin.
3. For **'bating of hides'** in the **'leather industry'**, whereby the enzymes cause adequate alterations in the hides to provide a finer grain and texture, greater pliability, besides an overall improved general quality.
4. Proteases also find their usage in the textile industry to afford **proteinaceous sizing.**
5. In the **'silk-industry'** proteases help in the liberation of the silk fibres from the naturally occurring protenaceous material wherein they are actually imbedded.
6. Proteases (*e.g.*, papain) are also employed as a meat tenderizer.
7. As an active and vital component in most **spot-remover** preparations for removing foodspots in the **dry-cleaning** industry.
8. Other areas in which proteases are employed include: food industry, brewing industry, film industry, waste-disposal (processing) management, and manufacture of protein hydrolyzates.
9. Pharmaceutical industry also does make use of **proteases** in the manufacture of certain highly specific products for helping the suffering mankind.

In conclusion, one may add that the *fungal proteases* usually present a wider pH activity range than do either *bacterial proteases* or *animal proteases.* Besides, to a certain degree this definitely gives rise to a wider range of usages particularly meant for the **fungal proteases.**

Classification of Proteases: Based on a broad survey of literatures it is now possible to classify the **proteases** into *five* distinct categories, namely:

i. Alkaline proteases,
ii. Neutral proteases,
iii. Acid proteases,
iv. Fungal proteases, and
v. Bacterial proteases.

These *five* different types of proteases shall now be discussed individually in the section that follows:

5.4.6.1 Alkaline Proteases

A good number of *organisms* and *fungi* prominently excrete **alkaline proteases.** However, the **most predominant producers** are as given below:

Organisms: *Bacillus strains* : *e.g., B. amyloliqueficans; B. firmus; B. licheniformis; B. megaterium; and B. pumilis;*

Streptomyces strains : *e.g., S. fradiae; S. griseus; and S. rectus;*

Fungi: *Aspergillus strains* : *e.g., A. fleavus; A. niger; A. oryzae; and A. sojae;*

Examples: The various examples of **alkaline proteases** are:

1. **Bacillopeptidases:** These refer to the enzymes used exclusively in *detergents* derived from *Bacillus* strains.
2. **Subtilisin Carlsberg:** It is obtained from *B. licheniformis.*
3. **Subtilisin BPN and Subtilisin Novo:** They are obtained from *B.amyloliquefaciens.*

Interestingly, all the *three* aforesaid enzymes do contain **Serine** strategically located at the active site of the molecule. In addition to these observations they are not inhibited by EDTA (ethylene diamine tetraacetic acid) an organic ligand, but are adequately inhibited by DFP (diisopropyl fluorophosphate).

Detergent Enzymes: In general, the **proteases** of this type essentially possess a number of vital and important characteristic features for enabling their usage as **detergent enzymes,** such as:

- Reasonable stability at high temperature
- Fairly stable in the alkaline range *i.e.,* between pH 9–11
- Adequate stability in association with chelating agents *e.g.,* **EDTA,** and **perborates.**

It has been observed that their stability in the presence of surface-active agents is rather at a low ebb; hence, limits their shelf life significantly.

Salient Features of Alkaline Proteases: These are as follows:

1. Enzyme concentrates are marked commercially in a **micro-encapsulated form** because the *dry enzyme powder* may cause **serious allergic reactions** on exposure.
2. Suitable encapsulated product may be prepared by melting a wet paste of enzyme at 50–70°C along with a specific hydrophobic substance *viz.,* **polyethylene glycol (PEG);** and then converted into small tiny particles.
3. These tailor-made solidified tiny spherical particles (globules) are not hazardous **to health** even when incorporated directly into the detergent.
4. Efforts are already on top-gear towards the development with regard to two extremely feasible and viable aspects, namely: (*a*) in **granular product** form; and (b) in '*immobilization of enzymes*' in **fibrous polymers.**

5.4.6.2 Neutral Proteases

Evidently, both **bacteria** and **fungi** are responsible for the excretion of **neutral proteases.** Of course, the various organisms that may produce these neutral proteases include are as follows: *Bacillius cereus; B. megaterium; B. subtilis; Pseudomonas aeruginosa; Streptomyces griseus; Aspergillus oryzae; A. sojae,* and *Pericularia oryzae.*

Salient Features of Neutral Proteases: The various salient features of **neutral proteases** are as stated below:

1. These are comparatively unstable and *cations* like: Ca^{2+}, Na^+; *anions* like: Cl^-, should be incorporated adequately so as to attain maximum stability.
2. The pH range of activity, in terms of percentage, is significantly narrow; besides, the **neutral proteases** are not stable appreciably to elevated range of temperatures as may be observed in Fig. 5.16.

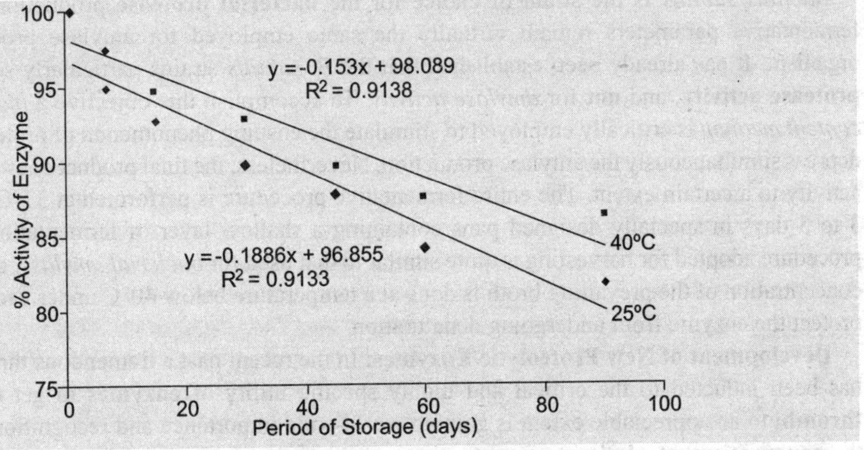

Fig. 5.16 *Temperature Stability Profile of a Neutral Protease*

It is pertinent to mention at this point in time that the **neutral proteases** get rapidly inactivated in the presence of the **alkaline proteases** (see section 5.4.6.1). Keeping in view these critical limitations, they do possess extremely restricted **industrial application(s).** However, these are employed extensively in the *food industry* for the manufacture of **bread rolls** and **cream-crackers;** besides, in the **leather industry.**

5.4.6.3 Acid Proteases

The **acid proteases** essentially include **rennin*-like proteases** obtained from fungi which are mostly employed in the commercial production of **'cheese'.** Besides, there are several other acid proteases that are similar to the mammalian **pepsin.** Generally, these enzymes do exhibit a pH optimum ranging between 2 to 4.

Acid proteases are used in a variety of manner in pharmaceutical and food industries as given below:

- In pharmaceutical preparations
- In digestion of '**soy protelin**' for soy-sauce production
- Cleavage of wheat gluten in the baking industry.

5.4.6.4 Fungal Proteases

A number of *fungi* give rise to the production of **fungal proteases** in an appreciable good yield. Thus, the large scale production of **fungal protease** has legitimately made use of a large cross section of fungal species; such as: *Mucor delemar; Aspergillus flavus; Aspergillus oryzae; Aspergillus wentii; Amylomyces rouxii.*

The most preferred media for the copious growth of fungus is the **wheat bran;** of course, certain other media are also exploited under specific fermentative parameters very much akin to those employed for amylase production. It has been duly observed that the various fungal proteolytic enzymes (proteases) are overwhelmingly present in the medium particularly at the **sporulation stage.** Subsequently, the proteases are meticulously recovered by adopting almost identical methods to those used for the **mold amylases.**

In fact, submerged fermentation procedures for the production of **fungal proteases** have been investigated duly at length, and there exists sufficient evidences to prove that such fermentations could turn out to be commercially viable and feasible in the near future.

5.4.6.5 Bacterial Proteases

Bacillus subtilis is the strain of choice for the **bacterial protease** production. However, the fermentative parameters remain virtually the same employed for amylase production by this organism. It has already been established that the *B. subtilis* strains particularly selected for **high protease activity**, and **not** for *amylase activity.* To accomplish this objective a *high carbohydrate content medium* is critically employed to stimulate the ensuing phenomenon of protease activity and depress simultaneously the amylase production. Nevertheless, the final product does contain amylase activity to a certain extent. The entire fermentative procedure is performed at 37°C for duration of 3 to 5 days in specially designed pans containing a shallow layer of fermentation medium. The procedure adopted for harvesting is quite similar to that used for *bacterial amylase,* except that usual concentration of the prevailing broth is done at a temperature below 40°C under vacuum in order to protect the enzyme from undergoing denaturation.

Development of New Proteolytic Enzymes: In the recent past a tremendous thrust and impetus has been inducted to the critical and highly specific utility of **enzymes** to get rid of **vascular thrombi** to an appreciable extent is gaining world-wide importance and recognition. Nevertheless, the **pancreatic proteolytic enzymes** (or **pancreatic proteases**) essentially serve as a '*vital adjunct*' to the treatment and management of **cystic fibrosis**. In the same vein, obviously the elucidation phenomenon of the pathways whereby enzymes explicitely exert anti-inflammatory activity profile would not only further enhance a greater in-depth understanding of the inflammatory mechanism, but also might lead to more efficacious enzyme preparations as well as dosage forms.

In the light of the aforesaid statement of facts the on-going development of newer breed of proteases (proteolytic enzymes) by the fermentative process immensely increases the scope and possibility of achieving these objectives squarely. However, there is another potentially exciting area is the apparent potentiation of '*drug penetration' vis-à-vis* observed *'clinical response'* when administered concomitantly with **proteolyic enzymes.** In case, this altogether new hypothesis or phenomenon is duly proved, confirmed, and established, it may ultimately pave the way to a rather more effective and vigorous *'therapy of antibiotics'* by virtue of the fact that an increased penetration of the drug of tissues of difficult access, or the greater pharmacological response at relatively lower dosage of drugs that are toxic in nature, with a resultant positive reduction in side-effects.

Besides, there is another equally vital area in the pretreatment of proteins exclusively for dietary and therapeutic purposes.

Examples: There are some typical examples to substantiate the above findings and observation, namely:

- Peptones for injection
- Digestion of lean beef with **pepsin** and **pancreatin proteases** for incorporation into dietary supplements
- **Trypsin** treated dermal collagen grafts after proper cross-linking with glutaraldehyde were not rejected.

Assay for Protease Activity: A solution of purified **casein** in water is prepared with the help of NaOH solution, adjusted the pH of 8.7, and diluted to a specified volume. A solution of the preparation under test is duly prepared in water by trituration and dilution. To the casein solution (previously warmed to 55°C) the unfiltered test solution is added, heated rapidly to 55°C, and maintained at this temperature for 20 minutes, and finally cooled to room temperature. To another casein solution unfiltered test solution, previously boiled and cooled, was added, heated to 55°C, cooled subsequently and incubated as above. To each solution then phenolphthalein and formaldehyde solutions were added duly, and titrated with standard alkali to pH 8.7. The difference between the aforesaid two titrations must not be less than 4.5 mL.

Thrombolytic Agents: The *'fibrinolytic system'** essentially comprises a group of proteins that interact complexly to afford the lysis of *thrombi,* besides to keep the fibrinolytic factors in check as far as possible. Plasminogen plays a major key role in the virtual activation of *fibrinolysis*. Indeed it is a *proenzyme* which is being converted to the active enzyme, *plasmin,* with the help of the following *two* important factors, namely:

a. **Intrinsic Factors:** *i.e.,* interactions among circulating intrinsic factors, such as: prekallikrein, kininogens, Factor XII, XIIIa, and

b. **Extrinsic Factor:** *e.g.,* Vitamin B_{12}.

There are some auxiliary factors also, such as: plasminogen proactivator, and the endothelial tissue which releases plasminogen activator, more precisely as tissue plasminogen activator-designated as **tPA**. The fibranolytic activity is kept in adequate control and check by such inhibitors as: $C1^-$ *inactivator*, α2-macroglobulin, and α2-antiplasmin. Importantly, once formed, plasmin cleaves fibrin into its corresponding split products.

It has been amply demonstrated and proved that both recombinant forms of **tPA**, namely: **Streptokinase** (SK), and **Urokinase** (UK) have significantly exhibited enormously lesser tendencies to produce haemorrhage as they exclusively get bound selectively to *fibrin* and not to the prevailing circulating *clotting factors*. In this manner, they are quite a bit selective for the **intended target** *i.e.,* a previously formed clot. Further evidences reveal that these are not absolutely free of the ensuing *'bleeding risk'*; however, as they invariably attack the many available **microclots** which are constantly being formed at the very sites of endothelial breaks, and hence clinical opinion is certainly divided over

Whether there prevails an appreciable advantage over SK and UK in this particular aspect. In true sense, target selectively affords a definite breeding problem, wherein the prevailing clots have a tendency to form around the IV catheters being employed for infusion, hence **heparin** is also usually infused to avoid this effect. Besides, their existing short-lives actually favor rethrombosis unless heparin is co administered. In fact, **anistreplase** and the other recombinant **tPA** products are appreciably much more expensive in comparison to SK or UK.

In the above context it is important to study a few typical examples of latest **thrombolytic agents,** namely: *alteplase, anistreplase,* and *reteplase*. These enzymes shall now be treated individually in the section that follows:

A. Alteplase (Recombinant) [Activase(R)]

It is a purified glycoprotein of a single, continuous chain containing 527 amino acids, with three carbohydrate side-chains. The biological potency is duly estimated by the help of an *in vitro* **clot-lysis assay** expressed in International Units [IU] as tested against a WHO standard.

Preparation: It is prepared by employing the complimentary DNA (cDNA) for natural human tissue-type plasminogen activator obtained from a **human melanoma cell line. Alteplase** gets secreted into the culture medium by an established cell line (Chinese hamester ovary cells) into which the DNA for alteplase has been meticulously inserted genetically. Ultimately, it is duly harvested, purified by chromatography, and lypholized. It is obtained finally as a white to off-white powder.

Therapeutic Applications: The therapeutic applications of **alteplase** are as given below:

1. It is indicated for thrombolysis in patients with acute myocardial infarction (MI), to improve upon the ventricular function, minimize the incidence of congestive heart failure, and reduce the rate of mortality.
2. It is also recommended in patients having acute massive pulmonary embolism, once the diagnosis has been adequately established by standard objective means and ways *e.g.,* **pulmonary angiography** or **lung scanning.**
3. In 1998, **activase (R)** was duly approved by US-FDA for the management and control of acute *ischemic* stroke in adults, for improving neurological recovery, and minimizing the incidence of disability.

B. Anistreplase [Eminase (R)]:

Preparation: Eminase ([R]) may be prepared by carrying out p-anisoylation of primary **human lys-plasminogen SK complex** (1:1) from **Group C β-haemolytic streptococci.** It is obtained as a white to off-white powder.

Therapeutic Applications: The various therapeutic applications of **anistreplase** are as stated under:

1. It is usually indicated for thrombolysis in patients exhibiting symptoms consistent with myocardial infarction (MI).
2. Randomized, controlled studies comparing it with either placebo or heparin-treated patients adequately demonstrated that Eminase(R) remarkably lowered the rate of mortality.

C. Reteplase [Retavase(R)]; 173–527-Plasminogen Activator (human tissue type):

Preparation: Reteplase is produced by recombinant DNA technology in *Esherichia coli*, and the protein is isolated as inactive inclusion bodies. It is converted into its respective active form by an *in vitro* folding process, and purified subsequently by chromatography. Potency is expressed in Units (U) employing a reference standard which is specific for **reteplase** and is not comparable with units used for other thrombolytic agents.

Figure 5.17 illustrates the diagrammatic representation of reteplase.

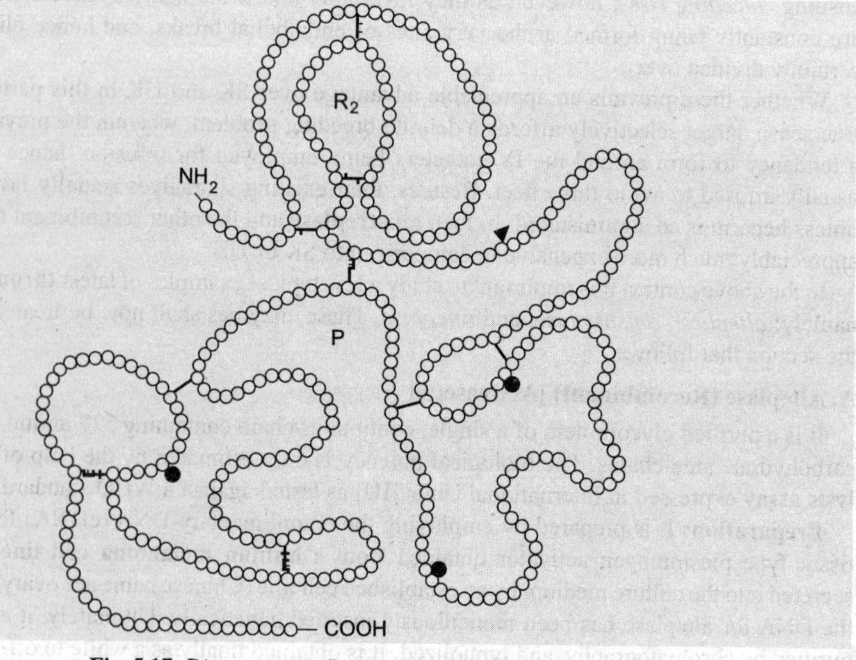

Fig. 5.17 *Diagrammatic Representation of Reteplase*

Therapeutic Applications: The various therapeutic applications of reteplase are enumerated below:

1. It is indicated mostly for the management and control of acute myocardial infarction (MI) specifically in adults for the improvement of ventricular function, reduction in the incidence of congestive heart failure, and above all considerable reduction of the rate of mortality intimately associated with myocardial infarction.
2. The genetically engineered deletion variant of human tissue plasminogen activator (tPA) is also recommended in pulmonary embolism.

5.5 Immobilization of Bacteria and Plant Cells

It has already been described earlier that **immobilization** particularly refers to — *'the imprisonment of a biocatalyst in a distinct phase which necessarily permits only exchange, but is clearly sepa rated from the bulk phase wherein the substrate, effectors, and inhibitor molecules are adequately dispersed and monitored.'*

5.5.1 Immobilization of Bacteria

The immobilization of bacteria (organism) may be explained by the help of fermentation of E. coli. for the production of **cytidine deaminase.**

It is well known that **cytidine deaminase** is extensively distributed among microorganisms, where its physiological role is confined to scavenge specifically exogenous and endogenous cytidine. However, in the particular instance of enteric bacteria, for instance: *E. coli.* and *Salmonella typhimurium,* the enzyme is appreciably inducible to high levels, thereby permitting these organisms to grow rapidly with *cytodine* as an exclusive source of nitrogen**. Therefore, it is worthwhile and also logical to look into *E. coli* as a source of large quantities of enzyme for actual usage in the production of **'Lamivudine'** [Epivir(R); Zeffix(R)], an **antiviral drug.**

Lamivudine

It has been demonstrated that cytidine deaminase production by *two* variants of *E. coli* strains **JM 10^{3}** and **B**, with and without cytidine are as follows;

S.No.	Strain of (E. Coli)	Scale	(–) Cytidine	(+) Cytidine
1.	JM103	50 mL	0.02	0.21
2.	B	50 mL	0.01	0.13

Based on the above findings one would expect the actual production to be approximately 10 folds as great in the presence of cytidine. In order to obviate the need to add cytidine to the fermentation broth, a constitutive mutant was virtually sought. Munch-Petersen *et al.* (1972) suggested that in *E. coli* both **cytidine deaminase** and **uridine phosphorylase** are coordinately expressed under the direct control of the **CytR repressor**. It has been observed that the expression of both genes is duly induced by **cytidine**, but not by **uridine.** As a result, the specific mutants which may grow progressively upon uridine are likely to have a defective CytR gene; and, therefore, will express both enzymes constitutively.

Nevertheless, the enzyme production by the constitutive mutant was just sufficient to support biotransformation process at a resonable **substantial scale;** however, for **production scale**, one may even require a still better source and type of enzyme. Such a challenging and herculein task was duly accomplished by **cloning** the **cytidine deaminase gene** (cdd) onto a multicopy plasmid under the control of the λPL promoter. Subsequently, the ensuing plasmid pPLcdd E was strategically introduced into *E. coli* TG1 (Amersham) by transformation, thereby attributing resistance to tetracycline. Thus, the recombinant strain [*E. coli* TG1 {p PLcdd E}, 3804 E] afforded ultimately an extremely high level of **cytidine deaminase production.** Importantly, the specific activity was found to be raised comfortably up to **80 times** than that accomplished with the constitutive mutant.

5.5.2 Immobilization of Plant Cells

Immobilization of plant cells has recently been developed as an alternative (substitute) methodology to the age-old suspension cultures for the exclusive production of **secondary metabolites.** *i.e.,* such metabolites which are known to be very necessary to plant life, many of them providing a defense mechanism against bacterial, viral, and fungal attack analogous to the immune system of animals.

Immobilized Plant Cells for Agriculture: In the recent past the enormous application of *'microbial inoculants'* have gained a tremendous momentum in the ever expanding domain of agriculture that could be anchored to the following *four* solid supporting facts, namely:

a. Apparent noticeable increment in **symbiotic** or **associative nitrogen fixation,**
b. Biological control and management of soil-borne plant pathogens,
c. Spectacular reduction in **aflatoxin** contents, and
d. Biodegradation of **xenobiotic** compounds.

It is, however, pertinent to emphasize at this juncture that in these bioactive processes, the critical survival of microbes under **biotic** as well as **abiotic** prevalent stresses emanated in the soil poses a **major limitation.** It has also been amply advocated that immobilization of microbial cells *via* various modes *e.g., entrapment, encapsulation* etc., in these specific instances has been proved to cater for adequate protection against these prevailing stresses.

Examples: The **two** typical examples are as given below:

a. Microbial cells entrapped in alginate:

These cells did survive against the environmental hazards of the soil; whereas, the actual survival of '*free cells*' (*i.e.,* the untrapped ones) was minimized astronomically under the prevailing drying/welting cycles in soil parameters, and

b. Algal Biofertilizers:

In this particular instance, the **algal biofertilizers** the phenomenon of immobilization not only displayed a positive edge in efficacy but also afforded a definite advantage.

Tissue Culture: Tissue culture refers to the growth of tissue *in vitro* on artificial media exclusively for experimental research. It is indeed a stark reality that tissue culture has immensely facilitated the techniques of microbial genetics as applicable specifically to the *higher plant cells.* One may strategically induce genetic variability in a relatively large homogeneous population of plant cells by adequate exposure to either chemical or physical **mutagens.** Thus, it is now quite possible to prepare various suspensions of appropriate cell cultures of higher plants, and maintain them more or less exactly in the same state for as long as one may desire. As a result, each single cell may prove to be as good as a potential bacterial cell for affording induction and followed by isolation of mutants and variants.

Nevertheless, the importance of cell culture depends upon the meticulous development of methodologies for enabling the isolation of a broad spectrum of cultured cell strains having apparent characteristic features that are entirely different from those of cells in the original cultures. Therefore, in order to isolate such obvious variant cell strains, established techniques in microbial studies may have to be enforced judiciously in cultured plant cell systems.

Application of Mutagens to Plant Cells: It is regarded to be an especially important methodology to enhance the ensuing frequency of variant strains in population of cells so that they may be easily identified and conveniently selected. The vigorous and constant search for **'chemicals'** that are virtually effective upon a broad spectrum of plant cell is invariably considered to be an important aspect of plant somatic cell mutant isolation.

In order to ascertain whether or not a particular substance is mutagenic exclusively depends upon the expression of an easily observed characteristic feature, such as: resistance to a *specific nucleic acid precursor analogue* termed as **6-azauracil**, present profusely different in **parent cells** and the subsequent **variants** derived from them after due treatment with the agent. Interestingly, the parent cells growing in culture are highly sensitive to this compound, whereas the variants which are apparently resistance to it, may be observed explicitely; and this difference forms the fundamental basis of its **'assay'.**

It has been established beyond any reasonable doubt that the ensuing *'difference'* is caused due to a highly deficient enzyme present in the **variant cells,** which is known as **uracilphosphoribosyl transferase,** and this actually affords a *'cidal action'* upon the cells. There are, in fact, *two* predominant strains of cells duly obtained from *two* altogether different species of plants, namely:

a. Haploid *Datura innoxia*, and

b. Diploid *Happolopappus gracilis*

That are found to be exerting resistance to this particular analogue have been meticulously isolated and exhibited to lack the aforesaid enzyme *i.e.,* uracilphosphoribosyltransferase.

Salient Features of Mutagens to Plant Cells: Following are some of the salient features of mutagens to plant cells:

1. **Higher plants** *e.g., Nicotiana tabacum,* and **ferns** *e.g., Todea barbara; Osmunda cinnamomea* helped in a big way for carrying out such studies.
2. Several varieties of **auxotrophic mutants** that essentially require *amino acids* and *vitamins* have been skillfully raised in *Todea barbara.*
3. Mutants that absolutely requiring *amino acids, purines,* and *vitamins* have been isolated with utmost success in *Nicotiana tabacum.*
4. Mutants that offer resistance to **Streptomycin** — an antibiotic; **8-Azaguanine** and **5-Bromo-2′-deoxyuridine** — base analogues have been isolated in higher plants as well.

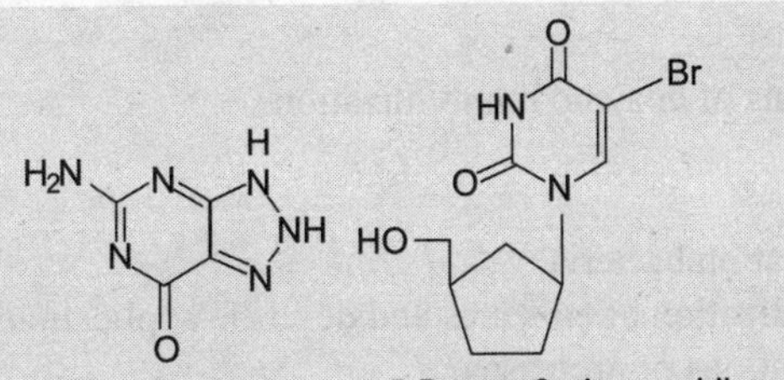

8-Azaguanine 5-Bromo-2 -deoxyuridine

5. **Auxotrophic** and **resistance mutants** are of utmost importance in carrying out the analyses of **genetic linkage, complementation,** and **recombination.**

6. **Inhibitors*** do play a major and pivotal role in the decephering of various metabolic pathways *in vivo*. Thus, by using different metabolic inhibitors one may conveniently affect virtually complete blockade of the *cellular metabolism* at a specific site; and, therefore, by critically examining the fall out of such blockages it becomes a lot easier to know exactly the nature of the pathway and also the factors responsible for controlling the entire process.
7. **Inhibitors** also help to control several cardinal functionalities, for instance; a specific step in DNA and RNA, protein anabolism (syntheses), and metabolic process of an organism.
8. **Mutants** also throw sufficient in-depth knowledge with regard to appropriate selection of products emanated due to *'fusion'* occurring between cells of variant genetic backgrounds (or **antecedents**).
9. **Mutants** solve a host of fundamental biological intricated problems to a great extent.
10. **Mutants** recovered carefully from cultured plant cells are really of **tremendous biotechnological importance**, and may serve as the basis of unfolding a good number of complex *agricultural, industrial* and *nutritional* problems speedily and logically.

Example: The wildfire disease in Tobacco is caused due to *Pseudomonas tabaci*. In fact, the tobacco cells that are specifically resistant to **wildfire toxin** have been recovered amongst a **mutagenized haploid cell population.** Therefore, *disease resistant tobacco plants* may be accomplished in *two* ways, namely:

i. Direct selection for resistance to a pathogen in the culture itself, and

ii. Appropriate selection of toxin resistance as a generalized means for producing particularly the disease resistant varieties.

Questions

1. Elaborate the various techniques involved in enzyme immobilization with suitable example. (JNTUA-May 2009)
2. Write note on hyaluronidase and streptokinase. (JNTUA-May 2009)
3. Explain various factors affecting enzyme kinetics. (JNTUA-May 2009)
4. Write short notes on immobilization of plant cells and tissue culture. (JNTUA-May 2009)
5. Medical prosthetics. (JNTUA-May 2009)
6. Write on production methodology of activase. (JNTUA-Nov 2010)
7. Explain various techniques of enzyme immobilization and factors affecting enzyme kinetics. (JNTUA-Nov 2010)
8. Protease. (JNTUA-Nov 2010)
9. How enzymes are classified? Explain. (JNTUA-May 2009)
10. Discuss about enzyme streptokinase along with its applications. (JNTUA-May 2009)
11. Humulin (JNTUA-Nov 2010)
12. Monoclate (JNTUA-Nov.2010)
13. Write the applications of enzyme immobilization. (JNTUA-Nov 2010)
14. Pencillinase (JNTUA-Nov 2010)
15. Hyaluronidase. (JNTUA-Nov 2010)
16. Describe immobilization bacteria. (JNTUA-Dec 2009)
17. Explain the immobilization of enzymes and describe applications. (JNTUA-Dec 2009)
18. What are the applications of proteases? (JNTUA-Dec 2009)
19. Describe the microbial production of protease enzyme. (JNTUA-Dec 2009)
20. Production of streptokinase by immobilized enzyme technology. (MGRU Apr-2004)
21. Mention ELISA test. (MGRU Apr-2004)

22. ELISA. (MGRU 2004)
23. Immobilization of enzymes. (MGRU 2004)
24. Write in short about the applications of animal cell tissue culture. (MGRU 2004)
25. Briefly explain amylase production. (MGRU 2003)
26. Discuss the procedure involved in extraction of enzymes from micro organisms. (MGRU 2004)
27. Explain the different methods of enzyme immobilization with examples. (MGRU 2004)
28. Write the salient features of enzyme immobilization?
29. Define carrier matrices? Explain their characteristic features?
30. Explain an enzyme immobilization with adsorption method?
31. Define hydrogels? How it is involved in the enzyme immobilization?
32. Write advantages of covalent bonding in enzyme immobilization?
33. Define an entrapment in enzyme immobilization with examples?
34. Define an encapsulation in enzyme immobilization with examples?
35. Write the advantages of enzyme immobilization?
36. Write the disadvantages of enzyme immobilization?
37. Define enzyme kinetics?
38. What is an enzyme activity?
39. Explain the factors affecting on enzyme kinetics?
40. What is Michaelis-Menten constant? Write the significance of Km value?
41. Write the kinetic characteristic features of enzymes?
42. Write the pH activity on enzyme kinetics?
43. Define optimum temperature? How the temperature affects on enzyme activity?
44. Define Turnover number?
45. Define specific constant?
46. Define rate enhancement of an enzyme activity?
47. Explain salient features of hyaluronidase?
48. Explain salient features of penicillinase?
49. Explain salient features of streptokinase?
50. Classify an amylase and explain its applications?
51. Write a short note on production of fungal α-amylase?
52. Write the classification of proteases?
53. Explain about alkaline proteases?
54. Explain about acid proteases?
55. Explain about alteplase?
56. What are secondary metabolites? How it is produced from the immobilization of plant cells?
57. Write short notes on immobilization of bacteria?
58. Write short notes on reteplase?
59. Write short notes on anistreplase?

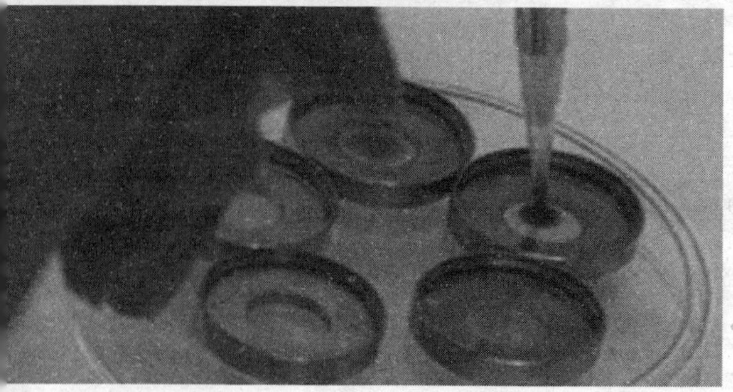

CHAPTER

6

Advent of Biotechnology

6.1 Introduction

The ever expanding advances in the domain of **'biosciences'**, related to both applied and fundamental; besides, the astronomical development of highly specialized disciplines, namely: Biochemistry,

Bioengineering, Genetics, Microbiology, Immunology, Molecular Biology and the like that have virtually converged the man's thinking towards one single objective aimed at utmost harvesting of economic benefits together with improved quality of life and environment. Based upon the most glaring and diversified applications of the aforesaid avenues and advances in the scope and knowledge of various disciplines helped in giving birth to a new terminology altogether known as **'Biotechnology'**, that essentially forms a bridge amongst biological sciences, physical sciences, and technological achievements.

In fact, this newer terminology came into being in mid 1970s, thereby superceding the earlier not-so-clear and ambiguous nomenclature *'bioengineering'*. Later on, this very term has been duly segregated into *two* different phrases as detailed below:

Biomedical Engineering: *i.e.,* the design and actual production of such products as: heart values, body scanners, pacemakers, artificial hips, artificial knee-joints etc.

Biochemical Engineering: *i.e.,* such chemical engineering phenomena that are based on organisms, biological substances, *viz.,* design of **'bioreactors'**, control product recovery, and purification.

The latest definition of **'biotechnology'** is as given below: *'the specific applications of scientific and engineering principles to the processing of materials by biological agents to provide goods and services'*.

Importantly, such agents invariably include a broad spectrum of biological substances, for instance: *enzymes, whole cells,* and *multicellular organisms.* Precisely in mid 1983, the word **'biotechnology'** almost attained the status of a *'buzzword';* and since then earned the reputation of a *'high technology'* symbol and *'god father'* image by institutions engaged in imparting tertiary education *viz.*, universities, IITs, etc.; besides, the corridors of the reputed corporate sectors. Undoubtedly, the impact was indeed so heavy and severe that the Government of India immediately decided to establish a separate department under the banner **'Department of Biotechnology' (DBT).** The main objective of this newly created department *i.e.,* DBT was to promote not only the educational institutions but also to boost up the adequate, meaningful, productive, result-oriented research programmes in the private industrial sectors as well. In a silent tone, it was a step well taken towards the legitimate and strategic advancements in the fields of biotechnology to catch up the progress and accomplishments already made in the Western World.

It is, however, pertinent to mention here that an extremely important aspect of biotechnology *i.e.,* **'genetic engineering'** is virtually becoming a topic of surmountable general interest and dire need by virtue of its long-term scope and possibilities in carrying out the legitimate alterations and improving the genetic heritage of agricultural plants, farm animals, and even human beings. However, the enormous inherent potential puts forward a number of vital and **important ethical, moral and ecological valid questions** that remain to be answered logically, apart from posing a **formidable scientific challenge.**

Nevertheless, the limit, horizon, and boundary of **'biotechnology'** is much wider in comparison to *'genetic engineering'*; and precisely the main emphasis in genetic engineering is exclusively and strategically concerned with the articulated manipulation of **bacteria** and **yeasts** rather higher organisms. **Biotechnology** may, with certain wisdom, knowledge, and skilful manipulative procedures be treated and regarded as a highly specialized 'single emerging area', albeit one having reasonably acceptable grey edges.

Biotechnologists in today's scenario deserve and command a much coveted and ever increasing recognition in a wide range of manufacturing and service industries thereby exploiting their acquired and specialized knowledge and expertise in various established biotechnological methodologies that apparently reduce costs effectively when compared to the age-old traditional procedures.

6.2 Advances In Biotechnology

In the light of the aforesaid *'advents in biotechnology'* a wide-spectrum of grey and prospective areas has emerged in the recent past that has inculcated a much deserved built-in confidence. A few vital and important examples are stated under:

i. Alcohol production,
ii. Algal biotechnology (Food),
iii. Biological fuel generation,
iv. Bioengineered plant materials,
v. Bioextractive metallurgy,
vi. Biopharmaceuticals (Pharmacobiotechnology based drugs)
vii. Cheese production,
viii. Indonesian Temph,
ix. Immunotoxins,
x. Japanese Enzymes
ix. Vegetative products, and
x. Newer approach to sewage treatment.

The aforesaid aspects shall now be treated briefly in the section that follows:

6.2.1 Alcohol Production

In general, the requirements for a glaring cost-effective fermentation of *organic feedstock's* for the fermentative production of **'alcohol'** from plant carbohydrates are as enumerated under:

- Reasonably lower transportation costs of raw materials.
- Low costs involved for conversion of **polymers** *viz.*, wood, cellulose, hemicellulose, starch etc. into their corresponding mono- and disaccharides.
- Application of *'mixed cultures'* so as to catabolize specially altogether different types of substrates and to convert them into the desired metabolite.
- Usage of highly characteristic **thermophilic strains** to minimize and save costs for cooling, to bring about excessive conversion rates, and also to lower drastically contamination risks.
- High energy consumption and demand for aeration, **anaerobic** methods are invariably preferred.
- Amenable to a feasible continuous process.
- Low recovery and concentration costs.

It is however, pertinent to state at this juncture that **'ethanol'** for utilization as a *chemical feedstock* was solely generated *via* fermentation in the early era of industrial microbiology. Interestingly, with the passage of time for many years it has been duly produced *via* chemical means instead, primarily through the catalytic hydration of ethylene ($CH_2 = CH_2$). Again in the recent past adequate and legitimate attention has turned towards the copious production of **ethanol** urgently required both for *fuel* and *chemical* utilities by the phenomenon of fermentation exclusively.

Examples: In 1986, three major countries in the world produced the following quantum of **'industrial ethanol':**

USA : 2.5×10^9 L
Germany : 1×10^8 L
Brazil : 1.1×10^{10} L

Agriculturally rich and intensive areas in Brazil, United States, and South Africa are under vigorous and intensive investigations with respect to the viable production of ethanol from various carbohydrates *e.g.*, **starch** and **sucrose.** The cardinal objective of such research oriented activities is to maximize exploitation of **'ethanol'** as a substitute for automobile fuel (*i.e.*, mixed usually with 'gasoline'). Of course in certain countries the 'ethanol' obtained from fermentative procedures is used exclusively to produce **petrochemicals** and **ethylene.**

Efficiency of energy conversion by fermentation to **'ethanol'** varies appreciably depending solely upon the type of 'raw material source' used.

Examples: Under optimal parameters the efficiency of energy yields is as stated under:

Carbohydrate Source	Efficiency of Energy Yield (%)
Cassava	50
Corn	25
Potatoes	59
Sugar beet	86
Sugar Cane	66

Biosynthesis of Ethanol: Bacteria and yeast possessing enormous potential have been employed for commercial production of ethanol, such as: the most abundantly used —

Organism (Bacteria) : *Zymomon l as mobilis*, and
Yeast : *Kluyveromyces fragilis; Saccharomyces cerevisiae*

It has been amply demonstrated that under **aerobic fermentative parameters** and also in the presence of **reasonable high glucose concentrations,** the yeast *Saccharomyces cerevisiae* no doubt grows very well but fails to yield any ethanol at all. Nevertheless, under strict **anaerobic conditions** the following steps occur sequentially as shown in Fig. 6.1 below:

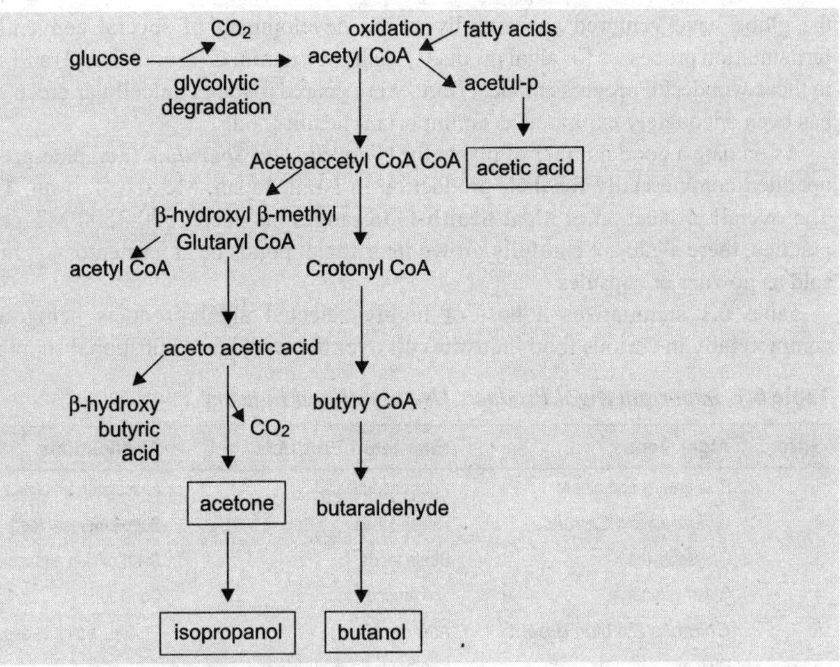

Fig. 6.1 *Biosynthesis of Ethanol*

Explanations: The various steps involved in the biosynthesis of ethanol may be explained as under:

Step 1: Growth of said yeast cells slows down.

Step 2: Pyruvate from '*glycolytic pathway*' gets split under the influence of enzyme '*pyruvate decarboxylase*' into corresponding **acetaldehyde** and **carbon dioxide.**

Step 3: Ultimately ethanol is produced from acetaldehyde by reduction with alcohol dehydrogenase ($NADH_2$).

Ethanol Tolerant Mutants: It has been duly established that by using **pure sugar solutions** one may accomplish ethanol concentration upto a maximum level of 10% only ; whereas, the skilful application of specifically designed **ethanol-tolerant mutants** one may even produce 12-13% ethanol, which are currently being scaled-up to full fledged production. Importantly, in recent years the widely acclaimed bacterium *Zymomonas mobilis* has, in fact, proved to be of tremendous potential advantages, namely:

i. Osmotic tolerance to higher sugar concentrations (upto 400 $g.L^{-1}$).

ii. Relatively enhanced ethanol tolerance (upto 130 $g.L^{-1}$).

iii. Increased specific growth rate in comparison to yeast (growth rate being, μ of 0.27 compared to 0.13 for yeast i.e., almost twice in laboratory culture studies).

iv. Anaerobic carbohydrate metabolism is invariably performed *via* the **Entner-Doudoroff pathway,** wherein only one mole of ATP is produced per mole of glucose consumed, thereby minimizing the quantum of glucose remarkably which gets converted to **biomass** rather than *ethanol* ultimately.

6.2.2 Algal Biotechnology (Food)

It has been established beyond any reasonable doubt that **algal mass cultures** do symbolize an overwhelmingly successful **food production program** thereby forging together agriculture and industrial fermentation meticulously. Since the past half-a-century a plethora of entrepreneurs across the globe have ventured successfully in the development of several conventional heterotrophic fermentation processes for algal products, such as : vitamin C (ascorbic acid) and steroids. In addition to these wonderful progress made, efforts were geared towards unicellular green algae *Chlorella* that has been adequately exploited as an important health food.

As on date a good number of plants for *Chlorella* and *Spurulina* (*i.e.,* blue-green algae) are being operated commercially for their production in Israil, Japan, Mexico, Taiwan, Thailand, and USA. The overall production of **algal health food** ranges between 2500-3500 MT per annum. In actual practice, there algae are carefully grown in artificial ponds or in fermentors, spray dried, and finally sold as powder or capsules.

Table 6.1 summarizes a host of highly selected algal products being used currently and commercially in various food industries all over the world as a nutritional supplement.

Table 6.1 *Important Algal Products Useful in Food Industry*

S.No.	Algal Genus	Emanated Products	Applications
1.	Blue greens and others	Pharmaceuticals	Anticancer antibiotics
2.	*Chlorella* and *Spirulina*	Health foods	Supplementary food
3.	Chrysophytes	Birala feeds	Seed raising aquaculture
4.	Chlamydomonas	Soil innoculum	Condition
5.	*Chlorella* and *blue greens*	Amino acids	Proline, arginine, aspartic acid
6.	Diatoms	Xanthophylls	–
7.	Dunaliella	β-Carotene	Food supplement and food colour
8.	Green algae	Vitamin C and E	Vitamin supplement
9.	Greens and Diatoms	Vegetable and Marine oils	Foods, feeds and supplement
10.	Red algae and blue-greens	Phycobiliproteins	Food colouring, Research

It has been revealed that the algal productivities in outdoor cultures evidently changes with suitable and favorable environmental climates. Thus, one may accomplish peak production ranging between 35–40 g^{-2} per day, and hence over a 300-day growing season per annum, an average overall productivity of 25 g^{-2} per day (or equivalent to 75 MT ha^{-1} per annum) is feasible. This essentially requires the effective utilization of productive algal species as well as preferred favourable conditions.

Nevertheless, one may have to observe the following parameters rigidly for all outdoor algal cultures for biotechnological production of food products, namely:

a. Applicability of highly selective experimental/plant parameters that critically favour dominance of one species,

b. Cultivation of algae which spontaneously crop up and dominate in ponds, and

c. Usage of well-defined and elaborated methodologies adopted for the prevention of ensuing contamination.

6.2.3 Biological Fuel Generation

It has been a great achievement for India to retain the world's third largest producer of **ethanol** *via* fermentative procedures next to USA and Brazil. India validly runs more than 125 distilleries across the country with an installed capacity of approximately 750 million liters per annum. However, the average yield of **ethanol** per MT of molasses ranges between 225-235 L depending on the content of residual cane sugar present in molasses. The major portion of **ethanol** is used up in various industrial applications, a reasonable proportion in making alcoholic beverages, and a certain quantum is utilized in the production of so called **'power gasoline'** as an automobile fuel energy. Industrial usage of ethanol encompasses a variety of products, such as: PVC, polyethylene (PE), synthetic rubber, solvents, pharmaceuticals, preservatives, and organic chemicals.

In a host of **'developing countries'** *e.g.,* Indian sub-continent, South-East Asia, African continent etc., the most judicious and practicable utility as **'diesel fuel'** is gaining wide recognition and tremendous popularity over the usual *petroleum variants.* Therefore, most approximately in these specified countries, the strategic conversion of *'biomass'* into **ethanol** (C_2H_5OH) and **methane** (CH_4) probably do not muster enough **primary interest** rather than to **device and develop** newer methods for the production of possible **diesel fuel substitutes** *via* intensive research and dogged determination, for instance: *alkanes, butanol* and *vegetable oils.* Besides, one may also exploit certain *available biomass sources* solely for **'diesel fuel generation',** such as : woody biomass yielding turpentine, extraction of oilseeds producing fuels, selected aquatic biomass (*viz.,* water hyacinth), and specific oil producing microorganisms (*viz., Botryococcus*). In fact, some of the vegetable oils do have the potential for being utilized as perspective (substitute) fuel in *'tractors'* that run on diesel only. Thus, the dual advantage of fast-growing, high yielding vegetable oils for use both as a **'food'** and a **'diesel fuel'** may turn out to be a certainly more attractive, feasible, and viable option that needs to be implemented rapidly.

Figure 6.2 illustrates the various aspects of **'biomass fermentative procedures'** thereby yielding much desired and valuable by products, namely: fuel oil, CO_2, and sugarcane bagasse.

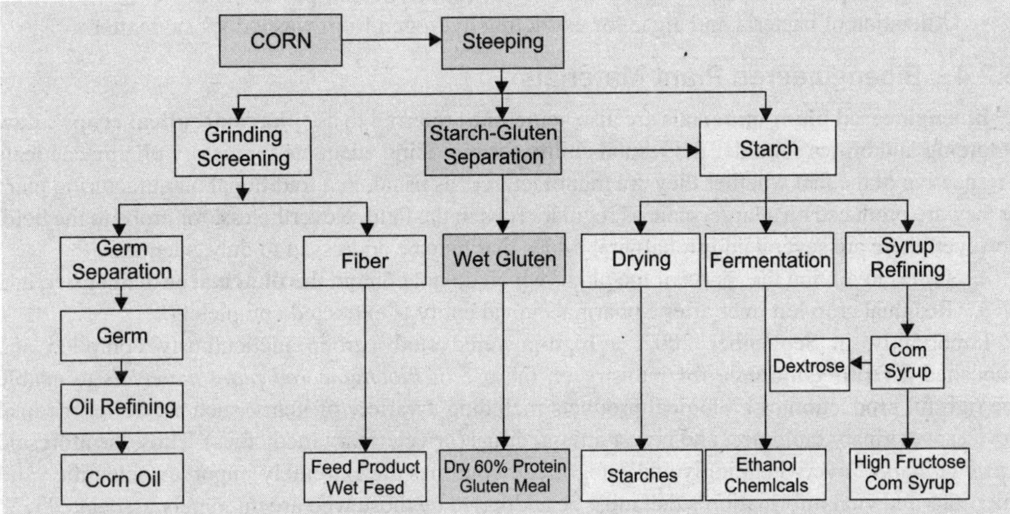

Fig. 6.2 *Sequential Conversion of Biomass into Value-added Products, Energy, and Industrial Feed Stocks.*

Growing Fuel: Biomass refers to solar energy stored in organic matter. The natural growth of plants and trees in the universe makes use of the phenomenon of *photosynthesis* thereby help in the conversion of energy from the sun in the form of CO_2 into **carbohydrates** *e.g.,* **cellulose, starches,** and **sugars.** In fact, the carbohydrates represent the organic chemical entities which exclusively make up the **'biomass'**. Eventually, when plants meet their fatal end, the very phenomenon of *'decay'* invariably gives rise to the *'energy'* stored in carbohydrates and discharges CO_2 back into the atmosphere. Hence, **biomass** designates a *'renewable source of energy'* by virtue of the fact that the growth of newer plants and trees replenishes the prevalent supply of carbohydrates.

Several millions of years, natural processes occurring in the earth meticulously transformed organic matter into present day's reserve of **fossil fuels,** otherwise termed as **non-renewable sources of energy,** which essentially comprise of *natural gas, crude oil,* and *coal* deposits; and these *three* components are being consumed regularly as on date across the globe with a ray of apprehension that they may not get exhausted one day leaving the world's consumers in peril and distress.

Interestingly, the actual usage of **'biomass'** for energy exploitation fails to enhance CO_2 emissions overwhelmingly; and, therefore, does not contribute significantly towards the possible risk of **'global climatic alteration'.** Contrarily, the legitimate consumption of **biomass** in this universe by mankind to generate energy is invariably regarded as a measure to dispose of nature's waste materials, perhaps as a scavenger, which may otherwise would create serious environmental risks.

In the very beginning of this new millennium (*i.e.,* 2001) United States only utilized **biomass sources** upto 3% of all energy consumed ; supplied more than 50% of all renewable energy utilized; represented nearly 10% of all electric generating capacity from renewable sources. However, in a global scenario **biomass** catered for more than six folds the combined energy provided by **geothermal, solar,** and **wind energy** sources. In true sense, globally **biomass** rightly and urgently meets almost 14% of the world's energy requirements efficaciously in the service of the mankind.

It is, however, pertinent to state here that the **'biomass energy'** presently refers to making exclusively '*fuel*', for instance: renewable **diesel** from plants, and **ethanol** ; but may also encompass incinerating plant materials and waste products *viz.,* skillfully tapping natural gas from garbage dumps, rice husk, and sawdust. Some newer emerging techniques include:

- Gasifying plant material to make fuel for electric plants
- Energy crops and fast growing trees for use in converted coal-power plants.
- Utilization of bacteria and algae for extracting hydrogen from waste disposal matter.

6.2.4 Bioengineered Plant Materials

Bioengineered plant materials are also sometimes referred to as **'pharmaceutical crops'.** Law enforcing authorities shoulder the responsibility for providing adequate regulatory pharmaceuticals irrespective of the fact whether they are manufactured, as usual, in a traditional manufacturing plant or they are produced on a large-scale as regular crops in the field. Nevertheless, for crops in the field, however, there are several additional vital issues that may be addressed to duly, such as:

a. Issues involving the 'parts of the plant' which do not contain the **pharmaceutical entity,** and

b. Residual crop left over after a pharmaceutical entity is extracted completely.

Importantly, in September 2002, a high-powered study group meticulously compiled and published a **Draft Guidance** for industry on the use of *bioengineered plant materials* to enable the rightful production of biological products including a variety of items, such as: newer medical devices, veterinary biologies, and newer animal drugs (or veterinary medicines). Thus, the aforesaid *'draft guidance'* overwhelmingly and categorically outlines the extremely important scientific valid questions and vital information's that must be addressed by those who are intimately associated with *bioengineered plant materials* to produce medical as well as veterinary products.

6.2.5 Bioextractive Metallurgy

The enormous thrust in current microbiological processes have significantly exploited, engaged, and adapted by the mineral industry are not only reasonably simple as well as practicable with regard to the specific engineering design, but also their actual effectiveness pertaining to their sensitivity to seasonal variations and sudden abrupt changes in the overall *'chemistry of the entire system'.*

Salient Features: The various salient features in *bioextractive metallurgy* are as follows:

1. Latest developments in the field of research focused towards the uptake of metals by *three* specific organisms, namely; *S. cerevisiae, R. arrhizus,* and *P. aeruginosa* render it possible, probable, and feasible that these microorganisms may be employed in particular precise processes for the recovery of metals from waste-water streams.
2. It has been duly established that the prevalent accumulation of metals by the host of microorganisms, irrespective of the method used, is certainly non-specific in nature.
3. Interestingly, the particular organisms essentially possessing **cellular components** are found to be extremely metal specific.

4. **Metallothionein** — a protein rich in S-containing amino acids, considered to be one of the best-recognized metal binding agents, provides a rich sulphhydryl (— SH) chelation site (*i.e.,* acts as the binding site).

Example: *Synechococcus* — *i.e.,* a marine cyanobacterium having a comparatively, small quantum of specific **'cadmium binding metallothionein'**, has the capability of binding an average of 1.28 atoms of Ca^{2+} per molecule of protein.

5. The most recent progress and accomplishment in the genetic manipulation of microorganisms in the domain of industrial purposes is geared up towards the *'leaching processes in metal bearing ores'*, and also the *'leaching involved in metal-contaminated waste waters'*.

Futuristic Programming: There are *seven* cardinal futuristic programming aspects in the **bioextractive metallurgy**, namely:

a. *Microbial genesis* of **methane** (CH_4) from organic residues in natural environments or **sulphur** (S) from sulphates,
b. *Volatilization* or *immobilization* of polluting toxic elements, for instance: arsenic (As); mercury (Hg),
c. Microbial disulphurization of coal,
d. Microbial removal of methane from coal mines,
e. Utilization of *aliphatic-hydrocarbon consuming bacteria* in **detecting petroleum deposits** (*i.e.,* exploration of natural petroleum deposits); besides various microbial processes for obtaining **'petroleum products'** from *tar sands* and *oil shale,*
f. Microbial processing and removal of **pyrites** (as impurities) from pottery clay, and
g. Immobilization of manganese (Mn), and recovery of Mn and radium (Ra) from the tailings *via* the application of microorganisms employing **bioaccumulation** or **accretion** or **bioconversion.**

6.2.6 Biopharmaceuticals (Pharmacobiotechnology Based Drugs)

Biopharmaceuticals may be defined as — *'complex macromolecules derived from recombinant DNA technology, cell fusion or such processes that essentially involve genetic manipulation.*

Examples: Biopharmaceuticals include: recombinant proteins, therapeutic monoclonal antibodies (MABs) and nucleic acid-based therapeutics (*viz.,* DNA-based medicines), genetically engineered vaccines, and gene therapy vectors.

In 1982, the first and foremost drug ever produced via genetic engineering was the wonder drug known as **'human insulin'**. Almost within a span of two decades (by mid-2000), **eighty four biopharmaceuticals** were duly approved for marketing by US-FDA, of which around forty were introduced between mid-1997 and mid-2000. In USA, the worldwide sales of these specialized drugs shot upto USD 15 billion by the end of 1998. Interestingly, USA distinctly represented almost 46% of the market in comparison to mere 36% for the *usual conventional drugs* by virtue of the following cardinal factors, such as:

- earlier regulatory approval (US-FDA)
- easier market acceptance
- much greater pricing flexibility than other countries on the globe.

No doubt, the **biopharmaceuticals** do represent rather small 5% of the world's prescription drug sales, they normally account for six of the world's top 50 best selling drugs. It is quite important to have a clear and distinct concept in mind between the following *two* important aspects, namely:

a. *Biotechnology* — as a new process technology, and
b. *Biotechnology* — as a *'drug discovery'* research tool.

Obviously, the *first* makes use of **'genetic engineering'** almost exclusively in the specialized and critical manufacture of only **large molecular weight drugs** *e.g.,* insulin, vaccine etc., which are rather difficult and impracticable to be produced either by synthesis or by extraction.

Evidently, the second aspect involves the meticulous search for **newer therapeutic targets**, with a large emphasis on the focus upon certain specific **small molecular weight drugs** which could easily and conveniently interact against those targets by the help of biotechnology based research tools, such as:

- cloned receptors as screens, and
- gene knock-out technologies

In the most specialized formation of transgenic organisms to determine protein function.

It is indeed pertinent to mention at this point in time that the **pharmaceutical industry** across the globe shall definitely hold and maintain its ever dominant status with regard to the discovery of '*small molecules*' *via* the meticulous application of **biotechnology** in drug discovery; whereas, the conceptualized ideas, development, and ultimate manufacture of *highly specific protein-based drugs* certainly need an altogether completely different degree of core competencies.

Biopharmaceuticals *i.e., biotechnology based drugs* may be broadly categorized into *two* heads, namely:

a. Approved medicines, and
b. Medicines under development.

The *two* different categories of biotechnology medicines shall be exemplified in the section that follows:

Approved Medicines: A few typical examples of **'approved medicines'** by several drug authorities are enumerated below:

S.No.	Algal Genus	Emanated Products	Applications
1.	Blue greens and others	Pharmaceuticals	Anticancer antibiotics
2.	*Chlorella* and *Spirulina*	Health foods	Supplementary food
3.	Chrysophytes	Birala feeds	Seed raising aquaculture
4.	Chlamydomonas	Soil innoculum	Condition
5.	*Chlorella* and *blue greens*	Amino acids	Proline, arginine, aspartic acid
6.	Diatoms	Xanthophylls	–
7.	Dunaliella	β-Carotene	Food supplement and food colour
8.	Green algae	Vitamin C and E	Vitamin supplement
9.	Greens and Diatoms	Vegetable and Marine oils	Foods, feeds and supplement
10.	Red algae and blue-greens	Phycobiliproteins	Food colouring, Research

Medicines under Development: Certain specific examples of such **'medicines under development'** are as stated under:

S.No.	Name of Product	Company	Indication (s)
1.	**Recombinant human platelet derived growth factor—BB (PDGF)**	Chiron (Emeryville, CA)	Wound healing;
2.	**Immuneron (Interferon gamma)**	Biogen (Cambridge MA)	Multiple sclerosis;
3.	**Cento RX (Mab)**	Centocor (Malvern, PA)	Anti-platelet prevention of blood clots ;
4.	**Myoscint (Mifarmonab)**	Centocor (Malvern, PA)	Cardiac imaging agents ;
5.	**Vax-Syn(R) HIV-1 (gp 160)**	Micro Gene Sys(Menden, CT)	AIDS ;

6.2.7 Cheese Production

Milk is regarded perhaps one of the first and foremost agricultural products which gets rapidly infected by the organism *Lactobacillus* and sour it by converting the milk-sugar *lactose* into the corresponding **lactic acid**. **Cheese** is, therefore, **one of the first fermented food products**. Since, then with the advent of tremendous innovative ideas and concepts with respect to the development of this spontaneous process received a substantial thrust to make *cheese* and allied products across the globe. In this context, the Netherlands, Denmark, Germany, and France were recognized in the world towards the development as well as production of a variety of processed cheese. Thus, cheese making is a milestone in the history of food processing and technology.

Technically, **cheese** refers to the dairy product, duly obtained from microorganisms, is produced from the Casein (*i.e.,* milk protein) of the milk. Initially, the protein gets curdled by the acid produced by the presence of streptococci in the milk. However, the process of curdling is adequately accelerated by the incorporation of **rennin** *i.e.,* an enzyme specifically derived from the inner stomach living of the calf. The acidic curd is separated from the liquid whey, which is employed to make '*whey powder*', and the curd is treated further to obtain a large variety of processed cheese.

6.2.8 Indonesian Temph

The **'Indonesian Temph'** is widely used vegetarian dish, quite rich in Vitamin B_{12}; and is usually prepared from *soyabeans* that are duly soaked and fermented. In general, the fungal fermentation with *Rhizopus* sp. is invariably preceded by a typical bacterial acid fermentation when soyabean is soaked. The fermentative process gets completed when the beans are virtually transformed into a **'compact cake'** by the mold *mycelium.* The resulting cake is sliced, and subsequently deep-fried in vegetable fat or simply cut into various pieces and used in soups as a replacement/substitute of meat. In actual practice, however, the fresh **Indonesian Temph** having an extremely pleasant dough-like flavour, may be dipped in shrimp, fish or soy sauces both before and after deep frying.

The usual commercial **Indonesian Temph** is, in fact, a very rich source of vitamin B_{12}, produced specifically by an unidentified bacterium that eventually grows upon the soyabeans along with the mold simultaneously. Importantly, the synthesis of vitamin B_{12} fails to commense if the *temph* is produced by carrying out the innoculation with **pure mold.** Interestingly, the well-known **Indonesian Temph** represents a very fine vegetarian blend of both **protein** and **vitamin** $\mathbf{B_{12}}$.

6.2.9 Immunotoxins

Immunotoxins refer to such toxin agents that may be attached to antibody molecules and, because of this enhanced toxicity, used to combat tumour cells. In fact, this technique has been adequately employed for the elimination of malignant tumours present in the bone marrow.

In other words, **immunotoxins** may be prepared by attaching **toxins**** to the monoclonal antibodies (MABs) strategically. A good number of **immunotoxins** have been duly made by attaching meticulously MABs to:

Bacterial Toxins : *e.g., Diphtherial Toxin (DT); Pseudomonal exotoxin* (PE40);

Plant Toxins : *e.g.,* Ricin A; Saporin;

Initial investigative immunotoxin clinical trials have adequately revealed that certain degree of early promise with regard to the shrinking of a few cancerous (*i.e.,* malignant) tumours *e.g.,* **lymphomas**. However, certain more intensive and extensive studies need to be performed before this altogether newer type of cancer treatment could be employed more widely and meaningfully.

It has been duly established that toxins may affect both *normal cells* and *cancerous cells* equally. Perhaps one may put forward a logical explanation that the particular MABs normally employed to take up the appropriate toxins to the targeted malignant cells may ultimately get attached to the respective antigens on certain '*normal cells*' as well. Immunologists are seriously engaged to identify some antigens that do occur predominantly and exclusively on these malignant cells. As on date, a few such antigens have already been reported.

It is, however, pertinent to mention here that the inherent large size of most immunotoxins virtually limits the extent to which they may actually penetrate right into some tissues. Keeping in view this remarkable revelation scientists have intensified their efforts in making the very size of the **immunotoxins** rather *smaller* and *lighter* (in weight) as well by utilizing carefully certain segments of the MABs. This line of action would certainly permit the **'drug substances'** to have an easy access to penetrate into the interior of cancerous tumors.

Interestingly, the 'clinical trials' of some immunotoxins are already in progress actively for curing such dreadful human ailments *viz.*, brain tumors, lymphomas, and certain types of leukemia's.

Example: Gemtuzumab Ozogamicin [*Synonyms:* Mylotarg: CMA-676; CDP-771;]: It is an immunoconjugate of N-acetyl-r-calicheamicin, *q.v.*, with the humanized mouse monoclonal IgG4k antibody, hP 67.6, directed against the human CD33 antigen located on the surface of normal and leukemic mycloid cells, but not on normal hematopoietic stem cells. It is actually designed to deliver antibodytargetted chemotherapy for the treatment of acute myclocytic leukemia (AML).

6.2.10 Japanese Enzymes

It is since quite well-known that the Japanese have, for ages, been making use of several enzymes *via* solid-state cultures of a good number of microbes upon a variety of known cereals, for instance: *barley, wheat, soyabeans* and *rice.* However, this highly localized and specialized process in Japan is widely known as **Koji Method,** which made use of a variety of species belonging to *Aspergillus, Monascus,* and *Rhizopus.* Interestingly, the **Koji Method** is employed primarily as a prevalent source of enzymes in the manufacture of *shoyu, miso,* and *sake* (a wine produced from rice).

Methodology: The *Koji Method* essentially involves the following steps in a sequential manner:

1. The substrate (*i.e.,* cereal) is soaked in water, drained, and heat-sterilized followed by immediate cooling.
2. The soaked and sterilized cereal is incubated along with the suitable mold.
3. The resulting substrate is then placed in **trays** or in large **shallow tanks** in a room maintained at an appropriate temperature or alternatively in an ordinary room with natural temperature variance.
4. The mold is permitted to grow adequately within a span of 3-4 days with frequent turning of the material either by hand or by mechanical means.
5. In the course of the above **'ripening process'** the substrate is adequately utilized as a source of a host of *enzymes.* Most commonly the resulting substrate is inoculated simultaneously with more than one strain of mold.

Industrial Applications: The wonderful **Koji Technique** is nothing but a reflection of the so called *ancient biotechnological innovative process* for the exclusive enzyme production, which has since been scaled up to the industrial level:

Examples:

a. **Microbial Rennet:** To manufacture microbial rennet this is used to prepare 'curd' in the cheese industry (see section 6.2.7).

b. **Feed Preparation:** It has also been used successfully to produce '*feed*' made from liquid animal waste mixed suitably with corn (maize).

6.2.11 Vegetative Products

There are several vegetative products made from commonly/indigenously harvested cereals, such as: *cassava, millet, rice etc.,* which are specific to a particular country and used as their **staple food**.

Examples: The various typical examples are as given below:

a. African Porridges: In several segments of the African continent one comes across **naturally fermented porridges** which essentially forms their **'staple food'**. The West African **'GARI'** (used in Nigeria, Ghana etc.) is invariably prepared from acid-fermented cassava porridge. In the course of fermentation, usually carried out at 35°C), any **cyanide-containing carbohydrates** present are duly hydrolyzed thereby removing the cyanide almost completely as hydrocyanic acid (HCN). In this manner the **cassava** is rendered acidic in nature and the characteristic flavour of **gari** is given out. The entire fermentative procedure takes almost 3 to 4 days, and caused due to the organism *Corynebacterium manihot* that eventually hydrolyzes the ensuing starch exothermally and gives rise to *lactic acid* and *formic acid*. Subsequently, yeast like fungus *Geotricum candidum* gets developed when the product turns acidic which ultimately oxidizes the acid, and gives rise to the characteristic *gari* flavour and aroma. In usual practice, the fluid content is squeezed out from the ferment, and the starchy residue is carefully dried in a shallow pan over fire with constant stirring to obtain finally a gelatinized granular powder; alternatively, the wet starchy residue is consumed directly as *'fufu'*. African also makes use of *maize* and *sorghum* profusely for fermentation so to obtain these acidic porridges as their staple food. Nevertheless, such **low-cost technologies** have been used since time immemorial in different zones in Africa, depending solely upon their cultural preference and linking.

b. Injeera: Ethiopia and Iretria (East Africa) makes use of **millet** more or less in the same manner as stated in

1. Above, except that the wet fermented dough is shaped in the form of **'chapati'** (a flatthin bread) and baked in coal-fired/electric round ovens. Fresh injeera may be used for 3 to 4 days. It is one of the most liked staple food amongst the **Ethiopians** and the **Iretrians** alike.

c. Indian Idli: **Idli** is a very common, age-old, fermented South Indian dish prepared from rice and a small amount of dehulled *black grams* (Moong dal) or even sometimes *lentils*. Idli is now being eaten all over India, just like **Pizza** in the West. It is slightly acidic steamed puffed soft bread which is quite rich in protein and easy to digest.

In usual procedure, both cereals (rice) and pulses* (black gram, or lentil) are soaked over night separately in the ratio of 3:1. The soaked rice and pulse are ground separately either by specially designed hand-operated grinding pestle and mortar made of stone or electrically operated grinding devices. Generally, rice is ground coarsely, and pulse ground finely. The ground products are mixed adequately into a big vessel, salt added as per taste, and then incubated overnight. During this process the batter becomes acidic and it is leavened by CO_2, primarily generated by *Leuconostoc mesenteroides*. However, the presence of *streptococcus faecalis* does help in attributing the desired strength of acidity that gives **Idli** the real texture, flavour, taste, and around.

The leavened and acidified batter is now cooked in a specially designed metal cups under steam when it gets puffed up and eventually becomes soft and spongy in texture.

6.2.12 Newer Approaches to Sewage Treatment

In actual practice, the urbanized countries in the world discharge an enormous volume of industrial and domestic sewage which need to treat biologically so that the treated sewage could be used for irrigation purposes usefully and effectively or may be discharged to certain extent into a running stream of water (river, rivulet etc.).

The latest methods available for the adequate sewage treatment are of *three* major types, namely:

a. Classical aerobic activated sludge process either with surface aeration or with oxygen introduced by forced compressed air,

b. Aerobic treatment process, and

c. Anaerobic digestion process.

All the above *three* methodologies shall only be discussed briefly in the section that follows:

6.2.12.1 Classical Aerobic Activated Sludge Process

Figure 6.3 vividly illustrates the classical aerobic activated sludge process with surface aeration or one may even introduce forced compressed air to cause the desired aeration. The main purpose of injecting air in the on-going aerobic process is to minimize drastically the BOD and COD of the untreated sewage material to make it fit for disposal either for irrigation utilities or gradual disposal in a current of fresh running water. The sedimentation basin as shown in Fig. 6.3 are two in number, the *first* — is called the primary sedimentation basin ; whereas the *second* — is termed as the secondary sedimentation basin. The sludge obtained from the second sedimentation basin is recycled into the raw sewage as well as the aeration basin to augment the activation of the sludge to lower the COD and BOD of the sewage material being introduced initially.

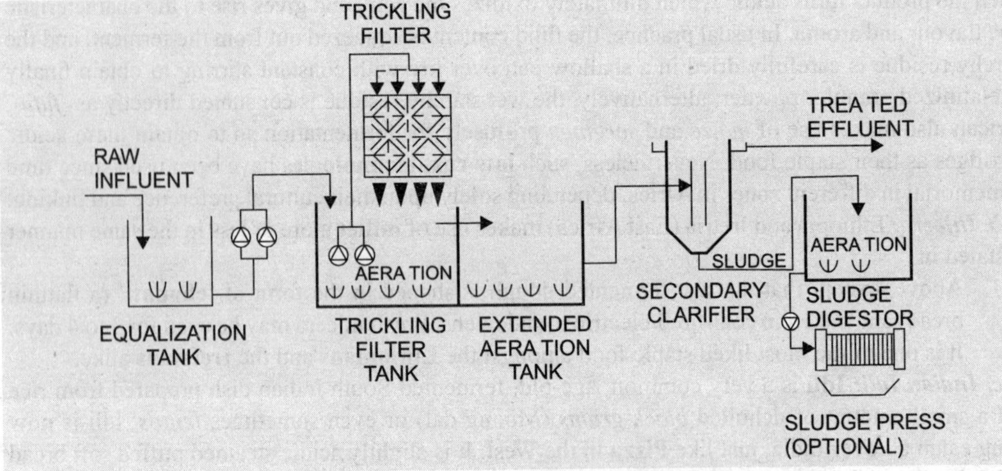

Fig. 6.3 *Classical Aerobic Activated Sludge Process*

Disadvantages: The various disadvantages of the aerobic systems are as follows:

1. Being an open construction the effective process control is restricted enormously,
2. No measure to control the growth of uncontrolled population of organisms, and
3. Gives rise to severe environmental pollution caused due to odour emission, and fog formation.

Figure 6.4 depicts explicitly the process which evidently uses the anaerobic digestion. In this particular instance, the biological process either commences occasionally directly up the raw sewage or rather more frequently upon the *solid material* (*i.e.*, sludge) usually recovered from sedimentation from the *'aerobic sedimentation processes* described earlier (see Fig. 6.3).

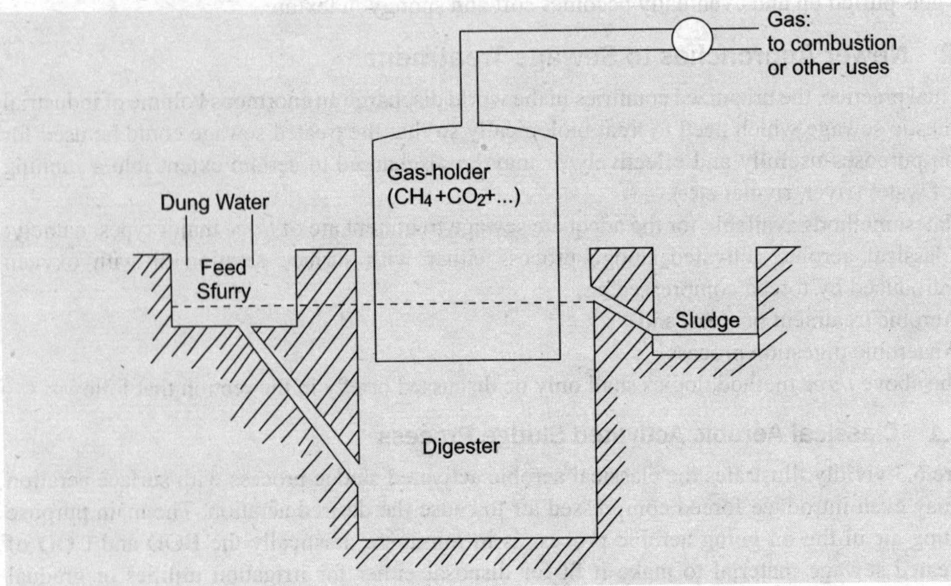

Fig. 6.4 *Diagrammatic Sketch of a Sludge Digester*

It is a stark reality that usual developments that took place in **'sewage treatment'** operations during the past century or so have been accomplished primarily and predominantly in an absolute empirical manner. Since the advanced *aerobic* and *anaerobic* sewage treatment processes are being studied on a more scientific footing, it is felt overwhelmingly that optimization shall certainly lead to the ultimate maximized success in the positive improvement in these newer processes. In fact, the earlier elaborative investigations were solely and primarily emphasized with regard to an in-depth understanding of the C-metabolism; however, the futuristic approach shall be focused and anticipated exclusively at a rather more divergent field including S, N and phosphate metabolism, because ultimately the complete elimination of these elements from **'treated sewage'** shall be the **'prime statutory demand and requirement'** as well. Besides, strategic and critical accumulations of heavy metals (e.g., Pb^{2+}, Hg^{2+}, Ag^{+}, Bi^{2+}, Cu^{2+}, As^{3+}, Sb^{3+}, Sn^{4+}) in the *stabilized sludge* are being increasingly recognized as a matter of serious concern. Perhaps *'bioextractive metallurgy'* (see section 6.2.5) may even prove to be an effective measure in this process also.

Bulking: Another vital, critical, and important problem is the prevailing phenomenon of **bulking** in sludge, that essentially prevents and checks the ensuing settling process particularly taking place in the **'clarification basins'.** It has been duly observed and revealed that **bulking** is prevalently caused due to the development of **filamentous microorganisms** which fail to settle down adequately and completely.

Bulking may be controlled effectively in certain specific instances by adopting the following means and ways:

a. Introduction of **'floatation processes'** — in domestic sewage treatment and disposal operation this technical solution is proved to be *quite expensive* and hence not viable economically, and

b. Introduction of a '*microbiological solution*' — may prove to be an ultimate satisfactory answer in the delivery of a **clear effluent** from the final settling basins.

Special Point: In the past several decades it has been observed that there has been a drastic and remarkable decrease in the content of **'organic material'** present in industrial effluents. Indeed this spectacular and wonderful accomplishment was duly possible due to the concerted efforts of extensive application of research and development amalgamated with an appreciable volume of expenditures with regard to newer treatment installations.

Questions

1. Production of industrial alcohol. (MGRU 2004)
2. Explain the production and recovery of alcohol by fermentation process. (MGRU 2002)
3. Explain the production and recovery of alcohol by fermentation process. (MGRU 2001)
4. Write the biosynthesis of ethanol?
5. Explain some of the algal health foods with example?
6. How can you generate the biological fuel?
7. What is fossil fuel? Predict the fossil fuel to future use?
8. Write notes on non-renewable source of energy?
9. What is biomass? How to control the global climatic alteration?

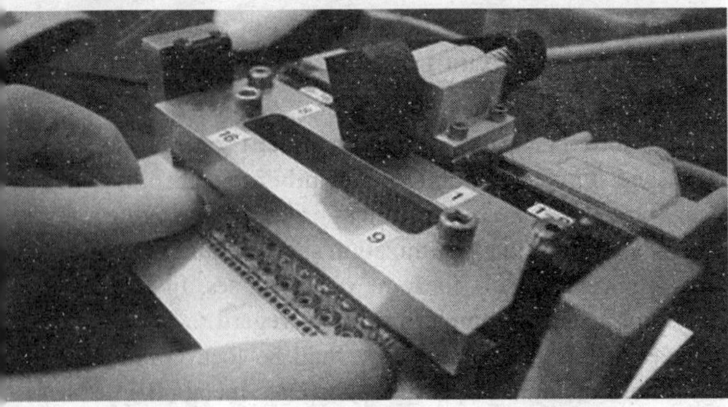

CHAPTER

7

Biosensor Technology

7.1 Introduction

Biosensors or **Enzyme Electrodes** invariably refer to such devices that sense and analyze biological information(s), namely; blood pressure (BP), temperature, heart rate, sophisticated determination of chemical and enzymes in body fluids.* The device may be used either in the laboratory or placed strategically within the body.

The quantum jump in various highly specialized fields of medicine, agriculture, industry, environmental control and monitoring, and latest trends in biotechnological advancements in research has absolutely necessitated the on-going routine analyses by the aid of specific physico-chemical computer-based analytical instruments that are exclusively conducted for the precise estimation and simultaneous monitoring the levels of certain **analytes.** Importantly, the conventional physical methodologies usually engaged for such **'routine analysis'** do not involve the usage of either any living **organisms** or molecules belonging to the **biological origin.** Therefore, to circumvent such an uncommon situation researchers have meticulously utilized either **living cells** or **biological molecules** to develop feasible, reliable, practicable, repeatable, reproducible, precise, and above all highly sensitive devices which are known as **'biosensors'.**

Biosensors distinctly and predominantly regarded and proved to be much more **superior** and **sensitive** in comparison to various known physico-chemical analytical instruments strictly based upon the following statement of facts, such as:

1. **Biosensors** do have the specific immobilized biological material in close contact of an appropriate transducer in order that the *biochemical signal* is rapidly converted into an *electrical signal*,
2. Immobilization of biomolecules allows reutilization of such molecules, that are rather expensive, and ultimately permits simplification of the entire assembly of apparatus,

3. **Biological-sensing element** is strategically positioned in a small specified zone and is also extremely sensitive which categorically facilitates the analysis of substances in rather small amounts feasible, and
4. **Biosensors** are designed and developed on specific need base analogy; hence they could be *highly specific* or *broad spectrum.*

Generalized Biosensor: One may also expatiate **biosensor** as a suitable probe, device, or electrode that upon making contact with an appropriate sample, adequately converts the presence of the desired **analyte** into a suitable corresponding measurable electrical signal. In actual practice, however, the precise concentration in the sample is duly interpreted in terms of the electrical signal *via* an appropriate combination of:

- Biological recognition system
- Electrochemical transducer, and
- Computer aided facilities.

Figure 7.1 gives the diagrammatic sketch of a generalized biosensor.

Microbial cell represented and exploited as one of the typical alternative biological recognition Systems; besides, other known systems invariably make use of **enzymes, immune protein, organelles**, and **tissue section.** Nevertheless, the microbial cell essentially possesses a dual characteristic feature, namely: (*a*) undergoes **immobilization;** and (*b*) **biochemical signal** gets converted to a corresponding measurable **electrical signal.**

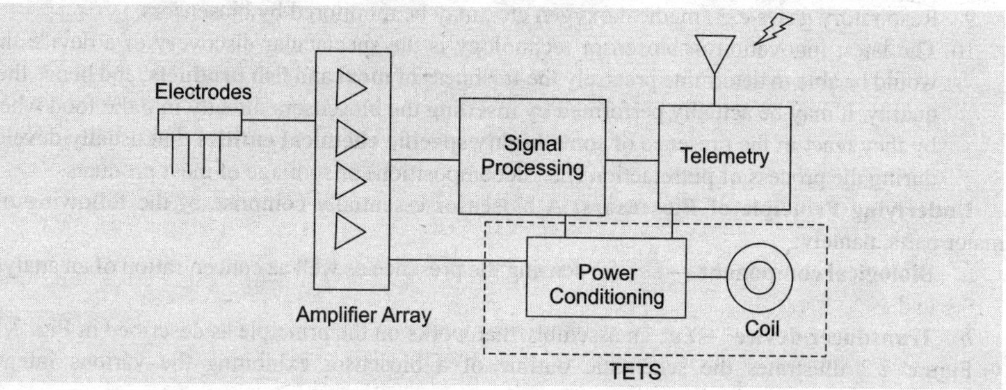

Fig. 7.1 *Diagramatic Sketch of a Generalized Biosensor*

Electrochemical Sensors: Electrochemical sensors have been prepared by following these steps in a sequential manner:

1. Immobilization of biological reagents upon the metallic surfaces.
2. **Avidin** binds *biotin* as well as *biotinylated reagents* that may be employed for analytical purposes.
3. A target strand of the specific viral DNA has been detected and identified successfully by making use of this altogether new approach essentially utilizing a particular **avidin-coated quartz crystal microbalance.**
4. In the particular event when two vital components *viz.*, a **biotin-oligonucleotide conjugate** and an **enzyme-oligonucleotide conjugate** are carefully incubated with a specific sample under investigation, it gives rise to the formation of a *biotin-DNA enzyme hybrid* in the presence of the **target strand.**
5. Avidin-coated surface is subsequently exposed to the respective sample. Thorough washings remove any possible *'unbound substance'*, and then the substrate is incorporated carefully.
6. The resulting *'product of enzymatic reaction'* happen to be an insoluble substance that eventually gets deposited.

7. Consequently, the ultimate critical increase in mass specifically alters the prevailing *microbalance frequency* directly in proportion to the concentration of the viral DNA.

Applications of Biosensors: The various vital and important applications of **biosensors** may be enumerated as under:

1. In the particular field of medical diagnosis enzymes are being employed prominently.
2. Various monitoring programmes in an industrial set-up is accomplished by the help of enzymes meticulously so as to obtain the optimum yield of the desired product(s).
3. Based on the highly specific nature of reactions, broad range of reactions which may be catalyzed effectively biosensors play a vital role in clinical analysis. Precisely, in the domain of clinical analysis enzymes are utilized specifically as reagents in the measurement of particular metabolites; and importantly these are invariably determined *in situ* in *body fluids* and *tissues* respectively, which may serve as a definite guideline or indicator of prevailing pathogenic parameters or metabolic disturbances.
4. Biosensors help in a big way for monitoring of various pollutants in water.
5. Biosensors afford the remote sensing of admixtures of mine gases in adverse environments.
6. In fermentation industries *e.g.*, alcohol from molasses, the monitoring of final desired products and cell cultures are duly ascertained by biosensors.
7. Biosensors also help in monitoring of **toxic gases** *e.g.*, in chemical industries, in war etc.
8. Biosensors do help in the assay of the concentration of ions.
9. Respiratory gases *e.g.*, medical oxygen etc., may be monitored by biosensors.
10. The latest innovation in biosensor technology is the spectacular discovery of a device that would be able to determine precisely the freshness of **meat** and **fish products**, and hence their quality. It may be actually performed by inserting the biosensors directly into the food where by they react in the presence of some **highly specific chemical entities** that usually develop during the process of putrefaction (*i.e.*, decomposition) or spoilage of meat products.

Underlying Principle of Biosensors: A biosensor essentially comprise of the following *two* major parts, namely:

a. **Biological component** — *i.e.*, for sensing the presence as well as concentration of an analyte, and

b. **Transducer device** — *i.e.*, an assembly that works on the principle as described in Fig. 7.1.

Figure 7.2 illustrates the schematic outline of a biosensor exhibiting the various integral components associated with it.

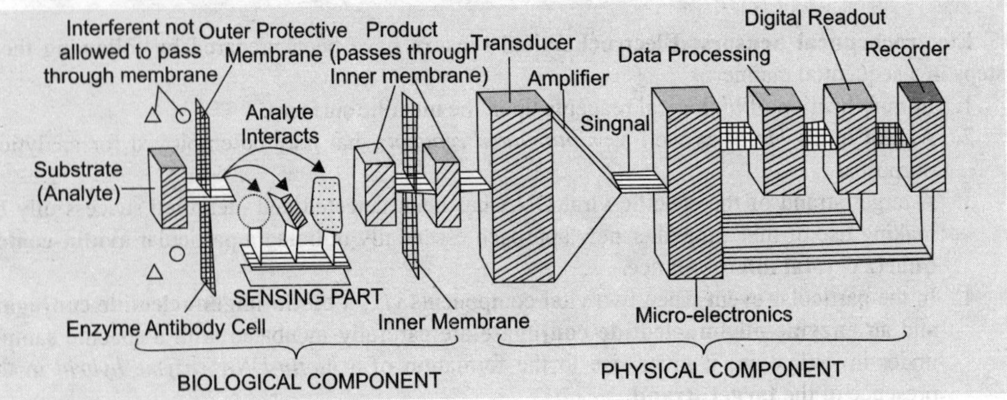

Fig. 7.2 *Schematic Diagramatic Sketch of a Biosensor Depicting its Various Vital Components*

Methodology: The various operational steps in the working of a **biosensor** (Fig. 7.2) are as detailed below:

1. The sample containing the analyte is first passed through a membrane so as to eliminate carefully most of the interfering molecules.
2. The *purified sample* is then made to interact with the **biological sensor** to yield the *desired product that* may be represented as an appropriate chemical entity or heat or electric current or charge.
3. The '*product*' subsequently passes through another membrane and ultimately gains an access to the transducer, that eventually converts the **biochemical signal** into the corresponding **electrical signal** which may be adequately amplified and read finally either on a *digital panel* or recorded on a suitable **recording device.**
4. Steps (1) through (3) distinctly affords the measurement of the concentration of a substrate *in situ* (*i.e.*, without any processing whatsoever), and thereby avoiding any consumption (wastage) of the sample under assay.

7.2 Types of Electrodes used in Biosensors

Biosensors invariably employ *two* distinct types of electrodes, such as:

a. Electrochemical electrodes, and

b. Microbial electrodes.

These *two* specialized variants of electrodes shall now be treated individually in the section that follows:

7.2.1 Electrochemical Electrodes [Enzymes Electrodes]

Electrochemical electrodes (or **Enzyme electrodes**) are a new type of *detector* or *biosensor* that has been exclusively designed for the **potentiometric** or **amperometric** assay of substrates, for instance: alcohol, amino acids, glucose, and lactic acid.

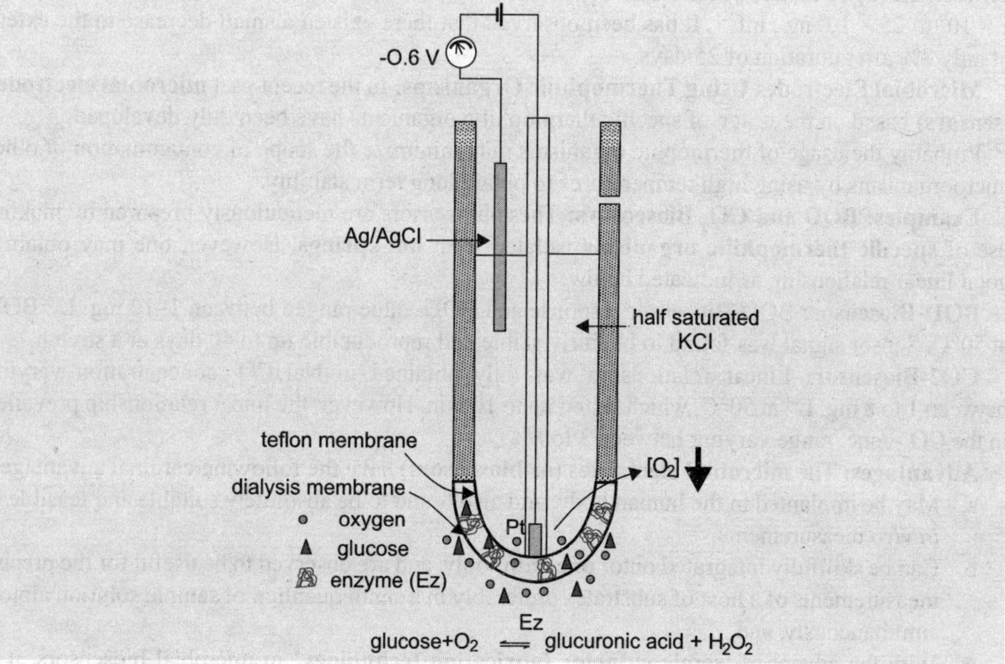

Fig. 7.3 *Diagramatic Representation of a Simple Biosensor Combining an Electrochemical Electrode and an Enzyme Immobilized onto a Semi permeable Membrane*

Figure 7.3 illustrates the specific design of the **electrochemical electrode** which is essentially composed of a given *electrochemical sensor* in close contact with a **thin-permeable enzyme membrane** that is capable of interacting specifically with the given substrates. Interestingly, the embedded enzymes strategically located in the membrane produce H^+ ions, oxygen (O_2), NH_4^+ ions, carbon dioxide (CO_2) or ever other small molecules depending solely on the enzymatic reactions taking place, that are rapidly detected by the particular sensor meticulously. Besides, the magnitude of the response gives the precise estimations of the prevailing concentration of the substrate.

Nevertheless, the *biological component* present in a **biosensor** may invariably be **an enzyme** or a **multi-enzyme system that** could also be an *antibody* or *organelle* or *microbial cell* or even *whole slices of tissue.*

7.2.2 Microbial Electrodes

Microbial electrodes (biosensors) have been designed meticulously for the estimation of **glucose, lactic acid, acetic acid,** and assimilable carbohydrates (sugars). A microbial sensor (electrode) essentially comprise of a microorganism immobilized membrane (or bacterial collagen membrane) and a pair of electrodes (*viz*., **Lead**-anode; and Platinum-Cathode). In fact, several types of sophisticated **microbial electrodes** have been duly developed, tested, and applied skillfully to the precise measurements of *biological substances* (Fig. 7.4).

Principle: The underlying principle of a **microbial electrode** (or **sensor**) is entirely based upon the fact whether the change in respiration or the quantum of produced metabolites do exert any affect on the ensuing assimilation of substrates by the prevailing microorganisms. Besides, the meaningful application of **auxotrophic mutants** may also selectively help in the assay of a wide spectrum of substances.

Examples: Design of vitamin B_{12} sensor by making use of immobilized *Escherichia coli-215*. The *E. coli-215* strain specifically needs vitamin B_{12} for its usual normal growth. Linear relationship between these two factors *i.e.,* vitamin B_{12} and normal growth, was duly obtained between the range 5×10^9 to 25×10^9 ng . mL^{-1}. It has been observed that there existed a small decrease to the extent of only 8% after duration of 25 days.

Microbial Electrodes Using Thermophilic Organisms: In the recent past **microbial electrodes (sensors)** based on the usage of specific thermophilic organisms have been duly developed.

Probably the usage of thermophic organisms may minimize the scope of contamination of other microorganisms by using high temperatures to obtain long term stability.

Examples: BOD and CO_2 Biosensors: These biosensors are meticulously prepared by making use of **specific thermophilic organisms** isolated from **hot-springs**. However, one may obtain a good linear relationship as indicated below:

BOD-Biosensor: BOD-Biosensor response and BOD-value ranged between 1–10 mg. L^{-1} BOD at 50°C. Sensor signal was found to be fairly stable and reproducible up to 40 days at a stretch.

CO2-Biosensor: Linear relationship was duly obtained in $NaHCO_3$ concentration varying between 1 to 8 mg. L^{-1} at 50°C, which lasted up to 10 min. However, the linear relationship prevailed in the CO_2-conc. range varying between 3 to 8%.

Advantages: The **microbial electrodes (or biosensors)** have the following cardinal advantages:

a. May be implanted in the human body, and also found to be absolutely suitable and feasible to *in vivo* measurements,
b. Can be skillfully integrated onto **'one chip'** only, and are observed to be useful for the precise measurements of a host of substrates preferably in a small quantum of sample solution almost simultaneously, and
c. With the advent of **'semiconductor fabrication technology'** in microbial biosensors, it is now quite convenient and possible to develop **disposable transducers** for the *biosensors via* mass production.

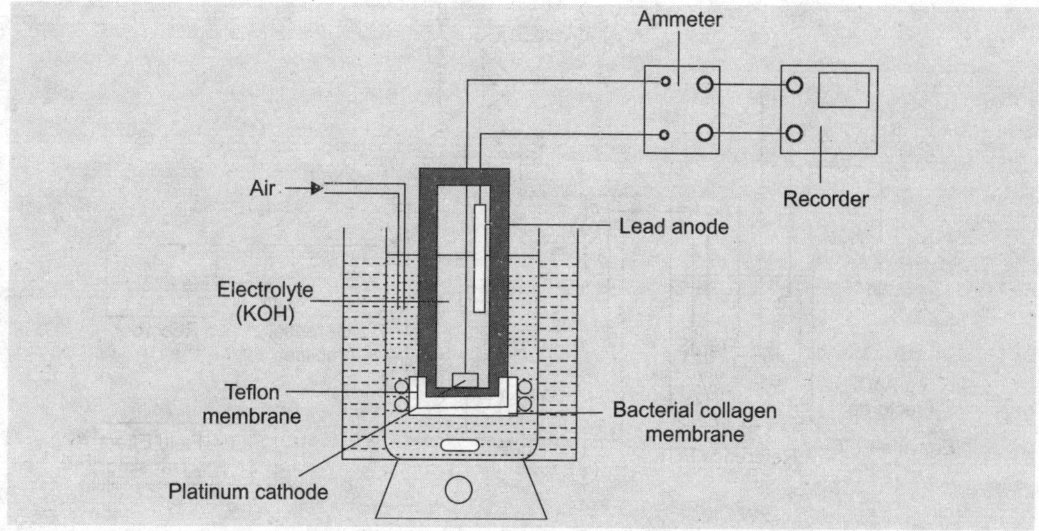

Fig. 7.4 *Diagramatic Sketch of a Microbial Electrode*

7.3 Biosensor Variants

In the last two decades there has been a phenomenal advancement in the specific domain of **'biosensor technology'**, thereby giving rise to the remarkable introduction of an array of **biosensors** to carry out the assay of biological product(s) *in situ,* namely:

i. Alcohol biosensor,
ii. Amorphous silicone biosensor,
iii. Glucose and carbon dioxide biosensor,
iv. Hypoxanthine biosensor,
v. Inosine biosensor,
vi. Image biosensor,
vii. Integrated multi-biosensor,
viii. Urea biosensor
ix. Thermistor containing biosensor,
x. Bioaffinity Sensor, and
xi. Opto-electronic biosensor.

These aforesaid biosensor variants shall now be treated separately as under:

7.3.1 Alcohol Biosensor

An elaborative research with respect to an **alcohol-sensitive micro-biosensor** employing an **ion-sensitive field effect transistor (ISFET)** in conjunction with the enzyme system prevailing in the cell-membrane has been duly reported. In this particular instance the cell-membrane of acetic-acid producing organism essentially possesses a complex-enzyme system that takes care of the oxidation of ethanol to acetic acid *via* acetaldehyde.

The alcohol biosensor system comprises of a membrane-bound alcohol dehydrogenase (ADH) enzyme, aldehyde dehydrogenase (ALDH enzyme), and an efficient electron-transfer system positioned strategically in the assembly. Thus, the designed complex enzyme system may be utilized judiciously for suitable application using an ISFET.

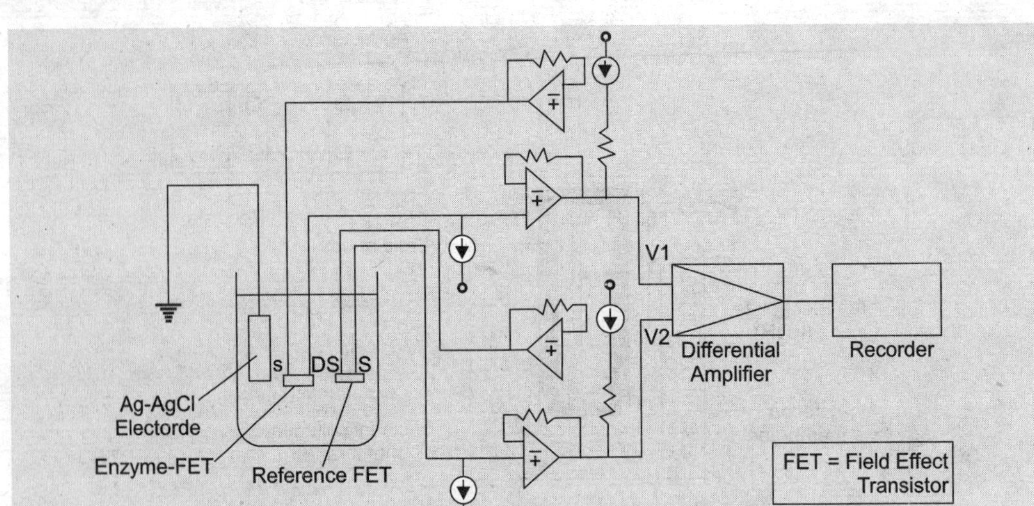

Fig. 7.5 *Diagramatic Representation of an Alcohol-Biosensor System*

7.3.2 Amorphous Silicon Biosensor

It has been amply demonstrated that an innovative ISFET design and assembly may be produced efficiently by making use of an amorphous silicon wafer (*i.e.,* a very thin slice) for the respective substrate. Interestingly, a plethora of such latest devices meticulously designed from amorphous silicon have attained virtually a world-wide recognition by virtue of their enormous utilities potential. In actual practice, a host of **substrates** *e.g.,* plastic, glass may be employed effectively for supporting the amorphous silicon. Likewise, **transistors** may also be designed and fabricated using a variety of different devices, such as: needle of a hypodermic syringe as depicted in Fig. 7.6.

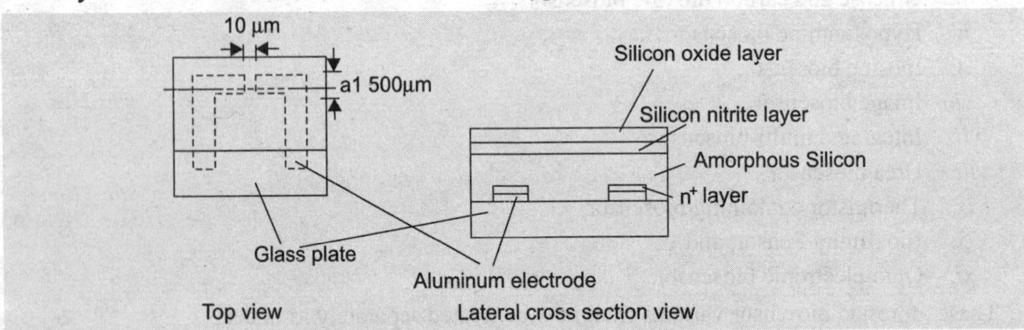

Fig. 7.6 *Structural Design of Amorphous Silicon ISFET*

7.3.3 Glucose and Carbon Dioxide (CO_2) Biosensor

It has been reported that **glucose biosensor** may be fabricated by immobilizing gold (Au) on the *sensitive portion of the mico-oxygen-electrode* by carefully cross-linking with bovine-serum albumin (BSA), and gibberellic acid (GA). Now, the enzyme immobilized membrane is articulately produced by carefully introducing the aforesaid sensitive portion of the micro-oxygen electrode into the mixture containing 2 mg of Au, 20 µ*l* of 10% BSA solution, and 10 µl of 25% GA solution. The glucose biosensor gives a positive response as soon as the glucose solution is injected into the buffer solution, and attains a steady status within a span of 5 to 10 minutes. The aforesaid biosensor practically afforded an absolute linear response for the corresponding glucose concentrations ranging between 0.2 and 2 mM, that is fairly comparable to the usual and conventional glucose sensors.

Suzuki *et al.* devised a unique microbial CO_2-sensor by making use of the above mentioned micro-oxygen electrode. Interestingly, an autotropic bacterium known as S17 that could grow exclusively in the presence of **'carbonates'** as a C-source is employed. Subsequently, the bacterial whole cells are immobilized upon a micro-oxygen electrode meticulously. Thus, the sensitive area of the oxygen electrode is carefully immersed in a 0.2% (w/v) sodium alginate solution in an aqueous medium and containing S17 whole cells, removed thereafter, and immersed almost instantly into a 5% $CaCl_2$ solution to give rise to the formation of **organism immobilized calcium alginate gel.** The formation of photoresist duly commences by the gas-permeable membrane over the bacteria immobilized gel. The photoresist is exposed to UV radiation just for a few minutes which has a response time between 2–3 minutes. In fact, CO_2 was provided by the acidification of sodium bicarbonate ($NHCO_3$), and its due concentration may be governed by CO_2-concentration. However, the linear relationship could be accomplished during the phase of reduction in current, and $NHCO_3$ concentration ranging between 0.5 to 3.5 mM; but above 3.5 mM no appreciable enhancement in response could be seen.

Figure 7.7 depicts the diagrammatic sketch of a micro-oxygen electrode, wherein the detail descriptions of the gold (Au)-electrode, gas-permeable membrane, and the agarose gel in 0.1 M KCl have been shown explicitly.

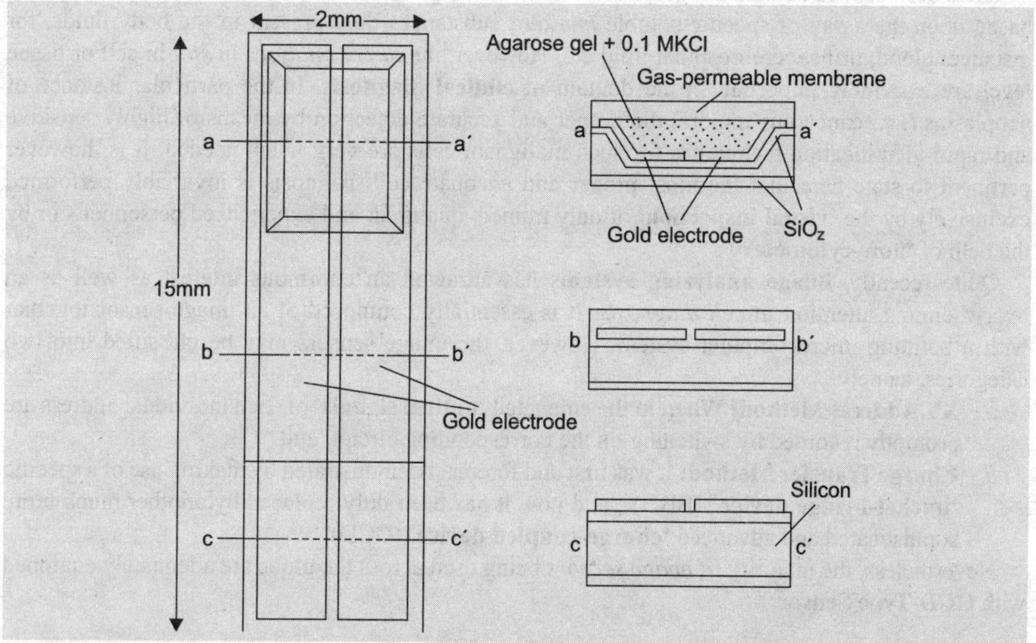

Fig. 7.7 *Diagramatic Sketch of a Micro-Oxygen Electrode*

7.3.4 Hypoxanthine Biosensor

Furuya *et al.* (1968) reported the fermentation of inosinic acid (5′-IMP) by using the strainKY13012, whereby the production of hypoxanthine continued during the initial 2 to 3 days. Subsequently, hypoxanthine gets decreased as IMP accumulation commences. Importantly, with Mn^{2+} as a limiting factor, abnormal cells having distinctly lowered permeability are generated. They excrete hypoxanthine which gets phosphorylated to 5′–IMP extracellularly. Besides, 5′–IMP is also synthesized *de novo* in the subsequent fermentation phase and is ultimately excreted directly into the culture medium. Thus, the liberated hypoxanthine is measured on the basis of the reaction invariably catalyzed by xanthine oxidase (XO). The change in pH caused due to the formation of uric acid is normally detected by employing a **Si-ion-sensitive field effect transistor** (Si-ISFET).

7.3.5 Inosine Biosensor

Nevertheless, the *inosine biosensor* is duly fabricated almost is the same pattern as that of *hypoxanthine biosensor* but instead making use of **nucleoside phosphorylase** and **xanthine oxidase** meticulously co-immobilized upon Si-ISFET at the same time. After a lapse of 90 seconds from the injection of **inosine solution,** the overall voltage slowly enhances and reaches an almost steady condition within nearly 7 minutes. Thus, the xanthine generated by the decomposition of inosine catalyzed by the enzyme nucleoside phosphorylase is then oxidized to the corresponding uric acid by the aid of xanthine oxidase (XO). The oxidation of hypoxanthine to uric acid by the help of xanthine oxidase (XO) is eventually initiated almost immediately after injection. Importantly, the response to inosine bears a definite time lag of 90 seconds after injection. Obviously, the ensuing phenomenon is solely attributed to the prevailing three step reaction. However, exclusively based upon this time lag the inosine sensor may help in the precise determination of **inosine** as well as **hypoxanthine** almost simultaneously.

7.3.6 Image Biosensor

It has been proved beyond any reasonable doubt that a plethora of **'clinical analyses'** are entirely based upon the assay of specific soluble *marker** substances duly present in the body fluids, for instance: blood, urine, cerebrospinal fluid etc. However, the *direct analyses in situ* in cell or tissue level are extremely important in the domain of **clinical diagnosis.** In the particular instance of neoplasms (*i.e.,* cancerous tumors) the proper and accurate detection by means of highly sensitive and rapid identification techniques for such malignant cells are very much needed. It is, however pertinent to state here that the most proper and adequate cell diagnosis is invariably performed exclusively by the **'visual inspection'** of duly trained, qualified, and experienced personnel's or by the help of **'flow-cytometery'**.

Quite recently, **image analyzing systems** has attracted an enormous interest as well as an overwhelming attention in *cell diagnosis.* It is essentially composed of an image sensor together with a befitting microcomputer system. However, the image sensors may be classified into two categories, namely:

a. **XY Address Method:** Wherein the emanated **'optical signals'** of each individual address are promptly recorded by switching on the corresponding circuit, and

b. **Charge Transfer Method:** It was first and foremost demonstrated by making use of a specific **'bucket-bridge device'** (BBD) ; and now it has been duly replaced by another much more sophisticated and advanced **'charge-coupled device'** (CCD).

Nevertheless, the majority of *image sensors* being used across the globe are adequately equipped with **CCD-Type Sensor.**

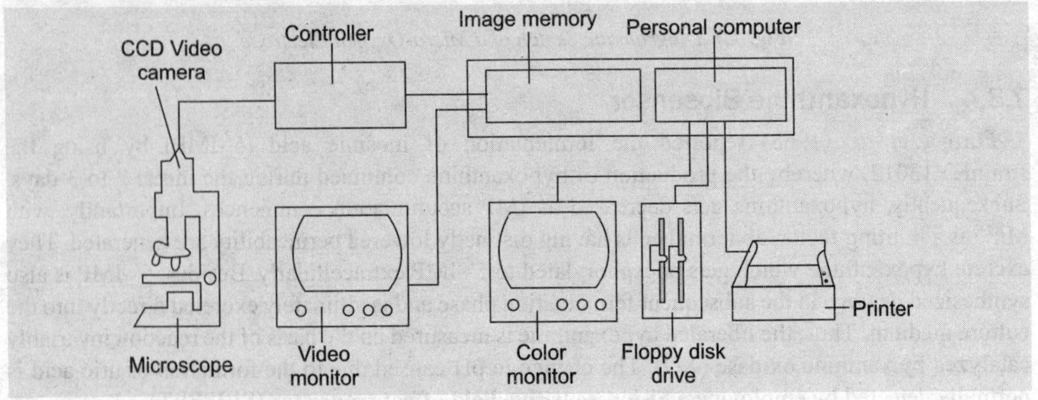

Fig. 7.8 *Schematic Diagram of an Imaging Sensor System*

Figure 7.8 depicts the schematic diagram of an imaging sensor system in which CCD-type video camera has been utilized.

The CCD is nothing but an **'integrated semiconductor chip'** which essentially consists of a series of **photodiode array tubes** and **charge transfer circuits.** Precisely, the ensuing electrical charges being accumulated at each phototube are transferred systematically to the output terminal by carefully controlling the electric potential in the chip. However, the output pulse height invariably correlates with the desired brightness aptly observed at the corresponding photodiode. Therefore, ultimately a visual image focused on the CCD may be adequately subject to conversion into a succession of analogue pulses.

Because, the battery of photodiodes are virtually spaced and arranged with a separation of 10 μm approximately, one would expect the same extent of image resolution. There are, of course, a plethora of distinct advantages to the unique and wonderful **solid state CCD image sensor** in comparison to a conventional *vidicon device.*

Advantages of CCD-Type Sensor: The various glaring advantages of CCD-Type Sensor are as follows:

- Compactness in dimension (size)
- High degree of sensitivity
- Lesser extent of distortion
- Afterimage problem eliminated completely
- Consumption of reasonably low power
- Extended and long operational life span.

7.3.7 Integrated Multi-Biosensor

In fact, there are almost **twenty** vital and prominent constituent elements that are predominantly required to be analyzed simultaneously. In order to accomplish such an extremely important task for the precise detection as well as quantification of various substances present invariably in *minute quantities* and that too in *small sample solution* simultaneously, it is not only an absolute necessity but also equally vital to develop an **integrated multi-biosensor.** In the recent past, a number of well conceptualized and designed integrated multi-biosensors surfaced that categorically employed ISFET* and microelectrodes meticulously. This unique combination of multi-biosensors based upon the variants of ISFETs and electrodes were very painstakingly coated with **specific enzyme immobilized membranes.** It is, however, pertinent to state at this point in time that to develop a particular enzyme immobilized membrane fabrication technique should adhere to the following requirements very strictly:

a. Enzyme immobilized membrane must be deposited precisely upon the **small functional electrodes** or the **gate region,**

b. Deposited enzyme immobilized membrane must ever peel off from the highly sensitive surface zone while in actual operation,

c. Enzyme membrane variants may be designed and prepared meticulously without any mixing whatsoever, and

d. Fabrication technologies are prominently applicable to a **'wafer'**, which is fairly comparable with IC process.

7.3.8 Urea Biosensor

The **urea biosensor** invariably comprise of a **urease immobilized membrane** in addition to a pH electrode. It is a well established fact that **urease catalyzed reaction** essentially gives rise to Ph alterations; and, therefore, enables the utilization of ISFET as a **transducer.** However, one may conveniently fabricate a precise **micro urease biosensor** as per the details provided as under:

1. An ISFET is carefully placed inside a vacuum chamber (or enclosure), and the organic compound 3-APTES (*i.e.,* 3-amino-propyltriethoxysilane) is duly vaporized at 80°C, 0.5 Torr for 30 minutes, immediately followed by glutaraldehyde (GA) interaction very much under identical experimental parameters.

The resulting **chemically modified ISFET** was duly covered with **cellulose acetate membrane** very cautiously containing 1, 8-amino-4-aminomethyl octane along with glutaraldehyde. Consequently, the ISFET was carefully immersed into the *urease solution*. Thus, the **urea biosensor** provides the desired linear relationship prevailing between the two vital components, namely: (*a*) initial rate of the output gate voltage; and (*b*) log of urea concentration. However, the value of **log urease concentration** varies between 16.7 to 167 mM, which may be used upto 20 days but with marginal degradation of the prevailing enzyme activity.

7.3.9 Thermistor Containing Biosensor

Thermistor refers to an apparatus for quickly determining very small changes in temperature. Materials that alter their resistance to the flow of electricity as the temperature changes are invariably used in these devices. In fact, even a small temperature change ranging between 0.1 to 0.001°C may be recorded precisely in the normal course of biochemical reactions. Gronow *et al.* (1988) reported the meticulous development of thermistors for immobilizing enzymes, such as: **cholesterol oxidase, glucose oxidase, invertase, tyrosinase,** and the like. It is pertinent to take cognizance of the glaring fact that the **thermistors** are invariably and gainfully used for the explicite studies with regard to antigen antibody reactions with utmost sensitivity *i.e.,* upto 10–13 mol. dm^{-3} in the specific instance of **Enzyme Linked Immuno Absorbant Assay (ELISA).**

7.3.10 Bioaffinity Sensor

The **bioaffinity sensors** are quite a recent development. They particularly help a lot in the measurement of the concentration of the ensuing **determinants** *i.e.,* resulting substrates (analytes) exclusively based upon *equilibrium binding,* thereby depicting an extraordinary high degree of selectivity. Kumar and Kumar (1992) amply proved and demonstrated that the **'bioaffinity sensors'** are of highly diverse characteristic features due to the usage of a variety of extremely specific substances, such as: **radio labeled, enzyme-labeled,** and **fluorescence labeled.** The principle of **'bioaffinity sensor'** is depicted vividly in Fig. 7.9.

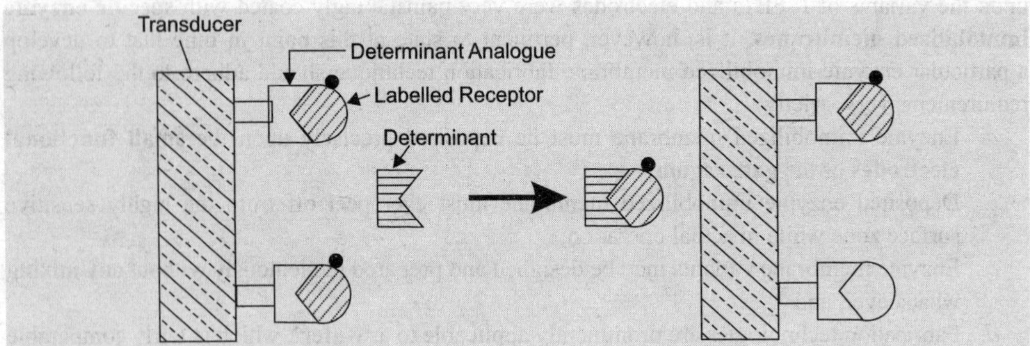

Fig. 7.9 *Principle of Bioaffinity Sensor*

Interestingly, in the **bioaffinity sensor** a *receptor* is strategically radiolabelled and subsequently allowed to get bound to an appropriate determinant analogue immobilized duly onto the surface of a transducer. It has been noticed that as soon as the prevailing concentrations of a determinant are adequately enhanced, the ensuing **'labeled receptor'** yields an intimately *bound complex with the respective determinant.*

7.3.11 Opto-Electronic Biosensor

The **opto-electronic biosensors** usually make use of either **enzymes** or **antibodies** that are strategically immobilized on the surface of a membrane. Gronow et al. (1988) suggested a means to measure colour whereby the *opto-electronic biosensor* is adequately immobilized onto a membrane having the enzyme and a specific dye. It is an established fact that a substrate (*i.e.,* an analyte) gets catalyzed duly to give rise to a definite product thereby causing a change in the pH of the medium. Importantly, this brings about a change in the particular **dye-membrane-complex.** Ultimately these apparent alterations in colour are precisely measured by the help of a *light-emitting diode* and a *photodiode.*

7.4 Biochips (or The Biological Computer)

Biochip is the wonderful outcome of modern-day-research with a befitting amalgamation of **microchips** and **biotechnology.** With its unique invention as well as discovery there lies an enormous scope in the most innovative idea for the development of **biological computers** in the near future.

Nevertheless, until the evolution of the **'wonder silicon microchips',** the actual setting up and installation of computers in research laboratories was not only expensive but also space consuming. Nowadays, one may even have either a **laptop** or a **desktop** computer.

Principle: The most vital and important a characteristic feature of macromolecules (*e.g.*, proteins) is their inherent ability of taking shape automatically into a predetermined 3D-structure. Therefore, this particular property of proteins largely helps in the intricate process of **biochip designing** by virtue of the fact that the circuits may be conveniently crammed within the 3D-protein structure. Besides, the designing of biochips may be accomplished by using a semi conducting organic molecule strategically inserted inside a protein frame-work; whereby the newly formed entire unit is meticulously attached upon a protein support as shown in Fig. 7.10.

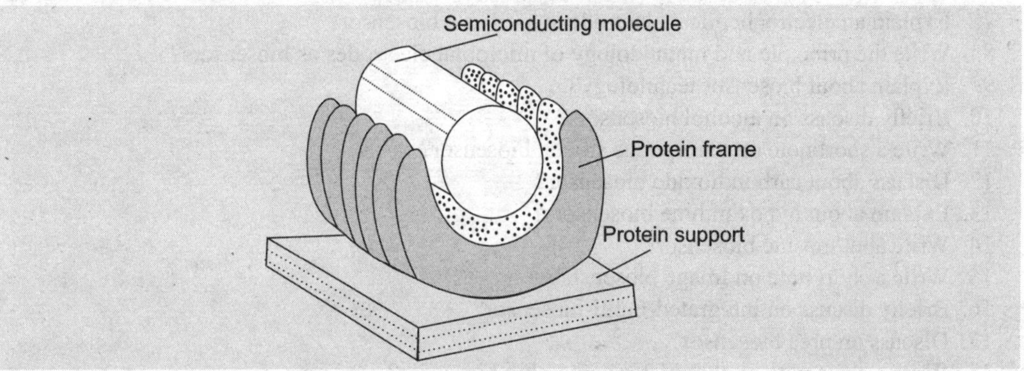

Fig. 7.10 *Diagramatic Sketch of a Biochip*

It has been duly observed that in the particular instance of biochips the electrical signals (or impulses) may pass *via* the ensuing *semi conducting organic molecule* exactly in the same manner as in the case of *silicon microchip*. Thus, the **biochip** has several glaring advantages over the silicon microchip as enumerated under:

a. In the case of **'biochip'** the total width of electrical circuits must not be more than that of one protein molecule, which is in fact smaller in comparison to possibly the smallest *'silicon microchip',*

b. Problems encountered on account of **'electron tunelling'** would be to a certain degree less predominant in a *'biochip model'* than a *'silicon-microchip model'*, and

c. Protein molecule invariably exhibits much less electrical resistance; and, therefore, comparatively less amount of heat shall be generated in the course of generation of electrical signals. As a result, one may be able to squeeze in a lot more circuits together which otherwise is not possible with *silicon microchips.*

Applications of Biochips: The various prominent applications of the **biochips** are as described under:

1. In general, the **biochips** may practically respond to natural nerve impulses eventually, thereby appearing as if it looks more natural when implanted judiciously into the **artificial limbs.**
2. It may also render a great help indeed to the **blind** or **deaf** persons. It may be designed so meticulously that it would not only sense light and sound but also convert them to the corresponding electrical signals. Consequently, these emanated signals after reaching brain cells would distinctly stimulate light and sound more effectively and efficiently.
3. Biochips may also be used possibly as a **heart-heat modulator.** Perhaps it might ease out and thus solve the problems of actual users of rather expensive **'pace-makers'.***
4. Biochips may be suitably designed to serve the urgent basic needs of military personnel's accordingly. Thus, these and render them virtually immune to the not-so-healthy and disastrous after-effects of the prevailing **electromagnetic waves** emanated enormously on account of the **nuclear explosion.**

Questions

1. Applications of gel electrophoresis in biotechnology. (RGUHS–Oct 2007)
2. Define the terms bioreactor and biosensor. (MGRU 2003)
3. Write the application of biosensors. (MGRU 2003)
4. Define biosensors?
5. Write the applications of biosensors?
6. Explain the types of electrodes used as biosensors?
7. Explain an electrochemical electrode is used as a biosensor?
8. Write the principle and methodology of microbial electrodes as biosensors?
9. Explain about biosensor technology?
10. Briefly discuss on alcohol biosensors?
11. Write a short note on amorphous silicon biosensor?
12. Discuss about carbondioxide biosensor?
13. Explain about hypoxanthine biosensors?
14. Write abut inosine biosensor?
15. Write a short note on image biosensor?
16. Briefly discuss on integrated-multi-biosensor?
17. Discuss on urea biosensor?
18. Write a short note on thermistor containing biosensor?
19. Write about bioaffinity sensors?
20. Discuss about opto-electronic biosensor?
21. Define biochips?
22. Write the applications of biochips?

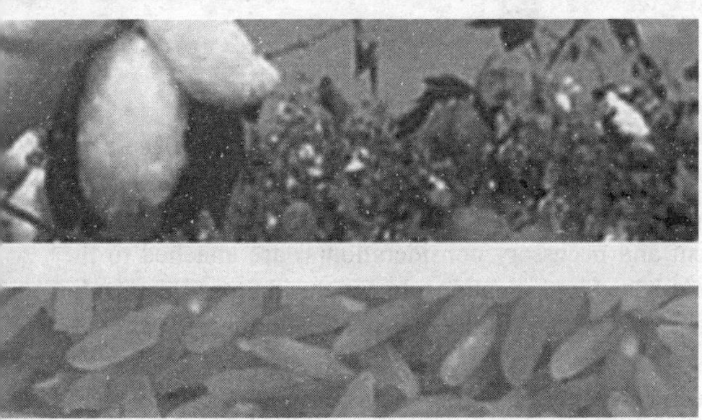

CHAPTER 8

Regulatory Issues in Biotechnology

8.1 Introduction

The rapid and geometrical progress accomplished duly in the last two decades have virtually necessitated the dire need and absolute requirement for the introduction of certain basic ideologies and also the prevention for the *massive misuse of biotechnological outputs* across the globe so as to avoid a precarious and threatening situation. Besides, these may also give rise to a lot of intentional mischief caused by such '*transnational companies*' actively engaged in the ruthless margin and persuit of pretty lukrative profits. Thus, one of these prime and major concerns is the extremely rapid '**pace of genetic erosion**'. Perhaps, it may ultimately lead to an ugly and grave situation whereby the '**basic genetic material**' would be available to only a few *multinational companies* in their respective so called **gene banks**. Therefore, earnest concerted efforts across the globe, particularly the third-world countries; must be geared into quick preventive and remedial action(s) by articulately preserving and saving the '*genetic diversity*' in its own environment rather than the usual **gene bank** or **germplasm bank** by aggressively mobilizing the much needed involvement of people.

It is worthwhile to mention at this point in time that the inhabitations of this beautiful world are swiftly proceeding from the prevailing '**green revolution**' to '**gene revolution**'. Hence, it has legitimately and gainfully gave birth to a host of newer **transgenic plants and animals, seeds, embryos,** and **sperms** that are well preserved for *timely-storage* and *future-usage*. The particular day is not too far when the farmers may have to solely rely and depends upon the '*genetically engineered seeds*'. However, there is still ample doubts and apprehensions whether such seeds would be 100% compatible for the prevailing sustainable agricultural practice '*absolutely free*' of any possible inherited **chemical poison** towards the safety of mankind.

Genetically Modified Organisms (GMOs) must not only be researched meticulously but also be intimately monitored so as to ensure that the hazardous effects to their users, if any, besides adverse effect(s) on the environment will not take place even to a remote extent. In addition, adequate, sincere, and earnest concerted efforts either by the respective arms of the governments or duly recognized nongovernment organizations (NGOs) must be undertaken that thorough absolutely urgent and necessary consideration(s) are attached to the various social and ethical aspects of such broad-based investigations. In conclusion, people must be made fully aware of the real and actual impacts of GMOs and the genetically engineered products without mincing words.

Examples: Certain efforts have already been carried out in a few countries in the world as given below:

1. Germany. The German Green Party has already called for a **5-year moratorium** on the respective commercial release of GMOs.

2. India. Gene compliance has been initiated as a '*public complaint*' against the very ideological concept for the '**patenting of life-forms**', and the '**misuse of biotechnology**'.

3. Great Britain. In UK, the **UK-genetics forum** is bitterly complaining for partially irresponsible applications of biotechnology.

4. USA. A plethora of '**agencies**' are vehemently opposing the intentional and deliberate release of GMOs.

8.1.1 Biosafety

Biosafety may be defined as — '*the policies and procedures invariably adopted to ensure the environmentally safe applications of biotechnology*'.

Biosafety Levels (BSL) usually refers to a classification system used to indicate the safety precautions required for those investigating microorganisms, especially viruses known to be dangerous or lethal to those exposed to them. In fact, there are *four* BSLs with BSL-4 requiring the highest level of security.

By virtue of the ever-growing concerns rapidly arising from the host of **genetically modified organisms (GMOs)** across the entire world the various international organization *viz.,* UNIDO/WHO/FAO/UNEP has legitimately constituted an Informal Working Group on **Biosafety**. Later on, in the year 1991, this specific working group duly prepared the '*Voluntary Code of Conduct for the Release of Organisms into the Environment*'. Soon-after the **International Centre for Genetic Engineering and Biotechnology (ICGEB)** was duly constituted, established, and recognised across the globe. ICGEB indeed played an extremely responsible and overwhelmingly important role with regard to the issue concerned with **biosafety** as well as the environmentally sustainable application(s) of **biotechnology**. Besides, ICGEB duly organizes **'animal workshops'** on **biosafety** together with the vital risk assessment for the legitimate release of GMOs. Evidently, it collaborates to the maximum extent with the management of UNIDO's **Biosafety Information Network and Advisory Services (BINAS)**, with a prime objective in monitoring the global development in the regulatory issues concerned exclusively in **biotechnology**.

With effect from September-1998, ICGEB has successfully provided an excellent world-wide facility *via* an *on-line bibliographic data-base on biosafety*, and risk assessment for the environmental release of GMOs. Interestingly, this particular '**database**', which is easily accessible *via* the website of ICGEB, also caters for numerous valuable information(s) on **biosafety** to its Member States. In fact, the Member

States also enjoy *via* ICGEB a plethora of genuine help and support in developing their own individual *national biosafety framework*. However, since February-1999, ICGEB has promulgated and adopted the much desired and widely acclaimed '*legal binding biosafety protocols*' by its signatory countries.

Keeping in mind the above fast-track development in the ever-increasing domain of '**biotechnology**' a good numbers of countries are at present actively engaged in the spectacular development of a n*ational framework* to modulate research and development taking place in the field of '**biotechnology**'. Persley *et al.* (1992) has explicitly described the various necessary steps absolutely urgent and necessary to establish rightfully a **'national biosafety system'** that essentially builds upon the prevailing regulatory experience, namely:

- Plant Quarantine Acts,
- Environmental Protection Acts, and
- Worker Health and Safety Regulations.

India has the privilege of setting up its own **'comprehensive national biosafety systems'** and the Philippines also established one. In order to have their optimum utilization and productive output these systems are essentially attached to a network of an **Institutional Biosafety Committee,** meticulously coordinated by a live wire of an *apex national biosafety committee.*

In the present prevalent scenario India has duly instituted the **Recombinant DNA Advisory Committee** located in the Department of Biotechnology (DBT) under the Government of India. The aforesaid *'Advisory Committee'* has duly prepared a set of *Recombinant DNA Safety Guidelines* that embraces broadly all areas of research and commercial scale operations involving **genetically engineered organisms.** Importantly, the highly important and specific guidelines for the institutional mechanism for implementing them essentially comprise of the following cardinal aspects:

a. Recombinant DNA Advisory Committee, under the authority of DBT, to formulate and update the '*biosafety guidelines*',

b. Institutional Biosafety Committees, located at all centers, must be grossly engaged in exclusive genetic engineering research and production activities,

c. Review committee on Genetic Manipulation under DBT, to guide and advise the *institutional biosafety committees,*

d. Genetic Engineering Approval Committee functioning under the Department of Environment to review and approve activities essentially making use of the large-scale genetically engineered organisms as well as their resulting product(s) in *research* and *development (R & D), industrial production, environment release,* and *field applications.*

Biotechnology does possess the great potential to handle and solve at least a few of the several vital emerging conflicts prevailing between the fundamental human requirements and the environmental concern significantly and efficaciously. Nevertheless, without the adequate support and due attention to the **'biosafety'** aspects closely, it may obviously give rise to newer problems enormously. As on date, only a very few developing countries in the universe have formulated definitive regulatory mechanism(s) so as to avoid this potential conflict effectively.

Feeding an Ever-Increasing World Population. Present day scenario vehemently demands that every bit of land available must be brought under regular cultivation so as to accomplish the major global herculian task of **feeding an ever-increasing world population.** Consequently, the environment is being subjected to an intense galloping and increasing impact of innumerable approved herbicides and pesticides mechanized aerial/manual sprays, fertilizer leaching, and above all the natural soil erosion phenomenon. Importantly, with the passage of time it would certainly and seriously compromise with the prevailing sustainability of the overall agricultural production across the globe. The advent of **'modern biotechnology'** predominantly makes use of the various developed scientific tools of molecular biology to produce highly specialized crop plants with precise combinations of the *'genetic traits'*. The ultimate objective and fond hope rests on the fact that **'future crops'** having essential pesticide resistant characteristic features shall emerge that can minimize the reliance on the organic chemical entities to a great extent. There are, in fact, two vital aspects, namely:

a. *Nitrogen-fixing enhancements* — to moderate the fertilizer usage, and
b. *Increased crop productivity* — to obviate the urgent immediate requirement for clearance and cultivation of more land.

Keeping in view the enormous advantageous potential of **'biotechnology'**, one must address to the following *two* aspects vividly:

i. Environmental cost involved, and
ii. Assurance that commercial usage of technologically advanced end-products may not eventually boil down to any sort of compromising with the environment.

Quintessence of Biosafety. A plethora of *'bioscientists'* do strongly opine that **genetically modified crop plants** may be cultivated with the least possible scope of any adverse consequences to the existing global environment. However, there are certain valid aspects to ponder, such as:

- Comprehensive knowledge of biological complexity neither possible nor available
- Unpredictable fate of organism being incorporated into the environment
- Extremely important and wise to evaluate possible consequences well in anticipation.

Therefore, the above glaring facts duly represent the **quintessence of biosafety.** It may be adequately defined as — *'the governmental policies and procedures adopted to ensure completely the environmentally safe applications of biotechnology'*. Thus, when it becomes a part and parcel of the **'governmental review programmes'**, it is always pertinent to ascertain the extent of risk involved of the emerging new products before these are actually subjected to **'test in the field'.**

Nevertheless, **modern agricultural biotechnology** needs to be implemented cautiously and carefully *via* well-defined **appropriate regulatory mechanisms** so as to reasonably resolve such usual encountered ideologies and conflicts as:

- Need for food Vs desire to conserve the environment.
- Promise of biotechnology *vis-à-vis* uncertainty of adverse effects on environment.

8.1.2 Topic of Concern [Website of ICGEB]

Topic of concern may be broadly classified into *five* major categories that are prominently related to the environmental release of the genetically modified organisms (GMOs) as stated under:

8.1.2.1 Risks for Human Health

- Toxicity Vs food quality/safety
- Allergies
- Pathogen's drug resistance *i.e.,* antibiotic resistance

8.1.2.2 Risks for Environment

- Persistence of gene/transgene/transgene products
- Resistance of target organisms or susceptibility of non-target organisms.
- Increased usage of chemicals in agriculture
- Transgene instability
- Unpredictable gene expression

8.1.2.3 Risks for Agriculture

- Weeds or super weeds
- Change in nutritional value
- Reduction of cultivars and loss of biodiversity

8.1.2.4 Risks for Interaction with Non-target Organisms

- Genetic pollution *via* pollen or seed dispersal
- Horizontal gene transfer

- DNA uptake *i.e.,* transfer of foreign gene to microorganisms
- Generation of new line viruses by recombination DNA technology

8.1.2.5 General Concerns

- Higher cost of agricultural production
- Loss of familiarity
- Ethical issues.

8.1.3 Biosafety Guidelines and Regulations

It is, however, pertinent to state here that several countries have adequately formulated the specific **Biosafety Guidelines** for rDNA manipulations with the following aims and objectives, namely:

a. To reduce the usual probability of infrequent release of GMOs, and

b. To prevent and check the intentional release of such GMOs into the prevailing environment.

The meticulous promulgation of **'the Recombinant DNA Safety Guidelines'** by the Department of Biotechnology (DBT), in India, have duly entrusted the authority to exercise powers conferred *via* the **Environmental Protection ACT 1986,** for several important functional activities, such as: *manufacture, usage, import, export, and storage of hazardous microorganisms/genetically engineered organisms, and cells.*

Importantly, all these guidelines are duly being implemented *via* the following *three* articulated mechanisms, for instance:

i. **Institutional Biosafety Committees (IBSCs)** — to monitor the on-going research activity at institutional level,

ii. **Genetic Engineering Approval Committee (GEAC)** — to permit the large scale application of GMOs at the commercial level, and open the field trials of *transgenic substances viz.*, agricultural crops, industrial products, health-care products, etc., and

iii. **Review Committee on Genetic Manipulation (RCGM)** — to allow the risky activities in the research laboratories under the direct supervision of DBT.

8.1.4 Operation/Function of Biosafety Guidelines and Regulations

It is worthwhile to mention here that virtually all the **'academic institutions'** and **'industrial organizations'** actively involved in genetic *engineering activities* should have essentially the properly constituted Institutional Biosafety Committees (IBSCs). Besides, with the adequate prior approval and granted permission of RCGM such **'research activities'** may be performed in India by making use of **transgenic materials.** A few such typical examples are stated as under:

i. A company imported the *'transgenic mustard seeds'* having the expression of **Barstar** and **Barnase genes** from Belgium to study and evaluate the exact performance of the said characteristic seeds upon the Indian Soils and its environment,

ii. Another company imported seeds of *'transgenic cotton'* essentially containing the **Bt gene** to carry out specific trails in **'glass-house'** by adopting the procedure of **back-coating with Indian cotton-lines**, and also to evaluate resistance of the transgenic plant materials to bollworms in India,

iii. A pharmaceutical organization duly carried out intensive and extensive experimental trials for the production of **Recombinant Hepatitis B Vaccines,** and **Human α-Interferon** by employing *yeast* and *E. coli* respectively, and

iv. A company imported the *recombinant strains of yeast expressing Hepatitis B surface antigen protein.* The company was duly granted approval and permission to perform elaborative experiments for pilot-scale production of **'Recombinant Hepatitis B Vaccines'** at IMTECH (Chandigarh).

8.1.5 Development of Herbicide Resistant Crops

Biosafety legitimately shares the ultimate responsibility and takes cognizance of both the potential for the plethora of undesirable consequences emanating from new technological advancements as well as the absolute requirement for appropriate measures to significantly minimize these consequences.

Example: Genetic engineering of crops is invariably claimed to have defended a host of the world's genuine problems specially to meet the '**hunger**'. Therefore, specific emphasis with respect to the present day *agricultural research* is mainly focused towards the **development of herbidicide resistant crops.**

Consequently, the crux of the problem suggests explicitly that the actual and genuine beneficiaries of the above cited new technology may not be identical as those forced to assume the ensuing risks involved. The promulgation of an **internationally binding safety protocol** has been initiated and instituted to avoid such *glaring imbalances*; besides, to contain adequately the outcome of ecological risks as well as socio-economic impacts of genetically engineered organisms together with their probable risks to human-health.

Valid cardinal and vital reasons for essentially including the genetically modified organisms (GMOs) under the regulation of a biosafety protocol are as enumerated under:

1. The potential for transgenic crops to become weeds and unwanted plants, to become channels *via* which new genes move to wild plants, and to facilitate the creation of new viruses that may cause newer plant diseases.
2. The potential of genetic engineering to contribute to the erosion of agricultural biodiversity by either of the two ways, namely:
   a. Creation of crops that essentially compete with wild plants and other traditional varieties, and
   b. Transfer of new crop's genes into the more primitive varieties.
3. The potential of genetic engineering to upset (imbalance) the prevailing '*ecosystems*' in manners that may not be properly understood or adequately remediated.
4. The potential for adverse social and economic impacts in developing countries from the products emanated from genetic engineering. Production of such *substitutes* for export crops has already led to tremendous loss of livelihoods and export earnings in certain countries in the world.
5. In some countries there is no facility and provision to ensure the safety of genetically modified organisms (GMOs), to monitor and regulate their entry at the border, and to take appropriate remedial measures in the event of certain untoward mishap(s).
6. The existence of a *transboundary ecological dimension* to genetically engineered organisms. Even when there is no human intent to export, living organisms may spontaneously *mutate, multiply,* and *migrate.*
7. Genetic engineering is based on the *'idea'* that characteristic features of organisms are determine uniquely by stable genes, such that the transfer of genes automatically gives rise to the transfer of the '**desired characteristics'.** Importantly, this genetic *determinism** fails to take into consideration the complex interactions amongst the genes that are duly involved in the overall development of all characteristics of an organism ; and, therefore, frequently masks the genuine inability to predict the ensuing consequences of transferring a gene from one type of organism to another.

A good number of **International Organizations** *viz*., EC, FAO, UNEP, and UNIDO are not only interested but also genuinely keen to look into **biosafety aspects,** such as:

- Biosafety and its impact on the use of *'biotechnology'* in the developing countries so as to assess the various needs in order to ensure that the *agricultural* and *environmental* applications of biotechnology move forward devoid of any undue risks or excessive costs.

- Real public concerns arising obviously from certain newer biotechnological product(s) causes lots of apprehensions that need to be resolved and confidence gained, in case biotechnology is to make its greatest impact and maximum contribution to the much needed welfare of society.
- A few developing countries have evolved and formulated their own stringent **'national biosafety systems'** thereby incorporating definite well-defined guidelines for:

a. Experimental *modus operandi,* and
b. Small-scale release of genetically modified organisms (GMOs).

However, the **'National Guidelines'** operative in India, are mainly based upon the **United States-National Institute of Health (NIH)** guidelines.

It is indeed pertinent to mention here that an evidently much greater and extended focus upon the benefits and risks involved in the specific release of an **'alien organism'**, in comparison to the process engaged for its production. It has been duly observed that there are certain critical and absolutely vital biological considerations with regard to the *'intended releases'* for which adequate strategies require to be devised exclusively to ensure the stability of its legitimate and safe introduction.

Example: The potential for the usual overexposure of the novel **Bt genes** for affording *'insect resistance'* ultimately leading to the rapid development of resistance.

8.2 Intellectual Property Right (IPR) and Protection (IPP)

Intellectual property right (IPR) usually refers to that segment of **'law'** that specifically is related to **patents, copy-rights, trademarks, trade secrets,** and **above all the plant variety protection**. Therefore, in order to boost up, encourage, and stimulate local innovative ideas and research activities, private and public sector collaborative strategies (*viz.,* private organization and academic institutions), to attract lucrative investment(s) from foreign countries it has become almost an absolute necessity to plan out clear national policies, articulated regulations, and superb understanding of IPR, which are as vital and important as the **'biosafety regulations'.** As to date there exist hardly any **'internationally accepted guidelines for the total management and control of IPR';** and, hence the proper and judicious utility of IPR has turned out to be a much debatable and controversial issue across the globe.

Consequently, the industrialized countries in the world are invariably demanding a much stronger, valid, and legitimate protection keeping in view the various provisions of IPR that usually change appreciably amongst them. It has been duly observed that particularly the '*developing countries*' do possess a strong anxiety of fear and apprehension that usually the **'strict IPR protection'** may, in fact, give rise to serious hinderance rather than promoting innovation within the country due to the glaring fact that a major segment of such IPRs are normally tilted and granted to the so-called foreign partners/institutions.

Van Wijk and Junne (1992) rightly pointed out several '*short-protection terms*' as applicable to the developing nations with regard to the IPR regulations, such as:

- Strong compulsory licensing provisions,
- exclude many products from protection,
- National IPR policies invariably forbid the patenting of **products** *viz.,* pharmaceuticals, microorganisms, and animal and plant species, and
- IPR protection for **processes** which evidently produce **'novel products'** is normally granted permission.

Importantly, one may observe that the **'IPR related laws'** were duly formulated from time to time both at **national** and **international** levels. However, USA has been inclined towards the promulgation and adoption of a strong and uniform *'IPR related laws'* across the entire globe.

Highlights of IPR-Related Laws. The various highlights of the **'IPR-related laws'** are as enumerated under:

i. Development of specific crop varieties is the others intellectual property right (IPR).

ii. IPR is duly protected by **'plant breeders rights'** (PBRs).

iii. PBRs are only available in *'developed countries'* and not in India (a developing country like many others).

iv. Principle of PBRs recognizes and advocates the 'gospel truth' the **'ultimate pact'** that farmers and rural communities have actually contributed enormously to the creation, conservation, exchange, and knowledge of genetic/species utilization of genetic diversity.

v. Both IPR and IPP adequately granted by the Government to the respective plant breeders to exclude others from producing, reproducing, or commercializing materials of a particular plant specimen for a duration ranging between 15-20 years. However, this *'specific plant variety'* must enjoy the status of being **new** and **never found before.**

In conclusion, one may remark that **'biotechnology'** has indeed played a pivotal and significant role in the adequate execution of well-defined, highly specific, and value-added sophisticated processing, designing, and production of valuable commercial products that may be used in a larger cross section of the society and the country as well *viz.*, agriculture environment, industry, pharmaceuticals, medical, and health care system(s) etc. Nevertheless, the involvement of the so called **'technology transfer in biotechnology'** is so minimal; and, therefore, requires nothing but a simple and minimum amount of technical and legal capability that is invariably found to be lacking amongst the *'developing countries'* currently. Hence, there is an urgent need to expand the trained personnel's in *biotechnology* is such developing countries.* It is earnestly hoped and believed that in the immediate future the **generich** *vis-à-vis* **technologically poor developing countries** should make a concerted effort to join hands together, and reach to a memorandum of understanding (MoU) to exchange vital help in different mutal programmes in the years yet to come.

8.2.1 Types of IPR-Protection

In general, the **intellectual property right (IPR) protection** may be accomplished duly by different means and ways, namely: **patents, copyrights, trade secrets,** and **trade marks.**

All these above mentioned aspects shall now be treated individually in the section that follows:

8.2.1.1 Patents

Patent may be defined as — *'a special right to the inventor that has been granted by the respective Government through legislation for trading new articles'*.

Nevertheless, a **patent** is regarded as a personal property that may be legitimately either **'lisenced'** or **'sold'** by the individual person or organization very much like any other property.

Examples

1. **USA.** The maximum limit of **'patent'** extends upto 17 years.
2. **EU.** Certain European countries the **'patent'** is granted solely to the inventors so that they may adequately develop newer articles beneficial to the society to which they belong or represent.
3. **India. Indian Patent Act (1970)** permits the **'process patents'** and not the **'product patents'**, which extended upto 5 years from the date of *grant* and 7 years from the date of filing the patent application.

Importantly, with effect from 1st January-2005, the uniform internationally accepted **Patent Laws'** have been promulgated with broadly and universally accepted guidelines.

Interestingly, a patent essentially consists of **three** essential segments, namely:

a. **Grant.** The grant is invariably filled and completed at the patent office, and this is not published. It is more or less a signed document that represents actually the agreement which solely grants patent right to the inventor.

b. **Specifications.** The specifications as well as claims are published as a single document which is made public at a minimum charge from the respective patent office.

c. **Claims.** This particular segment exclusively defines the *'scope of the invention'* to be protected by the **patent** which may not be utilized in practice by others at all.

Examples: The most important aspect that needs the utmost understanding and discussion is the simultaneous operations of **Federal/and State Patent Laws,** which may be expatiated from the following examples, such as:

a. **US-FDA** — has regulatory purview pertaining to the **patented pharmaceuticals** before allowing them for actual use.

b. **Environment Protection Agency in US** — discharging their responsibilities under the jurisdiction of **Federal Insecticide, Fungicide, and Rodenticide Act** only allows the release of *genetically engineered microbial pesticides.*

c. **Department of Biotechnology (DBT) in India** – has duly formulated **'the recombinant DNA safety guidelines'** so as to exercise powers conferred *via* the *Environmental Protection Act (1986).*

d. **Genetic Engineering Approval Committee (GEAC)** — under the Ministry of Environment and Forest has the powers to permit the commercial usage of GEMs at large-scale level; besides, open field trials of **'transgenic materials'.**

8.2.1.2 Copyrights

In actual practice, the **'copyright protection'** is nothing but a kind of expression of ideas.

Example: **Copyrights of Books:** In fact, the author(s), editors, publishers or both publisher and author/editor do have the provision of **copyrights.** Under this protection the materials (*i.e.*, contents) of the book cannot be either reproduced or reprinted without the prior written permission from the legal copyright holders. It is, however, pertinent to state at this point in time that evidently **patents** and **trade secrets** exclusively provide protection to the fundamental know-how, whereas **copyrights** essentially protect the expressed materials *viz.*, materials in printed, taped forms or video recorded. Interestingly, the biotechnological derived materials subject to copyright duly encompass such products as: **photo-micrographs, database of DNA sequences, and any published forms.**

8.2.1.3 Trade Secretes (Know-how)

Trade secret invariably refers to the *'private proprietary information'* which solely benefits the **'owners'**. However, it may be of any kind *e.g.,* **process technique, product yield** etc.

Example: Coca Cola Beverage. The coca cola company had adequately maintained and covered its **'best kept trade secrets'** of its original formula, form more than 100 yeras and more than 135 countries in the world, under this specific provision of the law. In US, the limit of **'trade secrets'** extends upto 2 years, while the same holds good in India upto 5 years. In the event when the **'trade secrets'** become known (or public) on or before the **stipulated granted period,** the '*intellectual*' is duly paid compensation, and the *unauthorized users (defaulters)* are punished by the law enforcing authorities adequately.

Importantly, the *'trade secrets'* in the field of *'biotechnology'* may essentially comprise of several parameters, such as : **hybridization conditions, cell-lines, processing, designing, consumer's list,** and the like.

8.2.1.4 Trade Marks

The **trade mark** is an identification symbol that is exclusively employed in the course of trade to not only enable the *'actual consumer'* to distinguish but also to identify precisely the genuinity of trader's products from identical goods/products of the other traders. The consumer invariably takes the advantage of these **trade marks** to choose exactly whose goods they intend to buy. In case, the traders are quite reasonably satisfied with the purchase of a particular item (and its '*brand*'), they may simply place a repeat order by making use of the **trade mark.**

Examples: There are indeed several examples which may be cited as given below:

KODAK : for photography goods;
IBM : for computers;
ROLEX : for wrist-watches;
REEBOK : for shoes;
ADIDAS : for sports shoes;
RAYMONDS : for suiting materials;
GALLENKAMP : for laboratory equipments;
ZODIAC : for readymade clothes;
SAMSONITE : for suitcases, and sky-bags;

It is worthwhile to mention here that according to OECD (1989) there are *five* cardinal advantages of patents and other forms of IPR, namely:

1. Encouraging and safeguarding the interest of intellectual and artistic creations,
2. Disseminating newer ideas, concepts, and technologies both rapidly and widely,
3. Promoting the investment,
4. Providing the genuine consumers with the result of creation and invention, and
5. Providing enhanced opportunities for the distribution of the above effects across the countries in a manner proportionate to national levels of economic and industrial development.

8.2.2 Status and Implication of IPR

The present day status and implications of IPR may be elaborated and expatiated under the following six points, namely:

i. **Intellectual property protection (IPP)** systems are not just arbitrarily fixed but they do evolve with the passage of time. As on date, the patent system in several countries essentially comprise of parts/segments of plants, whole plants, and plant varieties.

ii. Based upon the negotiations in the World Intellectual Property Organization (WIPO), bilateral consultations, and in General Agreement of Tariffs and Trade (GATT) the industrialized countries invariably strive for worldwide adaptation of IPP to the newer emerging technologies.

Thus, USA, Japan, and EU usually pressurize the developing countries (*e.g.,* India) to expunge (remove) completely the provisions in their patent laws which specifically exclude from patent protection such critical matter as '*living material*'. Besides, the prevailing plant breeder's right (PBR) might serve as a viable alternative for patent protection for plant varieties to certain developing countries in the world ; however, GATT does not take into consideration this alternative aspect at all.

iii. The major function of IPP in biotechnology is to promote profusely biotechnological innovation, application, and development. In case, the *developing countries* are left with no other choice than to enforce establishment of IPP for **biotechnological inventions** or for **plant varieties,** then the function of IPP shall be confined primarily to the promotion of the biotechnological innovation in the *industrialized countries.* In other words, IPP with respect to plant material as adopted by developing countries may certainly promote innovation in agricultural research in these countries, only in a situation when the introduction of IPP is directly and intimately related to their stage of development.

Nevertheless, there may arise three distinct situations with regard to the status and implications of IPR which shall be discussed briefly in the sections that follows:

Situation-I. *i.e., where intellectual property protection would not be appropriate:*

In case, practically little *breeding* or *biotechnological research activity,* occur, it is absolute little interest for any country to go in for either plant breeder's right (PBR) or patent protection in these fields.

Importantly, for plant breeding systems, critically characterized by an absolute open exchange of finished varieties, unimproved base materials, and breeding lines, there is no necessity to go in for the adoption of '*intellectual property protection (IPP)*' specifically for the plant material. It also holds good in the instance where local propagation of varieties is invariably encouraged as is the case in majority of developing nations.

Nevertheless, in the event when the component of the **'domestic IPP'** for the plant material is absent, a nation is quite free from any restriction whatsoever to import technical know how and varieties, to make use of the acquired knowledge abundantly, and also to propagate it freely and commercialize the **'end material'** within the borders of that nation.

Situation-II. *i.e., where plant breeder's right (PBR) may seem to be appropriate:*

In this particular instance, the prevalent **'breeding activity'** has undergone a development much beyond its preliminary stages; and. therefore, the implementation of a legal system pertaining to intellectual property protection (IPP) particularly for the plant material as a viable avenue of stimulating and encouraging private investment would remarkably promote local private plant breeding activities in favour of the development of market oriented agriculture research. The much acclaimed principle of the **'breeders exemption'** ultimately guarantees the *'free and fair'* utilization of genetical material (without any compulsion) of the so called protected variety towards the gainful creation and legitimate commercialization of new varieties. Of course, the **'farmer's privilege'** certainly provides the farmers certain degree of freedom in order to save ample quantum of seed essentially needed for the next crop production.

There is absolutely little doubt that the free importation of *'foreign improved varieties'* would definitely go a long way in involving as a necessary consequence for bringing in severe cutthroat competition for those specific varieties bred by domestic breeders. Alternatively, it may give rise to a positive impact upon the well established market oriented agriculture since farmers most probably may not depend exclusively either on *public* or on *local private* breeding activities to obtain the **improved varieties.**

Nevertheless, the plant breeder's right (PBR) system may prove to be effective only when the following conditionalities are fulfilled, such as:

- Farmers should be able to purchase modern varieties of seeds,
- Independent '*quality control*' and '*testing facilities*' must be available,
- Various approved channels to spread the information should always be available freely, and
- Users and holders of proprietary rights should be in a position to rely on an approved and recognized legal and technological infrastructure to protect their legitimate interests.

Situation-III. *i.e., where granting of patent protection might be appropriate:*

Importantly, the '**patent protection**' could be accomplished expeditiously only *via* an extremely superb and high level of research and development activities in **'biotechnology'**.

However, the domestic entrepreneurs (companies) may largely benefit from the **patent ability** of their biotechnological inventions, whereas **patent protection** certainly encourages foreign organizations to enable their knowledge and wisdom duly available in the entire world.

It may be worthwhile to state here that the legitimate right of the foreign companies to a reasonable remuneration for an inventor may not be a subject of a probable controversial debate; however, the granting of *utility patents of plants* involves and attracts sufficient risk that may have an access to a common pool of plant genetic resources, essential for *'plant breeding'* may become restricted ultimately. As a result, the ultimate patent protection of plant material would cause a tremendous hinderance in the overall agricultural development across the globe.

iv. Two vital and important aspects, namely: plant breeder's right (PBR) on plant varieties, and patent protection for the numerous biotechnological inventions should necessarily provide the *'public research institutes'* with substantial additional funding and also adequately protect their work against free commercialization. It is, however, emphasized amply that the *'ultimate quest'* for the strategic legal protection may not entail any delay whatsoever in providing improved plant material or technology needs for the futuristic growth. In the same vein, the availability across the national boundaries of inventions or innovations or varieties derived primarily from the on-going programmes of the prevailing **international agricultural research centers (IARCs)** must not be subjected to any sort of restrictions or limitations.

Importantly, whenever public institutes do lodge an application for IPP of their research product, it must be regarded that any step taken forward in the commercialization of the ensuing *subsidized public research* would lead to encounter possible opposition on the private sector related to their unfair trade practices.

v. *Intellectual property protection (IPP) for plant material specially in industrialized countries may adversely affect the agricultural export from developing countries.* It has been duly observed that the extension of the underlying scope of *plant breeder's right (PBR) protection* as explicitly applicable to almost all material of the protected specimen, besides any prolongation of the period of protection, may have an altogether adverse consequences to the farmers belonging to the developing nations because of the complete blockade of the export material of a specific variety gaining entry to a developed nation where this variety is entirely protected. Furthermore, the authorized certificate holders may prohibit this export operation:

a. Unless the farmers employed purchased seed, and

b. Unless the farmers pay hefty royalties for their multiplication of seeds legally.

vi. In a broader perspective the industrialized *(i.e.,* developed) countries avoid exerting undue presure upon the developing nations to protect and preserve the intellectual property embodied in plant material thereby ignoring, as far as possible, the consequences for the ensuing vast and noteworthy agricultural development taking place in these nations. In nutshell, the intellectual property protection (IPP) meant for plant material exclusively deserves to be adopted if it strategically promotes the much desired national agricultural development.

In Conclusion, one may add that the various rules and regulations, including the **plant breeder's right** (PBR) as well as the **patent legislation,** should be judged from that perspective solely.

8.2.3 Protection of Biotechnological Inventions

The **'use claim'** represents a type of *'patent claim'* which has turned out to be a much-talked about conspicuous feature of the **European Patents** where the invention is an altogether '*new use*' for an already known product. Thus, the prevailing **European patent system** enjoys this particular kind of a claim that has unnecessarily given rise to certain newer and controversial concepts and ideas for an universally accepted **'patent law'**.

Examples:

a. **Medicament.** *First,* medical usage for a known substance may be duly protected by a 'product for use ......' claim, whereas, a *second* medical indication (usage) essentially necessitates the need for a special form of actual '**use**' claim.

b. **Microbiological Field.** The specific discovery of a hitherto not-reported property (*i.e.,* characteristic feature) may, in certain particular circumstances, be adequately covered by an appropriate *'use'* claim, irrespective of the fact that the actual '*mode of usage*' is not new.

A few glaring examples are enumerated as under:

Product	Manufacturer (Country)	Remarks
Hepatitis C Virus	Chiron (USA)	In Great Britain the Patents Court have duly
Hepatitis B Virus	Biogen (Switzerland)	Decided the fate of these two products recentiy.
Tissue Plasminogen Activator (tPA)	Gentech (USA)	In Great Britain the Patents Court rejected the patent on recombinant tissue plasminogen activator (tPA) for want of inventiveness.
HcV-Vaccine	Chiron (USA)	Unfortunately, the claim of this vaccine was held **invalid** due to the lack of sufficient disclosure how to prepare such a vaccine.

Interestingly, the various countries who are the bonafide signatories to the convention, PBRs are invariably guided and governed by an international convention known as the International convention of the Union for the Protection of New Varieties of Plants (UPOV). However, in 1991, UPOV has been thoroughly revised in order to strengthen the prevailing scope of the rights as well as to overcome the defects of the earlier versions of the present treaty. The cardinal and prime aim of the entire terms of reference contained in the latest version of UPOV categorically highlights two most important aspects, namely:

a. Peaceful co-existence of PBRs for plant varieties, and

b. Peaceful co-existence of patent rights for transgenic plants.

Questions

1. What is gene bank? How do you maintain the gene bank?
2. What is GOM? Write the advantages & disadvantages of about it?
3. Define biosafety?
4. Write a short note on ICGEB?
5. Discuss on biosafety guidelines and regulations?
6. Briefly explain on intellectual property rights and protection?
7. Explain plant breeder's rights?
8. What is patent? Discuss on how do you get patent for a new product?
9. Explain on copyrights?
10. Discuss on trade secretes?
11. Discuss on trade marks?

CHAPTER 9

Safety in Biotechnology

9.1 Introduction

The potential for the better and deep understanding of '**biotechnology**' is such that the more one believes in and practices whole-heartedly this wonderful ever-emerging domain of science and technology, the more one actually accomplishes and delivers.

In the recent past, the manner, the speed, the momentum gained by the astronomical expansion and growth of this particular technology related to biosciences across the globe it has become absolutely necessary to introduce, implement, and promulgate certain '**biotechnological precautions**'. Nevertheless, these specific biotechnological precautions may be categorized under the following heads, namely:

i. Biological precautions,
ii. Chemical precautions, and
iii. Personal precautions.

The above mentioned *three* types of **biotechnological precautions** shall now be treated individually in the section that follows:

9.1.1 Biological Precautions

The various **biological precautions** may be summarized as given below:

1. The following are the *suggested* host bacteria, vectors for DNA, and DNA inserts

Host Bacteria: *Escherichia coli*, K-12 strains (MM294), HB101, JM series.

Vectors for DNA: *p*AMP, *p*KAN, *p*UC, *p*BR322, and M13.

DNA Inserts: Bacteriophage Lambda, T4, and *E. coli* sequences.

2. Sterilization. The sterilization of bottles, laboratory glass-wares *e.g.,* tubes; conical flasks, Petri-dishes, pipettes etc., and solutions should be duly carried out in autoclaves at 15 psi for duration of 15 minutes at 121°C.

Caution: Do not sterilize either DNA or bacterial cultures by autoclaving or direct heating.

3. Decontamination: In order to maintain perfect sterility on the laboratory bench work areas they should be properly wiped down using a 10% **Bleach Solution** (*viz.*, chlorinated lime or Calcium hypochlorite), both before and after working with DNA or microbes. For obtaining best results one must always make use of freshly prepared **Bleach Solution** every day. Importantly, the work surface areas should be invariably decontaminated at least once per day and also after every accidential/non-intentional spills while working in the laboratory.

4. Disposal of Organisms: The **disposal of organisms (bacteria)** may be accomplished by adopting any one of the following *three* procedures:

a. Place them in a **'biohazard bag'**, and autoclave it at 15 psi for 30 minutes at 121°C, and

b. Soak them in a 10% **'bleach solution'** for at least 60 minutes.

5. Disposal of Solid and Liquid Wastes: All accumulated solid and liquid wastes are first collected, autoclaved at 15 psi and 121°C for 30 minutes or by soaking in a bleach solution (10%) for 60 minutes before disposal.

Important: While autoclaving materials for disposal care must be taken to loosen all bottle caps and also to open the mouth of bags so as to enable to steam to escape easily and conveniently.

6. Storage of DNA and Microorganisms: Dedicated refrigerators exclusively meant for the adequate storage of DNA and microorganisms must be provided; and these materials should **not** be stored with food or beverages.

7. Storage of DNA: DNA should be kept frozen in a specially designed **non-frost-free freezer**. Special care must be taken that DNA not be allowed to undergo '*defrost*' between uses in the laboratory due to the fact it may lead to cleavage of long molecules.

8. Storage of Microorganisms: Microorganisms may be stored as **slants** or **stabs** at room temperature, whereas the **sealed plates** can be stored conveniently in a refrigerator. New cultures of bacteria must be propagated at least once in a mouth of maintain adequate **'live cells'**.

9. Management of Spills on Bench Top: In the event when either **bacteria** or **DNA** are spilled on a bench top while working always wear surgical sterile gloves and absorb the spill with either *paper towels* or *bench-protector paper*. It is an usual practice to manage and contain the spills by working from the otuer periphery of the spill, apply disinfectant or 10% bleaching solution, and wipe toward the center of the spill. However, step (5) stated above should be followed while carrying out the usual disposal of the paper towels/bench-protector paper duly.

9.1.2 Chemical Precautions

There are several vital and important **chemical precautions** which should be followed strictly and rigidly as far as possible as stated under:

1. It is invariably recommended that **DNA isolation procedures** should be chosen in such a manner so as to avoid the possible usage of either *phenol* or *chloroform* ; because, the former usually burns the skin on contact while the latter is toxic in nature.
2. **Homidium Bromide [Ethidium Bromide]:** Due to the possible carcinogenic and mutagenic effects of homidium bromide, the National Association of Biology Teachers (NABT) recommends that pre-college level teachers should make use of either **methylene blue** or **stain gels**. Since, methylene blue is inherently a mild toxic chemical entity one must put on sterile surgical gloves at all times when staining gels are used.

Caution: Students must not make use of either Homidium Bromide or handle gels stained with homidium bromide.

3. **Methylene Blue:** It can be employed maximum upto four times before discarding the same.
4. **General Precautions:** Certain **'general precautions'** may have to be followed while working in a laboratory, such as: to minimize formation of aerosols; to avoid forcing the last drop of fluid from the tip of a pipette; to avoid skin contact with ethanol and isopropanol.

9.1.3 Personal Precautions

There are a good number of personal precautions that one may have to adhere to strictly as detailed under:

1. Naked Flame and Inflammable Solvents: An individual has to observe special care and precaution while working near an open flame (or naked flame). To accomplish this all highly inflammable liquids/solvents must be kept or stored far away from the naked flame(s). The alcohol bottles/containers should be stoppered or covered duly when they are not in use. Synthetic dress materials, hats, dangling earnings, long hair styles etc., should be avoided in the laboratory.

2. Minor cuts in fingers, hands must be adequately protected by wearing sterile latex surgical gloves.

3. Protection of Eyes: Each and every student must put on the '*safety laboratory goggles*'*.

4. Apron or Laboratory coats. It is a safety as well as a professional practice to wear apron or laboratory coat, preferably white and made from cotton only, so as to prevent possible contamination or soiling of clothes from chemicals etc.

5. Nose and Mouth Mask: Always make use of preferably sterile disposable **'nose and mouth masks'** besides wearing gloves when one gets engaged in the handling of ingredients required for *culture media* or weighing and preparations of *antibiotic solutions*.

Caution: In the preparation of solution sodium lauryl sulphate (or sodium dodecyl sulphate, SDS) for carrying out the isolation of bacteria, always use a dust mask since SDS is an irritant.

$CH_3(CH_2)_{10}CH_2OSO_3Na$

Sodium dodecyl Sulphate

9.2 Biosafety

In the recent past the mankind has encountered several most severe and quite dangerous challenges pertaining to a plethora of problems associated with the **biosafety** *i.e.,* **safety in biotechnology**.

The absolute and dire necessity of biosafety has emerged by virtue of the spectacular and galloping advancements in the field of biotechnological advancements, as may be observed from the following successful accomplishments, namely:

1. Development of genetic engineering biotechnology: **Examples:** Creation of first successful man-made human chromosomes in the body of a mouse, cloning mammal (sheep), various genetic-engineering based drugs (*e.g.*, streptokinase, human insulin etc.), and animals having better characteristic features. Ultimately, all these wonderful achievements would certainly promote in the near future a good number of spectacular avenues in the domain of **'industrial biotechnology'.**

2. Transgenic Organisms: The marker transgenic or genetically modified organisms* is undergoing a very rapid development across the globe. Certain countries in the world already have the privilege to make use of these organisms profusely in various divergent fields, such as: medicine, production of food and beverages, and agricultural products.

Examples: (a) Introduction of transgenic plants (1996-1997): Various transgenic plants, viz., *herbicide, pest,* and *virus*-resistant varieties of potatoes, tomatoes, soyabean, maize, rapeseed, cotton, sugarbeet and the like were duly introduced actually right into the agricultural fields.

Interestingly, the total land area covered in USA in the year 1997 stood at 8 million hectares, which extended up to 24 million hectares in 1999 i.e., almost a 3 fold increase in just 2 years span.

Note of Caution: *In the face of an enormous apparent economic benefits derived evidently from the direct usage of such organisms, scientists/researchers do believed it absolutely necessary and important to seek broad based public attention and equally critical cognizance to the underlying importance with regard to* ***certain dire preventive measures*** *and* ***total elimination*** *of possible impacts of their introduction, and above all their harmful/ adverse effect to public health and environment.*

In conclusion, one may add that 'uncontrolled release of transgenic organisms into the environment may ultimately lead to serious 'ecological imbalance', and thereby give a 'red alert' to the ***biological diversity****.*

(b) Outlining the potential risks involved: The various array of potential risks involved essentially include the following cardinal aspects, namely:

- Transfer of tailor-made (*i.e.,* specifically designed genetic structures into the genotypes of the existing organisms.
- Origination of rather more viable dreadful organisms that may be capable of ousting other organisms of their respective ecological niches**.
- Unavoidable emergence of biologically active compounds and proteins that is obviously harmful for humans and animals. Importantly, as to date the leading countries of the world have gone much ahead with respect to the critical development of systematic and methodical **'advanced systems'** for carrying out.

Scientific research into **biosafety**. However, the analyzing aspects and prospects of the biotechnological development are duly balanced in the right perspective by the concerned **national legislative bodies** covering usage of biotechnology and its products. Nevertheless, various international organizations, namely: UNIDO, the European community, do contribute their earnest and meaningful timely efforts for the immediate strategic introduction/implementation of such highly sophisticated systems to the countries of the Eastern Europe including Ukraine.

9.3 Pathogenic Microorganisms and Fungi

A plethora of microorganisms and fungi do cause diseases in human beings. Therefore, it would be duly justified if both of these causative organisms are treated individually as given below:

9.3.1 Pathogenic Microorganisms

It has been duly proved and established that if a microorganism exerts an obvious adverse effect upon another organism i.e., causing specific diseases in humans, most probably by gaining an entry inside and then damaging its cells or affecting it with a chemical substance produced by it, it is invariably termed as **pathogens**. In other words, such organisms can also be referred to as the causative organism of that particular disease *e.g., Salmonella typhi causes* typhoid in the humans; *Giardia lamblia*— causes water borne diseases.

Diarrhoea may be caused by a wide range of *bacteria, viruses*, and *parasites* that invariably invade the gastrointestinal tract (GIT).

Examples: Certain common pathogenic organisms are: *Escherichia coli; Salmonella sp.*; Rotavirus; *Giardia* sp.; and *Cryptosporidium*.

9.3.2 Pathogenic Fungi

It is known universally that **fungi** essentially comprise of **moulds, yeasts**, and **higher fungi**. It has been observed that almost all **fungi** are *eukaryotic* in nature, and do possess sterols but not the least **peptidoglycan in their cell membrane**. These belong to the class of **chemoheteromorphs***, and a majority of them are **aerobic** in nature. Besides, quite a few *fungi* are also **saprophytes**** and found in soil and water, and eventually acquire their food and nutrition via absorption. These *fungi* produce characteristically both sexual and asexual spores. More than one hundred thousand species of *fungi* have been duly isolated, identified, and hence recognized across the globe; of which nearly 100 cause infections to the humans.

Moulds are also collectively referred to as a '*mycelium*' which essentially composed of a number of microscopic branching hyphae.

Yeasts represent invariably the **unicellular organisms** that are found to be either spherical or ovoid in shape and appearance. Yeasts do undergo replication by the phenomenon of **budding** rather than **binary fission**. The exact mechanism of budding in yeasts may be explained whereby the *cytoplasm* and *dividing nucleus* from the parent cell is initially a continuum with the bud or the daughter yeast, before a new cell wall gets deposited so as to make a distinct separation of the ensuing two cells. However, in certain specific instances these '**buds**' do not undergo detachment completely, and thereby may give rise to the formation of short-chain of cells usually known as '**pseudohypha**'. Mostly, yeasts are *single cells* and invariably generate rather smooth *bacteria-like colonies* when grown on the laboratory agar media; but unlike bacteria they do possess an altogether distinct nucleus, and, therefore, these are essentially **eukaryotes**.

Example: *Saccharomyces cerevisiae* is a typical example of yeast which solely gives rise to the production of **ethanol** under *anaerobic fermentative conditions*.

Various Diseases Caused due to Pathogenic Fungi: In fact, there are several **fungal infections** or **mycoses** that are exclusively categorized under different heads based upon the degree of tissue involvement and mode of entry right into the respective host.

Examples: Following are certain typical examples of fungal infections that are usually observed in the humans, namely:

a. ***Superficial***—i.e., found to be solely localized to the skin, nails, and the hair.
b. ***Subcutaneous***—i.e., infections are exclusively confined to `the dermis, subcutaneous tissue, and the adjacent areas.
c. ***Systemic***—i.e., deep rooted infections confined to the various internal organs in the humans.
d. ***Opportunistic***—i.e., infections that are caused exclusively in the **immunocompromised subjects**.

There are *two* main types of **fungi** which are prone to cause dreadful diseases in the human beings, namely:

i. Pathogenic Fungi, and
ii. Opportunistic Fungi.

These two types of *fungi* shall be discussed briefly in the section that follows:

Pathogenic Fungi: The primary pathogenic fungi cause inections that usually take place in previously healthy humans, and eventually come into being via the ensuing respiratory route.

Examples: Histoplasmosis, blastomycosis, coccidio-mycosis, and paracoceidiodomycosis. *Histoplasma capsulatum* is the causative fungi for **histoplasmosis**. The organism happens to be **dimorphic** in nature, and is more or less endemic in several parts of the globe. It is invariably found in the soil and its growth could be enhanced considerably due to the very presence of the excreta of birds and bats.

Lungs represent the main site of infection; however dissemination right into various other internal organs, such as: liver, heart, CN-system can also occur abundantly.

Opportunistic Fungi: These **fungi** specifically, attack the immunocompromised subject usually having a history of serious immune or metabolic defect or have undergone a recent surgery.

Examples:

a. Aspergillosis. *i.e.,* the different diseases caused by the mould **Aspergillus** sp., and exert its action due to the formation of a large number of **spores**. **Aspergillus fumigatus** invariably affect the lungs, sun uses, inner ear, and rarely the eyes.

b. Candiosis. i.e., mostly occur in immunocompromised patients. *viz.,* those undergoing the chemotherapeutic treatment.

Candida albicans mostly proliferates and disseminates throughout the entire body.

c. ***Cryptococcosis.*** i.e., largely a systemic infection caused by the yeast **Cryptococcus neoformans**. The most common manifestation caused by this organism is a *subacute* or *chronic type of meningitis* emenating from the inhalation of the organism.

Questions

1. Write about disinfection. (MGRU Apr-2004)
2. How will you prevent vortex formation. (MGRU Apr-2004)
3. What are all the biosafety methods that should be adopted in a microbiology lab. (MGRU 2003)
4. What are the precautions in biotechnology field?
5. Explain the biological precautions in biotechnology?
6. Discuss on chemical precautions of biotechnology?
7. How can protect from pathogenic organisms?
8. Define biosafety?
9. How can protect from pathogenic fungi?

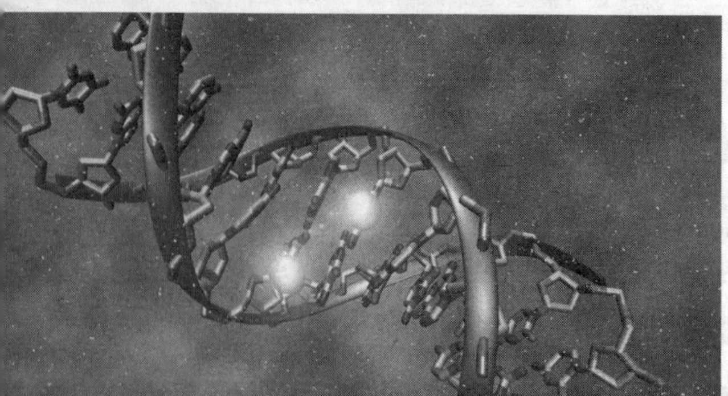

CHAPTER

10

Bioinformatics and Data Mining

10.1 Introduction

The most latest conceptualized development and tremendous galloping advancement in the domain of 'biotechnology' are **bioinformatics and data mining** which are collectively also termed as '***in silico biology***'. In true sense and perception these actually designate two altogether new emerging areas of research that specifically and essentially involve computer-aided management of data which is being generated, stored, and utilized exclusively for innumerable applications related to '**biotechnology**'.

It is, however, pertinent to mention at this point in time that currently '**bioinformatics and data mining**' are invariably regarded as two absolutely '*independent areas*', but there prevails an enormous scope, possibility, and probability that these two aforesaid areas will soon get merged and will ultimately and eventually turn out to be more or less indistinguishable. The present global trend is to exploit overwhelmingly these two areas of research under the able guidance, wisdom, and command by academicians, biotechnology-based organizations, and above all the international and national consortia to utilize the copious volumes of highly valuable and informative data, that are being fast accumulated (stored) in **massive databases** in the best possible useful manner.

Examples: There are glaring examples to expatiate the above statements of facts, namely:

1. Voluminous data accumulated on '**molecular markers**' and '**molecular maps**' of the genomes of a large number of animals and plants were generated exhaustively during the period 1980 to 2000, and
2. Proposed '**drafts**' of the much talked about '*human genome sequences*' were released in February – 2001 after getting a joint endorsement from the well-known **Human Genome Project**, and a famous **genomics** related organization called '**Celera genomics**'.
3. The New Millenium witnessed the complete sequencing of the genomes of *four* **eukaryotes**, namely:

- *Saccharomyces cerevisiae* — a budding yeast,
- *Coenorhabditis elegans* — a nematode,
- *Drosophila melanogaster* — a fruit fly, and
- *Arabidopsis thaliana* — a higher plant.

4. Early – 2002 gracefully observed the report with regard to the genome of the **fission-yeast** *Schizosaccharomyces pombe*.
5. In April – 2002, the '*Draft Proposals*' of **rice genome sequences** have been duly submitted by *three* agencies almost separately: *viz*., **Monsanto** (USA); **Syngenta** (USA); an individual group in China.

Special Notes:

a. Availability of these sequences have been made *via* the 'databases', and are being utilized fully for assigning meaning to each of these sequences, and

b. Copious volumes of data with respect to proteins, their amino acid sequences, and 3Dstructures may now be produced at a much faster accelerated place, which are further exploited towards the discovery of genes, and also for assigning specific roles and functions to these prevailing genes.

Keeping in view the impeccable emergence of '**bioinformatics technology**' exclusively based upon a host of most modern '**computational tools**' overwhelmingly provided by the epoch making revolution in *information technology* (IT), for instance : statistical software, graphics simulation modes, and database management, in order to rationally organize and critically analyze information's emanated by the not-so-mysterious biological systems with particular reference to biotechnology, information's about cells, and above all the prevailing biological molecules. Another extremely vital and important outcome of the prevailing '**innovative information revolution**' is the INTERNET *via* which the scientists and researchers across the globe broadcast this information profusely and predominantly.

It has been established beyond any reasonable doubt that the intensive as well as extensive ability to collect, store, analyze, utilize, and adequately distribute biological information(s) solely derived from DNA-protein-sequencing-mode analyses throws an ample in-depth fundamental knowledge to modern biotechnology. To accomplish this ultimate goal and objective the world has basically adopted an almost unanimous decision to ease out the critical funding strategies by combining together the *renowned biotechnological organizations* (companies) and *famous academic institutions* to help each other.

Interestingly, the real long-term aesthetic values of **bioinformatics** and the inherent strengths of data mining capabilities does not rest so much upon the '*developing tools and means*', but resides exclusively in the proper exploitation of the accumulated enormous knowledge of information(s) into a **broad range of spectacular products**, such as: therapeutics, animal and plant 'bioreactors' in the shape of genetically modified organisms (GMOs), newly discovered genes, and the like.

Nevertheless, the various technologies cited above ranging from monoclonal antibody technology (MAB-technology) to deoxyribonucleic acid chips (DNA-chips) have indeed catered for not only a massive quantum of extremely valuable information's, but also a large excess of **spectacular product variants**. In fact, the fundamental methodology essentially required for the adequate fool-proof organization and analyses of critical raw data with definitely go a long way to enable one to muster sufficient knowledge, better understanding, and accomplish a wide range of spectacular product variants. In nutshell, **bioinformatics technology** provides adequately vital tools and useful methods for organizing consistently a plethora of such activities as: accessing, processing, and integrating tones of valuable data from various sources.

In addition to this unique and remarkable uniformity, in absolute conjunction with the universal language of life at the very fundamental molecular level legitimately, gainfully, and broadly enables international collaboration amongst the scientist fraternity conducting research in plants, animals, or even microorganisms anywhere on this planet. Therefore, bioinformatics technology may increasingly help the scientists working in this particular domain to **map genomes, identify genes**, establish definite protein structure, simulate critical protein interactions, discover altogether newer therapeutic entities, design medicines, aimed at the targets, and to have an access strategically towards the ultimate effects of virtual mutations on gene function.

In the light of the dire necessities and emerging needs for the application of computers in biosciences, a new journal was aptly introduced in 1984, entitled as:

Computer Applications in Biosciences (CABIOS) by the Oxford University Press, London, which was eventually renamed as **Bioinformatics**. In the recent past, the terminology **'in silico biology'** designated as a relatively new area of biology that is solely confined to the various solutions based upon the usage of '*computers in biology*'.

Perhaps the 21st century may have the most opportune moment to see the extremely vigorous tidal wave of progress in the era of data accumulation that could be exploited judiciously as given below:

- updated sequence information about genes and proteins,
- functional annotations of genomic sequences,
- population variations,
- disease correlations, and
- Other information pertaining to biotechnology.

Since one and a half decade, precisely 1990, the various milestones vividly depicting the major events that occurred in the field of **'bioinformatics'** are as stated under:

1.	1990	BLAST: Fast sequence similarity searching
2.	1991	EST: Expressed sequence tag (sequencing)
3.	1993	Sanger Centre, Hinxton (UK)
4.	1994	EBI: European Bioinformatics Institute, Hinxton, U.K.
5.	1995	First bacterial genome completely sequenced
6.	1996	First yeast genome completely sequenced
7.	1997	PSI-BLAST*
8.	1998	Worm (multicellular) genome (*C. elegans*) completely sequenced.
9.	1999	Fruitfly (*D. melanogaster*) genome completely sequenced
10.	2000	Thale cress (*A. thaliana*) genome sequenced
11.	2001	Draft genome sequences of human (*H. sapiens*)
12.	2002	Draft genome sequences of rice (*Oryza sativa*)

10.2 Sequential Growth In Bioinformatics

Bioinformatics stretched its wings over the endless boundaries of spectacular success, worldwide recognition, and remote communication at every nook and corner in this world. There are certain historical landmarks in the sequential growth in the development of bioinformatics that need to be mentioned in this particular context; and, therefore, these are as enumerated under:

1. ***Staden Package.*** It solely involved the DNA sequencing and analysis.
2. ***PROPHET.*** It was primarily developed in USA as national computing resource for *'Life Science Research'* specially tailor-made to fulfil the dire and urgent requirements of basic data analysis and their consequent effective management. In actual practice, PROPHET essentially involved a host of such activities as : precise analyses of raw data, production of

graphics, simulation models, and detailed investigation with regard to molecular structure of macromolecules embracing nucleic acids (*viz.*, DNA, RNA) and an array of proteins.

3. ***BIONET [Abbreviation of: Biology Network]. Amos Bairoch*** (1980s) founded in Europe a user-friendly club christened as **BIONET**, for those who were intimately associated with the study of '*life-sciences*' using microcomputers to enable them share their acquired knowledge, wisdom, and experiences for the use of '**computers**', and **exchange software packages** amongst themselves to enlighten and broaden the horizons of ever-increasing in-puts in **Bioinformatics**.
4. ***NAPDB [Nucleic Acid Protein Data Bank].*** NAPDB package was duly released in 1984 with a **big bang**. It was accompanied by two EMBL's* nucleotide sequence databases at the time of its distribution, and a protein databank of 1200 sequences.
5. ***COMPSEQ.*** Amos Bairoch in mid 1984 altered the name of NAPDB to **COMPSEQ** after disposing of the '**exclusive rights**' another established organization known **GENOFIT**. In mid 1985, COMPSEQ first released a PC-compatible version with thirty three programmes. In 1986, the popularity of COMPSEQ even spread outside Europe.
6. ***PC-GENE.*** A California-based software company known as **Intelli-Genetics** bought over the '**exclusive rights**' of COMPSEQ from GENOFIT in late 1980s. **PC-GENE** is appropriately provided with an unique protein and nucleic acid sequence analysis package that could be utilized in *two* different ways, namely:
   a. *Translation* of a given 'gene sequence' into an amino acid sequence of a protein even including its secondary emanating structures, if any, and
   b. *Critical comparison* of a given 'gene sequence' with the sequences already available in the database.

PC-GENE continued to acclaim its wide popularity and befitting acceptance in the number of programmes offered and number of its genuine users simultaneously. Eventually, it came up with a good number of successive releases, for instance:

- Major new version with several new functions in 1989 having an altogehter *seventy-six programmes*, and
- Last 6.85 version released in 1995 essentially possessed *eighty-two programmes*.

7. ***PROSITE. Amos Bairoch***, in mid-1980s, succeeded in the development of a so-called '*dictionary of sites and patterns in proteins*', which was exclusively aimed at creating a database of protein sequences and structural correlations.
8. ***SEQUANELREF.*** It was evolved as a combination of PROSITE with another software, SEQUANELREF, that could help in carrying out the analysis and adequate comparison of sequences which were already available in PROSITE.
9. ***SWISS-PORT.*** It came into being in 1986 as a '*protein databank*', that is found to be still well known and popular amongst its users for providing an extremely important and vital source for protein sequence and structure.
10. ***SWISS-2D-PAGE.*** Early 1990s witnessed the epoch making discovery and emergence of **proteomics** databases, **SWISS-2D-PAGE** that essentially carried the valuable data strategically positioned on *two dimensional polyacrylamide gel-electrophoresis* (**2D-PAGE**) maps of proteins from a wide spectrum of tissues belonging to a number of organisms.
11. ***Networking Tools and Web Services.*** From 1991 to 1995 one has observed the meaningful development in the direction of **networking tools** *e.g.,* WAIS and Gopher; and **Web Services.** *e.g.,* **ExPASY** that particularly eased out the channel of remote communication.

It is, however, pertinent to mention at this juncture that with effect from 1995 onwards the highly specialized latest dimensions to biotechnology emerged as a full bloom altogether new discipline invariably termed as '**bioinformatics**'. Thus, many tertiary institutions of higher learning in India and abroad promulgated well defined academic curriculum to impart independent and advanced courses in the field of '**bioinformatics**'.

10.3 Web Services

Bioinformatics tools which are being used at present in the elaborated investigations and studies related to '**biotechnology**' and '**molecular biology**' are nothing but the innovated and modified versions of the tools that were duly developed and employed at the earlier stages several years ago (which have now been rendered as more or less obsolete). It is worthwhile to state here that a good number of these tools are available '*free of cost*' and may be downloaded from the corresponding plethora of **websites** or **web-services**. Besides, there are several other cardinal and useful other **bioinformatics tools** that are required to be licensed on requisite payments as they belong to certain individual companies or establishments. Table 8.1 records certain important web sites (services) invariably employed in the field of '**bioinformatics**'.

Table 10.1 *Certain Important Web Sites Invariably Employed for Bioinformatics.*

S.No	Subject	Source(s)	Internet Link [WEB-SITES]
1.	**Nucleic acid sequence**	Gen Bank	http:// www. ncbi. nih. gov : 80/enterz/query/fcgi ? bd = Nucleotide.
2.	**Genome sequence**	SRS at EMBL/FBI	http://srs. cbiac.uk.
		Entrez Genome	http://www.ncbi. nlm. gov: 80/entrez/ query.fcgi ? bd = Genome.
		TIGR database	http://www.tigr.org/tbl/
3.	**Protein sequence**	Gen Bank	http://www.ncbi.nlm.nin. gov : 80/entrez/query. fcgi ? bd = Protein
		Swiss-Port at ExPASY	http://www. expasy.ch/spro/
		PIR	http://www. ndrf.georgetown. edu
4.	**Protein structure**	Protein Date Bank	http://www.rcsb.org/pdb/
5.	**Post translational modifications**	RESID	http://www. ndrf. georgetown.edu/pirwww/search/ textresid.html
6.	**Biochemical and biophysical information**	ENZYME BIND	http://www. expasy. ch/enzyme http://www.ncbl.nlm.nih. gov :80/entrez/ query.fcgi ? db = structure.
7.	**Biochemical Pathways**	Path DB KEGG WIT	http://www./ncgr.org/software/pathdb http:/www.genome.ad.jp/kegg/ http://www.wit.mcs.anl. gov./WIT2 http.//www.industry.epi.ac.uk./valan/ Microarray
8.	**Microarray**	Gene Expression Links	http.//www.ebi.ac.uk.
9.	**Other Interesting Sites**	European Bioinformatics Institute DNA Database of Japan	http.//www.nig.oc.jp./home.html

Figure 10.1 Illustrate explicitly the major freely available **databases** and **data mining tools** that are frequently used across the globe profusely and abundantly.

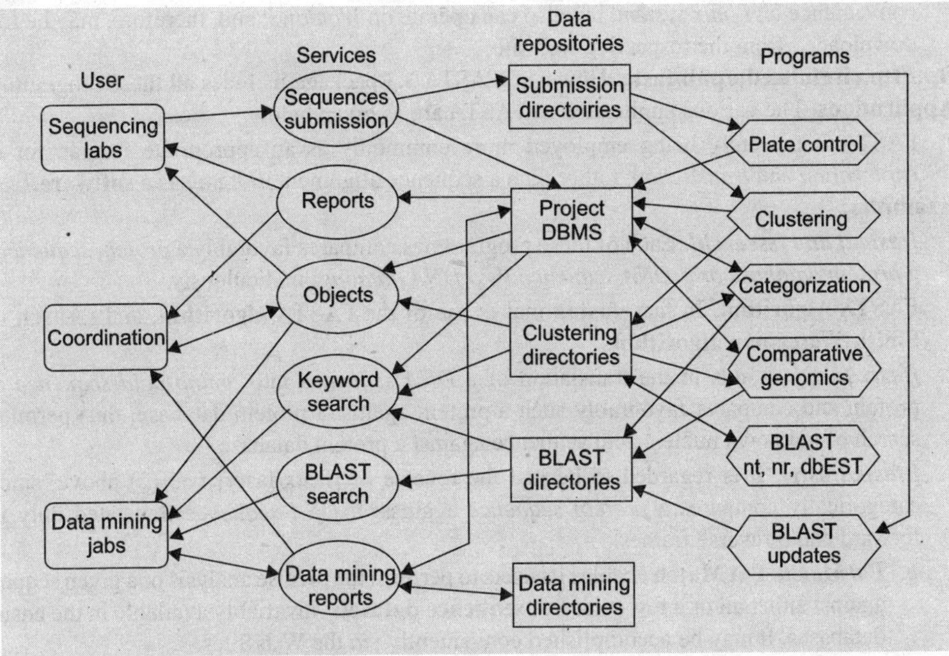

Fig. 10.1 *Major Freely Available Databases and Data Mining Tools.*

10.4 Alignment Tools

There are, in fact, *two* types of **alignment** tools that are used extensively in the exploitation and utilization of databases, namely:

a. Local sequence alignment tools, and

b. Multiple sequence alignment tools

These two types of alignment tools shall now be discussed individually in the section that follows:

10.4.1 Local Sequence Alignment Tools

The **local sequence alignment tools** specifically permit and help one to identify the exact location of **query sequence*** (or **input sequence**) amongst the available sequences in the database. Hence, it really aids in finding out the **'identity'** of a *query sequence*. Besides, it also helps in the discovery of: (a) **structural genes**; and (b) **regulatory sequences**; even though the *query sequence* contributes merely a segment of the parent gene or of a polypeptide duly encoded by this particular gene.

Advantages. The various glaring advantages of the **local sequence alignment tools** are as follows:

1. Conserved repetitive sequences, such as: short-sequence repeats (SSRs) or retrotransposons may be searched conveniently in the databases.
2. Help in carrying out intensive and extensive basic studies e.g., **'taxonomy and evolution'** to enormous usages in '*crop breeding*' and '*human health care*'.

A few typical as well as specific examples of the '*local sequence alignment tools*' are as given below:

a. **The FASTA Family.** FASTA is nothing but a package invariably employed for local sequence alignment that particularly predates BLAST (i.e., basic local alignment sequence tools). It essentially comprises of search programmes which are found to be analogous to the main BLAST-modes. In fact, the FASTA programmes mentioned here may be compiled with great convenience on *Linux system*, but also can operate on *Windows*; and, therefore, may be freely downloaded from the respective web site:

ftp://ftp.virginia.edu/pub/fasta. However, FASTA 3.3 package includes all these programmes.

Applications. The various application of FASTA are as given below :

1. FASTA is presently being employed more commonly as an appropriate format, for data *exploration* and *transaction*, rather than a sequence alignment tool *i.e.,* as a **software.**

Examples:

1. ***[fastaa] and [ssearch].*** Each of these programmes compares favorably a *protein sequence* Vs a *protein database or a DNA sequence Vs a DNA database* meticulously.

   FASTA Algorithm. In fact, **fastaa** makes use of the **FASTA algorithm**; and **ssearch** uses **Smith-Waterman algorithm.**
2. ***[fastx/fasty].*** It aids in the translation of a *DNA sequence* into *amino acid sequence* of a protein and compares favourably such a protein against a protein database, thus permitting search of unknown nucleic acid sequence against a protein database.
3. ***[tfastx/tfasty].*** It is regarded to be just the reverse of [fastx/fasty] *i.e.,* (2) above, since it categorically compares a *protein sequence* againsat a *DNA sequence* translated duly in 3 forward and 3 reverse frames.

   b. ***Pat Match.*** **Pat Match** enables its users to perform the precise analysis of a given sequence against either all or a few selected **'sequence datasets'** invariably available in the ensuing databases. It may be accomplished conveniently *via* the Web Sites.

However, the *datasets* that are commonly in use for this purpose essentially include the following ranges of applications, namely :

1. Protein sequences and their respective structures.
2. Genomic DNA sequences.
3. Bacterial artificial chromosomes (BACs).
4. EST sequences.

In fact, **Pat Match**, was initially developed in 1999 as an *Arabidopsis* **database**, which enables its users to find motifs by entering a '*regular expression pattern*' or simply a '*string of less than 20 characters*'.

c. ***BLAST [Basic Local Alignment Sequence Tool].*** In true sense, BLAST is invariably encountered in *two* versions, namely: (a) *earlier versions*; and (b) *later versions*. Now, these two identified versions of BLAST shall be treated individually in the section that follows:

1. BLAST-Earlier Versions. The most dynamic, reliable, and popular tool for searching and subsequently identifying **'sequence databases'** is accomplished by a package termed as BLAST. The earlier versions are solely based on an algorithm, which is strategically located at the core of a plethora of **'on-line sequence search servers'**. It acts judiciously by carrying out pair-wise comparisons of such sequences with specific emphasis upon seeking reasons of **'local similarity'**, in lieu of the global alignment having almost all sequences. Importantly, BLAST categorically permits pair wise: DNA-protein, DNA-DNA, protein-DNA, and protein-protein alignments employing the corresponding databases. In actual practice, however, BLAST users may engage and submit up to almost 20,000 nucleotides in **multi- FASTA** format and the prevailing programme carry out the desired search in the database for identical sequences. One may gainfully make utilization of the following '*earlier versions of BLAST*' efficaciously:

i. ***BLAST p.*** It compares favorably an *amino acid query sequence* against a protein sequence database,

ii. ***BLAST n.*** It amply compares a *nucleotide query sequence* against a nucleotide sequence database, *iii.* ***BLAST x.*** It effectively compares a *nucleotide query sequence* translated in all reading frames against an ensuing protein sequence database,

iv. ***t BLAST n.*** It compares efficaciously a protein query sequence against a nucleotide database that has been duly translated in all reading frames,

v. ***t BLAST x.*** It compares gainfully the six frame translations of a nucleotide query sequence against the corresponding six frame translations of a nucleotide sequence database,

vi. ***BLAST z.*** It compares adequately long stretches of nucleotides usually more than 2 kb (*i.e.*, kilo base pairs),

vii. ***BLAST bgp.*** It categorically permits the usage of *two* almost new BLAST modes *viz*. (a) **PHI BLAST**—that specifically makes use of protein motifs *e.g.,* found in PROSITE plus other motif databases predominantly, so as to enhance the possibility of locating **'biologically significant matches'**; and (b) **PSI BLAST**—that utilizers particularly an interactive alignment technique to detect and identify *weak pattern matches,* and

viii. ***bl2 seq.*** It clearly permits a distinct comparison of *two* known sequences specifically making use of **BLAST p** and **BLAST n** programmes (*viz., 'i'* and *'ii'* above)

2. ***BLAST—Later Versions.*** A constant vigorous and concerted effort is on towards the development of newer and latest versions of BLAST to meet a variety of definitive aims and objectives in order to enhance progressively the *'penetration strength'* of the prevailing programme.

Precisely, the later versions of BLAST were duly introduced in the year 2001-2002 having certain new sequence alignment tools which are extremely beneficial for extracting useful and newer information(s) derived specifically from the query (input) sequence adequately.

The various tools being introduced under the **BLAST-later** versions are described briefly as under:

i. ***Vee Screen.*** It evidently provides an output, that lists all segments pertaining to the query which intimately match any of the sequence present in the **Univec database** including those of plasmids, phage, cosmids, BACs, PACs, and YACs.

ii. ***IgBLAST.*** It predominantly facilitates the analysis of immunoglobulin sequences in **Gen Bank**. It essentially records the *three* basic **germlines,** such as : (*a*) V-genes; (*b*) two Dgenes; and (*c*) two J-genes, that distinctly exhibit the nearest possible match to the prevailing query sequence,

iii. ***Mega BLAST.*** It is indeed a **'multiple alignment tool'** with the aid of which a set of ESTs is conveniently compared with a set of genes along with quite identical EST sequences that are invariably grouped together in the form of *'clusters'* for further investigations associated with EST mapping,

iv. ***SNP BLAST.*** It essentially provides an output that enlists all available high confidence SNPs available in the SNP database (db SNP) in the sequences that usually correspond to the query sequence, and

v. ***Power BLAST.*** It represents an altogether new network blast application for the automatic analysis of *'genomic sequences'*. It essentially combines blast searching with probably additional screening phenomenon for *'low complexity regions'* and *'repeats'*. Importantly **Power BLAST** gives rise to one to several alignment outputs displaying alignment of the *query sequence* along with all *matching sequences,* quite contrary to the earlier versions that might yield just only one-to-one alignment output.

d. ***Par Align [http://dna.uio.no/search/].*** The year 2001 witnessed the introduction of **Par Align** programme which is characterized by initial exploitation of *'parallelism'* to perform a very rapid computation of the exact optimal ungapped alignment of all diagonals existing in the alignment matrix. As a result, **Par Align** is proved to be more effective than the programmes of the so called *BLAST family* with respect to **speed**. Besides, a good number of facilities that are adequately available in **BLAST** are indeed not available in **Par Align** by virtue of the fact that parallelism essentially gives rise to division of a **'major tasks'** into relatively **'small tasks'** which are critically carried out in parallel to enhance the speed overwhelmingly.

e. ***Protein Engine and Transeq [http//www.ebi.ac.uk/].*** **Protein Engine** and **Transeq** *i.e.,* the *two* programmes are readily available as vital and important tools on **EBI** (European Bioinformatics Institute) **homepage**. Infact, these two programmes are first and foremost employed for translating the *DNA sequences* into the corresponding *language of proteins.* Consequently, the protein sequences thus obtained may be used for carrying out further sequence similarity searches; besides, the detailed investigation of 3D-structures duly encoded by the query DNA sequence. Interestingly, **t BLAST x** may also permit the usage of a **DNA query sequence** for looking at the very corresponding protein segments encoded by it. It has been duly observed that **t BLAST x** fails to utilize the entire amino acid sequence encoded by the query sequence.

f. ***INTERPRO.*** The **INTERPRO** helps to analyse the protein sequences that have been obtained directly either from proteins or from those duly predicted on the basis of genomic sequences from several organisms.

Example. Predicted gene products were duly analyzed from the genomes of four organisms, namely: **nematode** (*C. elegans*), yeast, *Arabidopsis*, and *fruitfly* to actually determine the valid and important differences present in conserved protein domains.

10.4.2 Multiple Sequence Alignment Tools

The main objective of the **multiple sequence alignment tools** is to ascertain *via* a planned investigation to study groups of related **genes** or **proteins** to infer and establish *'evolutionary broad relationships'* prevailing between genes. In addition it also helps to discover patterns that are usually shared amongst various groups or functionally and structurally related sequences.

A few important multiple sequence alignment tools are employed in the study of genes are discussed as under:

a. CLUSTALW [http://www.ebi.ac.uk]. **CLUSTALW** refers to a programme specially designed for accomplishing progressive multiple sequence alignment. The underlying principle usually employed in this programme is that of a **phylogenetic* analysis,** and essentially involves the various steps as detailed under:

1. First of all a *'pair-wise distance matrix'* with respect to all the requisite sequences need to be aligned is generated and a specific **'guide tree'** is made creatively by making use of the *neighbour-joining algorithms,*
2. Consequently, each and every most intimately related pairs of sequences attached to the ultimate branches of the specific **'guide tree'** are adequately aligned to each other,
3. The relatively less related sequences are subsequently alignment to obtain a definite profile; and finally all such *'profiles'* are duly aligned to each other until a complete **dendogram** is achieved.

Summararily, the **CLUSTALW** programme is very much identical to such other programmes as: NSYS, UPGMA, that essentially make use of **molecular marker** or **morphological** data for the ultimate creation of *distance matrix* and the *dendogram,* except that it particularly uses either DNA or: protein sequences.

It has already been established beyond any reasonable doubt that **CLUSTALW** may also be exploited for pairwise global protein or nucleic acid sequence alignments existing amongst ORFs with a significant **BLAST** alighment (E < 10– 10). It would meticulously provide a significant degree of divergence particularly for each of the large number of pairwise comparisons that may be properly utilized for an elaborated and exhaustive **comparative genomics research.**

b. PHYLIP. **PHYLIP** comprises of thirty most crucial programmes which implement different **phylogenetic analysis algorithms,** and hence recognized as an indispensable package.

Highlights of PHYLIP are as follows;

i. Each programme almost runs individually.

ii. Large segment of programmes invariably look for an *input file* [called **'infile'**], and write an *output file* [known as **'out-file'**]; instead of entering parameters *e.g.*, E-value, number of returns required etc., as required with **BLAST**.

The sequence of DNA and protein analysis is frequently and abundantly carried out by the help of **PHYLIP programmes** as detailed below:

i. **PROTPARS** — concludes phylogenesis* from protein sequence inputs,

ii. **PROTDIST** — helps in the computation of an evolutionary distance matrix from protein sequence input,

iii. **DNAPARS** — infers phylogenesis from DNA sequence input,

iv. **NEIGHBOR** — concludes phylogenesis from distance matrix data employing either pair wise clustering or the NEIGHBOR joining algorithms, and

v. **DRAWGRAM** — draws a rooted phytogenetic tree based upon output from one of the phylogeny inference programme.

c. Bio Numeric Version 2.0. Importantly, the **Bio Numeric Version 2.0** refers to an unique software package available off-line to have the download facilities against payment. In order to perform an elaborated study with regard to a *genetic similarity* or *diversity,* one may handle the available experimental data in two ways, namely :

i. In the form of Gel or Capillary Electrophoresis patterns, High Performance Liquid Chromatography (HPLC) profiles, and autoradiograms, and

ii. In the form of ensuing nucleotide sequences of DNA/RNA and amino acid sequences of proteins respectively.

Mechanism: The **Bio Numeric Version 2.0** first and foremost constructs a similarity matrix by making use of any one of the *available algorithms.* The resulting similarity matrix is used for constructing a **dendogram** by the aid of one of the most suitable available techniques, for instance: UPGMA, Single Linkage, Neighbour-joining, Ward, and Complete Linkage.

10.5 Data Mining

Data mining may be defined as — *'the non-trivial retrieval of implicit, previously unknown and potentially useful information from various sources of data'. Importantly,* **data mining** exclusively complements and overwhelmingly expands *bioinformatics***, so that both the former and the later are apparently distinct in nature, but there is every possibility, change, and ample scope that eventually they may ultimately merge together. Though at present they do have their own distinct identity, but sooner or later eventually **data mining** and **bioinformatics** will turn out to be absolutely undistinguishable.

It may be observed explicitly that **data mining** is solely practised in the field of **'biotechnology'** intimately involving various branches of **'life sciences'** *viz.,* biology, microbiology, agriculture, and above all the health care system. Besides, **data mining** may also be extended legitimately and exploited in other areas not related to life-sciences, such as: banking, database providers, engineering, financial institutions, government agenicies, manufacturing, marketing, telecommunications, travel industry, and service industries. In fact, the copious and massive information's generated from the above sources could be utilized to its maximum extent by means of a good number of highly specialized software's already in actual use across the globe.

The ever fast developing **'Biopharmaceutical Industry'** in the world is profusely using enormous quantum of databases that are virtually flooded with a plethora of vital information's, retrieved from a variety of **data mining** methodologies, such as:

1. Annotated databases of the disease profiles
2. Molecular pathways involved in dreadful human diseases
3. Quantitative structure activity relationships (QSARs)
4. Precise chemical structures of combinatorial libraries of compounds
5. Results of mandatory 'clinical trials' of new molecules

*(Data mining is employed to help the '**pharmaceutical industry**' in general and '**biopharmaceutical industry**' in particular to exploit and utilize this valuable information gainfully and fruitfully).*

10.5.1 Applications of Data Mining

With the advent of tremendous volume of highly informative, valuable, useful data generated and stored so efficienctly there exists a **'big challenge'** to the **biopharmaceutical industry** with respect to the critical and precise decision towards the development of absolutely viable **'targets and lead compounds'**. Thus, **data mining** goes a long way to simplify and focus on these complex sets of data in an absolutely efficient and intuitive manner. In fact, there are quite an appreciable number of *'organizations'* that cater for **'data mining services'** for a variety of specialized applications. Importantly, there are *six* predominant and well-known approaches with regard to the **'data-mining'** applications, namely:

a. **Influence-based mining.** *i.e.,* intensive search for cause and effect relationships between *data sets* and *pharmacogenomics,*

b. **Affinity-based mining.** *i.e.,* data mining system distinctly identifies data points thereby making the approach more meaningful and useful, which is rather important to distinguish **'accidental/incidental'** motifs *vis-à-vis* those of definite biological significance,

c. **Time-delay data mining.** *i.e.,* to identify patterns which are specifically combined or rejected as the data set gets voluminous in future,

d. **Trends-based data mining.** *i.e.,* alterations are investigated minutely which essentially take place in specific data sets over a certain period (time); and examining the trends instituted,

e. **Comparative data mining.** *i.e.,* various data collected at different sites *vis-à-vis* different time periods are compared to detect and identify the extent of ensuing dissimilarities, and

f. **Predictive data mining.** *i.e.,* it largely complements and expands traditional bioinformatics.

10.6 Selected Organization Vis-A-Vis Interest In Bioinformatics

Table 10.2 records the names of various **pharmaceutical** and **biotechnology** based organizations, country of origin, software/database provided, facilities supplied, and web sites attached as under:

Table: 10.2 *Selected Organizations vis-a-vis Interest in Bioinformatics*

S.No	Organization	Country of Origin	Software/ Data Base	Facilities Supplied	Web Site
1.	Base 4 Bioinformatics	Canada	Pharmatrix	Specific requirements of pharma and biotech industries	www.base 4.com
2.	Bio Systematia	UK	Bionumeric	Analysis of data from gels, nucleic acid sequences and phenotypes.	www/biosystema tica.com
3.	Cellomics	USA	A Database	Optimization of drug discovery	www.cellomics.com

4.	Double Twist	USA	An Integra ted portal	Retrieve and interpret data for genomic discovery.	www.doubletwist.com
5.	cBioinformatics	USA	Several Softwares	Bimolecular and genetic analysis	www.cbioinformatics.com
6.	Genaissance Pharmaceuticals	USA	DecoGen Browser	Access to databases for querying, viewing reports and performing analysis	www.genaissance. com
7.	Genetics computer GP	USA	Wisconsin package	Sequence comparison, fragment assembly, gene finding, pattern recognition, DNA/RNA analysis, protein analysis	www.gcg.com
8.	Genomica	USA	Innov. Quot ient Discov. Manager	- Analysis and searching for homologies among known genes and proteins.	www.genomica com
9.	Genset	USA	BioIntelli-gence	DNA sequence data in company's Netgene and Signal Tag databases.	www.genxy.com
10.	Hyseq	USA	HyGnostocs	Sequencing and analyses of genes relevant to diseases.	www.hyseq.com

10.7 Wonders Of Bioinformatics And Data Mining

Since the emergence of **bioinformatics** and **data mining** a good deal of extremely useful information's has been duly generated from the analysis of copious volumes of *experimental data.* Hence, a total and absolute dependence upon the stored *experimental data* may at times prove to be a serious limitation of the two specialized branches of **bioinformatics** and **data mining.** It has also been adequately reported that both of these emerging oceans of knowledge and wisdom could even create **'wonders'** on being exploited independently devoid of any laboratory experiments. And this altogether newer emerging field of specialization is invariably termed as **'in silico biology'.**

Examples. Various diversified latest applications have been suggested, tried, and tested in an elaborated manner *viz.*, eletronic PCR, electronic-restricted digestion, electronic southern hybridization, and in silico FISH.

Interestingly, in an overwhelmingly large instance, one may arrive at real wonders in outcome when these two aforesaid tools are successfully and gainfully used for analysing the data invariably generated from experimental work namely: **genomics, metabolomics, proteomics,** and **transcriptomics**—based research projects.

In reality, there are several on-going projects of great value, importance, and utility, such as: **human genome project, whole genome sequencing project,** which otherwise might not have even seen the light of the sunshine without the judicious and prompt handling of the sequencing data by the *wonders* of the prevailing tools of **bioinformatics.**

It is, however, pertinent to state here that the most useful information's generated, collected, and stored *via* the excellent wings of **bioinformatics** and skills of **data mining** tools employing the relevant databases may be expanded, exploited, and even extended towards the wonderful designing of more advanced well-meaning experiments.

Examples. Emergence of molecular markers e.g., STS, SSR, SNP and ESTP based on **bioinformatics;** and subsequently used for *genotyping* a broad-spectrum of experimental designs. It has proved to be an effective means of bioinformatics tools for *biotechnology*, thereby minimising the routine bench-work to an appreciable extent.

10.8 Bioinformatics Information Centres In India

Keeping in view the astronomical advancements in the emerging domain of **bioinformatics** there are nine well planned **Distributed Information Centre (DICs)** have been duly established together with fourteen **User Centers.** The names, exact locations of the city, of the nine DICs are as given under:

S.No	Name of Institutions	City
1.	Indian Institute of Science (IISc)	Bangalore
2.	Madurai Kamraj University	Madurai
3.	Bose Institute	Calcutta
4.	Jawaharlal Lal Nehru University	New Delhi
5.	Poona University	Pune
6.	Centre for Cellular and Molecular Biology (CCMB)	Hyderabad
7.	National Institute of Immunology (NII)	New Delhi
8.	Institute of Microbiological Technology (IMT)	Chandigarh
9.	Indian Agricultural Research Institute (IARI)	New Delhi

It is worthwhile to mention here that the above mentioned DICs are directly linked with one another, and also with the Central Information Network at the Department of Biotechnology (DBT), New Delhi that has an access to the various International Databases in Biotechnology.

Questions

1. Define in silico biology?
2. What are massive databases?
3. Write the applications of bioinformatics?
4. What is PROPHET?
5. Explain about BIONET?
6. Explain the web services in life sciences?
7. Discuss about FASTA with applications?
8. Define BLAST and write the various applications in life sciences?
9. Discuss on multiple sequence alignment tool?
10. Explain phylogenetic analysis algorithms?
11. Discuss bio numeric version 2.0?
12. Define data mining?
13. Write the applications of data mining?
14. Write the wonders of bioinformatics and data mining?
15. Write the bioinformatics information centres in India?